Medical Devices for Pharmacy and Other Healthcare Professions

Medical Devices for Pharmacy and Other Healthcare Professions

Edited by
Ahmed Ibrahim Fathelrahman,
Mohamed Izham Mohamed Ibrahim, and
Albert I. Wertheimer

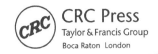

CRC Press
Taylor & Francis Group
Boca Raton London

CRC Press is an imprint of the
Taylor & Francis Group, an **informa** business

First edition published 2022
by CRC Press
6000 Broken Sound Parkway NW, Suite 300, Boca Raton, FL 33487–2742

and by CRC Press
2 Park Square, Milton Park, Abingdon, Oxon, OX14 4RN

Library of Congress Cataloging-in-Publication Data
Names: Fathelrahman, Ahmed Ibrahim, editor. | Mohamed Ibrahim, Mohamed Izham, editor. | Wertheimer, Albert I., editor.
Title: Medical devices for pharmacy and other healthcare professions / edited by Ahmed Ibrahim Fathelrahman,
  Mohamed Izham Mohamed Ibrahim, Albert I. Wertheimer.
Description: First edition. | Boca Raton : Taylor and Francis, 2022. | Includes bibliographical references and index.
Identifiers: LCCN 2021033224 (print) | LCCN 2021033225 (ebook) | ISBN 9780367430894 (hardback) |
  ISBN 9781032168241 (paperback) | ISBN 9781003002345 (ebook)
Subjects: LCSH: Medical instruments and apparatus. | Drugs.
Classification: LCC R856 .M434 2022 (print) | LCC R856 (ebook) | DDC 610.28/4—dc23
LC record available at https://lccn.loc.gov/2021033224
LC ebook record available at https://lccn.loc.gov/2021033225

ISBN: 978-0-367-43089-4 (hbk)
ISBN: 978-1-032-16824-1 (pbk)
ISBN: 978-1-003-00234-5 (ebk)

DOI: 10.1201/9781003002345

Typeset in Times
by Apex CoVantage, LLC

Publisher's note: This book has been prepared from camera-ready copy provided by the authors.

To the late Professor Mohamed Azmi Ahmed Hassali (1974–2021)
for his contribution in Pharmacy Practice and Social Pharmacy
disciplines, and Dr. Yasser A. Ibrahim (1961–2021), one of the
contributors of this book who passed away before completing
his chapter.
Ahmed Ibrahim Fathelrahman

To my beloved father, Mohamed Ibrahim (1941–2018)
Forever missed
Thanks for everything
Mohamed Izham Mohamed Ibrahim

This book is dedicated to my wife Joaquima Serradell who has
attended alone far too many concerts, plays, and other events, while
I spent time on this endeavor. Thank you Joaquima.
Albert I. Wertheimer

Contents

SECTION I Medical Devices for Specialized Services and Purposes

SECTION II Medical Devices for Clinical Specialties

Foreword

Not every pharmacist encounters medical devices as part of their daily practice—but with rapidly advancing technology and a growing number of products entering the market, many more soon will. That's why all pharmacists would be wise to keep a copy of *Medical Devices for Pharmacy and Other Healthcare Professions* on their bookshelves to be ready to serve the patients who depend on these devices.

This resource is just right for both experienced practitioners and beginners. My colleagues, Drs. Ahmed Ibrahim Fathelrahman, Mohamed Izham Mohamed Ibrahim, and Albert I. Wertheimer, have created a robust, handy guide for everything that's most important to know about medical devices. It also takes a deeper dive into medical devices' context within disparate health landscapes.

Medical devices—from the ubiquitous to the groundbreaking—pose untold opportunities for our changing profession and new methods to provide life-changing patient care. Pharmacists' skills in the evaluation of medications' efficacy, safety, affordability, and associated outcomes are a natural fit with optimizing the use of medical devices. Just as important is our experience counseling patients, responding to their concerns, and answering their questions in settings that are most compatible with daily life.

This is especially important given the evolution in healthcare delivery and the ways patients consume care. They're taking more control over their health, and healthcare technology is key to that. Our patients may use medical devices for the diagnosis, treatment, monitoring, and prevention of disease states, but realizing their full potential requires proficient operation and a deep understanding of their purposes and capabilities.

Just like they do with medications, patients need access to a health professional who can communicate complex information, use data to personalize care, and demonstrate proper usage of equipment. Booking an appointment with a primary care physician or specialist to get those services is impractical and can lead to suboptimal use and noncompliance. It's a no-brainer that patients should get them from the provider they see most, know best, and can reach most easily, especially those in rural and underserved areas.

With resources like *Medical Devices for Pharmacy and Other Healthcare Professions* at hand, pharmacists will be prepared to meet their needs, whether that means educating ourselves or ensuring our counseling is thorough, successful, and digestible. We are already armed with the framework to get the maximum value out of these devices. This book can help fill in the blanks.

I'm grateful that Drs. Ahmed Ibrahim Fathelrahman, Mohamed Izham Mohamed Ibrahim, and Albert I. Wertheimer are working to help us answer every question our patients and our fellow providers ask us. I'm excited to see the technological marvels to come and how they will affect pharmacy practice. Above all, I'm motivated to learn everything I can. Thankfully, I can grab this book and immediately benefit from its authors' knowledge and expertise—and so can you.

Scott Knoer, MS, PharmD, FASHP,
Executive Vice President and CEO of the
American Pharmacists Association

Preface

A profession can only survive for as long as the public feels that it adds value and utility. When it fails to deliver valued services, it declines or dies. For example, the blacksmith who attaches iron shoes to the bottom of horses' feet is nearly nonexistent, since there is a very limited need for these services today. This is the similar fate of the cooper, a person who makes wooden barrels. Today, large volumes of liquids are usually housed in glass or plastic containers and the only major use of wooden barrels is found in wine-making. The practicing pharmacist does not often become concerned or involved in many contemporary medical devices, but that is no reason why they should be ignorant about the topic.

Today, more than ever, the pharmacist is a full member of the health team and many of the pharmacist's patients are using cardiac pacemakers, TENS pain reduction devices, insulin pumps, and a host of other devices used in nearly all specialty areas of medicine and surgery. We cannot afford to be left behind and must stay current in the medical device area, even if devices come into play on intermittent, infrequent occasions. A physician may ask the pharmacist which medical device or technology would be most effective to improve medication adherence; or a pharmacist may be asked by a patient if he can clean his insulin pump, how he can keep it safe in hot weather, and which insulin smart pump would be more suitable for traveling. We must be prepared to answer questions such as these. It is acceptable to ask the patient to wait a few minutes while we check a reference source, since no one expects a pharmacist to be able to precisely answer every single question instantaneously.

This book is the answer to how the pharmacist and other healthcare providers can be familiar with the most common medical devices in current use. It is not enjoyable reading and was not intended to be read in one sitting. In actuality, it is better used as a nearby reference source that can be called upon when a device-related question arises. The editors hope that it will make the pharmacist reader as well as other healthcare providers as knowledgeable as possible about this important, evolving area of technology.

Moreover, this book can be used as a reference book for clinical training offered to pharmacy and medical students as a part of clinical skill lab settings. The images and illustrations provided in the book will be useful for students in becoming familiar with the features and designs of various devices and understanding how to operate them and interpret their readings and measures appropriately.

Ahmed Ibrahim Fathelrahman, Izham Ibrahim, and Albert I. Wertheimer

Editors

Ahmed Ibrahim Fathelrahman is currently an associate professor at the Department of Clinical Pharmacy, College of Pharmacy, Taif University, Saudi Arabia. Prior to that from September 2017 to August 2021, he was an assistant professor at the same department. From September 2011 to August 2017, he was an assistant professor and head of department of Pharmacy Practice, Qassim University, Saudi Arabia. Before joining Qassim University in 2011, he worked with the Ministry of Health, Sudan for 13 years in different units and departments such as the Central Medical Supplies Public Corporation (CMS) Sudan (1997–2000); the Revolving Drug Fund, Khartoum State (2000–2005); the General Directorate of Pharmacy and the Khartoum State Drug Information Centre, the Ministry of Health, Khartoum State (2005–2010), and the General Directorate of Planning and Development of the Khartoum State Ministry of Health (2010–2011). Ahmed Ibrahim Fathelrahman is the main author or co-author of more than 50 articles and titles that represent publications in international peer-reviewed journals, books, book chapters, or conference presentations besides other works published in some local journals. Ahmed Ibrahim Fathelrahman is a reviewer for a variety of international peer-reviewed journals from the fields of pharmacy, public health, tobacco control, and toxicology, and he acted as a member of review committees of various international scientific meetings regularly organized by international societies such as the International Society of Pharmacoeconomics and Outcomes Research (ISPOR) and the Society for Research on Nicotine and Tobacco (SRNT). Ahmed Ibrahim Fathelrahman was also an editorial board member of Heliyon, an open-access multidisciplinary journal published by Elsevier. In April 2016, he produced together with Professor Mohamed Izham Mohamed Ibrahim from Qatar University and Professor Albert I. Wertheimer from College of Pharmacy, Nova Southeastern University, USA, an edited book published by Elsevier Science entitled *Pharmacy Practice in Developing Countries: Achievements and Challenges*. In 2018, they produced another edited book published by Elsevier Science entitled *Pharmacy Education in the Twenty First Century and Beyond: Global Achievements and Challenges*. Ahmed Ibrahim Fathelrahman was a winner of the Young Investigator Scholarship of the APACT 8th Asia Pacific Conference on Tobacco or Health, Taipei, Taiwan (17–20 October 2007); Universiti Sains Malaysia (USM) Research Fellowship (September 2007–December 2009), and the Sanggar Sanjung Award for Best Publication, Universiti Sains Malaysia, 2010. Ahmed Ibrahim Fathelrahman worked as a member of research ethics committees of each of the following: the Ministry of Health Khartoum State, the Community Medicine Council of Sudan Medical Specializations Board, the College of Pharmacy at Qassim University, and Al-Qassim Region, Saudi Arabia. Ahmed Ibrahim Fathelrahman supervised the research of more than 30 medical or pharmacy students in Sudan and Saudi Arabia at levels of Bachelor, Doctor of Pharmacy, Master of Science, Medical Doctor, and Fellowship.

Mohamed Izham Mohamed Ibrahim is a Professor of Social and Administrative Pharmacy at the College of Pharmacy, Qatar University. He obtained his PhD in Pharmacy Administration from the Philadelphia College of Pharmacy & Science (PCPS), Philadelphia, USA, in 1995. His research areas, publication and consultancy, are in the area of social and administrative pharmacy that focus on pharmaceutical policy and supply management, pharmacoeconomics, pharmacoepidemiology, sociobehavioral aspects of pharmacy, and pharmaceutical management and marketing. Dr. Izham has supervised and participated in over 100 MSc and PhD graduate students from 15 countries in Africa and Asia. He has published 15 books and more than 250 articles. He won the 2015 Qatar University Scopus Medical and Health Sciences Scientist Award. He has also functioned in multiple consultant roles to the government in Malaysia, Sudan, Mongolia, Qatar, and non-governmental bodies at national and international levels (World Health Organization, Health Action International). He was formerly the Coordinator of Health Campus Program at Universiti Sains Malaysia; Director of the Corporate and Sustainable Development Division, Chancellery Department, Universiti Sains Malaysia; the founding Program Chairman for Social and Administrative Pharmacy Program, Universiti Sains Malaysia; the Deputy Dean of Research and Postgraduate Studies, School of Pharmaceutical Sciences, Universiti Sains Malaysia; Professor and Founding Chairman, Pharmacy Practice Department, College of Pharmacy, Qassim University, Al-Qassim, KSA; and Founding Associate Dean for Research and Graduate Studies Affairs at College of Pharmacy, Qatar University. His last post was the Head of Research and Graduate Studies—Pharmacy, QU Health at Qatar University.

Albert I. Wertheimer is a professor at Nova Southeastern University, College of Pharmacy, in Ft. Lauderdale, Florida, USA. He has made major contributions to the field of social and administrative pharmacy. He has guided over 100 PhD students and more than that number of MSc students. He is an author or editor of 44 books, numerous book chapters, and about 430 articles in scientific and professional journals. Professor Wertheimer has lectured or consulted in over 70 countries. He is the editor-in-chief of the *Journal of Pharmaceutical Health Services Research*, published quarterly by the Oxford University Press.

Contributors

Kadir Alam, PhD
Associate Professor, Department of Clinical
Pharmacology and Therapeutics
B.P. Koirala Institute of Health Sciences
Dharan, Nepal

Mohammed Aldubayee, MD, MHSc, CDE
Associate Dean, Office of Research, College of Public
Health & Health Informatics and Associate Professor,
King Saud bin Abdulaziz University for Health Sciences
(KSAU-HS)
Deputy Chairman, Department of Pediatrics, King
Abdullah Specialized Children's Hospital (KASCH),
King Abdulaziz Medical City, Ministry of National Guard
Health Affairs
Riyadh, Saudi Arabia

**Ahmed Al-Jedai, PharmD, MBA, BCPS, FCCP, FAST,
FASHP, FCCP**
Professor
Alfaisal University Colleges of Medicine and Pharmacy
Therapeutic Affairs, Ministry of Health
Riyadh, Saudi Arabia

Haafiz Allah-Bakhsh, MD
Consultant Pediatric Gastroenterologist and Pediatric
Transplant Hepatologist
King Abdullah Specialized Children's Hospital
Ministry of National Guard—Health Affairs
Riyadh, Saudi Arabia

Mohammed Alshennawi, BPharm, MBA
General Director, General Administration of
Pharmaceutical Care
Therapeutic Affairs, Ministry of Health
Riyadh, Saudi Arabia

Ahmed Awaisu, PhD, MPharm (Clinical), BPharm
Professor and Head, Department of Clinical Pharmacy and
Practice
Qatar University College of Pharmacy, QU Health
Doha, Qatar

**Amir Babiker, MBBS (U of K), FRCPCH (UK), CCT
(UK), MSc Endocrinology and Diabetes (UK)**
Associate Professor, King Saud Bin Abdulaziz University
for Health Sciences (KSAU-HS), Ministry of National
Guard Health Affairs (MNGHA)
Consultant Paediatric Endocrinologist, King Abdullah
Specialized Children's Hospital (KASCH)
King Abdulaziz Medical City, Riyadh (KAMC-R),
Ministry of National Guard Health Affairs (MNGHA)
Riyadh, Saudi Arabia

Hazem Fathy Elewa, RPh, PhD, BCPS
Associate Professor and Head of Clinical Training,
Department of Clinical Pharmacy and Practice
Qatar University College of Pharmacy, QU Health
Clinical Pharmacy Specialist, Hamad Medical Corporation
Doha, Qatar

Elhassan Hussein Eltom, MPharm, MBA
Lecturer of Pharmacology and Therapeutics, Department
of Pharmacology
Faculty of Medicine, Northern Border University
Arar, Saudi Arabia

Ahmed Ibrahim Fathelrahman, MSc, PhD
Associate Professor, Department of Clinical Pharmacy
Taif University College of Pharmacy
Taif, Saudi Arabia

Farhat Naz Hussain, MPharm
Teaching Assistant, Department of Pharmaceutical
Sciences
Qatar University College of Pharmacy, QU Health
Doha, Qatar

Mohamed Izham Mohamed Ibrahim, BPharm, PhD
Professor of Social and Administrative Pharmacy,
Department of Clinical Pharmacy and Practice
Qatar University College of Pharmacy, QU Health
Doha, Qatar

**Mohammed Abdelrahim Idris, FRCP, FSBN, FSBTN,
SCE Nephr (UK)**
Consultant Nephrologist/Transplant Nephrologist
King Fahad Medical Military Complex
Dhahran, Saudi Arabia

**Nor Fatin Farhani Mohamed Izham, MB, BCh, BAO
(NUI, RCSI)**
Senior House Officer
University Hospital Limerick
Limerick, Ireland

**Syed Furrukh Jamil, MBBS, FRCPCH, CCT (UK),
PgC Medical Education, FHEA, CHSE**
Consultant Pediatrician, King Abdullah Specialized
Children's Hospital, King Abdulaziz Medical City
Joint Appointment Assistant Professor, King Saud Bin
Abdulaziz University for Health Sciences
Ministry of National Guard—Health Affairs
Riyadh, Saudi Arabia

Bhuvan KC, MPharm (Clin), PhD
Lecturer, School of Pharmacy
Monash University Malaysia
Jalan Lagoon Selatan
Bandar Sunway, Selangor, Malaysia

Asmita Priyadarshini Khatiwada, BPharm, MPharm
Research Assistant, Department of Pharmaceutical and
Health Service Research
Nepal Health Research and Innovation Foundation
Lalitpur, Nepal

Mohamad Haniki Nik Mohamed, BPharm (Hons), PharmD
Professor, International Islamic University Malaysia
Kulliyyah of Pharmacy, Pharmacy Practice Department
Jalan Sultan Ahmad Shah, Bandar Indera Mahkota
Kuantan, Pahang, Malaysia

Mohamed Awad Mousnad, BPharm (Hons), MSc, PhD
Consultant of Pharmacoeconomics and
Pharmacoepidemiology, Assistant Professor, Faculty of
Pharmacy, International University of Africa
Khartoum, Sudan

Subish Palaian, PhD
Associate Professor, Department of Clinical Sciences
Ajman University College of Pharmacy and Health Sciences
Ajman, United Arab Emirates

Rishi Ram Poudel, MBBS, MS (Ortho)
Consultant in Musculoskeletal Oncosurgery,
Musculoskeletal Oncology Unit
Nepal Cancer Hospital and Research Centre Department
of Surgical Oncology
Harisiddhi, Lalitpur, Nepal

Silvia E. Rabionet, EdD
Associate Professor and Chair of the Sociobehavioral and
Administrative Pharmacy Department
Nova Southeastern University College of Pharmacy
Ft. Lauderdale, Florida

Sajin Rajbhandari, MBBS, MD
Assistant Consultant, Department of Medical Oncology
Nepal Cancer Hospital and Research Centre Pvt. Ltd.
Harisiddhi, Lalitpur, Nepal

Salina Sahukhala, BPT
Physiotherapist, Physiotherapy Unit
Nepal Cancer Hospital and Research Centre
Harisiddhi, Lalitpur, Nepal

Sowndramalingam Sankaralingam, MBBS, MSc, PhD
Associate Professor, Department of Clinical Pharmacy
and Practice
Qatar University College of Pharmacy, QU Health
Doha, Qatar

Binaya Sapkota, BPharm, PharmD
Coordinator and Lecturer, Department of Pharmaceutical
Sciences
Nobel College Faculty of Health Sciences
Sinamangal, Kathmandu, Nepal

Sunil Shrestha, BPharm, PharmD
Ph.D. Student
School of Pharmacy, Monash University Malaysia
Jalan Lagoon Selatan, Bandar Sunway, Selangor, Malaysia

Abderrezzaq Soltani, MPharm, PhD, PgCert, FHEA
Department of Clinical and Pharmaceutical Sciences
University of Hertfordshire School of Clinical and
Pharmaceutical Sciences
Hatfield, UK
Assistant Professor | Academic Quality Assurance
Vice President for Medical and Health Sciences Office
Qatar University
Doha, Qatar

Albert I. Wertheimer, PhD, MBA
Professor, Sociobehavioral and Administrative Pharmacy
Department
Nova Southeastern University College of Pharmacy
Ft. Lauderdale, Florida

Monica Zolezzi, BPharm, MSc, ACPR, PhD
Associate Professor and Coordinator, Structured Practical
Experiences in Pharmacy (SPEP) Program, Department of
Clinical Pharmacy and Practice
Qatar University College of Pharmacy, QU Health
Doha, Qatar

1 Introduction

Medical Devices History, Current Perspectives, and Shortages

Ahmed Ibrahim Fathelrahman and Mohamed Izham Mohamed Ibrahim

CONTENTS

BACKGROUND

The Global Harmonization Task Force (GHTF) is an expert group set up in 1992 jointly by regulatory authorities and the medical device industry.[1] In 2005, GHTF approved a definition of medical devices that received wide acceptance among stakeholders. The definition reveals the variety of forms and application of medical devices. According to GHTF, "A medical device is any instrument, apparatus, implement, machine, appliance, implant, in vitro reagent or calibrator, software, material, or another similar or related article that does not achieve its primary intended action in or on the human body solely by pharmacological, immunological, or metabolic means and that is intended for human beings for:

* The diagnosis, prevention, monitoring, treatment, or alleviation of disease.
* The diagnosis, monitoring, treatment, alleviation of, or compensation for an injury.
* The investigation, replacement, modification, or support of the anatomy or a physiological process.
* Supporting or sustaining life.
* Controlling conception.
* Disinfecting medical devices.
* Providing information for medical or diagnostic purposes using in vitro examination of specimens derived from the human body."

To understand what medical devices are, we need to distinguish between them and medications and pharmaceutical products from one hand, and distinguish between them and other consumers' products from another hand. According to Monsein, consumers' products are not medical devices if used for general purposes but are neither dedicated to nor intended or promoted for medical applications.[2] For example, a screw is considered a medical device when it is promoted for holding bones together rather than holding pieces of wood together.[2] On the other hand, medical devices are different from drugs in that they do not achieve their principal action through chemical action or metabolization in or on the body. For example, plaster cast used for bone healing is considered a device, while a topical ointment used to promote bone healing is considered a drug.[2] However, the differentiation between medical devices and drugs is not always easy, mainly because of the widespread use of several products straddling the borderline between a device and a drug, such as insulin pens and implantable drug delivery devices.[1]

HISTORICAL OVERVIEW ON THE USE OF MEDICAL DEVICES IN MANAGEMENT, CONTROL, PREVENTION, AND MONITORING OF DISEASES

There are several milestones in a long journey that witnessed the evolution and the revolution in the medical devices industry. Although some historians have backdated their appearance in the world to as far as 7000 BCE by the ancient Egyptians and Etruscans, the official appearance of medical

DOI: 10.1201/9781003002345-1

TABLE 1.1

Important Milestones in Modern Medical Devices History According to the WHO[1]

No.	Important event	Years
1	First modern stethoscopes	1800–1850
2	X-rays discovery	1895
3	First cardiograph	1903
4	First modern respirator	1927
5	First cardiac catheterization	1928
6	First metallic hip replacement surgery	1940
7	First kidney dialysis machine	1945
8	First artificial hip replacement	1950
9	First commercially available artificial heart valve	1951
10	First successful external cardiac pacemaker	1952
11	First totally internal pacemaker	1960
12	First computerized axial tomography scanner	1970
13	First laparoscopic procedure	1972
14	First pulse oximeter	1972
15	First regulatory system for medical devices in the US	1976
16	First magnetic resonance imaging device for full body scan	1977
17	First multichannel cochlear implant	1978
18	First permanent artificial heart	1982
19	First implantable cardioverter defibrillator	1985
20	First robot-assisted surgical procedure	1985
21	First European Union regulatory system	1993

devices in modern history was in the 1700s.[3] According to the World Health Organization (WHO), the important milestones in medical device development started with the development of first modern stethoscopes (1800–1850), followed by X-rays discovery (1895).[1] Table 1.1 shows 21 important milestones in modern medical devices history.

THE TREMENDOUS DEVELOPMENT IN MEDICAL DEVICES TECHNOLOGY DURING THE LAST DECADES

Over the last five to six decades, the pharmaceutical and healthcare market witnessed a vast and fast development in medical devices. This was driven by certain factors, including a) the tremendous advancements in science and technology, b) changes in some health philosophies and the widespread existence of newer concepts such as teamwork and collaboration among healthcare providers, health promotion, and the self-care concept, and c) the globalization that produced populations with comparable cultures, health needs, challenges, and awareness about health and diseases. This last factor in producing one large global market with similar demand encouraged manufacturers to be involved in the large-scale production of products with variable user-specific characteristics to satisfy customers everywhere. The advancement in technology resulted in the production of sophisticated devices with a variety of capabilities. The information technology and informatics brought the

healthcare team together and facilitated their collaboration to take care of patients and communities. The manufacturers used the new environment that encourages more patient involvement in caring for their health and produced devices for self-monitoring of various diseases and health conditions.

It has been estimated that the number of medical devices with different types, purposes, and versions reached about 1.5 million, divided into about 10,000 various categories.[1] Due to the rising concerns about self-care, the number of medical devices introduced to the community pharmacy to be operated there or sold to patients for home use increases quickly every year. This has put a particular concern about the pharmacists' essential role in managing and controlling the sale and use of such devices. Previously, medical devices were likely to be seen inside hospitals and other facilities providing monitoring, diagnosis, and treatment to the patients. Nowadays, medical devices are commonly seen in community pharmacies and as household products.

REGULATION OF MEDICAL DEVICES

Both drugs and medical devices are regulated in the United States by the US Food and Drug Administration (FDA). Although the regulation of drugs began in 1906, medical device regulations were not in place until 1938, when the Federal Food, Drug, and Cosmetic Act was approved.[4] However, such regulations were limited and intended only for controlling adulteration and misbranding in medical devices. An important amendment made in 1976 to fulfill some quality control standards in response to an increase in reports of injuries related to some medical devices.[4] At present, medical devices (like drugs) are required to comply with regulations regarding labeling, advertising, production, and post-marketing surveillance. However, if compared with regulations applied on drugs, medical device regulations are still limited.[4] For example, the demonstration of safety and efficacy in humans is required only with Class III medical devices (i.e., medical devices are classified into Class I, Class II, and Class III). In addition, no inspection is performed in the medical device industry.

THE GAPS IN KNOWLEDGE AND EXPERIENCE ABOUT MEDICAL DEVICE USE AMONG PATIENTS AND HEALTHCARE PROFESSIONALS

An overview of the literature reveals a significant gap in knowledge and associated skills required for efficient medical device technique use among patients. Inadequate experience with device technique was also evident among healthcare professionals. Many studies on patients' awareness and appropriate operation of medical devices focused on the devices commonly used by patients, such as asthma inhalers and the simple devices like those used to measure liquid medications at home. The following are examples of such literature.

An experimental study by Van Der Palen et al from the UK revealed high but variable rates of errors among participants concerning various inhaler device techniques. Ellipta showed lower errors among patients than Diskus (Accuhaler), metered-dose inhaler (MDI), and Turbuhaler.[5] This is likely due to variation in the easiness of handling the devices. Such variation was replicated again in a study by von Schantz et al. from Finland.[6] The researchers compared only dry-powder inhalers Diskus, Easyhaler, Ellipta, and Turbuhaler. The percentages of participants showing correct device techniques were as follows: Diskus 48%, Easyhaler 19%, Ellipta 55% and Turbuhaler 16%. Patients' preferences of the devices seem to be related to the easiness of use and ability to use the device correctly.

Bryant et al. from New Zealand assessed the inhaler technique among patients presented to community pharmacies.[7] They found high rates of inappropriate performance with marked variation in the proportions of patients showing good techniques regarding turbuhaler and MDI with or without a spacer. Most participants received initial instructions from their doctors, but a lower proportion of them recalled having their inhaler technique rechecked.

Plaza et al. conducted a systematic review of the literature assessing errors in inhalers techniques among healthcare professionals.[8] Using the data from 55 studies involving more than 6,000 healthcare professionals, they estimated that the inhaler technique was considered correct in only 15.5% of cases (95% confidence interval; 12–19.3). The authors concluded that inhaler technique skills among professionals have worsened in recent years despite extensive training efforts. The authors raised the attention to the urgent need for efficient strategies to improve healthcare professionals' training in the appropriate use of inhalers.

Almazrou and associates conducted a study to assess Saudi mothers' experiences with measuring cups, syringes, and droppers for oral liquid medications.[9] One of the study objectives was to compare the accuracy of dosing across these devices. The researchers found low rates of accurate measurements among participants, with only 58%, 50%, and 51% of participants measuring an accurate dose of paracetamol using oral dosing syringe, dropper, and dosing cup, respectively. Participants measured more than the anticipated dose with the dosing cup and less than the anticipated dose with the dropper. Dosing correctness for each type of devices was significantly affected by the participants' education status. Most of them had not had previous counseling on the use of liquid medication measuring devices.

ACCESS TO RELIABLE INFORMATION ABOUT MEDICAL DEVICES

Having reliable information is very important in all aspects of patient management. Credible information and communication are critical points in evidence-based medicine and practice. Medical devices or equipment (e.g., wheelchair, blood glucose meter, X-ray machine, pacemaker, surgical gloves) and pharmaceuticals are important approaches used to manage patients in either in-patient, out-patient, or home care. Patients and healthcare providers use medical devices for medical purposes. There is a rapid increase in the array, variety, and complexity of medical devices. These devices are used for diagnosing, preventing, monitoring, or treatment of disease. There are also devices used as an aid, such as equipment for people with a disability (e.g., crutches, three-wheel walker). Generally, they have a mechanical or physical effect on the body of the users. Therefore, it is important to ensure that these medical devices are of quality, safe, and effective.

Accordingly, FDA classifies medical devices into three classes: Class I, II, and III.[10] These categories are based on the risk aspects, safety, and effectiveness; Class I has the lowest risk, while Class III has the highest risk. International and national regulatory agencies should manage safety issues using a medical device vigilance system. Information regarding malfunction or deterioration or inconsistency in labeling or instructions needs to be recorded in the system, which later will be helpful for users.

Other important information for users is the list of manufacturers, wholesalers, retailers of medical devices, and registered medical devices in the country. A website would be a good source of information for the community. It should contain information related to the regulations, clinical studies, quality auditing and surveillance, designated and authorized agency, advice and support for patients, healthcare professionals and industry, and educational materials for the public.

Table 1.2 lists a few sites that provide valuable and reliable information on medical devices.

TABLE 1.2
Source of Information Related to Medical Devices

Organization	Link
Government of the United Kingdom	www.gov.uk/guidance/medical-devices-information-for-users-and-patients#:~:text=A%20medical%20device%20is%20a,physical%20impairments%20become%20more%20independent
United States Food and Drug Administration (USFDA)	www.fda.gov/medical-devices
Australian Therapeutic Goods Administration (TGA)	www.tga.gov.au/medical-devices
European Commission	https://ec.europa.eu/health/md_sector/overview_en
European Medicines Agency	www.ema.europa.eu/en/human-regulatory/overview/medical-devices
National Medical Products Administration of China	http://english.nmpa.gov.cn/medicaldevices.html
Pharmaceuticals and Medical Devices Agency of Japan	www.pmda.go.jp/english/
Medtech Regulatory Special Interest Group (SIG)	www.med-technews.com/topics/medtech-regulatory-special-interest-group-sig/

MEDICAL DEVICES IN HEALTH PROFESSION STUDENTS' CURRICULA

Should we teach health profession students topics on medical devices and technologies? Should the aspects of medical devices and technologies be part of the curriculum? If yes, then what topics, and how should they be taught to students?

The latest medical technologies applied in the healthcare system include virtual reality, precision medicines, artificial organs, sensors, smart inhalers, health wearables, and many more. These technologies, which involve a fusion of biomedical and material sciences, will continue to be the key method used in patient management and the primary market in the future.

There are academic institutions that offer degrees at the undergraduate and graduate levels in health/medical technologies. These programs should be taught (e.g., skills and concepts) in multidisciplinary approaches involving experts in medicine, engineering, life sciences, physical sciences, and business.

There are a few methods of teaching that can be utilized in teaching medical device technologies to students. These include a combination of lecture materials, observational learning, problem-solving, hands-on training, experiential learning, medical simulations, industry guest expertise, texts and readings, and internet-based searches to develop their understanding of the problem and design their solutions. Such approaches are expected to successfully provide a significantly increased knowledge base and competence of medical device design.[11–13] According to May-Newman and Cornwall, teaching courses related to medical device design are very challenging and using traditional educational approaches might not be effective.[12] Some colleges provide training in the research, development, and manufacturing of medical devices. These programs and courses are open for healthcare professionals, engineers involved in biomedical product design and development, regulatory officers, manufacturing professionals, etc.

Individuals interested in the field can use their knowledge and skills to invent and design medical devices (e.g., producing prototypes). Others can also proceed to manufacture, test, and commercialize the product.

Colleges offering courses related to medical technologies include topics such as the following in their curricula:

- Fundamental knowledge of engineering, biomedicine, and biotechnology
- Regulatory aspects
- Principles of product design and development
- Microelectromechanical system fabrication techniques
- Manufacturing
- Technology innovation management
- Technology macroenvironment
- Quality aspects
- Safety aspects
- Entrepreneurship

Here are examples of colleges or institutes which offer programs in medical device technologies:

www.mtu.edu/engineering/graduate/certificates/medical-devices/

https://cse.umn.edu/tli/medical-device-innovation-curriculum

www.birmingham.ac.uk/postgraduate/courses/taught/chemical-engineering/healthcare-technology.aspx

www.auckland.ac.nz/en/study/study-options/find-a-study-option/medical-devices-technologies.html

www.strath.ac.uk/engineering/biomedicalengineering/strathclydeinstituteofmedicaldevices/

www.ncad.ie/postgraduate/school-of-design/msc-medical-device-design/

www.uclaextension.edu/engineering/bioengineering/certificate/medical-device-engineering

www.seas.harvard.edu/news/2014/05/medical-mechanics

https://extension.ucsd.edu/courses-and-programs/regulatory-affairs-for-medical-devices

www.tp.edu.sg/schools-and-courses/adult-learners/all-courses/skillsfuture-series/medical-device-school.html

ABOUT THE BOOK IN YOUR HAND

1. The primary readers are pharmacists and pharmacy personnel practicing in various settings, and pharmacy students worldwide. This book is intended to provide information, knowledge, and guidance on the safest and best way to use medical devices for the diagnosis, prevention, monitoring, and treatment of common diseases and conditions.

2. It is intended to be a comprehensive review of medical devices that pharmacists and pharmacy personnel may deal with in various working settings to provide pharmaceutical care, including hospitals, community pharmacies, and other settings and at points of care testing.

3. Devices under pharmaceutical care represent the core part of the book. They are presented according to a clinical specialty such as endocrinology, cardiology, orthopedics, and nephrology; and within each therapeutic area, devices are presented according to common conditions and diseases (e.g., diabetes devices and those for growth disorder under endocrinology), by purposes (e.g., blood pressure monitoring and pulse oximetry under cardiology), or according to body organs like the chapter on gastroenterology and hepatology devices.

4. This book contains a section on medical devices for specialized services and purposes that links devices used collectively while providing services such as smoking cessation and anticoagulation clinics, and those used for particular purposes such as those improving adherence.

5. This book is intended to provide descriptions of different devices, including but not limited to the important features, purposes of use, how to use or operate properly, maintenance, interpretation of their readings, and more.

6. This book is intended to be a practical and concise guide for pharmacists and users to simplify information about devices and provide the information needed for proper use.

7. This book is intended to act as an atlas that illustrates information textually and graphically using photographic pictures, diagrams, and drawings.

8. This book provides the available evidence on the effectiveness and cost-effectiveness and the latest information in medical devices.

9. Besides the medical devices that pharmacists come in direct contact with, each chapter on the particular therapeutic area includes some medical devices that are not related directly to pharmacy, but which pharmacists should know (devices that pharmacists might not come in direct contact with, but should know about if their patients have or use them so they can understand what they are experiencing such as pacemakers, defibrillators, left ventricle assist devices, deep brain stimulation devices for seizure disorders, bone density testing devices for osteoporosis, pulse oxygenation measurement, blood pressure and temperature devices, vascular filters, artificial heart valves, etc.

10. For devices that are usually used by patients or which patients need to know about (such as insulin syringes, insulin pens, and glucose monitoring devices) there is a special part in every chapter ready to be conveyed by pharmacists who want to educate and counsel patients entitled "Special tips for patient counseling."

WHO SHOULD READ THIS BOOK?

1. Pharmacists practicing in different settings as well as other interested practicing medical professionals
2. Pharmacy and medical students (e.g., can be used as a teaching source in pharmacy practice and clinical courses such as patient assessment, hospital pharmacy, community pharmacy, responding to symptoms, over-the-counter medications and devices, clinical skills lab, industrial pharmacy, etc.)
3. Pharmacy and medical educators
4. Administrative authorities in academic institutions and the inventory control departments in such institutions (medical and pharmacy colleges) as a primary list of instruments/devices and technologies needed for training in students' practical laboratories and clinical skills labs.

5. Nursing and nurse practitioner programs may be interested in a product such as this. Perhaps medical technology programs as well.

REFERENCES

1. World Health Organization. Medical devices: managing the mismatch: an outcome of the priority medical devices project. Geneva, Switzerland: World Health Organization; 2010.
2. Monsein LH. Primer on medical device regulation. Part I. History and background. Radiology. 1997 Oct;205(1):1–9.
3. Hutt PB. A history of government regulation of adulteration and misbranding of medical devices. Food, Drug, Cosmet Law J. 1989 Mar 1;44(2):99–117.
4. Sweet BV, Schwemm AK, Parsons DM. Review of the processes for FDA oversight of drugs, medical devices, and combination products. J Manag Care Pharm. 2011 Jan;17(1):40–50.
5. Van Der Palen J, Thomas M, Chrystyn H, et al. A randomised open-label cross-over study of inhaler errors, preference and time to achieve correct inhaler use in patients with COPD or asthma: comparison of ELLIPTA with other inhaler devices. NPJ Prim Care Resp Med. 2016 Nov 24;26(1):1–8.
6. von Schantz S, Katajavuori N, Antikainen O, et al. Evaluation of dry powder inhalers with a focus on ease of use and user preference in inhaler-naive individuals. Int J Pharm. 2016 Jul 25;509(1–2):50–8.
7. Bryant L, Bang C, Chew C, et al. Adequacy of inhaler technique used by people with asthma or chronic obstructive pulmonary disease. J Prim Health Care. 2013;5(3):191–8.
8. Plaza V, Giner J, Rodrigo GJ, et al. Errors in the use of inhalers by health care professionals: a systematic review. J Allergy Clin Immunol Pract. 2018 May 1;6(3):987–95.
9. Almazrou S, Alsahly H, Alwattar H, et al. Ability of Saudi mothers to appropriately and accurately use dosing devices to administer oral liquid medications to their children. Drug, Healthc Patient Saf. 2015;7:1.
10. US FDA. Classify you medical devices. 2020. Available from: www.fda.gov/medical-devices/overview-device-regulation/classify-your-medical-device (accessed 12 June 2021).
11. Sherman J, Lee HC, Weiss ME, et al. Medical device design education: identifying problems through observation and hands-on training. Des Technol Educ. 2018;23(2):154–74.
12. May-Newman K, Cornwall GB. Teaching medical device design using design control. Expert Rev Med Devices. 2012 Jan;9(1):7–14. https://doi.org/10.1586/erd.11.63.
13. Baura G and Berry T. AC 2011–1920: comprehensive teaching of medical devices. Washington, DC: American Society for Engineering Education; 2011.

Section I

Medical Devices for Specialized Services and Purposes

2 Medical Devices for Pharmacy-Based Anticoagulant Services

Hazem Fathy Elewa

CONTENTS

BACKGROUND

Oral anticoagulation therapy is used to prevent thromboembolism in patients with variety of disorders, including atrial fibrillation, prosthetic heart valves, coronary artery disease, and venous thromboembolism.[1,2] Warfarin is the mainstay oral anticoagulant medication and one of the most widely prescribed medications all over the world.[3] Because of the narrow therapeutic index of warfarin and large interpatient variability, close and consistent monitoring of anticoagulation is mandated to ensure optimal outcomes and minimize the risks associated with inappropriate management. International normalized ratio (INR) is a reliable surrogate marker that has been used for decades as an indicator for warfarin's therapeutic effect to ensure optimal outcomes for anticoagulated patients.[2] Guidelines recommend that healthcare providers involved in the management of oral anticoagulation therapy should do so in a systematic and coordinated fashion, incorporating patient education, systematic INR testing, tracking, follow-up, and good patient communication of results and dosing decisions.[4] The challenging management of oral anticoagulation therapy has led to the development of a variety of models including patient self-management, specialized anticoagulation clinics, and pharmacist-managed anticoagulation clinics.[5] Many studies have indicated that specialized anticoagulation clinics can reduce complications associated with inappropriate warfarin use and improve its efficacy.[6] Pharmacist-managed anticoagulation clinic represents a model that provides patients with more consistent management, closer monitoring,

more education, and awareness especially in regards to interacting drugs and food that can alter warfarin efficacy and safety.[5,7–9] Overall flow in specialized anticoagulation clinics starts with patient check-in, measurement of INR, patient interview and data gathering, assessment of warfarin therapy, making a therapeutic plan, and scheduling a follow-up appointment for the patient.[10] INR can be measured through venipuncture at the laboratory or through finger stick point-of-care (POC) testing. POC testing is considered to be a faster, more patient-friendly and reliable alternative to the venipuncture measurement of the INR.[11] Since the 1990s, POC devices started to be introduced as self-testing devices as well which allowed patients to measure their INR at home. In the practice of self-monitoring, a patient tests the INR at home then contacts the clinic to report it and gets instruction on appropriate dose adjustment, and in self-managing, a patient tests the INR at home then makes adjustment to the dose based on a predetermined instruction scheme.[12,13] Both INR venipuncture and POC instruments work essentially through the same mechanism by measuring primarily the prothrombin time (PT). The PT measures the recalcification and clotting time of a patient's plasma in the presence of thromboplastin (a potent tissue procoagulant extract).[14] Due to lack of standardization of commercial thromboplastin used by the different laboratories, PT results differ significantly from one facility to another. Based on international collaborative study, the use of INR was proposed and adopted by the World Health Organization (WHO) in the early 1980s.[15] INR system is defined as the ratio of the PT to the geometric

DOI: 10.1201/9781003002345-3

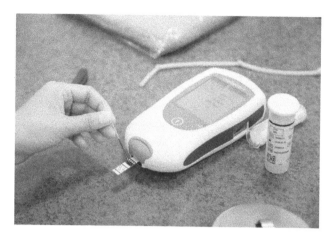

FIGURE 2.1 CoaguCheck System™ including testing, lancing device, and test strips.

Source: www.shutterstock.com/image-photo/khonkaen-thailand-january-27-2018-drop-1010736280

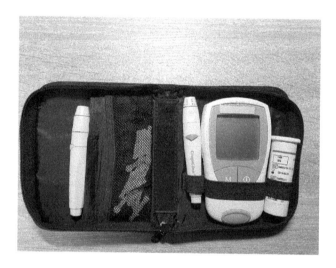

FIGURE 2.2 CoaguCheck System™ with a strip inserted into the device and the testing in progress.

Source: www.shutterstock.com/image-photo/heiligenhaus-nrw-germany-november-30-2018-1288429105

mean of prothrombin time of at least 20 adult normal subjects calculated in terms of the appropriate International Sensitivity Index (ISI). It can be calculated using the following formula, INR = (patient's PT/mean PT)^{ISI}. The ISI is a numerical value that calibrates the responsiveness of any given commercial thromboplastin system relative to the international standard. It takes into account the variability in results obtained using different commercial systems in calculating the results. With the INR system, results from different laboratories and countries can be compared with very minimal variabilities.

DEVICE DESCRIPTION

A typical portable POC INR test device is a battery-operated meter that has an electrical charging dock. It has a screen that displays the results and an opening for the testing strips. Meters are typically supplies with a lancing device, test strips, and standards for calibration. A test strip is inserted into the meter, then the lancing device is used to obtain a capillary blood droplet which is applied directly to the test strip. The meter reads the test strip and measures the time it takes the blood to form a clot then presents the results on the screen as INR (and PT in some meters). Among the most common POC INR test devices are CoaguCheck System™ by Roche Diagnostics, Hemochron™ by International Technidyne Corporation (ITC), and Alere™ by Abott.

HOW TO USE/OPERATIONAL REQUIREMENTS

The following steps will explain how to use the POC INR meter.

1. Turn on the device using the on/off switch. Alternatively, insert a test strip and the device will automatically turn –on.
2. Wash hands using warm water and soap. Dry hands thoroughly.
3. Apply alcohol swab to the finger that will be pricked by the lancing device.
4. Remove the test strip from the container and insert it into the designated opening in the meter.
5. Confirm that the code chip number displayed on the device screen matches the batch number on the test strip container.
6. Prick the tip of the finger with the lancing device and discard the lancet in a sharps or plastic container.
7. Wait until the device gives the signal that it is ready (For example: showing a figure of a blood drop on the screen, or beeping. The signal may differ from one device to another).
8. Apply the blood sample to the target area of the test strip within 15 seconds of pricking the fingertip.
9. Keep applying the blood to the strip until the device beeps signaling that the sample is being processed.
10. Wait until the INR results appear on the screen which may take 30–60 seconds, and record the result.
11. Remove the test strip and dispose of it appropriately.

INTERPRETATION OF READINGS

As previously explained, POC INR testing devices measure the PT/INR with some newer models equipped to measure the partial thromboplastin time (PTT) and activated partial thromboplastin time (aPTT). PT/INR measures the time it takes the blood to clot. Since INR is a ratio taking into account the PT of healthy individuals, a normal INR of a healthy subject is (or very close to) 1.[14]

INR is used in clinical settings to measure the anticoagulation effect of vitamin K antagonists such as warfarin. INR targets of 2.5 (2–3) or 3 (2.5–3.5) are the most common therapeutic targets used in the different thromboembolic conditions requiring warfarin therapy.[16] INR below therapeutic target indicates reduced anticoagulation effect of warfarin which may be associated with increased risk of thrombosis (especially with INR below 1.5). On the other hand, INR above therapeutic target indicates augmented anticoagulation effect of warfarin which may be associated with increased risk of bleeding (especially with INR above 4.5).[17]

IMPORTANT SAFETY ISSUES

Here are some important safety tips that should be followed to achieve adequate operation of the POC INR device.

1. The meter should be operated at room temperature.
2. The meter should be kept horizontal when testing is in process.
3. The meter should not be used near a strong magnetic field.
4. Avoid using a code chip from a box of test strips other the one that is actually used.
5. Avoid touching the test strip with wet hands.
6. Avoid removing the test strip while measurement is in process.
7. Do not delay the application of the blood onto the test strip by more than 15 seconds.
8. Blood sample application should be done all at once.
9. Avoid addition of more blood sample once the measurement is in process.
10. Avoid touching buttons on the meter while the device is testing.

STORAGE CONDITIONS AND MAINTENANCE

Meters should be stored at room temperature. Avoid storing the meter in damp or humid conditions (more than 85% humidity). Meters should be kept in a clean, dust-free area. Meters should be regularly cleaned especially if it is dirty or has any remaining blood spots. Use a swab or damp cloth for cleaning and avoid using sprays of any kind. The appropriate cleansing agents include 70% isopropyl alcohol and 10% hypochlorite solution (1 part bleach to 9 parts distilled water). Wipe the device from the outside after being turned off and avoid the accumulation of liquids near any openings. Dry the exterior with a lint-free cloth and wipe away any residual liquid or moisture. INR meters require routine performance of quality control (QC); however, devices differ in how often QC is required and how it is performed. Some devices have internal electronic QC run with every PT/INR check while others may require daily and/or weekly manual QC. QC is performed through the addition of one or more standard solutions that should yield certain readings in order to pass the QC. Refer to the individual meter manual for more detailed instructions.

IMPORTANT FEATURES AND SPECIAL ADVANTAGES

Here are some of the most important features and advantages of POC INR devices.

1. Most meters automatically store the results (up to 100 readings or more).
2. Most meters have the ability to scan the medical record number to store the results to the corresponding patient.
3. Most meters have the ability to interface with the electronic medical record system used at the healthcare facility and migrate the results to the corresponding patient medical record.
4. Compared to the conventional venipuncture INR performed in the laboratory, POC INR meters require much less blood volume (around 10 mcl), require less processing time and labor, and are more convenient for the patient.
5. POC INR meters can function with a capillary blood sample (retrieved through finger prick) which is less painful and more convenient for the patients than the venipuncture INR performed at the laboratory.
6. Many POC INR meters have also the ability to measure PTT and aPTT.

SPECIAL TIPS FOR PATIENT COUNSELING

Here are some important tips that should be considered by the practitioner performing the INR POC testing or communicated to the patient/family if performing self-testing.[18]

1. Make sure that the fingers are not too cold by massaging the hands, holding hands under the arm, or washing hands with warm water.
2. Avoid squeezing or "milking" the fingers to get sufficient amount of blood.
3. Avoid switching to another spot on the same finger or to a different finger if unable to get a sufficient amount of blood from the initial spot.
4. POC INR meter readings may be affected by some factors/medical conditions such as hematocrit, anemia, antiphospholipid antibody syndrome, malignancy, infection, and inflammatory conditions.
5. Laboratory INR may need to be performed occasionally to confirm INR readings in the conditions stated previously.
6. Laboratory INR is also recommended for confirmation of POC INR readings above 5 since INR readings may be less accurate above this value in most POC meters.
7. Encourage patients using self-testing meters to get their INR compared occasionally to laboratory INR values to confirm accuracy of their meters.

AVAILABLE EVIDENCE ON THE EFFECTIVENESS AND SAFETY

Warfarin is the cornerstone prevention and treatment of a wide variety of thromboembolic disease such as deep venous thrombosis, pulmonary embolism, and stroke. Because of the narrow therapeutic index of warfarin and large interpatient variability, close and consistent monitoring of anticoagulation through the INR is mandated to ensure optimal efficacy and safety.[19,20] Thus, it is very important to use INR testing devices with high accuracy and precision to ensure results' validity when making clinical recommendations for warfarin patients.[21] POC INR testing devices were introduced to the market in the 1990s to meet the increased demand for oral anticoagulant (warfarin) use. Due to the ease of their use by healthcare providers, convenience for the patient (requires only a finger prick) and short time from test to result, a majority of clinics managing warfarin patients rely heavily on POC INR testing devices. And while the precision and accuracy of the POC INR testing devices are slightly lower than that achieved with the automated INR laboratory instruments,[11,21] their clinical advantages have helped many patients to be more consistent with and adherent to their INR follow-up measurements. This in turn translates into better effectiveness and safety outcomes. It is worth mentioning, however, that it is very important to calibrate POC INR testing devices as instructed by the manufacturer and to routinely compare the POC INR testing device results with a laboratory test to eliminate potential imprecision errors.

ECONOMIC EVALUATION

As explained in the introduction of this chapter, there are various types of INR testing strategies: laboratory INR testing; POC clinic-based INR testing; POC self-monitoring home INR testing; and POC self-managing home INR testing. Although the same POC device may be used in the last 3 strategies, the strategy itself may yield different clinical and economical outcomes. In a cost utility analysis that was conducted comparing these 4 strategies by the Canadian ministry of health, it was found that the laboratory INR testing had the least cost ($7,033 per patient). On the other hand, self-managing POC INR testing strategy had the greatest number of quality-adjusted life-years (QALYs) (4.2136) but was only marginally higher than the laboratory INR testing (4.1957) with an additional cost of $233. This led to an incremental cost-effectiveness ratio (ICER) of $13,028 per QALY gained for the self-managing strategy. The POC clinic-based INR testing and the POC self-monitoring home INR testing were dominated by the self-managing strategy with total incremental cost of $575 and $968 more per patient and fewer QALY gains.[22]

As in any economic model, these results cannot be considered generalizable since they may differ based on the healthcare setting, country, payer perspective, frequency of INR checks, and time in therapeutic range.

CHALLENGES TO THE PHARMACISTS AND USERS

POC INR testing meters are not without challenges to the pharmacists and the users. Among the most common challenges are the following:

1. Capillary blood sample should be accessed within 15 seconds which may not be sufficient period of time especially for untrained users. In this case, another finger should be pricked and the initial test strip may need to be discarded if it came into contact with the initial blood sample.
2. Laboratory INR is also recommended for confirmation of POC INR readings above 5 since INR readings may be less accurate above this value in most POC meters.
3. POC INR meters reading may be affected by some factors/medical conditions such as hematocrit, anemia, antiphospholipid antibody syndrome, malignancy, infection, and inflammatory conditions.
4. Laboratory INR may need to be performed occasionally to confirm INR readings in the conditions stated here.

RECOMMENDATIONS: THE WAY FORWARD

While warfarin is still used for patients requiring treatment with oral anticoagulants, direct oral anticoagulants are now becoming more frequently used and there may be future POC testing devices to measure the effect of these drugs.

CONCLUSION

The aims of POC testing are convenience for the patient, faster test results to the healthcare provider, and potentially more timely clinical decision-making, all of which improve clinical outcomes and reduce healthcare resource use. The site of POC is not restricted to the bedside, but can occur in a variety of locations, as long as the technology is in close proximity to the patient: in a hospital, a doctor's office, a pharmacy, the patient's home, a community clinic, or an anticoagulation clinic.

REFERENCES

1. Nutescu EA, Shapiro NL, Ibrahim S, et al. Warfarin and its interactions with foods, herbs and other dietary supplements. Expert Opin Drug Saf. 2006;5(3):433–51.
2. Pirmohamed M. Warfarin: almost 60 years old and still causing problems. Br J Clin Pharmacol. 2006;62(5):509–11.
3. Nutescu EA, Spinler SA, Dager WE, et al. Transitioning from traditional to novel anticoagulants: the impact of oral direct thrombin inhibitors on anticoagulation management. Pharmacotherapy. 2004;24(10 Pt 2):199S–202S.
4. Guyatt GH, Akl EA, Crowther M, et al. Executive summary: antithrombotic therapy and prevention of thrombosis, 9th ed: American College of Chest Physicians evidence-based clinical practice guidelines. Chest. 2012;141(2 Suppl):7S–47S.

5. Nutescu EA. Anticoagulation management services: entering a new era. Pharmacotherapy. 2010;30(4):327–9.

6. Chiquette E, Amato MG, Bussey HI. Comparison of an anticoagulation clinic with usual medical care: anticoagulation control, patient outcomes, and health care costs. Arch Intern Med. 1998;158(15):1641–7.

7. Garton L, Crosby JF. A retrospective assessment comparing pharmacist-managed anticoagulation clinic with physician management using international normalized ratio stability. J Thromb Thrombolysis. 2011;32(4):426–30.

8. Young S, Bishop L, Twells L, et al. Comparison of pharmacist managed anticoagulation with usual medical care in a family medicine clinic. BMC Fam Pract. 2011;12:88.

9. Elewa HF, DeRemer CE, Keller K, et al. Patients satisfaction with warfarin and willingness to switch to dabigatran: a patient survey. J Thromb Thrombolysis. 2014;38(1):115–20.

10. Vazquez SR, Jennifer C, Gale H, et al. Anticoagulation clinic workflow analysis. J Am Pharm Assoc. 2009;49(1):78–85.

11. Tay HM, Lai YF, Kong MC, et al. Generational performance of three point-of-care testing devices compared with standard laboratory measurement of the international normalised ratio across extended ranges. J Clin Pathol. 2019;72(4):311–15.

12. Heneghan CJ, Garcia-Alamino JM, Spencer EA, et al. Self-monitoring and self-management of oral anticoagulation. Cochrane Database Syst Rev. 2016;7(7):CD003839.

13. Gardiner C, Williams K, Mackie IJ, et al. Patient self-testing is a reliable and acceptable alternative to laboratory INR monitoring. Br J Haematol. 2005;128(2):242–7.

14. Poller L. International Normalized Ratios (INR): the first 20 years. J Thromb Haemost. 2004;2(6):849–60.

15. WHO. Requirements for thromboplastins and plasma used to control oral anticoagulant therapy (Requirements for Biological Substances no. 30, revised 1982). 1983. Contract No.: no. 687.

16. Ageno W, Gallus AS, Wittkowsky A, et al. Oral anticoagulant therapy: antithrombotic therapy and prevention of thrombosis, 9th ed: American College of Chest Physicians evidence-based clinical practice guidelines. Chest. 2012;141(2 Suppl):e44S–88S.

17. Hylek EM, Skates SJ, Sheehan MA, et al. An analysis of the lowest effective intensity of prophylactic anticoagulation for patients with nonrheumatic atrial fibrillation. N Engl J Med. 1996;335(8):540–6.

18. FDA. Information for health care providers using INR test meters in a clinical setting. 2018 [updated 8 Feb 2018]. Available from: www.fda.gov/medical-devices/warfarin-inr-test-meters/information-health-care-providers-using-inr-test-meters-clinical-setting.

19. Elewa H, Jalali F, Khudair N, et al. Evaluation of pharmacist-based compared to doctor-based anticoagulation management in Qatar. J Eval Clin Pract. 2016;22(3):433–8.

20. Stoudenmire LG, DeRemer CE, Elewa H. Telephone versus office-based management of warfarin: impact on international normalized ratios and outcomes. Int J Hematol. 2014;100(2):119–24.

21. van den Besselaar AM. Accuracy, precision, and quality control for point-of-care testing of oral anticoagulation. J Thromb Thrombolysis. 2001;12(1):35–40.

22. Health CAfDaTi. Point-of-care testing of international normalized ratio for patients on oral anticoagulant therapy: systematic review and economic analysis. Ottawa: The Agency; 2014 July.

3 Self-Testing Medical Devices for the Detection, Diagnosis or Management of Health Conditions
A Public Health Perspective

Silvia E. Rabionet

CONTENTS

INTRODUCTION

Self-tests, also known as home tests, are typically sold over the counter (OTC) in pharmacies and allow users to test self-collected specimens and interpret the results in the comfort of their homes without the need of a trained or licensed health professional. These tests differ from home collection tests, which require mailing or taking the sample to a laboratory or clinic for processing analysis and interpretation.[1]

In this chapter I will present medical devices in the form of self-tests approved by the FDA for diagnosis and monitoring of illnesses that constitute public health threats and that have a global impact. Specifically, I will be presenting the evolution and current use of self-tests in monitoring diabetes and in identifying new cases of HIV and COVID-19. These testing technologies involve self-collection of a biological samples such as blood, oral fluid, or urine; self-testing of the sample; and interpretation of the results by the individual tested. The products include inserts of self-explanatory instructions provided by the manufacturer. I will also be discussing the impact that these devices can play in curtailing current epidemics and review some challenges associated with their widespread use. The discussion will consider their significance in creating the capacity for self-care. These discussions will be contextualized by describing the public health burden of the selected illnesses. Self-testing technologies have proven their diagnostic capabilities, but also are a powerful tool for clinical prevention, avoiding complications of diseases like diabetes, and preventing spread of infectious diseases like HIV and COVID-19.

DIABETES AND SELF-TESTING AND MONITORING

Diabetes is a chronic disease that leads to uncontrolled blood glucose. It occurs either when the pancreas does not produce enough insulin or when the body cannot effectively use the insulin it produces. It is estimated that 422 million people worldwide are suffering from diabetes. Diabetes has been associated with damage to the heart, blood vessels, eyes, kidneys, and nerves. According to the World Health Organization,[2] people with diabetes have a two- to three-fold increased risk of heart attacks and strokes. Poor blood flow and neuropathy in the feet increases the chance of foot ulcers and infections, eventually leading to amputations. It is the cause of 2.6% of global blindness due to diabetic retinopathy that results in accumulated damage to the retina. Diabetes is also among the leading causes of kidney illnesses and failure.[3,4]

Currently, more than 34 million Americans have diabetes, representing 10.5% of the United States population. This percentage increases with age, reaching 28.8% among people 65 and over. Approximately 90–95% of them have type 2 diabetes. People over age 45 are at a greater risk of developing diabetes, but increasingly more children and younger adults are also developing it. It is estimated that 7.3 million adults are not aware that they have diabetes.[5]

Diabetes management requires glucose level monitoring and adequate insulin dosing. For people who already have a diagnosis of diabetes, a home blood glucose test enables them to monitor their blood sugar levels. Self-monitoring blood glucose (SMBG) devices play an important role in the management of diabetes and in the reduction of risk of serious secondary clinical complications.[6] This can not only benefit individual patients but can result in reduced expenditures at the primary care level and in hospitalizations. Meter and reagent strip systems to monitor blood glucose were developed in the late 1960s, making it a viable first step for diabetes self-monitoring with instant clinical information. This technology has experienced significant development in design and dissemination over the past 60 years. The first portable glucose meter was the Ames Reflectance Meter and became widely available in 1970. They are regulated by the US Food and Drug Administration (FDA). The FDA issues warnings and educational material to encourage adequate use.[7,8] Figure 3.1 illustrates a SGBM meter.

SMBG is the most widely used method for monitoring how effectively the body is processing glucose in the comfort of the home. SMBG meters are portable devices that measure blood glucose concentration in a drop of blood using finger-stick blood samples and test strips. Over the past six decades, enormous progress has been made in glucose meters' technology. The size of SBGM meters have been reduced, and its accuracy has significantly improved. Many meters are now affordable and have integrated advanced data-handling capabilities and features to record daily doses of insulin, intake of carbohydrates, and workout history. Most meters allow for recording results on cellular smartphones, using apps. There is evidence of the impact of lower cost on increased use, enabling patients to monitor their blood glucose levels. Despite their benefits Clarke et al. argue that

> a number of barriers to optimal adherence to SMBG have been identified and include demographic factors, notably in ethnic minority groups, and significantly psychosocial elements such as anxiety, self-perception of diabetes and vulnerability to complications, and the quality of support available by the healthcare provider and family. Patients may be stressed by the responsibility of self-care and the demands of regular and possibly repeated painful finger-prick, or lack the motivation and discipline required.[9]

The advent of real-time continuous glucose monitoring (CGM) systems that measure glucose levels continuously constitute an important breakthrough and revolutionary development in diabetes self-home-care technology. They are especially beneficial for people with type 1 diabetes. However, the American Diabetes Association (ADA), the American Association of Clinical Endocrinologists (AACE), and American College of Endocrinology (ACE) have reported its benefit for people on intensive insulin treatment. CGM comprises a glucose-sensing device inserted in the abdomen or on the arm, electrochemically measuring glucose levels in subcutaneous tissues; it eliminates the need for continuous finger-sticks. The Guardian Real-Time System (Medtronic MiniMed) got FDA approval in 1999 as the first CGM device.[10] Since then, the accuracy of CGM technologies has remarkably improved, reaching the performance of SMBG devices. CGM devices currently in the market provide alerts to the patients helping them detect hypo- and hyperglycemic events. Some of the most commonly used systems with integrated alerts are the Dexcom G5 Mobile and G6, the Medtronic Enlite and Guardian, FreeStyle Libre 2, and the Senseonics Eversense (refer to Figure 3.2). Cappon et al. Claim, "CGM devices have been proved to improve safety and effectiveness of diabetes therapy, reduce hypoglycemia incidence and duration, and decrease glycemic variability. Furthermore, the real-time availability of blood glucose values has been stimulating the realization of new tools to provide patients with decision support to improve insulin dosage tuning and infusion."[11,12]

Research and development continue to provide innovative ways to advance autonomous devices. The healthcare systems need to promote their use and find alternatives for dissemination, reduce costs, and guarantee widespread availability of the newer technologies as they emerge. The data collected by these devices provide options for patient-provider communication and allow for the potential of improving the health and quality of life of the patient with diabetes. In addition, I claim that the collected data could be useful in making epidemiological decision at the micro and macro levels.

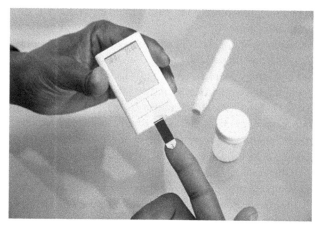

FIGURE 3.1 Glucose monitoring meter and strips.

Source: www.fda.gov/consumers/consumer-updates/how-safely-use-glucose-meters-and-test-strips-diabetes

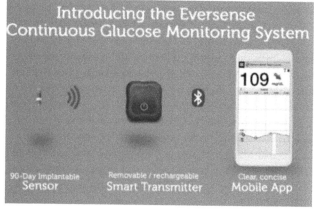

FIGURE 3.2 Example of a continuous glucose monitoring system.

HIV AND DIAGNOSTIC SELF-TESTING

The human immunodeficiency virus (HIV) attacks the body's immune system. HIV is found in blood, semen, pre-seminal fluid, vaginal fluid, rectal fluid, and breast milk. It is transmitted person to person, underscoring the importance of screening and awareness of having the disease. If HIV is not treated, it can lead to AIDS (acquired immunodeficiency syndrome). There is currently no effective cure for HIV. HIV disease continues to be a serious health issue for parts of the world. However, with proper medical care and adherence to antiretroviral therapy, HIV can be controlled.

Worldwide, there are about 1.7 million new reported cases each year. About 37.9 million people were living with HIV around the world, and 24.5 million are receiving antiretroviral therapy (ART). An estimated 770,000 people have died from AIDS-related illnesses since the start of the epidemic. In the United States it is estimated that 1.2 million live with HIV; of those about 14% (1 in 7) were unaware that they had HIV.[13]

Screening and early diagnosis is key for controlling the progression of the illness in individuals and for curtailing the epidemic at the population level. The gap in screening has been explained by lack of access to care, poor knowledge about risks, and the stigma associated with having HIV. Self-testing for HIV can be a powerful tool for closing the gap on early screening. Although the US Food and Drug Administration (FDA)-approved HIV home-collection tests have been on the market since 1996, various concerns have prevented the approval of a home test until recently, including that people that tested positive might delay contacting the healthcare provider. Since July 2012, the FDA approved the OraQuick® In-Home HIV Test for rapid home-testing, manufactured by OraSure Technologies, Inc. It remains the only approved test in the United States. There is authorization to sell in stores and online to people over 17 years or age. The FDA describes the OraQuick® In-Home HIV Test as "an in-vitro diagnostic home-use test for HIV (HIV-1 and HIV-2) in oral fluid. This test works by looking for your body's response (antibodies) to fighting the HIV virus. A positive result is preliminary and follow-up confirmatory testing is needed."[14] The FDA reported specificity of the test to be 99.8% (indicating one in 5,000 results may be a false positive. The FDA conducted a Monte Carlo mathematical simulation model of self-test use that demonstrated that 4,000 infections might be prevented in the first year of its use.[15]

After self-testing, linkage to healthcare clinical service should follow, independently of the results. Confirmatory tests are needed if positive, and if the confirmatory test is positive treatment should be offered. In the case of a negative test, the option to receive FDA-approved PrEP (or pre-exposure prophylaxis) drugs should be offered and evaluated.

The CDC recommends "that everyone between the ages of 13 and 64 years old be screened for HIV at least once as part of their routine health care." Home self-testing should facilitate and promote population level compliance of this recommendation. More frequent testing is recommended for people who have a higher risk of infection because of behaviors such as having sex without condoms, having sex with multiple partners, or using injectable drugs with shared needles.[16] For this test, the person must swab his or her gums to collect an oral fluid sample and use the materials in the kit (stick and tube with testing solution) to test the oral fluid sample and the results will be available in 20 to 40 minutes. The test is not reliable at detecting HIV infections within 3 months of onset of exposure. Refer to Figures 3.3 and 3.4.

Issues of global adoption, dissemination, implementation, and benefits of home self-testing have been widely

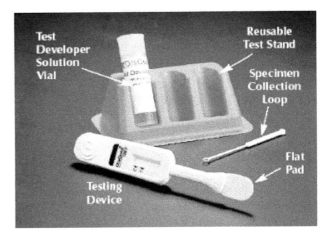

FIGURE 3.3 The contents of the The OraQuick® In-Home HIV Test.

Source: OraQuick Home HIV Test Kit (drugabusecontrol.com)

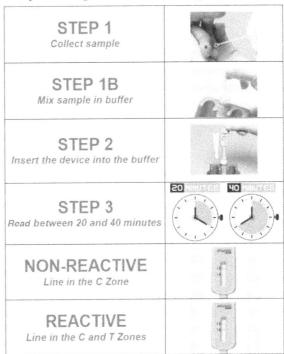

FIGURE 3.4 Educational step-by-step testing procedure.

Source: simple-finger-stick.png (633×805) (knscanada.com)

discussed in the scientific and lay literature.[17] Salient issues are the appropriate and coordinated linkage to culturally sensitive care, the generalized stigma associated with HIV, and the lack of mental health support. These issues are barriers that are shared by other interventions and innovations to address the HIV epidemic.[18] These issues underscore the need to continue workforce development, targeted health education, scaling of resources, and revised data-driven policies. The home self-testing technology is a promising tool for a coordinated response to HIV. In the United States, the product is sold in pharmacies, increasing the possibility of pharmacists' involvement while significantly contributing to screening as prevention from a population perspective. Pharmacists, with the right level of awareness and health education skills, can contribute to the dissemination, adopting, and appropriate use of home self-testing.

SELF-TESTING FOR COVID-19

Since 2019, the whole world has been addressing the COVID-19 epidemic, a dangerous disease caused by SARS-CoV-2 virus discovered in Wuhan, China. It is very contagious and has quickly spread around to all continents.[19] Since its onset there has been an untiring and constant race to address the health consequences and the social disruptions caused by the virus responsible for COVID-19.

In September 2021, the United States reported nearly 40.8 million accumulated diagnosed cases, and 656,318

deaths. Worldwide 173.4 million people have reported having COVID-19 and the deaths are quickly approaching 3.8 million. COVID-19 most often causes respiratory symptoms that can feel much like a cold, the flu, or pneumonia, but COVID-19 can also harm other parts of the body. Older adults and some specific groups, like minorities and people living in underdeveloped countries, have suffered a disproportionate burden of the disease.[20] The massive response has included preventive measures like mandated mask-wearing, social distancing, school and business closings, and travel bans, among others. Rapid and unprecedented resources have been devoted to biomedical research and the development of vaccines. The US FDA have provided emergency-use authorization to three different vaccines. Vaccination plans have been rolled out around the world, with different levels of success. Treatment protocols to address the multiple symptoms are constantly under revision, and some have avoided hospitalizations and deaths.

Within this context, we cannot minimize the role of testing and screening for COVID-19 as a diagnostic measure and as one of the pillars for reducing the spread of the virus. The FDA is actively authorizing COVID-19 tests understanding the importance of it as a public health measure, jointly with other prevention strategies. This includes emergency-use authorizations for COVID-19 tests in which some or all testing processes can be performed at home. A negative result means the test did not detect the SARS-CoV-2 virus, and a positive result means the test did detect the SARS-CoV-2 virus. The FDA

02/11/2021	Ellume Limited	Ellume COVID-19 Home Test 12/15/2020	Lateral Flow, Fluorescence, Instrument Read, Over the Counter (OTC) Home Testing, Screening	Home, H, M, W
04/12/2021	Abbott Diagnostics Scarborough, Inc.	BinaxNOW COVID-19 Ag Card Home Test 12/16/2020	Lateral Flow, Visual Read, Prescription Home Testing	Home, H, M, W
03/01/2021	Quidel Corporation	QuickVue At-Home COVID-19 Test 03/01/2021	Lateral Flow, Visual Read, Prescription Home Testing	Home, H, M, W
03/31/2021	Quidel Corporation	QuickVue At-Home OTC COVID-19 Test 03/31/2021	Lateral Flow, Visual Read, Over the Counter (OTC) Home Testing, Serial Screening	Home, H, M, W
04/01/2021	Abbott Diagnostics Scarborough, Inc.	BinaxNOW COVID-19 Antigen Self Test 03/31/2021	Lateral Flow, Visual Read, Over the Counter (OTC) Home Testing, Serial Screening	Home, H, M, W
03/31/2021	Abbott Diagnostics Scarborough, Inc.	BinaxNOW COVID-19 Ag Card 2 Home Test 03/31/2021	Lateral Flow, Visual Read, Over the Counter (OTC) Home Testing, Telehealth Proctor Supervised, Serial Screening	Home, H, M, W
06/04/2021	OraSure Technologies, Inc.	InteliSwab COVID-19 Rapid Test Rx 06/04/2021	Lateral Flow, Visual Read, Prescription Home Testing	Home, H, M, W
06/04/2021	OraSure Technologies, Inc.	InteliSwab COVID-19 Rapid Test 06/04/2021	Lateral Flow, Visual Read, Over the Counter (OTC) Home Testing, Serial Screening	Home, H, M, W

FIGURE 3.5   Individual EUAs for antigen diagnostic tests for SARS-CoV-2 authorized for home testing as of June 4, 2021.

Source: www.fda.gov/medical-devices/coronavirus-disease-2019-covid-19-emergency-use-authorizations-medical-devices/in-vitro-diagnostics-euas-antigen-diagnostic-tests-sars-cov-2

"cautions patients against using the results from any serology test as an indication that they can stop taking steps to protect themselves and others, such as stopping social distancing or discontinuing wearing masks."[21] Refer to Figure 3.5 for a list of current home tests approved by the FDA. It should be highlighted that this list is rapidly changing and expanding.

Currently, most of the OTC testing options are not covered by health insurances in the United States. Some COVID-19 collection kits are available for a $0 upfront charge if prescribed or if the person to be tested meets symptoms-related screening criteria for COVID-19 testing. They have not been designed to test the efficacy of the COVID-19 vaccination, a common misconception among the population. The role of the chain and independent pharmacies has been recognized during this pandemic and has been instrumental in the testing and screening. With the addition of OTC testing options that can be conducted from the comfort of home the pharmacies remain a critical component of the pandemic response nationally and internationally.

The applicability and accuracy of a self-testing strategy for SARS-CoV-2 from a population perspective merits further study, due to the newness of the technology and the changing patterns of the epidemic.[22] It has been argued by some that the expansion and investment in SARS-CoV-2 testing programs with more frequent and rapid tests across diverse communities, in conjunction with the self-isolation of individuals with confirmed infection. are essential for alleviating the COVID-19 pandemic.[23,24]

CONCLUSION

Self-testing for monitoring and diagnosis of diseases cannot be ignored as a prevention tool. As primary healthcare services patient-centered care and shared clinical decision making are accepted as best practices, the ability to empower patients with point of care tests becomes an indispensable tool. In the case of monitoring diabetes, patients have embraced the technology and its evolution in such a way that self-monitoring has become the norm. This is not necessarily the case when it comes to infectious diseases like HIV and COVID-19. Barriers associated with financing and linkage to care remain the greatest concerns.

Tests by themselves are not a solution to improve health. They have to be embedded in coordinated public health strategies that consider the social determinants of health. In order for the benefits of self-testing for chronic and infectious diseases to be maximized, there is a need to empower patients to understand and manage their self-diagnosis with appropriate resources. Patients need to trust the system, set clear health objectives, be transparent, share the results, and be skillful in communicating with health professionals. Furthermore, psychological support must be readily available to ensure that patients are prepared to receive their results and engage in appropriate management. Concurrently to the dissemination of the technology, there is a need to educate patients to use, understand, and manage the diagnostic results. To fully benefit from self-testing technology, there is a need for systemic approaches to improving health outcomes.

REFERENCES

1. Ibitoye M, Frasca T, Giguere R, et al. Home testing past, present and future: lessons learned and implications for HIV home tests. AIDS Behav. 2014;18(5):933–49. https://doi.org/10.1007/s10461-013-0668-9.

2. World Health Organization. Diabetes. Available from: www.who.int/news-room/fact-sheets/detail/diabetes (accessed 30 Apr 2021).

3. Bourne RR, Stevens GA, White RA, et al. Causes of vision loss worldwide, 1990–2010: a systematic analysis. Lancet Glob Health, 2013;1(6):e339–49. https://doi.org/10.1016/S2214-109X(13)70113-X.

4. Saran R, Li Y, Robinson B, et al. US Renal data system 2014 annual data report: epidemiology of kidney disease in the United States. Am J Kidney Dis. 2015;66(1 Suppl 1):Svii–S305. https://doi.org/10.1053/j.ajkd.2015.05.001.

5. Centers for Disease Control. Diabetes data and statistics. Available from: www.cdc.gov/diabetes/data/index.html (accessed 10 May 2021).

6. Centers for Disease Control. Monitoring your blood sugar. Available from: www.cdc.gov/diabetes/managing/managing-blood-sugar/bloodglucosemonitoring.html (accessed 10 May 2021).

7. US Food and Drug Administration. How to safely use glucose meters and test strips for diabetes. Available from: www.fda.gov/consumers/consumer-updates/how-safely-use-glucose-meters-and-test-strips-diabetes (accessed 5 May 2021).

8. US Food and Drug Administration. The FDA warns against use of previously owned test strips or test strips not authorized for sale in the United States: FDA safety communication. Available from: www.fda.gov/medical-devices/safety-communications/fda-warns-against-use-previously-owned-test-strips-or-test-strips-not-authorized-sale-united-states (accessed 5 May 2021).

9. Clarke SF, Foster JR. A history of blood glucose meters and their role in self-monitoring of diabetes mellitus. Br J Biomed Sci. 2012;69(2):83–93.

10. Gifford R. Continuous glucose monitoring: 40 years, what we've learned and what's next. Chemphyschem. 2013;14(10):2032–44. https://doi.org/10.1002/cphc.201300172.

11. Cappon G, Vettoretti M, Sparacino G, et al. Continuous glucose monitoring sensors for diabetes management: a review of technologies and applications. Diabetes Metab J. 2019;43(4):383–97. https://doi.org/10.4093/dmj.2019.0121.

12. Vettoretti M, Cappon G, Acciaroli G, et al. Continuous glucose monitoring: current use in diabetes management and possible future applications. J Diabetes Sci Technol. 2018;12(5):1064–71. https://doi.org/10.1177/1932296818774078.

13. Centers for Disease Control. HIV basic statistics. Available from: www.cdc.gov/hiv/basics/statistics.html (accessed 15 May 2021).

14. Centers for Disease Control. HIV basic statistics. Available from: www.cdc.gov/hiv/basics/statistics.html (accessed 15 May 2021).

15. Myers JE, El-Sadr WM, Zerbe A, et al. Rapid HIV self-testing: long in coming but opportunities beckon. AIDS. 2013;27(11):1687–95.

16. Centers for Disease Control. Getting tested for HIV. Available from: www.cdc.gov/hiv/basics/hiv-testing/getting-tested.html (accessed 15 May 2021).

17. Estem KS, Catania J, Klausner JD. HIV self-testing: a review of current implementation and fidelity. Curr HIV/AIDS Rep.2016;13(2):107–15.https://doi.org/10.1007/s11904-016-0307-y.

18. Wood BR, Ballenger C, Stekler JD. Arguments for and against HIV self-testing. HIV/AIDS (Auckland, N.Z.). 2014;6:117–26. https://doi.org/10.2147/HIV.S49083.

19. Centers for Disease Control. Basics of COVID-19. Available from: www.cdc.gov/coronavirus/2019-ncov/your-health/about-covid-19/basics-covid-19.html (accessed 11 June 2021).

20. World Health Organization. WHO Coronavirus (COVID-19) dashboard. Available from: https://covid19.who.int (accessed 11 June 2021).

21. US Food and Drug Administration. Coronavirus Disease 2019 testing basics. Corona. Available from: www.fda. gov/consumers/consumer-updates/coronavirus-disease-2019-testing-basics (accessed 4 June 2021).

22. Iruzubieta P, Fernández-Lanas T, Rasines L, et al. Feasibility of large-scale population testing for SARS-CoV-2 detection by self-testing at home. Sci Rep. 2021;11(1):9819. https://doi.org/10.1038/s41598-021-89236-x.

23. Du Z, Pandey A, Bai Y, et al. Comparative cost-effectiveness of SARS-CoV-2 testing strategies in the USA: a modelling study. Lancet Public Health. 2021;6(3):e184–91. https://doi.org/10.1016/S2468-2667(21)00002-5.

24. Boum Y, Eyangoh S, Okomo MC. Beyond COVID-19-will self-sampling and testing become the norm? Lancet Infect Dis. 2021 Apr 12;S1473–3099(21)00197–3. https://doi.org/10.1016/S1473-3099(21)00197-3. Epub ahead of print. PMID: 33857408; PMCID: PMC8041358.

4 Medical Devices for Management of Tobacco Use Disorder

Mohamad Haniki Nik Mohamed and Ahmed Ibrahim Fathelrahman

CONTENTS

DOI: 10.1201/9781003002345-5

GENERAL BACKGROUND

Smoking is a leading cause of preventable mortality and morbidity, mainly from various vascular and respiratory diseases and cancer. Despite available scientific evidence on the health hazards of cigarette smoking, its prevalence is still high in many parts of the world, especially in low- to middle-income countries.

Nicotine addiction involves being dependent on nicotine, a naturally found psychoactive substance in tobacco. Nicotine stimulates the central nervous system at the commonly delivered doses by tobacco products to exert pleasure; improve mood, memory, and concentration; reduce anxiety and appetite; and induce other short-lived feelings of well-being. The addictive nature of nicotine includes drug-reinforced behavior, obsessive use and reoccurring use after abstaining from it, withdrawal symptoms, physical dependence, and tolerance.[1]

Based on the *Diagnostic and Statistical Manual of Mental Disorders, Fifth Edition* (DSM-5), tobacco use disorder is diagnosed when an individual uses tobacco for more than a year, and a minimum of two (2) of the eleven (11) following sub-features appear:

1. More amounts of tobacco over a longer time-frame than planned
2. Inability to quit or lessen the amount of tobacco use despite efforts to do so
3. An excessive amount of time spent on attaining or using tobacco
4. Craving or a strong desire or urge to use tobacco
5. Relinquishing responsibilities because of tobacco use
6. Persistent use of tobacco despite its negative impacts both socially and in relationships
7. Abandoning career, social, and other activities to use tobacco
8. Use of tobacco in harmful situations/settings
9. Persistent use of tobacco even in the face of physical or emotional difficulties related to tobacco use
10. Tolerance, as defined by either the need for markedly increased amounts of tobacco to achieve the desired effect or a markedly diminished effect with continued use of the same amount of tobacco
11. Withdrawal, as manifested by either the characteristic withdrawal syndrome or the use of tobacco to relieve or avoid withdrawal symptoms

Tobacco withdrawal occurs when an individual experiences the following symptoms upon cessation, including craving, problems concentrating/focusing, anxiousness, headaches, weight gain (mainly due to increased appetite), reduced heart rate, difficulties sleeping (e.g., insomnia), agitation or mood disturbance, and depression. The symptoms spike in the first several days and gradually fade around 4 to 8 weeks of continued smoking abstinence.

According to the American Psychiatric Association, tobacco use disorder is separated into three categories: mild, moderate, and severe. If two or three symptoms from the criteria exist, the tobacco use disorder is considered mild. The disorder is classified as moderate when four to five of the symptoms from the criteria are met. With six or more of the criteria, the diagnosis of severe tobacco use disorder is made.[1]

Clinical intervention that can be offered to the smokers by the healthcare professionals can be divided into three levels depending on the intensity and service provided: very brief, brief, and intensive clinical intervention.[2] Brief clinical intervention by the healthcare professionals including pharmacists increases quit rates effectively.[3] Pharmacists must act to identify those who use tobacco and offer treatment to them.

One of the strategies is based on the 5A's approach (ask, advise, assess, assist, and arrange follow-up) intended to be brief and taking minimum time from healthcare providers (Table 4.1). Upon identifying a smoker, pharmacists can provide opportunistic advice for quitting, offer assistance, make a referral (e.g., to a quit-smoking clinic), recommend pharmacotherapy, and arrange a follow-up. This opportunistic advice focuses on increasing smokers' motivation to stop smoking to improve their quitting success rate.[4] Evidence shown that such brief intervention increases overall tobacco abstinence rates.[5] There is high-quality evidence that individually delivered smoking cessation counseling can assist smokers to quit. There is moderate-quality evidence of a smaller relative benefit when counseling is used in addition to pharmacotherapy and of more intensive counseling (longer and multiple sessions) compared to a brief counseling intervention.[6]

STEP 1: ASK ABOUT TOBACCO SMOKING

Pharmacists and other healthcare providers should ask all their patients about smoking status, and they should document such information as much as possible. This should be provided as convenient during customers' routine visits regardless of their intentions to quit and whether they ask for assistance or not. Changes in smoking status should be reported continuously at each visit as smokers progress from no intention through interest in quitting, to quit attempts, to quitting, to preventing relapse. All healthcare settings should adopt good systems for documentation to ensure that smoking status is perfectly recorded at every visit.[7,8]

STEP 2: ADVICE TO QUIT

The healthcare providers should offer all patients found to be smoking clear advice about quitting. Evidence shown that advice by healthcare providers including pharmacist improves quit rates. The length of person-to-person contact sessions has been found to be associated with successful treatment outcomes and such association has been described to represent a strong dose-response relationship.[8] Collaboration between healthcare providers in providing advice has a further-strengthening effect on such rates. Healthcare providers are encouraged to provide at least a brief intervention constituting concise cessation advice to all tobacco users. However, maximum effectiveness is achieved when intensive interventions are offered whenever possible because smokers' thoughts, perceptions, and emotions towards smoking and quitting are always inconsistent (Table 4.2).[9] Face-to-face treatment sessions repeated at least four times appears to be more effective in increasing cessation. Thus, when feasible, smoking cessation service providers should make efforts in arranging for at least four sessions with patients stopping tobacco.[10]

Pharmacists should be trained to deliver brief advice effectively in order to assist smokers. This training should provide them with knowledge and skills on various types of smoking cessation advice to trigger a quit attempt.[11]

STEP 3: ASSESS WILLINGNESS TO MAKE A QUIT ATTEMPT

Various models have been proposed regarding the motivation of smokers and their willingness to quit. The Transtheoretical Model of Change or "Stage of Change" model has been used to determine smokers' willingness to quit. This model suggests that the smoker goes through a series of phases during his/her smoking cessation process: pre-contemplative (the smoker does not contemplate quitting smoking), contemplative (the smoker begins thinking about quitting smoking within the next six months), preparative (the smoker is prepared to quit smoking), smoking cessation, and the eventual relapses that restart the cycle.[12] Those in the pre-contemplation and contemplation stages are considered to have a lower willingness to quit than those in the preparation stage. However, there is no sufficient evidence that motivating smokers based on stage of change model has successful outcomes, indicating that readiness or motivation to stop smoking may not be integral for quitting.[13]

Interestingly, motivational interviewing (MI) has been used as a counseling style that helps smokers explore and resolve their uncertainties about quitting. MI may modestly increase the likelihood of long-term smoking cessation when used with other smoking cessation intervention components or when compared with non-MI smoking cessation interventions.[14] However, there is also the possibility that MI may reduce quit rates relative to other smoking cessation interventions. Further evidence is likely to strengthen or weaken this idea.

Trained pharmacists involved with tobacco use disorder treatment should assist smokers regardless of the smoker's motivation at any given time. In addition to assessment of motivation level to quit smoking, pharmacists should also assess the level of nicotine dependence. The Fagerström Test for Nicotine Dependence (FTND) is still widely used to assess the level of nicotine dependence among cigarette smokers despite having some issues concerning its validity

and reliability.[15] The FTND incorporates two crucial questions, i.e., the Heaviness of Smoking Index (HSI), to assess the number of cigarettes smoked per day and the time to first cigarette (TTFC).[16]

A useful tool in assessment of smoking is the carbon monoxide (CO) analyzer. It is a simple, noninvasive, and relatively inexpensive method to assess recent tobacco smoking and also to validate smoking cessation.[17,18] Carbon monoxide is produced by incomplete combustion of organic materials, including tobacco leaves. The CO level detected in exhaled air by CO-oximetry can be used to evaluate the heaviness or intensity of smoking. In general, there is a direct relationship between the levels of CO and the number of cigarettes smoked.[17] It has been observed that the measurement of CO in exhaled air in smokers could be an indicative test of immediate and future harm to their health as a consequence of smoking[19] and this could increase their motivation to stop smoking, which could lead to smoking cessation in these patients.

However, available studies have provided mixed results regarding the effect of biomedical risk assessment as an aid for smoking cessation. A recent Cochrane systematic review concluded that moderate-certainty evidence limited by risk of bias did not detect an effect of feedback on smoking exposure by CO monitoring.[20] Nonetheless, it is still considered an important part of smoking cessation service given its practicality and affordability.

The measurement of CO levels in exhaled air by CO-oximetry is an inexpensive, noninvasive, and rapid technique that requires little technical training, making it a technique for risk assessment in smokers that can be easily applied in primary care and could serve as a reinforcement aid in smoking cessation intervention activities.

STEP 4: ASSIST IN QUIT ATTEMPT

First step in assisting smokers to quit is setting a quit date. The quit date is preferred to be set within two weeks from being interested in quitting.[21] Smokers' counseling is a core part in smoking cessation interventions. It can be offered individually, in a group, or via telephone. Using multiple approaches in delivering smoking cessation interventions increases abstinence rates; thus, it should be encouraged. However, evidence indicates that individual counseling results in better quitting outcomes than group or phone counseling and self-help.[10,22]

Telephone counseling can take on one of two approaches: either "proactive counseling" or "reactive counseling." Smokers receive regular calls from smoking cessation service providers on a scheduled basis when a proactive approach is followed. When a "reactive counseling" approach is desired, smokers seek help or advice via initiating calls to a helpline. Proactive services have been evaluated widely compared to reactive services because they can be controlled easier. According to an available evidence, behavioral counseling formats should include proactive telephone counseling elements.[23]

STEP 5: ARRANGE FOLLOW UP

Lapsing and/or relapsing are common occurrences among smokers attempting to quit. Lapsing refers to returning to the smoking habits temporarily before being able to quit again whereas relapsing refers to a permanent or long-term return to smoking. Continuous abstinence is accomplished when a patient stops smoking for at least six months. Within the first few weeks of quitting smokers are at higher risk of relapse. Thus, they should be offered a support from families, friends, and healthcare providers in the first week of quitting. Research indicated that abstinence for as long as twelve months is a strong predictor of long-term abstinence.[24]

Research suggest that the smoking abstinence rate and its effectiveness can be enhanced by using multiple treatment sessions. More than eight sessions within six months (intensive interventions) may result in a greater quitting rate. Nevertheless, fewer smokers might benefit from such interventions (i.e., having limited reach) and may not be viable in some primary care settings.[7] National Centre for Smoking Cessation and Training (NCSCT) of the UK recommends evidence-based behavior change techniques delivered via at least six (6) sessions while dealing with smokers looking for assistance with quitting as described here:[25]

First session:	1 or 2 weeks before Quit Date (Pre-Quit Assessment)
Second session:	Quit Date
Third session:	1 week after Quit Date
Fourth session:	2 weeks after Quit Date
Fifth session:	3 weeks after Quit Date
Sixth session:	4 weeks after Quit Date

Activities at each session differ accordingly, e.g., the earlier session is to get the smoker to commit to abrupt cessation (or gradual reduction with pharmacotherapy) while later on is about the "not a puff" rule to prevent lapse and relapse. As mentioned earlier, the CO breath analyzer can be used at each session to assess any recent smoking activity.[26] CO tests at every visit are helpful to show the patient objective proof of improved health after they have stopped smoking completely and to check whether they have stopped smoking.[26]

At the end of the 6-month follow-up post quit date, final verification of abstinence can be done using the CO breath analyzer and/or the cotinine level in body fluids. Cotinine is the primary metabolite of nicotine. When cigarette smoke is inhaled, nicotine is absorbed through the lungs and undergoes extensive metabolism in the liver. Typically, 70–80% of nicotine is metabolized into cotinine.[27] Cotinine detection is generally preferred over nicotine due to its longer average half-life, which is estimated to be 15–40 hours.[27,28]

In comparison, the average half-life for nicotine is only 2 hours.[27] Although samples for cotinine detection can be obtained from the blood, urine, or saliva, salivary cotinine test is preferred in the clinical setting since it is the most noninvasive and easiest to perform in the community pharmacy setting. Evidence shows that cotinine is the preferred method for determining smoking status over CO monitoring.[28,29]

Research suggests that intensive tobacco dependence treatment has more impact than brief treatment. Such intensiveness can be fulfilled via increasing the length of individual treatment sessions, increasing number of sessions, and incorporating specialized behavioral therapies. Intensive clinical interventions could be offered by any adequately trained healthcare provider who has the facilities available to offer intensive interventions suitable for any tobacco user ready to participate in them.[7]

TABLE 4.1
The "5A's" for Brief Intervention

1. Ask about tobacco use.
   - Identify and document tobacco use status for every patient at every visit, including the adolescents.
   - Where appropriate, ask the patient's caretaker about tobacco use or exposure to tobacco smoke in living and/or working environment.
2. Advise to quit.
In a clear, strong, and personalized manner urge every tobacco user to quit.
Advice should be:
   - Clear—for example: "I believe it is crucial for you to quit smoking immediately, and my staff and I can assist you," or perhaps, "Reducing the number of cigarettes while you are unwell or sick is not enough."
   - Strong—for example: "As your pharmacist, I know that quitting smoking is the most important action you can take to improve your condition/health now as well as in the future. We are here to help you quit successfully."
   - Personalized—Linking tobacco usage with existing health problems/illness, social norms, social rejection, and/or other social and economic consequences, motivation level/ readiness to quit, and/or the effect of tobacco use on kids and family members.
3. Assess willingness to make a quit attempt.
Is the patient willing to make a quit attempt currently?
   - Provide support if the patient is willing to make a quit attempt.
   - Offer intensive treatment or refer to intensive intervention.
   - Apply motivational interviewing using the "5 R's" (relevance, risks, rewards, roadblocks, and repetition) if the patient is unwilling to make a quit attempt yet.

4. Assist in quit attempt.
   - Offer counseling with pharmacotherapy (unless medication is contraindicated) for the smoker willing to make a quit attempt.

Preparations for quitting: STAR (Set, Tell, Anticipate, Remove)

   - **Set** a quit date. A quit date must be set as soon as possible or within two (2) weeks of the first session. Smokers may choose between abrupt quitting (cold turkey) or gradual reduction, i.e., cutting down the number of cigarettes gradually until the set date. Preferably, get the smoker to quit abruptly.
   - **Tell** family members, acquaintances, and coworkers about quitting to obtain understanding and support. In addition, assist smokers in getting extratreatment social support from self-help groups, if available. If there are other smokers (e.g., in the household), encourage them to quit together and request others not to smoke in his/her presence to reduce the risk of therapeutic failure and exposure to secondhand smoke.
   - **Anticipate** challenges to a proposed quit attempt, especially during the critical first few weeks. Challenges include nicotine withdrawal symptoms. Talk with the smoker about challenges/causes and how he or she will effectively conquer them. Offer exercises on problem-solving/skills.
   - **Remove** tobacco products from his or her environment. Preceding quitting, avoid smoking in sites where much of the patient's time is spent such as at work, in the house, or in the car.
   - Provide a supportive healthcare environment while reassuring the patient in his or her quit attempt.
   - Total abstinence is very important. Explain the "not a single puff" rule after the quit date to prevent lapse and relapse.
   - Discuss previous experiences with quitting. Identify what assisted and what prohibited quitting in the former attempts.
   - Discuss alcohol. The smoker should consider decreasing or abstaining from drinking alcohol during the quit attempt because it may cause lapse and relapse.
   - Advise the use of authorized smoking cessation medications, when indicated. Describe how such pharmacotherapies reduce craving and withdrawal symptoms, increasing smoking cessation success.
   - Provide supplementary materials and information, if available.

5. Arrange follow-up.
   - Timing is important. Follow-up appointments should be scheduled weekly until the quit date, if possible, and within the first week after the quit date.
   - Subsequent appointments are recommended every week within the first month, and then every 2 weeks for the second and third month, and every month after that up to 6 months.
   - Appointments should be in person whenever possible, or via telephone, etc.
   - Actions during follow-up:
   - Congratulate success.
   - If tobacco use has occurred, review circumstances and provoke a commitment for complete quitting.
   - Inform the smoker that any lapse that occurred can be viewed as a learning experience.
   - Identify obstacles already faced and foresee obstacles in the near future.
   - Assess medication use and any associated difficulties, including side effects.
   - Think of incorporating more intensive treatment; in the event of failure, a referral is recommended.

Source: Adapted from Fiore et al.[7] and NCSCT.[25]

TABLE 4.2
Elements of an Intensive Tobacco Dependence Intervention

Assessment	• The willingness of tobacco users to make a quit attempt using an intensive treatment strategy should be assessed.
	• Other assessments can deliver useful information in counseling (e.g., anxiety, addiction).
Program clinicians	• The involvement of various kinds of clinicians should be efficient.
	• Having a healthcare provider present to convey a solid message about quitting, information about health risks of smoking and benefits of quitting, and recommending and prescribing medications is a possible counseling strategy that should be endorsed.
	• Additional counseling interventions can be delivered by nonmedical personnel.
Program intensity	There is evidence of a strong dose-response relationship; thus, when possible, the program intensity should be as follows:
	• In terms of length, sessions should be extended to more than 10 minutes.
	• In terms of number, sessions should be at least 4.
Program format	• Group or individual counseling can be offered.
	• Counseling via telephone calls is effective and is complementary to the treatments provided in the clinical setting.
	• The provision of self-help materials and the use of cessation web sites are possible additional options.
	• Follow-up interventions should be scheduled.
Type of counseling and behavioral therapy	Counseling should include practical counseling (problem solving/skills training) integrated with social support during treatment.
Medication	• Every smoker should be offered cessation pharmacotherapy, when indicated. There is insufficient evidence of effectiveness among some groups like pregnant women, smokeless tobacco users, mild smokers, and adolescents.
	• The pharmacist should describe how medications assist in reducing withdrawal symptoms and craving, and as so improving quitting success.
	• Combining counseling and medication increases abstinence rates, as well as certain combinations of cessation medications when indicated.
Population	Intensive intervention programs can be offered to any tobacco user wanting to make such an effort.

Source: Adapted from Fiore et al.[7]

DEVICE 1: CARBON MONOXIDE BREATH ANALYZER

A) BACKGROUND

The incomplete combustion of organic materials is responsible for the production of carbon monoxide (CO). It is a colorless and odorless toxic gas that can be assessed from a breath or blood sample. However, it is less expensive and simpler if assessed from breathing. Devices used to measure CO in breathing are commercially available (based on measuring the rate of conversion of CO to CO2 when passing across a catalytically active electrode).[26] Spectrophotometry is used to measure blood carboxyhemoglobin (COHb). The specificity for CO level as a measure of smoking status is high among heavy cigarette smokers but low among light cigarette smokers.[26] There are environmental sources of CO of similar amounts to those found in light smokers. One limitation of using CO in breathing as an indicator of smoking status is the initial cost for the CO monitor. Measurement of CO cannot be applied to the detection of smokeless tobacco use such as electronic cigarettes because such technique does not involve a combustion mechanism, as will be described later in this chapter.

B) DEVICE DESCRIPTION/IMPORTANT FEATURES

There are several CO monitors available on the market (Figures 4.1 & 4.2); for example, from Micro Medical™ and Bedfont™. Some devices have multiple patient profiles for adults and adolescents and carbon monoxide breath testing for pregnant smokers, with the parts per million (ppm) reading and % COHb for the mother-to-be plus the fetal ppm reading and % FCOHb conversion.

Some of the device characteristics include quick response time, 1 ppm resolution, instant display of CO levels in ppm & % COHb, colour light indicators, capable of interfacing with

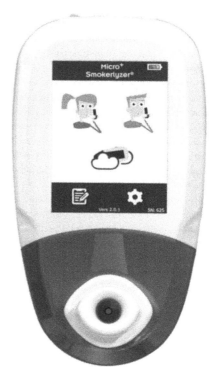

FIGURE 4.2 The Micro⁺™ Smokerlyzer® CO monitor

Source: From www.bedfont.com/micro

COBRA, a Windows-based software package for performing and storing real-time breath tests on PC.

C) PURPOSE/HOW TO USE

The healthcare provider should inform the patient that the device is used to assess the level of carbon monoxide (CO) in the expired breath air and correlate the value to that. He or she should follow manufacturer's instruction that come with these devices. However, the following procedure is

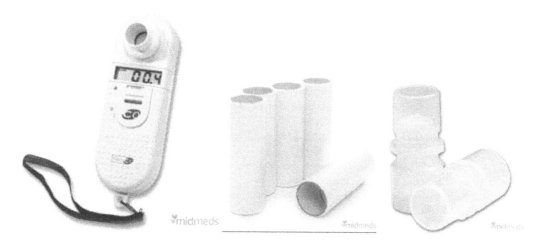

FIGURE 4.1 Carbon monoxide breath analyzer.

Source: Images from www.midmeds.co.uk/micro-medical-micro-monitor-carbon-monoxide-monitor-p-4735.html

applicable to all monitors to detect the level of CO in the expired breath air:

1. Both the patient and the healthcare practitioner providing smoking cessation service should use sanitizer gel (non-alcohol) on their hands before the test.
2. Attach a clean, disposable mouthpiece (a new one for each patient) to the monitor.
3. Turn the device on.
4. Ask the patient to take a deep breath.
5. The monitor will count down 15 seconds and beep during the last 3 seconds.
6. The patient needs to blow slowly into the mouthpiece, aiming to empty his or her lungs.
7. The parts per million (ppm) of carbon monoxide in the lungs will be displayed on the screen.
8. The mouthpiece should be removed by the patient (for infection control reasons) and disposed of in a refuse sack which is tied before being placed into another bag for collection (double bagging) to prevent domestic staff from touching the mouthpieces.
9. The CO monitor should be cleaned between tests using a non-alcoholic wipe.

D) IMPORTANT SAFETY ISSUES (CAUTIONS AND COMMON ADVERSE EFFECTS)

Ensure proper hygiene and safety measures are adhered to, especially to reduce or prevent transmission of microorganisms. Certain CO analyzers have specific devices for testing patients with certain infectious disease, such as tuberculosis (TB). In addition, analyzers from Bedfont™ can be fitted with D-pieces™ to filter out 99.9% of airborne bacteria along with single-use mouthpieces, for excellent and low-cost infection control.[1]

D-piece™ (www.bedfont.com/micro)

The D-piece™ incorporates a one-way valve to prevent air from being drawn back from the monitor. The mouthpiece itself is specifically designed with integrated filtration to remove > 99% of airborne bacteria, > 96% of viruses, and any moisture from the patient's breath. The D-piece™ should be changed every four weeks or more often if visibly soiled. An automatic reminder will appear on the screen every 28 days.

E) STORAGE CONDITIONS AND MAINTENANCE

Calibration of the device should be done using calibration gas (e.g., 20 ppm of 110 liters CO from Micro Medical™) every 3 to 6 months.

F) IMPORTANT FEATURES (CAPABILITIES AND LIMITATIONS) AND SPECIAL ADVANTAGES

Carryover effects may be possible; hence some manufacturers recommend "airing out" the device between uses.

G) SPECIAL TIPS FOR PATIENT COUNSELING

Ensure precautions are taken, including cleaning of the device to avoid potential transmission of respiratory infections, including SARS-CoV-2.

H) EVIDENCE OF EFFECTIVENESS AND SAFETY

The measurement of CO levels in exhaled air by CO-oximetry is used to assess the heaviness of smoking. A direct association has been identified between CO levels and the number of cigarettes smoked.[17] In addition, tobacco abstinence also can be identified via the CO level in exhaled air.[18] Moreover, CO levels in the patient's exhaled air predict immediate and long-term smoking-related health harm among smokers.[19]

I) ECONOMIC EVALUATION (COST-EFFECTIVENESS)

The assessment of CO levels in breathing by CO-oximetry is an inexpensive, noninvasive, rapid, and simple method that is easily applicable for smokers in primary care settings.[32] This makes it a suitable risk assessment technique and a supportive tool in quitting intervention activities.

J) IMPLICATION TO THE PHARMACY PROFESSION AND PHARMACY PRACTICE

Having an objective assessment of recent smoking is useful in the provision of smoking cessation service, particularly in relation to motivating smokers to make a quit attempt and maintain abstinence.

DEVICE 2: COTININE TEST KIT

A) BACKGROUND

From the product insert (Saliva NicAlert™, Confirm Biosciences):

NicAlert™ has been designed to quantify cotinine in saliva in vitro. It indicates whether a person has been subjected to any tobacco product during the last two days. A 10 ng/mL has been used as a cut-off level for the test. A false positive result can be obtained with secondhand smoke exposure. For quality control of the test, the manufacturer includes a positive and a negative control.

The sensitivity and specificity of cotinine for evaluating smoking status has been shown to be higher than CO monitoring.[29–31] The reference method used for measuring cotinine is gas chromatography/mass spectrometry (GC/MS) or liquid chromatography/masssSpectrometry (LC/MS).

B) DESCRIPTION/IMPORTANT FEATURES

The test is a sort of immunochromatographic assay that uses monoclonal antibody-coated gold particles and a series of avidity traps that allow quantification. There are gold particles coated with monoclonal antibodies to cotinine contained at the sample collection end of the strip. Cotinine is a nicotine metabolite with a relatively long half-life. The quantity of cotinine in the sample is determined by the apparent color change representing the distance the gold migrates on the strip.

c) How to Perform Testing

1. Once the NicAlert™ package is opened, lay the NicAlert™ strip down flat on a non-absorbent surface, like the specially marked area on the plastic-laminated instruction card (Figure 4.3).
2. The NicAlert™ Saliva Collection Kit contains the funnel, the saliva tube container, and the snap-on top for the saliva tube container; remove them from the package and set aside.
3. Place the funnel in the saliva tube container; instruct the patient to spit/deposit saliva into the funnel in a sufficient amount to fill at least one half of the saliva tube container. Then discard the funnel.
4. Spin on the top of the saliva tube container and squeeze 8 drops from the inverted saliva tube directly onto the white padded end of the NicAlert™ strip.

Caution: Handle any saliva sample as if it were a potential biohazard and discard appropriately after testing.

d) How to Read Saliva NicAlert™

1. Read the NicAlert™ 15–30 minutes after disappearance or fading of the blue band. Bands may darken over this period. Do not allow total disappearance of bands as so as lower readings such as a 0 may be obtained quickly (Figure 4.4).
2. The result is the lowest band. In at least one of the numbered zones (Levels 0–6) on the strip, there should be a reddish band. Note: The marking levels on the strip appear as a 66 ("6"), 55 ("5"), etc. This is to make the strip easier to read. If the color looks like an indistinguishable stain throughout the strip, the results are not valid, and the test must be repeated with a new NicAlert™ strip. Note: There is more than one level in which there is a reddish band or color in the strip. Different levels may have different shades or colors in them. The test result is indicated by the existence of a reddish band in the lowest-numbered level. It does NOT have to be the darkest band.

e) Test Limitations

Saliva NicAlert™ is to be used with human saliva. A positive result reveals the presence of cotinine in the sample which indicates an exposure to a tobacco product. A technical or procedural error or a sample adulteration or contamination may cause a wrong result. If the saliva seems

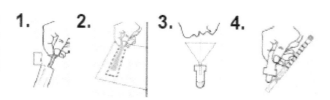

FIGURE 4.3 NicAlert™ saliva collection steps.

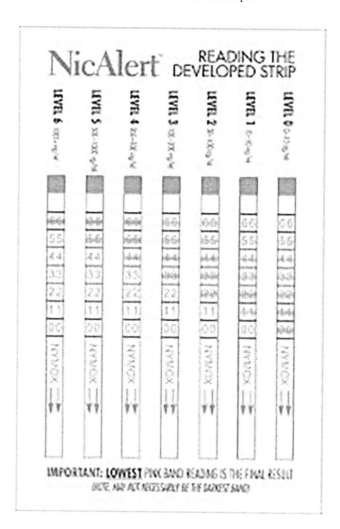

FIGURE 4.4 Reading the developed strip of NicAlert™.

TABLE 4.3

NicAlert™ Test Results and Different Cotinine Concentration Ranges

Level	Cotinine concentration (ng/ml)	Interpretation
0	0–10	Non-user of tobacco products
1	10–30	User of tobacco products
2	30–100	User of tobacco products
3	100–200	User of tobacco products
4	200–500	User of tobacco products
5	500–1000	User of tobacco products
6	>1000	User of tobacco products

to be unusual in appearance it should not be tested with saliva NicAlert™. The test result is only a preliminary (Table 4.3). This should be interpreted in the light of clinical consideration and professional judgment. A more specific alternative assay method is needed such as gas chromatography/mass spectrometry (GC/MS) to confirm a preliminary positive result.

F) TEST CHARACTERISTICS

Shelf life:

Based on stability testing, NicAlert™ strips have a validity that expires after at least two years if stored at room temperature.

Detection Limit

A measurement of 10 ng/mL is considered the limit of detection. Saliva controls were diluted to 20, 10, 8, 6, 4, 2, and 0 ng/mL cotinine and read in duplicate with NicAlert™ Strips.

Sensitivity and specificity of the test:

The saliva strip test results, averaged over the two operators, had a sensitivity of 99% and a specificity of 96% compared to smoking status determined by urine cotinine measurement by GC/MS (50 ng/mL cut-off).

Cross-Reactants:

Cotinine-negative saliva was spiked with chemicals related to cotinine at 100,000 ng/mL.
Nicotinic Acid—cloudy, no distinctive bands
Nicotinic Acid n-oxide—no cross-reactivity
Niacinamide—no cross-reactivity
Nicotine—trap level 3
3-OH cotinine is a known cross-reactant with cotinine in immunoassays. 3-OH cotinine was spiked into cotinine negative ("0" NicAlert™) urine at the following concentrations: 50 ng/mL, 150 ng/mL, 250 ng/mL, 750 ng/mL, and 1200 ng/mL. 3-OH cotinine showed a 12–40% cross-reactivity with cotinine in the NicAlert™ assay.

DEVICE 3: NICOTINE REPLACEMENT THERAPY

A) BACKGROUND

Nicotine replacement therapy (NRT) products are among the first-line agents for smoking cessation. NRT products gradually substitute the nicotine obtained from cigarettes and thus help reducing withdrawal symptoms associated with quitting. NRT is available on the market in a variety of formulations, including transdermal skin patches, chewing gums, inhalers/inhalators, lozenges (which allow for buccal absorption of nicotine), and oral and nasal sprays. Nicotine is delivered to the brain via oral preparation more quickly than skin patches, but more slowly and in less amounts than smoking cigarettes.[33]

Research suggests that all forms of NRT increase the probability of succeeding in quitting attempts. Overall, there is no difference in the effectiveness between different forms of monotherapy NRT, and the chances of successful abstinence improve by 50–70%.[26] NRT products are effective if used alone or provided with counseling, but pharmacotherapy with behavioral intervention yields the best results. Evidence shown that strengthening the volume of behavioral support for patients using a smoking cessation medication improves the probability of abstinence for longer by about 10% to 25%.[34]

NRT products generally do not require a prescription for pharmacists to dispense. Once the indication is established, and safety issues are ruled out, pharmacists can recommend the most suitable product(s) based on the patient's suitability and cost. Dosing is usually based on the severity of nicotine dependence. Based on the FTND score, more heavily dependent smokers usually need higher doses of NRT (e.g., the 4 mg NRT gum is preferred over the 2 mg).

Some NRT products have been studied as pre-quit medications, e.g., NRT patch. Data suggest that starting the use of NRT patches shortly before the planned quit date may increase the chance of success. Nicotine preloading appears to facilitate smoking abstinence by reducing urges to smoke, smoke intake before quitting, and urges to smoke after quitting.[35]

Side effects from using NRT are related to the type of product and the technique used and may include skin irritation from patches, irritation to the inside of the mouth from gum and lozenges, and in rare situations non-ischemic palpitations and chest pain.[36] Experimental and observational studies of NRT in patients with cardiovascular diseases report no rise in adverse cardiovascular effects than those receiving placebo.[37–39] A meta-analysis of studies evaluating NRT observed a rise in cardiovascular symptoms such as arrhythmia and tachycardia, due to the nicotine sympathomimetic action, but no rise in major cardiovascular effects (death, myocardial infarction, stroke).[40]

The NRT-associated adverse effects, serious adverse effects and withdrawals have been assessed infrequently in the literature, resulting in low- or very low-certainty evidence for all alternatives. There was no evidence of a presence of cardiac-related adverse effects, serious adverse effects, or withdrawals. Overall withdrawal effects have been reported significantly more frequently with NRT nasal spray than with the NRT patch in one study, and more frequently with 42/44 mg patches than 21/22 mg NRT patches in two studies.[41]

In patients who are quitting and getting behavioral support, there is moderate-certainty evidence that an increased behavioral support concentrating on adherence to smoking cessation medications can moderately enhance adherence. Adherence-based interventions may target the practicalities of taking medicines and improving attitudes towards medicines. However, there is no evidence on whether such interventions are working for patients who are quitting without standard behavioral support.[42]

B) DEVICE DESCRIPTION/IMPORTANT FEATURES

TABLE 4.4
Nicotine Gum

Precautions	**Pregnancy:** Smokers who are pregnant should be firstly persuaded to stop smoking without medications. Nicotine gum should be used during pregnancy only if the increased probability of smoking abstinence, with its expected benefits, outweighs the risk of nicotine replacement and potential associated smoking. In the same context, previous factors should be put into consideration for lactating women. **Cardiovascular diseases:** Although NRT is not an independent risk factor for acute myocardial events, it should be used cautiously in certain cardiovascular patient groups such as those within 1 to 2 weeks post-myocardial infarction, those with serious arrhythmias, and those with severe or worsening angina pectoris.
Side effects	Frequent side effects of nicotine chewing gum include hiccups, dyspepsia, mouth soreness, and jaw ache. These are usually mild and temporary and often can be relieved by modifying the patient's chewing technique.
Dosage	Nicotine gum is marketed as 2 mg and 4 mg. The 2 mg gum is advised for those who smoke fewer than 20 cigarettes each day. In contrast, 4 mg gum is recommended for patients smoking 20 or more cigarettes per day, or for time to first cigarette (TTFC) is within 30 minutes. The maximum recommended regimen of nicotine gum is 24 pieces/day for a duration up to 12 weeks. Dosage and duration of therapy should be tailored to suit each patient's needs.
Availability	A popular example is Nicorette Icy Mint Gum® 2 and 4 mg.
Prescribing instructions	**Chewing technique:** Patients should be advised to chew the gum slowly until a minty or peppery taste appears, then keep between cheek and gum to enable the oral absorption of nicotine. Gum should be chewed slowly and intermittently and kept for about 30 minutes or until the taste disappears. **Absorption:** Acidic food and drinks like juices, coffee, and soft drinks interfere with the buccal absorption of nicotine; thus, ingesting anything except water should be avoided for 15 minutes prior to and during chewing. **Scheduling of dose:** Patients often do not use enough gum to get the maximum effect: they do not chew enough pieces per day, and they do not use the gum for the recommended number of weeks. Directions to chew the gum on a scheduled basis (at least one piece every 1–2 hours during waking hours) for at least 1–3 months may be more beneficial than chewing the gum "when necessary."

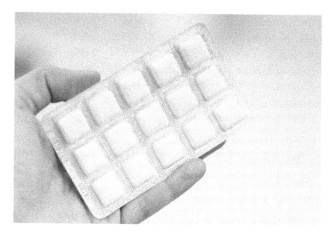

FIGURE 4.5   Nicotine gum.

Source: www.shutterstock.com/image-photo/pharmacist-holding-nicotine-gum-blister-pack-1598261977

TABLE 4.5
Nicotine Patch

Precautions	**Pregnancy:** Smokers who are pregnant should be firstly persuaded to stop smoking without medications. Nicotine patch should be used during pregnancy only if the increased probability of smoking abstinence, with its expected benefits, outweighs the risk of nicotine replacement and potential associated smoking. In the same context, previous factors should be put into consideration for lactating women. **Cardiovascular diseases:** As with nicotine gum.
Side effects	**Skin reactions:** About half of smokers using the nicotine patch have a local skin reaction. Such reactions are normally mild and self-limiting but may get worse over the course of treatment. Using 1% hydrocortisone cream or 0.5% triamcinolone cream and changing the site for patch application may lessen the local reactions. Fewer than 5% of patients may require discontinuation of nicotine patch treatment. **Other side effect:** Insomnia.
Dosage	Continuing treatment for at least 8 weeks gives the same efficacy as extended treatment periods. No difference in the efficacy between 16- and 24-hour patches use. Treatment should be tailored to the characteristics of each smoker such as prior experience with the patch, heaviness of smoking, level of addiction, etc. Patients who smoke 10 or less cigarettes per day should be started on a lower patch dose.
Availability	Popular examples include Niquitin® (21, 14, and 7 mg/24 hr) and Nicorette® (25, 15, and 10 mg/16 hr). **Niquitin®:** If smoking ten cigarettes or more a day, start with Step 1 (21 mg) and gradually move to Step 2 (14 mg) after six weeks and then Step 3 (7 mg) for two weeks, as directed on the pack, over ten weeks. If smoking less than ten cigarettes a day, start at Step 2 and follow the eight-week program described on the pack. **Nicorette Invisi®:** Use 25 mg for 8 weeks, then 15 mg for 2 weeks, and finally 10 mg for 2 weeks.

Prescribing instructions: Location: It is advised to place a new patch between the neck and the waist. preferably on the upper arm or shoulder in a hairless area.

Activities: Patients are not required to be restricted from any activity while using the patch.

Time: As soon as the patient wakes up, he or she should apply the patch. Patient should be advised to remove the 24-hour patch before bedtime or use the 16-hour patch if experiencing sleep disruption. Patients with a time to first cigarette of 30 minutes or less may benefit from applying the patch directly before sleeping. The plasma nicotine level is highest upon waking for up 6 to 8 hours post application of the patch.

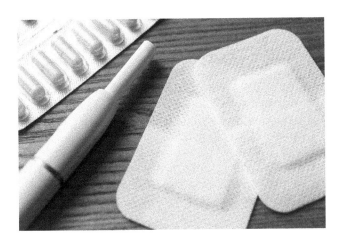

FIGURE 4.6   Nicotine patch.

Source: www.shutterstock.com/image-photo/nicotine-patches-pills-electronic-cigarette-on-1627428565

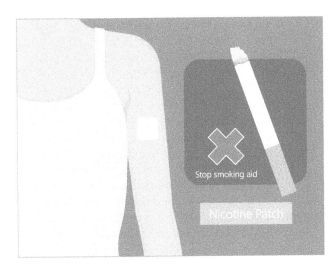

FIGURE 4.7   Common site for placing a nicotine patch.

Source: www.shutterstock.com/image-vector/nicotine-patch-stop-smoking-therapy-1758790004

TABLE 4.6
Nicotine Inhaler

Precautions	Pregnancy and cardiovascular diseases: As with nicotine gum.
Side effects	Local irritation reactions: Local irritation in the mouth and throat occurs in 40% of patients using the nicotine inhaler. Cough is observed in 32% and rhinitis is observed in 23% of patients. The severity of such symptoms is generally mild, and their occurrence is reduced with prolonged use.
Dosage	A dose from the nicotine inhaler consists of a puff or inhalation.

Each cartridge delivers 4 mg of nicotine over 80 inhalations. The recommended dosage is 6–16 cartridges/day. Recommended duration of therapy is up to 6 months. Instruct patient to taper dosage during the final 3 months of treatment. |
| Availability | 4 mg/cartridge |
| Prescribing instructions | Ambient temperature: The inhaler and cartridges should be kept at room temperature. Duration: Use is advised for up to 6 months with a gradual reduction in the frequency of use over the last 6–12 weeks of treatment. Absorption: Acidic food and drinks like juices, coffee, and soft drinks interfere with the buccal absorption of nicotine; thus, ingesting anything except water should be avoided for 15 minutes prior to and during inhalation. Best effects: Best outcomes are reached by frequent puffing. |

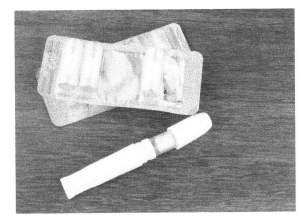

FIGURE 4.8   Cigarette nicotine replacement inhaler and cartridges.

Source: www.shutterstock.com/image-photo/cigarette-nicotine-replacement-inhaler-cartridges-1475197781

TABLE 4.7
Nicotine Lozenge

Precautions	• Post myocardial infarction, severe dysrhythmia, or cerebrovascular accident • Active oesophagitis, oral or pharyngeal inflammation, gastritis, gastric or peptic ulcer • Moderate to severe renal/hepatic impairment • Children < 18 years • Pregnancy

(*Continued*)

TABLE 4.7
(Continued)

Side effects	Nausea, vomiting, upper abdominal pain, diarrhea, dyspepsia, hiccups, stomatitis, flatulence, dry mouth, constipation, oral discomfort, headache, dizziness, tremor, sleep disorders such as insomnia and abnormal dreams, nervousness, palpitations, pharyngitis, cough, pharyngolaryngeal pain, dyspnoea, increased sweating, arthralgia, myalgia, application site reactions, chest pain, pain in limb, asthenia, fatigue
Dosage	2 mg and 4 mg
Prescribing instruction	It is advised that smokers of less than 20 cigarettes per day be prescribed up to 2mg and those who smoke more than 20 cigarettes per day be prescribed 4 mg.

Stepwise treatment for abrupt cessation:

Week 1–6: 1 lozenge every 1–2 hours.
Minimum: 9 lozenges per day.
Week 7–9: 1 lozenge every 2–4 hours.
Week 10–12: 1 lozenge every 4–8 hours.
Maximum: 15 lozenges perday.
Maximum duration: 24 weeks.

Gradual cessation:

Use a lozenge when there is a strong desire to smoke. Max: 15 lozenges perday. Patients should be asked not to swallow or chew the lozenge and they should not eat or drink while the lozenge is in the mouth.

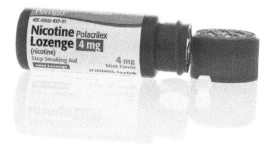

FIGURE 4.9 Nicotine lozenge.

Source: www.shutterstock.com/image-photo/winneconne-wi-29-june-2019-package-1446292061

c) Economic Evaluation (Cost-Effectiveness)

According to Jha and colleagues, NRT can be considered more cost-effective than other tobacco control interventions.[43] A recent report from the United States Surgeon General covering some literature on economic evaluation of smoking cessation interventions indicated cost-effectiveness of NRT.[44] Part of such literature is shown in Table 4.8.

d) Implication to the Pharmacy Profession and Pharmacy Practice

1. Pharmacists have been shown to positively impact tobacco use disorder management, from advising smokers about quitting to assisting them in using cessation medicines coupled with behavioral interventions. A systematic review and meta-analysis involving community pharmacy-delivered interventions for smoking cessation demonstrated effectiveness compared with control, ranging from 28% to 46% (for counseling and NRT) and 13.8% to 15% for counseling, vs 1.3% to 8% for control) at 6 to 12 months.[45]

2. Community pharmacists are strategically positioned, given their accessibility to smokers who may ask about quitting smoking medications or other health-related needs. The application of brief and intensive interventions is, however, variable, and many pharmacists cite time limitation as the main barrier to the provision of cessation service. This is despite the finding that most pharmacists acknowledged the importance of providing smoking cessation intervention as part of the pharmacy service.

3. Pharmacists may require additional knowledge and skills to deliver effective smoking cessation interventions. Training health professionals to provide smoking cessation interventions had a measurable effect on smoking, continuous abstinence, and professional performance.[46]

4. Both governmental and non-governmental organizations offer training programs, e.g., Association for the Treatment of Tobacco Use and Dependence (ATTUD) in the USA, Certified Smoking Cessation Service Provider (CSCSP) in Malaysia, and the National Centre for Smoking Cessation and Training (NCSCT) in the UK. Part of pharmaceutical care service provision includes dose adjustment or drug change, especially in drug-smoking interactions and smoking cessation.

5. Pharmacists are tasked with screening for drug-smoking interactions due to polycyclic aromatic hydrocarbons (PAHs) in tobacco smoke. PAHs are primarily responsible for hepatic enzymes CYP1A2 and CYP2B6 induction and, to a lesser extent, CYP3A4 and CYP2C19. The degree of enzyme induction shows significant inter-individual variability. It may be dose-dependent, with one study demonstrating dose-dependent increases in CYP1A2 induction with an increased number of cigarettes smoked per day. Genetic polymorphisms of the CYP1A2 gene and ethnic differences also contribute to interindividual variability in both smokers and non-smokers. Upon smoking cessation, enzyme induction rapidly recovers within days of cessation and reaches a new steady-state within one week. The effects of smoking and abrupt smoking cessation are clinically relevant in managing patients treated with a CYP1A2 substrate. Hence, pharmacists need to be cognizant of clinically significant smoking-drug interactions

TABLE 4.8
Cost-effectiveness of NRT

Perspective/setting	Comparison	Unit of measurement	Cost	Study
National health system perspective/ primary care settings	NRT added to brief counseling compared with brief counseling alone	Incremental cost per life-year saved	Ranged from $1,115 to $2,541 depending on the age groups	Stapleton et al. 1999
Health insurance perspective	NRT compared with usual care	Cost of NRT per additional quitter	$171	Salize et al. 2009
State program perspective	NRT compared with brief counseling	Cost of NRT per additional quitter	$3,781	Hollis et al. 2007
Program perspective	Adding free NRT to Quitline counseling	Incremental costs per life-year saved Incremental costs per quit attempt	$132 and $267 respectively	Fellows et al. 2007
Funding agency perspective	Adding free NRT to Quitline counseling	Incremental costs per quit attempt	$808	An et al. 2006
Payer perspective	Physician-based cessation counseling with nicotine patch compared with counseling alone	Incremental cost-effectiveness ratios (per QALY gained)	Ranged from $9,463 to $23,589	Fiscella and Franks 1996
Societal perspective		Incremental cost-effectiveness ratios (per QALY gained)	Ranged from $2,388 to $9,791	Cromwell et al. 1997
National health services perspective	NRT compared with counseling or advice alone	Incremental cost-effectiveness ratios (per life-year saved)	Ranged from $2,511 to $6,020	Song et al. 2002
Payer perspective	Counseling and NRT compared with brief physician counseling alone	Incremental cost-effectiveness ratios (per life-year saved)	Ranged from $1,267 to $42,160	Oster et al. 1986; Wasley et al. 1997; Gilbert et al. 2004; Cornuz et al. 2006
Societal perspective	Counseling and NRT compared with brief physician counseling alone	Incremental cost-effectiveness ratios (per QALY gained)	Ranged from $2,021 to $9,002	Feenstra et al. 2005
Payer perspective	The receipt of advice and motivation compared with usual advice from a pharmacist	Cost-effectiveness ratios (per life-year saved)	Ranged from $628 to $2,678	Crealey et al. 1998
Payer perspective	Incorporating four methods under pharmacist direction (quitting cold turkey, two kinds of NRT, and bupropion) compared with self-directed quit attempts	Cost-effectiveness ratios (per successful quit)	Ranged from $478 to $2,496	Tran et al. 2002

and pharmacokinetics and pharmacodynamic alterations.[47][47]

6. In addition, since post-cessation weight gain is common, pharmacists can assist smokers who are concerned about weight gain to choose the most appropriate management, e.g., to consider bupropion SR or NRT, in particular nicotine gum, which has been shown to delay weight gain after quitting along with other lifestyle changes in diet and exercise.[48][48]

E) CHALLENGES TO PHARMACISTS AND USERS

1. The time factor has always been cited as a barrier to fully implementing the 5A's (Ask, Advise, Assess, Assist and, Arrange follow-up) by pharmacists.

2. The use of such devices for at least 8 to 12 weeks also raises adherence among patients, especially those on a combination of products. In addition, despite data on cost-effectiveness of treating tobacco use disorder using such pharmacological

devices, accessibility to the products is still limited due to affordability issues, especially in the private sector, and to prioritizing treatment of other diseases, particularly in the government sector.

3. Moreover, emerging tobacco products, including heat-not-burn and electronic cigarettes, are often claimed as 'safer' alternatives for quitting combustible tobacco products. Some of these are sold illegally and create a challenge for evidence-based smoking cessation interventions by pharmacists.

DEVICE 4: ELECTRONIC NICOTINE DELIVERY SYSTEMS (E-CIGARETTES)

A) BACKGROUND

Such devices are battery-operated devices called electronic nicotine delivery systems and they have been widely known as e-cigarettes.[49] They are claimed to be used as a method of

POD system Infographics

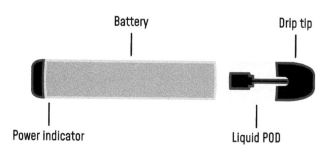

FIGURE 4.10 E-cigarette structure.

Source: Electronic Cigarette Infographics Pod System Parts Stock Vector (Royalty Free) 1512660923 (shutterstock.com)

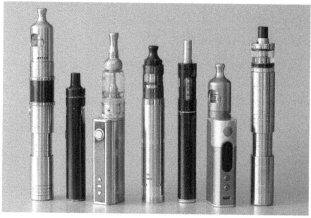

FIGURE 4.11 Different shape of e-cigarettes,

Source: Set Different Tube Ecigarettes Vaping Electronic Stock Photo (Edit Now) 1106352104 (shutterstock.com)

tobacco dependence treatment. However, they have become popularly used worldwide among youth and young adults resembling tobacco products. There has been long debate about their effectiveness in reducing nicotine dependence, safety, and how they should be regulated.

B) DEVICE DESCRIPTION

Despite availability of a huge number of shapes and designs ranging from cigarettes, to cigars, to pens, to USB looka-like designs, all e-cigarettes are composed of three main parts: a rechargeable battery, an atomizer, and a reservoir (Figures 4.10, 4.11 & 4.12).[49] The atomizer and the reservoir are collectively called cartomizer or cartridge.[49,50] In addition to the variability in shapes, there is a wide variability in characteristics of e-cigarettes.[49–52] Some e-cigarettes are disposable after the device stops producing and delivering nicotine, and some are refillable (i.e., with nicotine solution) and rechargeable. Some devices are activated automatically via airflow sensors when users start inhaling while others contain manual on/off switches. Some devices contain an element that regulates puff duration and or number of puffs that can be taken consecutively. Some e-cigarettes are provided with a flame-looking light-emitting diode at the end of the battery to resemble the appearance of conventional burning cigarette.

C) PURPOSE/HOW TO USE

Concentrated nicotine solution in the reservoir is evaporated upon activation of a heating coil inside the atomizer. Instead of having nicotine carried as a smoke due to burning of a tobacco product in case of conventional smoking devices (i.e., cigarettes, cigars, and pipes), an e-cigarette produces a vapor, plume, aerosol, fog, or mist which carries the nicotine delivered to the lungs.[51] Thus, the processes of inhalation and exhalation or production and intake of the aerosol is called vaping instead of smoking.[49]

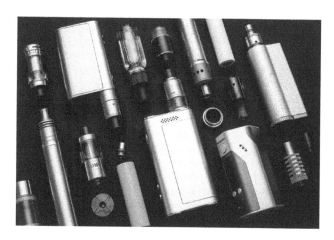

FIGURE 4.12 Different designs of e-cigarettes.

Source: Popular Vaping Device Modupgrade Parts Modern Stock Photo (Edit Now) 611469689 (shutterstock.com)

D) IMPORTANT SAFETY ISSUES[49,51,52]

1. The refill solution may contain minor amounts of concentrated nicotine solution of about 500 mg toxic enough to kill an adult if ingested. This is 10 times the lethal dose.
2. The filled solutions as well as the vapors contain minor amounts of heavy metals and at least 20 known carcinogenic and teratogenic chemicals.
3. The concentrated amounts of flavoring agents included in the solutions can produce cardiovascular and respiratory irritation and inflammation.
4. It has been stated that e-cigarettes resemble another tobacco product and that smokers move from traditional cigarette addiction to be addicted to them; and that they attract new tobacco users who have never been smokers or traditional tobacco users before. Furthermore, they resemble a gateway via which users shift to regular tobacco use.

E) Important Features

Ordinary tobacco smoke includes nicotine besides a huge number of substances and chemicals reaching more than 5,000 constituents either already present or produced via burning of a tobacco product,[53] while e-cigarette vapor contains pure nicotine. However, besides nicotine, there are other additives present in e-cigarettes including solvents (such as propylene glycol and vegetable glycerin) and flavoring agents.[49] Thus, despite presence of a smaller number of contents, e-cigarettes are not totally free from hazardous constituents. According to Kaisar et al., there are small amounts of heavy metals, and at least 20 known carcinogens and teratogenic compounds have been identified in the e-liquid as well as the aerosol.[49]

F) Evidence of Effectiveness and Safety

It is important to make a note that the available evidence on the effectiveness and safety of e-cigarettes is conflicting even among systematic reviews and meta-analyses, and such evidence should be handled with caution. Differences in findings of systematic reviews might be due to differences in inclusion and exclusion criteria of the reviewed research such as study design, length of study follow-up, subjects' characteristics, characteristics of compared group or nature of compared treatment (e.g., do nothing, conventional intervention, etc.), and primary or secondary end points. Type of analysis, comprehensiveness of literature coverage, presence of publication bias, and the criteria used for quality assessment of studies are other variables that might be responsible for the conflicting findings and differences. In the following. we present examples of such literature.

Rahman et al. conducted a systematic review and meta-analysis of 6 studies on e-cigarettes and smoking cessation.[54] They aimed to examine whether the use of e-cigarettes is associated with smoking cessation or reduction, and whether there is any difference in efficacy of e-cigarettes with and without nicotine on smoking cessation. Among findings was that nicotine-filled e-cigarettes were more effective for cessation than those without nicotine. Use of e-cigarettes was also associated with a reduction in the number of cigarettes used.

Kalkhoran and Glantz conducted a systematic review and meta-analysis of 38 studies on e-cigarettes and smoking cessation in real-world and clinical settings.[55] Cigarette smoking cessation was the primary end point. They compared odds of smoking cessation among smokers using e-cigarettes with smokers not using e-cigarettes. Among findings was that the odds of quitting cigarettes were 28% lower in those who used e-cigarettes compared with those who did not use e-cigarettes. The authors concluded that e-cigarettes are associated with significantly less quitting among smokers.

A study on potential deaths averted in USA by replacing cigarettes with e-cigarettes was conducted by Levy et al.[56] The study considered a strategy of switching cigarette smokers to e-cigarette use ("vaping") in the USA to accelerate tobacco control progress. The authors concluded. "Our projections show that a strategy of replacing cigarette smoking with vaping would yield substantial life year gains, even under pessimistic assumptions regarding cessation, initiation and relative harm."

Bullen et al. conducted a pragmatic randomized controlled superiority trial in Auckland, New Zealand.[57] They randomized smokers with quit intention into three groups receiving either e-cigarettes, nicotine patches, or placebo e-cigarettes (no nicotine). The follow-up period was 6 months and the primary end point was biochemically verified continuous abstinence. The authors reported that achievement of abstinence was substantially lower than they anticipated for the power calculation; thus, they had insufficient statistical power to conclude superiority of nicotine e-cigarettes to patches or to placebo e-cigarettes. The authors concluded that "e-cigarettes, with or without nicotine, were modestly effective at helping smokers to quit, with similar achievement of abstinence as with nicotine patches, and few adverse events."

Hajek et al. performed a randomized controlled trial of e-cigarettes compared with nicotine replacement therapy.[58] They randomly allocated adults attending UK National Health Service stop-smoking services to either nicotine-replacement products of their choice, including product combinations, provided for up to 3 months, or an e-cigarette starter pack (a second-generation refillable e-cigarette with one bottle of nicotine e-liquid), with a recommendation to purchase further e-liquids of the flavor and strength of their choice. Treatment included weekly behavioral support for at least 4 weeks. The primary end point was biochemically validated continuous abstinence for 1 year. The study conclusion was that e-cigarettes were more effective for smoking cessation than nicotine-replacement therapy when both products were accompanied by behavioral support.

Brown et al. conducted a real-world effectiveness study of e-cigarettes when used to aid smoking cessation.[59] The cross-sectional study included 5,863 adults who had smoked within the previous 12 months and made at least one quit attempt during that period with either an e-cigarette only (n = 464), NRT bought over the counter only (n = 1,922), or no aid in their most recent quit attempt (n = 3,477). The authors found that e-cigarette users were more likely to report abstinence than either those who used NRT bought over the counter [odds ratio (OR) = 2.23, 95% confidence interval (CI) = 1.70–2.93] or no aid (OR = 1.38, 95% CI = 1.08–1.76). They concluded that "among smokers who have attempted to stop without professional support, those who use e-cigarettes are more likely to report continued abstinence than those who used a licensed NRT product bought over-the-counter or no aid to cessation. This difference persists after adjusting for a range of smoker characteristics such as nicotine dependence."

In 2015, the Public Health England, which is an operationally autonomous executive agency of the Department of Health, published an evidence review report on e-cigarettes.[60] The report delivers the following key messages:

1. "Smokers who have tried other methods of quitting without success could be encouraged to try e-cigarettes (EC) to stop smoking and stop smoking services should support smokers using EC to quit by offering them behavioral support."

2. "Encouraging smokers who cannot or do not want to stop smoking to switch to EC could help reduce smoking related disease, death, and health inequalities."

3. "There is no evidence that EC are undermining the long-term decline in cigarette smoking among adults and youth and may in fact be contributing to it. Despite some experimentation with EC among never smokers, EC are attracting very few people who have never smoked into regular EC use."

4. "Recent studies support the Cochrane Review findings that EC can help people to quit smoking and reduce their cigarette consumption. There is also evidence that EC can encourage quitting or cigarette consumption reduction even among those not intending to quit or rejecting other support. More research is needed in this area."

5. "When used as intended, EC pose no risk of nicotine poisoning to users, but e-liquids should be in 'childproof' packaging. The accuracy of nicotine content labelling currently raises no major concerns."

6. "There has been an overall shift towards the inaccurate perception of EC being as harmful as cigarettes over the last year in contrast to the current expert estimate that using EC is around 95% safer than smoking."

7. "Whilst protecting non-smoking children and ensuring the products on the market are as safe and effective as possible are clearly important goals, new regulations currently planned should also maximize the public health opportunities of EC."

8. "Continued vigilance and research in this area are needed."

IMPORTANT NOTES TO THE READERS OF THIS CHAPTER ABOUT THESE MESSAGES

- It is important to highlight here that previous report messages are not presented here to act as a guideline for smoking cessation services. It is a sort of policy statement that is intended to be implemented in the context of practice of the practitioners to whom it has been directed. However, we present such key messages here as a matter of knowledge update or a lesson to inform those who may be interested to know what others say about e-cigarettes.
- It is important to highlight that an individual pharmacist practicing in a smoking cessation clinic should adhere to the local clinical practice guidelines adopted by the authorized scientific organizations or practice-regulating agencies in his or her country.

CHAPTER RECOMMENDATIONS (THE WAY FORWARD)

There is a need for more pharmacists certified as smoking cessation service providers and a pool of tobacco treatment specialists for hard-to-treat cases. Due to the mobility of patients, pharmacists must use available technology (web-based, mobile phones, apps, social media, etc.) to provide counseling and follow-up for patients. Further research into the delivery of effective smoking cessation using various behavioral and pharmacological interventions, including for special populations, to achieve higher quit rates and ensure safe use of medications is needed. Additionally, even though tobacco use disorder is a chronic relapsing addictive disease, high-quality evidence related to the devices for relapse prevention is still lacking.

LESSONS LEARNED/POINTS TO REMEMBER[44]

- Medical devices such as carbon monoxide breath analyzers, cotinine kits, and medications (nicotine replacement therapy products) approved as first-line agents for smoking cessation (gum, patch, lozenge, inhalator/inhaler, and mouth or nasal spray) are helpful in smoking cessation service.
- The evidence is sufficient to infer that smoking cessation improves well-being, including higher quality of life and improved health status.
- The evidence is sufficient to infer that smoking cessation reduces mortality and increases lifespan.
- The evidence is sufficient to infer that smoking cessation interventions are cost-effective.

CONCLUSIONS

Tobacco use disorder is still prevalent in many parts of the world, resulting in deaths and diseases that are avoidable. Article 14 of the WHO Framework Convention on Tobacco Control (FCTC) calls for quit smoking services to be more available and accessible, in tandem with other tobacco control strategies.

Pharmacist-delivered smoking cessation interventions combining behavioral support and first-line pharmacotherapy are practical and cost-effective, particularly when compared with usual care.

Pharmacists have a more significant role to play to deliver smoking cessation services effectively. This requires pharmacists to undergo extra training to obtain additional knowledge and skills towards becoming tobacco treatment specialists. Research is needed to ascertain the efficacy and safety of emerging products for smoking cessation and treatment of special populations.

REFERENCES

1. American Psychiatric Association. Diagnostic and statistical manual of mental disorders, 5th edn. Arlington, VA: American Psychiatric Association; 2013. p. 571–4.
2. De Bruin M, Viechtbauer W, Eisma MC, et al. Identifying effective behavioural components of Intervention and Comparison group support provided in SMOKing cEssation (IC-SMOKE) interventions: a systematic review protocol. Syst Rev. 2016 Dec;5(1):1–9.
3. Stead LF, Buitrago D, Preciado N, et al. Physician advice for smoking cessation. Cochrane Database Syst Rev. 2013;2013(5):CD000165.
4. Wee LH, West R, Bulgiba A, et al. Predictors of 3-month abstinence in smokers attending stop-smoking clinics in Malaysia. Nicotine Tob Res. 2011 Feb 1;13(2):151–6.
5. Tobacco TC. A clinical practice guideline for treating tobacco use and dependence: 2008 update: a US public health service report. Am J Prev Med. 2008 Aug 1;35(2):158–76.
6. Lancaster T, Stead LF. Individual behavioural counselling for smoking cessation. Cochrane Database Syst Rev. 2017(3).
7. Fiore MC, Jaén CR, Baker TB, et al. Treating tobacco use and dependence: 2008 update. Rockville, MD: US Department of Health and Human Services; 2008 May 27.
8. Aveyard P, Begh R, Parsons A, et al. Brief opportunistic smoking cessation interventions: a systematic review and meta-analysis to compare advice to quit and offer of assistance. Addiction. 2012 Jun;107(6):1066–73.
9. Hum WL, Bulgiba A, Shahab L, et al. Understanding smokers' beliefs and feelings about smoking and quitting during a quit attempt: a preliminary evaluation of the SNAP model. J Smok Cessat. 2013;8(1):17.
10. Cahill K, Stevens S, Perera R, et al. Pharmacological interventions for smoking cessation: an overview and network meta-analysis. Cochrane Database Syst Rev. 2013(5).
11. The New Zealand guidelines for helping people to stop smoking. Wellington: Ministry of Health; 2014. Available at: www.health.govt.nz/system/files/documents/publications/nz-guidelines-helping-people-stop-smoking-jun14.pdf (accessed 19 Jan 2019).
12. Prochaska JO, Velicer WF, Redding C, et al. Stage-based expert systems to guide a population of primary care patients to quit smoking, eat healthier, prevent skin cancer, and receive regular mammograms. Prev Med. 2005 Aug 1;41(2):406–16.
13. Riemsma RP, Pattenden J, Bridle C, et al. Systematic review of the effectiveness of stage-based interventions to promote smoking cessation. BMJ. 2003 May 29;326(7400):1175–7.
14. Lindson N, Thompson TP, Ferrey A, et al. Motivational interviewing for smoking cessation. Cochrane Database Syst Rev. 2019, Issue 7. Art. No.: CD006936. https://doi.org/10.1002/14651858.CD006936.pub4.
15. Korte KJ, Capron DW, Zvolensky M, et al. The Fagerström test for nicotine dependence: do revisions in the item scoring enhance the psychometric properties? Addict Behav. 2013 Mar 1;38(3):1757–63.
16. Heatherton TF, Kozlowski LT, Frecker RC, et al. Measuring the heaviness of smoking: using self-reported time to the first cigarette of the day and number of cigarettes smoked per day. Br J Addict. 1989 Jul;84(7):791–800.
17. Jarvis JM, Rusell MAH, Saloojee Y. Expired air carbon monoxide: a simple breath test of tobacco smoke intake. BMJ. 1980;2:484.
18. West R, Hajek P, Stead L, et al. Outcome criteria in smoking cessation trials: proposal for a common standard. Addiction. 2005;100:299–303.
19. Wald NJ, Howard S, Smith PG, et al. Association between atherosclerotic disease and carboxyhaemoglobin levels in tobacco smoke. BMJ. 1973;1:761–5.
20. Clair C, Mueller Y, Livingstone-Banks J, et al. Biomedical risk assessment as an aid for smoking cessation. Cochrane Database Syst Rev. 2019, Issue 3. Art. No.: CD004705. https://doi.org/10.1002/14651858.CD004705.pub5 (accessed 2 Feb 2021).
21. Cahill K, Lancaster T, Green N. Stage-based interventions for smoking cessation. Cochrane Database Syst Rev. 2010(11).
22. Michie S, Hyder N, Walia A, et al. Development of a taxonomy of behaviour change techniques used in individual behavioural support for smoking cessation. Addict Behav. 2011 Apr 1;36(4):315–19.
23. Stead LF, Hartmann-Boyce J, Perera R, et al. Telephone counselling for smoking cessation. Cochrane Database Syst Rev. 2013, Issue 8. Art. No.: CD002850. https://doi.org/10.1002/14651858.CD002850.pub3.
24. Nohlert E, Öhrvik J, Tegelberg Å, et al. Long-term follow-up of a high-and a low-intensity smoking cessation intervention in a dental setting—a randomized trial. BMC Public Health. 2013 Dec;13(1):592.
25. NCSCT Standard Treatment Programme. A guide to providing behavioural support for smoking cessation. Available from: www.ncsct.co.uk/usr/pub/ standard_treatment_ programme.pdf (assessed 24 Jan 2019).
26. SRNT Subcommittee on Biochemical Verification. Biochemical verification of tobacco use and cessation. Nicotine Tob Res. 2002 May;4(2):149–59.
27. Benowitz NL, Hukkanen J, Jacob P. Nicotine chemistry, metabolism, kinetics and biomarkers. Nicotine Psychopharmacol. 2009:29–60.
28. Raja M, Garg A, Yadav P, et al. Diagnostic methods for detection of cotinine level in tobacco users: a review. J Clin Diagn Res: JCDR. 2016 Mar;10(3):ZE04.
29. Abrams DB, Follick MJ, Biener L, et al. Saliva cotinine as a measure of smoking status in field settings. Am J Public Health. 1987 Jul;77(7):846–8.
30. Jatlow P, Toll BA, Leary V, et al. Comparison of expired carbon monoxide and plasma cotinine as markers of cigarette abstinence. Drug and Alcohol Depend. 2008 Dec 1;98(3):203–9.
31. Marrone GF, Paulpillai M, Evans RJ, et al. Breath carbon monoxide and semiquantitative saliva cotinine as biomarkers for smoking. Hum Psychopharmacol: Clin Experim. 2010 Jan;25(1):80–3.
32. Middleton ET, Morice AH. Breath Carbon monoxide as an indication for smoking habit. Chest. 2000;117:758–63.
33. Malaysia Clinical Practice Guidelines on Treatment of Tobacco Use Disorder. 2017. ISBN 978-967-0769-78-3.
34. Stead LF, Koilpillai P, Lancaster T. Additional behavioural support as an adjunct to pharmacotherapy for smoking cessation. Cochrane Database Syst Rev. 2015, Issue 10. Art. No.: CD009670. https://doi.org/10.1002/14651858.CD009670.pub3.

35. Przulj D, Wehbe L, McRobbie H, et al. Progressive nicotine patch dosing prior to quitting smoking: feasibility, safety and effects during the pre-quit and post-quit periods. Addiction. 2019 Mar;114(3):515–22.

36. Hartmann-Boyce J, Chepkin SC, Ye W, et al. Nicotine replacement therapy versus control for smoking cessation. Cochrane Database Syst Rev. 2018(5). https://doi.org/10.1002/14651858.CD000146.pub5.

37. Meine TJ, Patel MR, Washam JB, et al. Safety and effectiveness of transdermal nicotine patch in smokers admitted with acute coronary syndromes. Am J Cardiol. 2005 Apr 15;95(8):976–8.

38. Pack QR, Priya A, Lagu TC, et al. Short-term safety of nicotine replacement in smokers hospitalized with coronary heart disease. J Am Heart Assoc. 2018;7:e009424.

39. Mills EJ, Thorlund K, Eapen S, et al. Cardiovascular events associated with smoking cessation pharmacotherapies: a network meta-analysis. Circulation. 2014;129:28–41.

40. Cahill K, Lindson-Hawley N, Thomas KH, et al. Nicotine receptor partial agonists for smoking cessation. Cochrane Database Syst Rev. 2016, Issue 5. Art. No.: CD006103. https://doi.org/10.1002/14651858.CD006103.pub7.

41. Lindson N, Chepkin SC, Ye W, et al. Different doses, durations and modes of delivery of nicotine replacement therapy for smoking cessation. Cochrane Database Syst Rev. 2019, Issue 4. Art. No.: CD013308. https://doi.org/10.1002/14651858.CD013308.

42. Hollands GJ, Naughton F, Farley A, et al. Interventions to increase adherence to medications for tobacco dependence. Cochrane Database Syst Rev. 2019, Issue 8. Art. No.: CD009164. https://doi.org/10.1002/14651858.CD009164.pub3.

43. Jha P, Chaloupka FJ, Moore J, et al. Chapter 46: tobacco addiction. In: Jamison DT, Breman JG, Measham AR, et al., editors. Disease control priorities in developing countries, 2nd edn. Washington, DC: The International Bank for Reconstruction and Development/The World Bank Group; 2006.

44. U.S. Department of Health and Human Services. Smoking cessation. A Report of the Surgeon General. Atlanta, GA: U.S. Department of Health and Human Services, Centers for Disease Control and Prevention, National Center for Chronic Disease Prevention and Health Promotion, Office on Smoking and Health; 2020.

45. Brown TJ, Todd A, O'Malley C, et al. Community pharmacy-delivered interventions for public health priorities: a systematic review of interventions for alcohol reduction, smoking cessation and weight management, including meta-analysis for smoking cessation. BMJ Open. 2016;6:e009828. https://doi.org/10.1136/bmjopen-2015-009828.

46. Carson KV, Verbiest MEA, Crone MR, et al. Training health professionals in smoking cessation. Cochrane Database Syst Rev. 2012, Issue 5. Art. No.: CD000214. https://doi.org/10.1002/14651858.CD000214.pub2.

47. Lucas C, Martin J. Smoking and drug interactions. Aust Prescr. 2013;36:102–4.

48. Farley AC, Hajek P, Lycett D, et al. Interventions for preventing weight gain after smoking cessation. Cochrane Database Syst Rev. 2012, Issue 1. Art. No.: CD006219. https://doi.org/10.1002/14651858.CD006219.pub3.

49. Kaisar MA, Prasad S, Liles T, et al. A decade of e-cigarettes: limited research & unresolved safety concerns. Toxicology. 2016 Jul 15;365:67–75.

50. Grana R, Benowitz N, Glantz SA. E-cigarettes: a scientific review. Circulation. 2014 May 13;129(19):1972–86.

51. Riker CA, Lee K, Darville A, et al. E-cigarettes: promise or peril? Nurs Clin. 2012 Mar 1;47(1):159–71.

52. Glantz SA, Bareham DW. E-cigarettes: use, effects on smoking, risks, and policy implications. Annu Rev Public Health. 2018 Apr 1;39:215–35.

53. Talhout R, Schulz T, Florek E, et al. Hazardous compounds in tobacco smoke. Int J Environ Res Public Health. 2011 Feb;8(2):613–28.

54. Rahman MA, Hann N, Wilson A, et al. E-cigarettes and smoking cessation: evidence from a systematic review and meta-analysis. PLoS ONE. 2015 Mar 30;10(3):e0122544.

55. Kalkhoran S, Glantz SA. E-cigarettes and smoking cessation in real-world and clinical settings: a systematic review and meta-analysis. Lancet Respir Med. 2016 Feb 1;4(2):116–28.

56. Levy DT, Borland R, Lindblom EN, et al. Potential deaths averted in USA by replacing cigarettes with e-cigarettes. Tob Control. 2018 Jan 1;27(1):18–25.

57. Bullen C, Howe C, Laugesen M, et al. Electronic cigarettes for smoking cessation: a randomised controlled trial. Lancet. 2013 Nov 16;382(9905):1629–37.

58. Hajek P, Phillips-Waller A, Przulj D, et al. A randomized trial of e-cigarettes versus nicotine-replacement therapy. New England J Med. 2019 Feb 14;380(7):629–37.

59. Brown J, Beard E, Kotz D, et al. Real-world effectiveness of e-cigarettes when used to aid smoking cessation: a cross-sectional population study. Addiction. 2014 Sep;109(9):1531–40.

60. McNeil A, Brose LS, Calder R, et al. E-cigarettes: an evidence update. A report commissioned by Public Health England. Public Health England. 2015;111:14–15.

5 Medical Devices to Improve Medication Adherence

Mohamed Izham Mohamed Ibrahim and
Nor Fatin Farhani Mohamed Izham

CONTENTS

BACKGROUND

In disease management, adhering to medication is essential. Clinicians, healthcare systems, and other stakeholders (e.g., payers) have raised concerns with medication nonadherence because of growing evidence that it is prevalent. Nonadherence to medications is associated with adverse outcomes, waste of resources, and higher care costs.[1]

The long-term use of pharmacotherapy with multiple medications is required for the treatment of chronic illnesses, especially among the elderly (Figure 5.1). It is estimated that approximately half of the patients do not take their medications as prescribed.[2] Thus, while these medications effectively fight disease, their most significant advantages are often not realized. Numerous factors are contributing to poor medication adherence. These include those that are associated with patients (e.g., suboptimal health literacy, and lack of involvement in the treatment decision-making process), those that are associated with healthcare professionals (e.g., communication barriers, ineffective communication of information about adverse effects, prescription of complex drug regimens, and provision of care by multiple physicians), and those that are associated to healthcare systems (e.g., limited access to care, office visit time limitations, and lack of health information technology).[3,4] Ways to improve adherence must be multifactorial because barriers to medication adherence are multifaceted and diverse.

Medication adherence continues to be a vital element of the pharmacy practice. Pharmacists are in a strategic position between patients, payers, and other healthcare providers to overcome this problem. They need to focus particular consideration on interventions that may help patients continue or improve compliance. Pharmacists can (i) educate patients about the importance of adherence, (ii) identify ways to help patients avoid running out of medications (i.e., refill reminders), (iii) provide strategies for improving adherence with medication aids, such as pillboxes and dosing calendars, (iv) identify confounding factors that may adversely affect adherence, and (v) review medication regimens to identify possible simplification strategies.

In some countries and settings, pharmacists have direct access to patients. Pharmacists can influence patient medication adherence. Thus, they can recognize poor adherence, assist in removing barriers that may be evident, and help the inclusion of adherence interventions into the care plans of their patients.

Some healthcare professionals rarely come across the different types of medication adherence devices and technologies. This chapter focuses on highlighting medical devices and technology that can assist patients, caregivers, and healthcare providers in enhancing medication adherence.

DOI: 10.1201/9781003002345-6

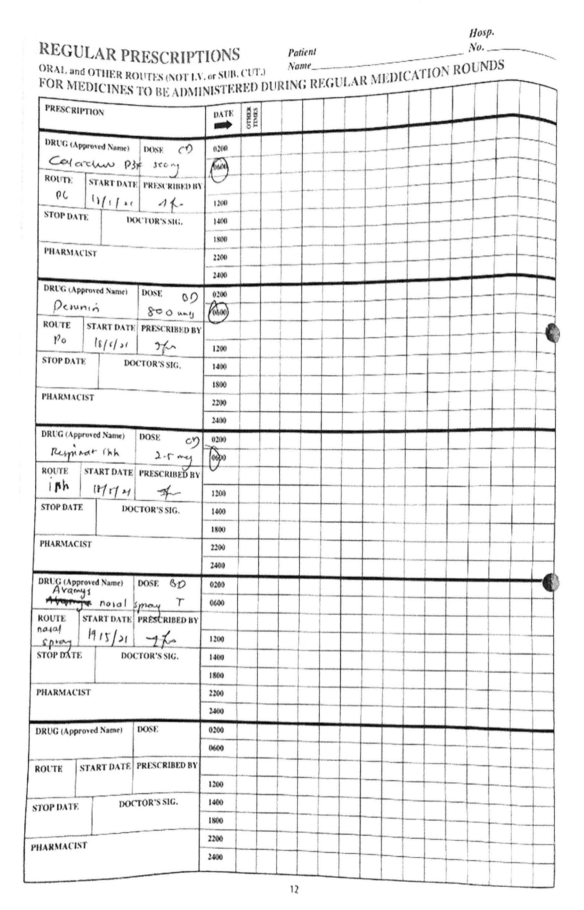

FIGURE 5.1　Lists of medications prescribed to a patient with chronic illness.

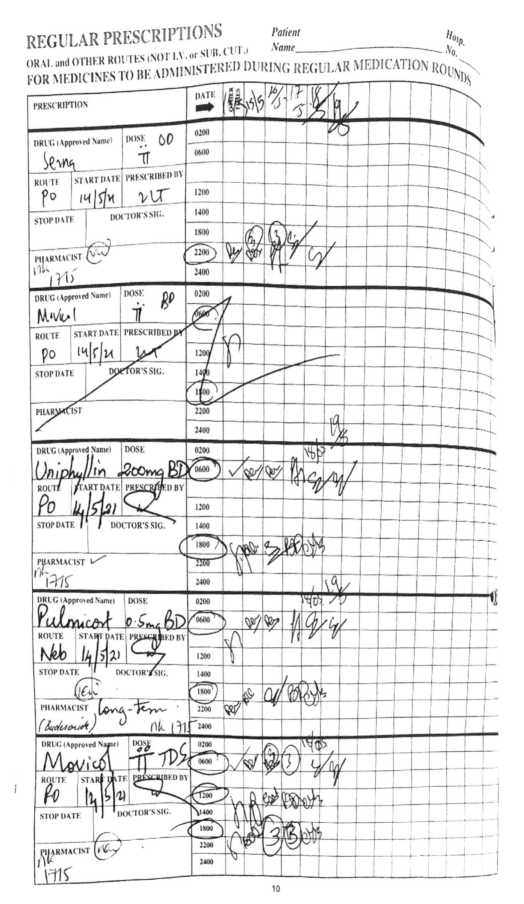

FIGURE 5.1 (Continued)

REGULAR PRESCRIPTIONS

ORAL and OTHER ROUTES (NOT I.V. or SUB. CUT.)

FOR MEDICINES TO BE ADMINISTERED DURING REGULAR MEDICATION ROUNDS

Patient Name _____   Hosp. No. _____

PRESCRIPTION		DATE ➡	OTHER TIMES	17/5	18						
DRUG (Approved Name) Lactulose 15ml	DOSE	0200									
		0600									
ROUTE PO	START DATE 14/5/21	PRESCRIBED BY	1200								
			1400								
STOP DATE	DOCTOR'S SIG.	1800									
		2200									
PHARMACIST MK 17/5		2400									
DRUG (Approved Name) Pantoprazole 40mg	DOSE	0200									
		0600									
ROUTE PO	START DATE 14/5/21	PRESCRIBED BY	0800								
			1200								
STOP DATE	DOCTOR'S SIG.	1400									
		1800									
PHARMACIST MK 17/5		2200									
		2400									
DRUG (Approved Name) Atorvastatin	DOSE 10mg	0200									
		0600									
ROUTE Po	START DATE 15/3/21	PRESCRIBED BY JR	1200								
STOP DATE	DOCTOR'S SIG.	1400									
MK 17/5		1800									
PHARMACIST need to clarify Patient upset not getting statin		2200									
		2400									

DRUG (Approved Name) Prednisolone.	DOSE 40mg	0200	17/5	18	19/5	21/5	23/5	7/5	29/5	29/5	31/5
		0600	40mg	35mg	30mg	25mg	20mg	15mg	10mg	5mg	
ROUTE po	START DATE 17/5/21	PRESCRIBED BY	8.00								
		1200									
STOP DATE 01/06/21	DOCTOR'S SIG.	1400									
		1800									
PHARMACIST R/v 5/7.	MK 17/5	2200									
		2400									

DRUG (Approved Name)	DOSE	0200	Pharmacist Med Rec 17/5/21
		0600	
ROUTE please R/v 1chart / hold	START DATE	PRESCRIBED BY	• Spiolto Respimat inhaler 2.5mcg II OD
		1200	• Calcichew D3 forte 500mg/400iu II OD
STOP DATE as needed	DOCTOR'S SIG.	1400	• desunin 800 units BD OD Rvd
		1800	
PHARMACIST		2200	PRN
Thanks Dr Clark #742		2400	• second inhaler 10mcg II @ 15pm

11

PRESCRIPTION SLIP
(Discharge / Outpatient)

MRN: 435412

NG TUBE: YES NO OTHER TUBE FEEDING
PREGNANCY: YES NO

VERBAL ORDER

ROUTE/ DOSAGE FORM	MEDICATION	DOSE
1	plavix	75mg
1	Bisoprolol	2.5mg
1	mecobalamin	500mcg
1	alpha calcidol	0.25mcg
1	Atorvastatin	40mg
1	Calcium Carbonate	1g
1	pantoprazole	40mg
1	Exforge (10/80 mg)	1tab
1	Empagliflozin	10mg
1	galvus met (50/1000)mg	1tab
1	glimepiride	2mg

DATE: 16/2/21 TIME: 2pm

DOCTOR'S SIGNATURE: DOCTOR'S NAME:

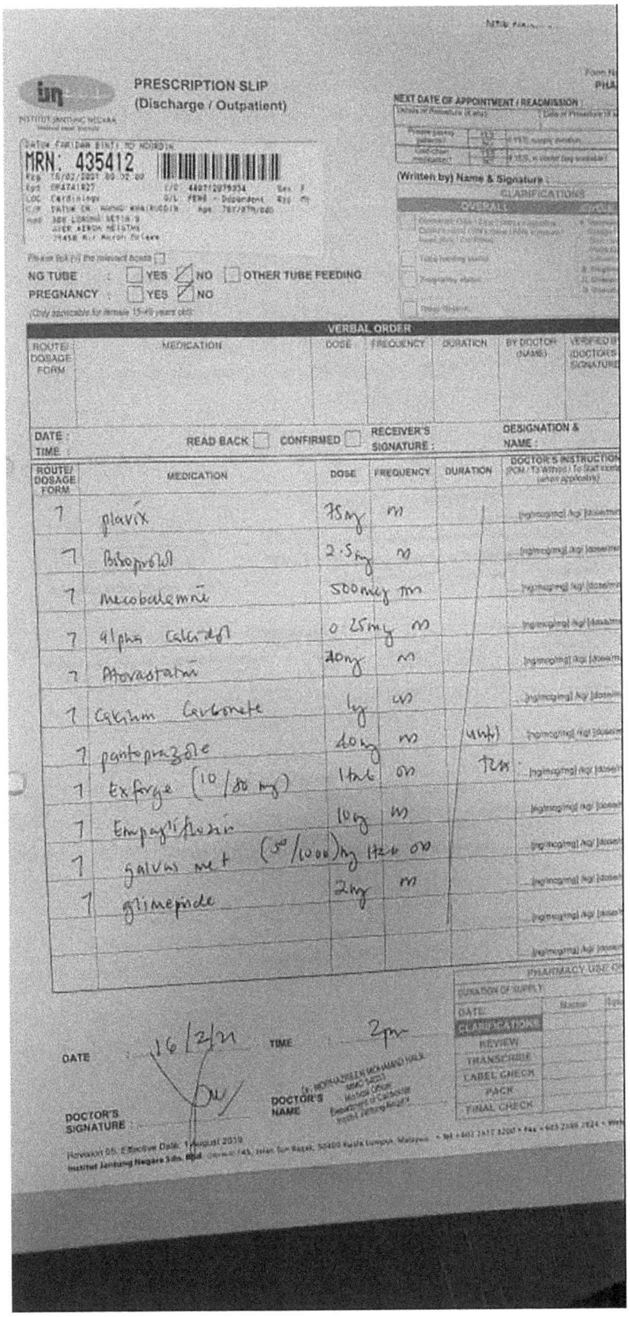

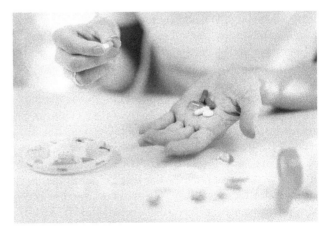

FIGURE 5.1 (Continued)

WHAT DOES MEDICATION ADHERENCE MEAN?

Dr. Koop said, "Drugs do not work in patients who do not take them."[5] Delamater (2006) and Meichenbaum et al. (1987) defined adherence as "active, voluntary, and collaborative involvement of the patient in a mutually acceptable course of behavior to produce a therapeutic result."[6,7] In addition, the World Health Organization defined medication adherence as "the degree to which the person's behavior corresponds with the agreed recommendations from a health care provider."[8] According to Caetano et al. (2006) and Cramer et al. (2008), two concepts are built within the behavior of medication adherence—adherence and persistence.[9,10] According to the Agency for Healthcare Research and Quality (na), medication adherence is "the patient's conformance with the provider's recommendation concerning timing, dosage, and frequency of medication-taking during the prescribed length of time" and persistence is defined as the "duration of time patient takes medication, from initiation to discontinuation of therapy."[11] In addition to the element of persistence within the concept of adherence, Masaus and Bahr (2012) have classified adherence into three phases: initiation, implementation, and discontinuation.[12] Any interventions carried out to tackle the problem of medication nonadherence by the healthcare providers, especially pharmacists, must target these components.

IS MEDICATION NONADHERENCE PANDEMIC?

Medication nonadherence is prevalent in many settings, i.e., primary care, nursing homes, the patient's home (Figure 5.2), and geographical areas. Many healthcare professionals have encountered elderly patients with multiple comorbidities who presented with paper bags filled with several different medication boxes—and they are all mixed up—different meds in a different box. It is worrying to see that between healthcare professionals, their general practitioner, and pharmacists—no one highlights to these elderly patients that they would benefit from having their medications placed at least in pillboxes or blister packs.

It has been reported that between 20% and 30% of medication prescriptions are never filled. Further, around 50% of chronic disease medications are not taken as prescribed, despite evidence that medical therapy improves the quality of life and prevents death.[2,13]

The WHO and the Organisation for Economic Co-Operation and Development (OECD) estimate that one out of two patients with chronic diseases does not use their

FIGURE 5.2 A pill organizer.

Source: www.shutterstock.com/image-photo/medicine-nonadherence-woman-holding-pills-hand-1854834133

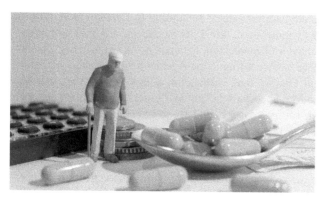

FIGURE 5.3 The overwhelming task of medication adherence, especially for the elderly.

Source: www.shutterstock.com/image-photo/decreased-medication-compliance-increased-patient-burden-1953931399

medication as prescribed.[14,15] In Europe alone, nonadherence is estimated to annually contribute to the premature death of 200,000 patients and excess healthcare costs of €125 billion.[15] The noncompliance problems in the Asian and African communities were also prevalent.[16]

Poor compliance to therapy is predominantly prevalent among older patients suffering from chronic illnesses, such as cardiovascular disorders, metabolic disorders (e.g., diabetes), respiratory disorders (e.g., asthma and chronic obstructive pulmonary disease) and neurological and central nervous system-related disorders (e.g., multiple sclerosis and Parkinson's disease).[17] (Figure 5.3)

The most common types of noncompliance include not having a prescription filled, taking an incorrect dose (too much or too little), taking the medication at the wrong time, forgetting to take one or more doses, and stopping the medication too soon.

According to Rubin (2005), adherence rates for type 2 diabetes patients are ranged from 65% to 85% for oral agents and 60% to 80% for insulin.[18] Factors that affect adherence in this population are comparable to those in patients with other chronic diseases such as treatment regimen complexity, understanding the treatment regimen, perception of the benefits of treatment, costs of medications, adverse effects, and emotional well-being.[18]

Macquart de Terline et al. (2019) revealed poor adherence to antihypertensive medications and the associated factors (i.e., traditional medicine use, socioeconomic status) in the sub-Saharan countries.[19] Uncontrolled blood pressure can be found in about half of people with hypertension (HTN).[20] Inadequate medication adherence is the significant cause of poor blood pressure control.[21,22] Inadequate medication adherence also is the leading cause of cardiovascular disease and is associated with high morbidity and mortality.[23] Among patients with presumed resistant HTN, 43% to 65.5% are medication nonadherent.[24,25] Kolandaivelu et al. (2014) reported that nonadherence to cardiovascular medications is pandemic and a leading risk factor for treatment failures and poor outcomes.[26] Ho et al. (2006) reported that

only 66% of patients in the PREMIER Registry reported taking key medications after experiencing an acute myocardial infarction.[27] In another report, Jackevicius et al. (2008) mentioned that only 78% of patients filled prescriptions within 120 days of acute myocardial infarction.[28]

Favorable health outcomes in psychiatric disorders such as schizophrenia, bipolar disorder, and depression failed to be achieved due to medication nonadherence.[29] The risk of relapse and hospitalization increases, and the quality of life reduces due to nonadherence to the treatment of severe mental illness.[30] According to Lacro et al. (2002) and Sajatovic et al. (2006), the rates of partial adherence or nonadherence with foundational psychopharmacologic treatments in serious mental illness vary, but are estimated to be at least 40–50%.[31,32] The estimates of medication adherence within the psychiatric population based on disease states vary, i.e., major depressive disorder: 28–52%; bipolar disorder 20–50%; schizophrenia: 20–72%; and anxiety disorders: 57%.[33,34,35,31,36] In a systematic review, it is reported that nonadherence to psychotropic medications is ethnicity-related and higher for Latinos than for Euro-Americans.[37] The matter gets worse when certain groups of patients like the elderly experience polypharmacy.[38]

Based on the point just discussed, these tools also help in reducing medication error: wrong tablets, wrong quantity, wrong time, etc. Time is significant for Parkinson's patients because they need to take their medications at the same appointed time every day.

MEDICATION NONADHERENCE: WHY DOES IT MATTER?

Medication adherence is experienced in both high-income and low- to middle-income countries (LMICs). It can affect quality and length of life, hospital readmission, health outcomes, and overall healthcare costs.[39,40,41] For example, the risk of hospitalization was more than double in diabetic, hypertensive, hypercholesterolemic, or congestive heart failure patients who were nonadherent to prescribed treatments compared with the general population.[42] Serious health consequences and loss of productivity are caused by poor adherence to prescribed regimens. Further, productivity loss can affect income and social well-being.[43] In the literature, the rates of nonadherence vary widely and can be very high, even in the strictly controlled setting. As mentioned earlier, several factors cause nonadherence. For example, chronic illness patients are less probable to follow prescription orders than those with acute conditions.[44] It is becoming ever more difficult and demanding for healthcare providers to meet quality measures related to medication use while dealing with large, diverse, and complex patient populations.

HOW TO PREVENT MEDICATION NONADHERENCE

There are several adherence-intervention approaches. Healthcare providers are only part of the patient care

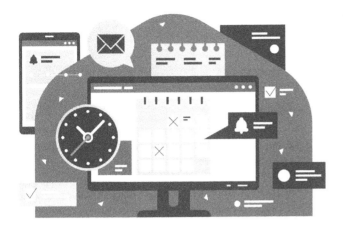

FIGURE 5.4 Scheduled electronic medication reminders.

Source: www.shutterstock.com/image-vector/electronic-screen-schedule-planning-information-vector-1594086256

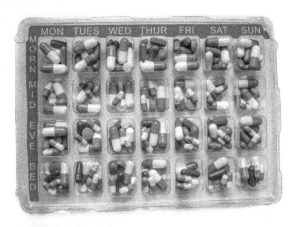

FIGURE 5.6A A pill organizer with detailed scheduling for time of day and day of week.

Source: www.shutterstock.com/image-photo/tablets-capsules-monitored-dosage-system-which-535504627

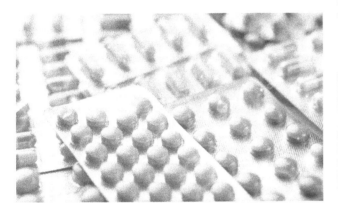

FIGURE 5.5 Adherence packaging in the form of easily trackable blister packs.

Source: www.shutterstock.com/image-photo/colorful-capsule-round-pills-blister-package-1669253995

equation. One of the focuses is patient-centered. The methods are electronic reminders (Figure 5.4), regimen simplification, adherence packaging (Figure 5.5), pillbox organizer (Figure 5.6), 90-day supplies, automatic refills, minimizing adverse effects, reducing medication cost, providing incentives, and ongoing communication.[45] Further, there are additional methods, i.e., in-person models, electronic mailed, faxed materials, phone calls, or electronic strategies such as electronic pillboxes, automated phone calls, computer-generated targeted interventions mobile text.

The focus of this discussion will be on devices and technologies that can improve medication adherence, e.g., intelligent delivery devices (pills, injectors, inhalers, wearable injectors) and smart accessories (blister packs, pill bottles/boxes, medication dispensers).[17]

The latest developments combine a drug with a smart adherence-monitoring tool, the so-called drug-device combinations. The US Food and Drug Administration (FDA)-approved drug-device combinations include a smart insulin

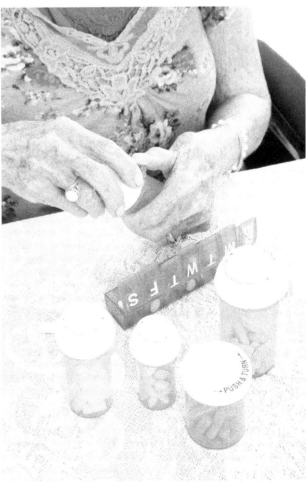

FIGURE 5.6B A pill organizer assisting the elderly.

Source: www.shutterstock.com/image-photo/senior-woman-sorting-her-pills-week-111130346

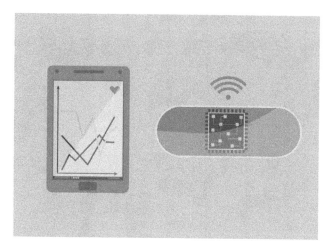

FIGURE 5.7   Smart adherence-monitoring tools.

Source: www.shutterstock.com/image-vector/smart-pills-future-medicine-pill-microchip-1154331838

pen, a smart pill (Figure 5.7), and a smart inhaler.[46] These integrated devices may help personalized disease management. They could also be relevant for doctors and payers to rule out nonadherence to first-line therapies before more expensive second-line therapies, such as the biologic agents, are used.[47]

While all these remarkable technologies and methods exist, unfortunately, access to these within certain areas or countries is not widely known. In clinical practice, patients on multiple different medications and complex drug regimens are primarily older people. While there are different methods of achieving compliance, unfortunately, older people are not well equipped with devices that can help them with these mobile applications.

DIGITAL TOOLS: INNOVATIVE STRATEGIES FOR IMPROVING MEDICATION ADHERENCE

Table 5.1 describes some of the tools and technologies used to enhance medication adherence.

There are several solutions used to enhance medication adherence, including hardware, software, and clinical solutions, or an integration of these.

HARDWARE SOLUTIONS

Some of the common solutions are pillboxes, pill bottle strips with toggles and reminder caps, and blister packaging. These are low-cost devices but are not effective in improving medication adherence. Choudhry et al. (2017) compared the effects of three low-cost reminder devices (i.e., pill bottle strip with toggles, digital timer cap, or standard pillbox).[48] They reported that these devices did not improve adherence among nonadherent chronic-condition patients. Technology advancements have enabled real-time electronic monitoring with internet-connected devices. These devices can alert patients, family members, and

healthcare providers of missed medications. These innovations will raise the cost and cause accessibility and affordability issues.

SOFTWARE SOLUTIONS

Due to the high cost of hardware solutions, scientists have moved to software solutions. Among the few mobile applications are MediSafe™ and HealthPrize™. These technology-mediated interventions are scalable solutions. The capability to use electronic health records is expected to help improve medication adherence; it can systematically collect, organize, access, and analyze health information. Through better connectivity among patients, their providers, and the healthcare system, health information technology can assist monitoring of quality metrics and improve medication management. The use of electronic prescribing and health information technology offers an important opportunity to assess and enhance medication adherence at the point of care and detect nonadherence. Electronic medical records can also assist in medication reconciliation by offering a way for members of an individual's healthcare team to retrieve information to reconcile medications during transitions of care, hospital admissions, and hospital discharges.[49] Clinical trials conducted to assess interventions based on cell phones, text messages, and electronic reminders on pagers indicate that electronic automated triggers alone are not effective for improving adherence towards pill refill. Besides, these technologies did not create substantial change in physician actions related to medication reconciliation.[41]

Patient-level adherence patterns can be determined by pharmaceutical database technology. This technology functions by filling newly prescribed medications and refills, which provides continuous contact with patients outside the hospital or clinic visits. Pharmacists are easily reached, knowledgeable on information sources, and accessible to discuss potential contraindications or concerns regarding medications with patients and caregivers. Cramer et al. (2008) suggested that data generated in the pharmacy permits identification and analysis of the proportion of days that patients have access to medication, as either a cumulative medication gaps metric or medication possession ratio.[50] In addition to these metrics, electronic data systems can be automated to produce phone call reminders to patients to refill their pills.

Another solution is applying telemonitoring systems for medication-related self-management. Patients are able to generate and respond to their data using the in-home telemonitoring systems. The patients or caregivers document and report symptoms, such as weight gain or shortness of breath, and associated medication dosing that the healthcare provider can review for evaluation of trends. Moreover, the telemonitoring system can provide reinforcement, medication-related education, and opportunities for review and reconciliation. It applies a two-way communication strategy

TABLE 5.1

Description of Medication Adherence Improvement Devices and Technologies

Device/Technology	Description and examples
Adherence packaging	A 31-day supply of medication is sealed in medical-grade packaging, indicating the prescription of the health provider and how the medication should be taken; formats include blister packs and pill boxes which compartmentalize medications into days and time of day for simplicity, accessibility and ease of use. Common attributes: Each package is a prescribed unit, and the primary package section is a blister and a secondary outer container made from paperboard or plastic. Other features include high product stability, barcodes or readable color schemes, child-resistant features, and track-and-trace features.
Automated phone calls or interactive voice response system	The system interacts with callers without input from a human other than the caller; it can play a pre-recorded message or other information.
Automatic refills	Prescription will be automatically refilled and mailed (usually a week) before the patient runs out of medication. Examples include MedaCube™, Pria™, Hero™, and Philips™.
Bio-ingestible sensors	These devices are pill-sized electronic chips that ping the patient's smartphone with data after the patient swallows them; the chip alerts the patient's smartphone and in some cases alerts the physician, with relevant data once it is in the patient's digestive tract. Patients wear a patch that relays this data from the sensors in the chip. Examples include MyTmed™ and Abilify MyCite™.
Cloud-based system	Patients and healthcare providers can connect; patients can get a video link to their pharmacist by using a mobile device. Example: iRetainRx™.
Electronic health records (EHR)	Patients and providers may systematically collect, organize, access, and analyze health information; patients may better understand health information. EHR is expected to help improve medication adherence. Examples include Epic Systems Corporation, Allscripts, Advanced MD, athenahealth.
Email	Providers may email messages to remind patients about medication-taking, refilling prescriptions, and other health advice.
Electronic pill monitors	Automated reminder greets patients and reminds them to take their medications; also provide alerts to physicians or other caregivers when preprogrammed drug-use schedules are missed. Example: MedSignals™.
Electronic pill bottles	Bottle records every time it is opened and transmits data via microchip. Example: MEMS®, Medication Event Monitoring System.
Electronic reminders (Figure 5.8)	Smartphone apps, watches with alarms, and text messages (SMS) remind people to take medications as prescribed. Examples include smartphone app MyMedTimes™ and PillDrill™.
E-pill Once-a-Day Reminder	This reminder is analog; a plastic dial easily affixes to a smooth surface, like a medicine cabinet or refrigerator; once the patient takes medication, he or she turns the dial to the current day of the week to record last dose of medication.
Faxed materials	Education materials and medication information can be faxed to patients.
In-home teledispensing and telemonitoring systems	System dispenses prepackaged medications on time with reminder alerts while tracking medications; medications are organized into pouches by day and time of administration, and labeled with participant's name, medication name, and dosage. Examples include spencer™ and MedMinder™.
Internet of Things (IoT) (Figure 5.9)	System uses digital activity trackers to monitor health; adds a medical adherence app to smart watches that helps users remember their prescription dosages on a periodic basis in the form of nudges or reminders; features include cloud storage of information, GPS, and RFID. Examples include smart medication transportation (transporting medication); drug checker system.
Interactive Voice Response (IVR) telemonitoring	A computer-based telephone system initiates calls, receives calls, provides information, and collects data from users.
Mobile health (mHealth)	Mobile technology acts as a healthcare delivery method via smartphones and wireless data transmission. Examples of such applications include Wechat and BBreminder.
Multicompartmental pillboxes	These pillboxes have several compartments with different alarms that beep and vibrate at scheduled medication times. Example: TabTime Vibe vibrating pill timer/reminder.
Medication adherence apps available on Apple® devices	There are approximately 400 of these apps; each has 1 or 2 features, commonly focused on behavioral strategies through alerts, precision patient engagement system, reminders and logs, personalized machine learning algorithms, complex medication instructions, cloud data storage, database of medications, and tracking of missed and taken doses; some apps are free. Examples and available devices: • Dosecast—iTouch®, iPhone®, iPad® • MedCoach—iTouch®, iPhone®, iPad® • Pill Monitor—iTouch®, iPhone®, iPad® • CARE4TODAY™—iTouch®, iPhone®, iPad® • CassianRx™—MediTrak®

(Continued)

TABLE 5.1
(Continued)

Device/Technology	Description and examples
Medication adherence apps available on Android® devices	Approximately 250 apps are available; each has 1 or 2 features, commonly focused on behavioral strategies through alerts, reminders and logs, complex medication instructions, cloud data storage, database of medications, and tracking of missed and taken doses; some apps are free. Examples and available Android versions: • Dosecast—Android® 1.6 and up • MedCoach—Android® 2.2 and up • RxCase Minder®—Android® 1.5 and up
Medication adherence tool—non-digital	This type of tool contains all essential information on current therapy, increases communication, takes a simple approach, provides a visual way to show all the medications that a patient needs, tracks evidence of effectiveness, and is portable. Examples include reminder charts, pill cards, educational videos, pill organizers, and pill cutter.
Mobile apps mobile text messaging	The system sends text messages directly to patients as a reminder to take medicines. Examples include Memotext's patient adherence software and Microsoft's online health portal.
Mobile games	These apps transform adherence into games and prizes by collecting compliance data and rewarding players (patients) for adherence. Examples include HealthPrize™, Pillboxie™, and Mango Health™.
Peer-to-peer pill reminders	A simple smartphone app can help manage numerous people's medications; also tracks prescriptions and reminds when it's time for a refill; will alert family members when a patient has not taken medications. Example: Medisafe™, an iOS and Android mobile app (and cloud-synced database).
Pharmaceutical database technology	The system identifies patient-level adherence patterns for filling newly prescribed medications and refills, providing a community-based point of contact with patients beyond the time constraints of hospital or clinic visits.
Phone calls	Phone calls can be made by either patient or provider; any related questions and concerns are welcome.
PillPack	Patients may transfer over medications and set up a start date; dosed-out medications start arriving at the patient's doorstep every two weeks, in plastic packages strung together on a roll. The service will contact the doctor to confirm the patient's medicine schedule, and again when the prescriptions are getting low. The service also has a smartphone app that allows users to set various reminders throughout the day.
Smart inhaler	A built-in sensor measures inhaler adherence and the adequacy of inspiratory flow; it also detects, records, and stores data on inhaler events. Electronic rings can be attached to compatible asthma devices for the monitoring of every actuation (such as SmartInhaler®), Asthmapdis, Doser, Akita, and ProAir Digihaler.
Smart medication cabinet system	System has a scheduled medication alarm; sensors detect if cabinet is opened and deactivate the alarm, then send report of compliance.
Smart package systems	System alerts patients via sound cues and provides tracking of dispensed medicines; small, electronic card affix to medication packaging records date and time of intakes when a button is pushed; Bluetooth features transfer data to mobile devices. Example: Time4Med™ device, a blister packages equipped with an e-label (a so-called Smart Blister).
Smart pill (see also bio-ingestible sensors)	Smart pills allows physician to monitor pressure, pH, and temperature in the GI tract; can also be an embedded microchip that record details; data is captured and transmitted. The "SmartPill" Ingestion Event Marker was cleared by the FDA in July 2012 for marketing as a medical device containing a formula of a digital period-sized sensor with aripiprazole, an antipsychotic agent; the same sensor is also combined in capsules with the oral chemotherapeutic agent capecitabine.
Smartphone-based electronic diary (e-diary) (Figure 5.10)	E-diaries keep a prospective documentation of medication intake, and offers digital reminders. Some of the challenges include accuracy of system and data, energy consumption, user acceptability, tampering and doubts about sustainability over long-term continued use.
Smart pill dispensers	These devices use home voice assistants for optimal outcome of medication adherence; these devices also incorporate remote access to medical professionals, and various other activation systems while dispensing medications. They can also relay video and audio signals to notify users. Although they can be expensive they can meet a variety of patient needs, but there is difficulty in tracking absolute adherence, such as for immunosuppressive medication.
Smart pills bottle	Sensors in the bottle cap detect when the bottle is opened; or sensors in the bottom of the bottle can identify the weight of the pills and calculate if the patient were adherent; fixed sensors can be mounted on pillboxes. Although they can be expensive, they can meet a variety of patient needs, but there is difficulty in tracking absolute adherence, such as for immunosuppressive medication.
Smart watch	Smart watches provide reminders and other useful content. Example: TransplantHero.
Teleconsultation (Figure 5.11)	This allows the healthcare provider to contact the patient directly via telephone, and to use mobile phones, computers, and applications to provide the necessary education regarding medication; teleconsultation allows providers to reach patients across great distances.

Note: This list may not be exhaustive; others devices and technologies maybe available.

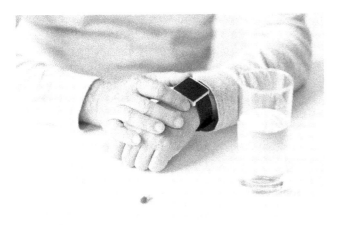

FIGURE 5.8   Smart watch.

Source: www.shutterstock.com/image-photo/age-medicine-health-care-people-concept-573837103

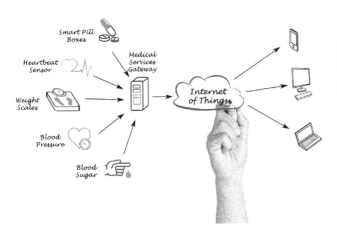

FIGURE 5.9   Telemedicine—Internet of Things (IoT).

Source: www.shutterstock.com/image-photo/diagram-telemedicine-313494767

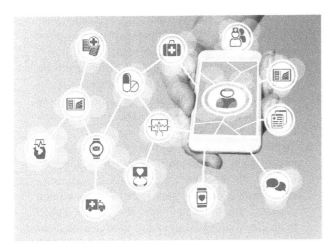

FIGURE 5.10   Smartphone (eHealth).

Source: www.shutterstock.com/image-photo/digital-mobile-healthcare-concept-hand-holding-451442275
www.shutterstock.com/image-photo/ehealth-concept-on-screen-529379551

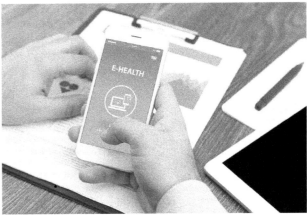

FIGURE 5.10   (Continued)

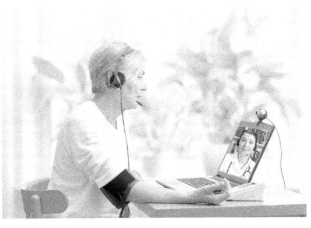

FIGURE 5.11   Teleconsultation.

Source: www.shutterstock.com/image-photo/senior-woman-her-living-room-front-1055436890

that supports accessibility and communication between patient and healthcare provider.

However, these solutions are not effective in tackling behavioral and environmental issues related to medication nonadherence.

CLINICAL SOLUTIONS

Sometimes patients lack understanding and they need to be educated. This intervention should be ongoing communication and needs reinforcement. Pharmacists can perform a clinical intervention such as medication therapy management (MTM), a systematic, patient-centered process to assess all the potential barriers to effective therapy. MTM is applied to optimize medication use. Pharmacists evaluate a patient's medications to confirm that each medication is appropriate for the patient, taken as ordered, and effective.[51]

TECHNOLOGY-ENABLED MULTIFACETED INTERVENTIONS

One way to increase the effectiveness of interventions to enhance medication nonadherence is to apply multiple solutions, e.g., technology-enabled multi-approach interventions. Multiple solutions are integrated to enhance adherence. Well-designed digital health solutions can enable more proactive care. Multi-approach interventions can drive medication optimization, coordinated care, and cost savings.

HOW CAN TECHNOLOGY IMPROVE MEDICATION ADHERENCE? THE EMERGING USE OF TECHNOLOGY

Aldeer et al. (2018) reviewed medication adherence monitoring technologies.[52] They classified these technologies into various categories: proximity-based (e.g., Radio Frequency Identification [RFID] technology), vision-based (e.g., smartphone camera), sensor-based (e.g., wearable, fixed, and ingestible sensors), and fusion-based systems (i.e., combination of techniques). Smart technologies can improve patients' health. Medication adherence will likely improve when motivated patients trust and use the technology.[53] However, technology alone will not solve the complicated adherence puzzle, partly because it does not work in isolation.[54] As mentioned earlier, ultimately, numerous factors contribute to nonadherence, whether it be patient-related, physician-related, or system-related factors such as limited understanding of disease and purpose of medications, lack of explanations regarding the importance of compliance by healthcare professionals, limited resources, or cost of drugs. The tools will not work in isolation, but will increase compliance, couple with implementing other strategies (e.g., behavioral models), and tackle other nonadherence problems (e.g., unaffordability or inaccessibility of medications).

There are hundreds of devices, technologies, and apps available to enhance medication adherence. The number in the market is increasing. However, how effective are these technology-based adherence devices?

Case studies:

1. A patient who had a heart attack—and had stenting a couple of years before—presented again with another heart attack (i.e., stents were blocked) due to nonadherence to medications. Generally, once a patient is discharged after a heart attack, he or she is on multiple medications (antiplatelets, beta blocker, statin, ACE inhibitors, etc.). Medication nonadherence is not necessarily due to lack of tools but more to lack of understanding the diseases and the importance of taking the medications as prescribed.

2. A study of electronic monitoring devices (EMD) was carried out on HIV-infected patients treated with highly active antiretroviral therapy (HAART).[55] Patients were asked to put their prescriptions in a container with an EMD and complete a questionnaire. The concomitant use of pillboxes was patients' key reason for not using the EMD as ordered. At the beginning of the study, patients

agreed to open the EMD cap when taking medications out of a pillbox; thus, the EMD would record the dose. Nevertheless, patients who used a pillbox for their medication storage occasionally forgot to open the EMD at the corresponding time. The use of pillboxes accounted for about 20% of missed EMD data. Of particular interest to pharmacists is the recommendation to avoid EMDs in populations that rely heavily on pillboxes. EMDs may not be valuable complementary interventions in these populations, since pillboxes are often used as adherence tools for patients with many medications.

3. Chaudhry et al. (2010) studied home-based telemonitoring in heart failure patients.[56] The trial indicated that patient engagement with the device was poor. At six months, almost half of patients were not using the device, although automated reminders were sent after two days of non-use. They concluded that expecting patients to start and use computerized, technology-based monitoring was not effective in improving medication adherence or adherence-related clinical outcomes.

4. Christensen and co-workers (2010) studied the impact of a reminder device and electronic monitoring on patient adherence with antihypertensive therapy.[57] It was a randomized cross-over design: patients who were on electronic adherence monitoring with a reminder and monitoring device were compared with patients who were on standard therapy. The findings indicated no difference in blood pressure, 6% improved medication adherence in the intervention group at six months, and at 12 months, 2% improved medication adherence in the intervention group.

5. The effect of a pharmacy-based health literacy intervention and patient characteristics on medication refill adherence in an urban health system was studied by Gazmararian and colleagues (2010).[58] They conducted three-part interventions: automated telephone reminder calls to refill prescriptions, picture prescription card for health literacy, and clear health communication training for pharmacists. No difference in the improvement of medication adherence before and after intervention between the study groups was found.

6. Tamblyn et al. (2020) applied computerized drug management systems in primary care settings to increase the detection and response to cardiovascular medication adherence issues.[59] They wanted to assess the automated alert intervention linked to an electronic medical record to trigger medication reconciliation by primary care physicians. The automated reminder did not show improved adherence to prescription refill or increased therapeutic dosing changes. Nevertheless, drug profile review increased in uncontrolled hypertensive patients. Additionally, there was no significant increase in

drug discontinuations due to side effects. After six months of follow-up, the researchers found no significant change in refill adherence.

7. Park and colleagues (2019) reviewed the published evidence on the mobile phone apps that targeting medication adherence.[60] They managed to identify around 700 apps from Apple and Android operating systems. Most of the apps used behavioral approach intervention to enhance adherence. Even though many consumers provided positive feedbacks, still there are limitations and room for improvement in the apps.

8. In 2020, Armitage and associates published a systematic review and meta-analysis on medication adherence effectiveness of mobile device apps.[61] They also evaluated the behavior change techniques used by the apps to improve adherence. The patients included were for any diseases and any duration. Based on the nine trials and slightly more than one thousand patients included, they concluded that mobile apps might positively affect medication adherence. The interventions delivered by smartphone apps are related to higher levels of self-reported adherence to prescribed medications. However, the long-term effectiveness of the interventions, i.e., sustainability, was not evident; thus, further studies are required.

Pharmacists need to consider a combination of in-person (such as MTM) and electronic technology interventions. Combinations of in-person with automated reminders or triggers have generated excellent outcomes for improving medication adherence and clinical outcomes, the accuracy of the active medication list, patient and caregiver satisfaction with information, and improvements in the person-centeredness of care or patient-provider relationship. Another important point to consider is the capabilities of patients handling these digital solutions. Hence, there are several factors to consider when addressing the suboptimal use of medication.

Table 5.2 describes the advantages and disadvantages in some of the devices and technologies used to improve medication adherence.

TABLE 5.2
Advantages and Disadvantages of Medication Adherence Devices and Technologies

Devices/Technologies	Advantages	Disadvantages
Smart device	Value for money	Sustainability (e.g., battery waste, technical robustness) and system implementation (e.g., privacy regulations, doctor and patient acceptability, and affordability)
Reminder devices like pillboxes, pill bottle strips with toggles, and reminder caps	Low cost; good when nonadherence is unintentional	Do not drive improvements; fail to provide immediate feedback, to alert patients about missed doses, or to track overall adherence
Real-time electronic monitoring with internet-connected devices	Real-time monitoring; alerting patients, healthcare providers, and family members of missed medication events	Need stability of electricity supply and network connectivity
Mobile apps (for Apple and Android)	Cost-effective, scalable solution; medication tracking, financial incentives, gamifying medication taking; targeting behavioral and educational aspects; alerting patients to take medication, tracking medication-taking, reminding to refill, indicating amount left, and storing medication information	Unable to demonstrate clinical outcomes in peer-reviewed journals; unable to address underlying behavioral or environmental issues
Digital health	Real-time insights; enable more proactive care; keep the user at the center	Data validation, sustainability, patient data protection
Smartphone	Daily text messages, reminders, monitors, medication logs, search functionalities, interactive education module, social support networks, constantly accessible, provides a repository for information, low cost, generates reminders with no connectivity, multilingual	Lack of self-management features
Oral medication monitors	Provide a long-term measure of adherence, data in real-time, can record data/time/frequency of container openings, up to 100% specificity between event monitoring and refill data, reveal medication-taking patterns	Number of actual medications ingested is questionable; due to the cost, it is not feasible for routine clinical practice; malfunction and loss of data, poor device durability, not convenient/conducive for traveling
Digital inhaler	Reliable data evident, able to detect medication dumping; creating sense of independence and accountability, increasing motivation	Mechanical failure, difficulty pressing the device, failure to record actual inhalation of medication, cannot download data to a computer program, inability to confirm if the right technique is used, expensive

Sources: (46, Zijp et al., 2019; 62, Xu, 2021; 63, Ingerski et al., 2011)

Note: This list may not be exhaustive; others devices and technologies maybe available.

TABLE 5.3
Medication Adherence Resources

Organization	Link
Agency for Healthcare Research and Quality	https://digital.ahrq.gov/ahrq-funded-projects/emerging-lessons/medication-adherence
Pharmaceutical Research and Manufacturers of America	https://catalyst.phrma.org/ask-about-adherence-new-resources-from-the-medication-adherence-alliance
American Association of Colleges of Pharmacy	www.aacp.org/sites/default/files/aacp_ncpa_medication_adherence_educators_toolkit_0.pdf
Network for Excellence in Health Innovation	www.nehi.net/writable/publication_files/file/medication_adherence_tools.pdf
Centers of Excellence for Relapse Prevention	https://easacommunity.org/files/Medication%20Adherence%20Scale.pdf
Center for Disease Control	www.cdc.gov/hiv/research/interventionresearch/compendium/ma/complete.html
Medication Adherence Alliance	http://managingyourmeds.org/
Royal Pharmaceutical Society of Great Britain	www.rpharms.com/resources/quick-reference-guides/medicines-adherence
College of Psychiatric and Neurologic Pharmacists	https://meridian.allenpress.com/mhc/article/2/8/229/36968/Toolbox-Medication-adherence-resources-for
National Council for Mental Wellbeing	www.thenationalcouncil.org/wp-content/uploads/2020/03/Medication_Adherence_Toolkit_Final.pdf?daf=375ateTbd56
Cochrane UK	www.evidentlycochrane.net/medication-adherence-evidence-review/
European Network to Advance Best Practices & TechnoLogy on Medication AdherencE (ENABLE)	www.cost.eu/actions/CA19132/#tabs|Name:overview
ISPOR—Special Interest Group	www.ispor.org/member-groups/special-interest-groups/
Medical Devices and Diagnostics	medical-devices-and-diagnostics www.ispor.org/member-groups/
Digital Health	special-interest-groups/digital-health

RESOURCES TO SUPPORT HEALTHCARE PROFESSIONALS AND PATIENTS/PUBLIC

Here are a few resources that can provide information and education materials to support individuals to enhance medication adherence (Table 5.3).

LESSONS LEARNED AND CONCLUSIONS

Medication nonadherence is an epidemic. The issue of nonadherence to medications is increasingly recognized as needing shared goal-setting between patients and healthcare professionals like pharmacists who are accessible to the patients. There are many reasons for not taking the medication as ordered, such as being busy and tending to forget, stopping treatment due to feeling fear or discomfort, doubt

about the benefit of the treatment, social stigma with the medicine, etc. Healthcare providers assume patients have knowledge, motivation, skills, and resources to adhere to the prescriptions dispensed. However, this is not always true. The use of technology-based interventions alone or passive delivery without an active, in-person component, are not effective in enhancing adherence rates or patient outcomes. Medication nonadherence is a complex issue. Studies have provided evidence that increasing digital health solutions will complement but not replace the benefits of in-person communication for medication-taking. The devices and technologies discussed in this chapter are expected to close the gaps in medication adherence, applying evidence-based approaches to deliver an integrated experience that drives medication optimization, coordinated care, and cost savings.

However, some of the devices and technologies are still under the clinical trial settings. As part of the review process, FDA and other national regulatory agencies need to consider risk-benefit aspects. Other considerations are insurance, reimbursement, and ethical issues. The key word here is "access." Some of the devices and technologies are costly. Are these covered in the insurance policy? Data and information on medication adherence are recorded in a Web-based portal and can be accessed by healthcare providers. The patient's autonomy, informed consent, decision-making process, privacy, and confidentiality are ethical challenges. Integrating hardware and software solutions into the therapy is for reminding and monitoring purposes and not specifically for therapeutic purposes.

The challenge of medication nonadherence is closely related to the psyche of patients. Thus, scientists and healthcare professionals must understand the science of behavioral health, and proven theories and models on how to enhance adherence. Their behavior is shaped and influenced by information they acquire and process, as well as their experiences. We need to identify patients at risk using technology and to target patients with poor adherence. We need to research and develop more cost-effective technology-enabled user-centric devices.

REFERENCES

1. Ho PM, Bryson CL, Rumsfeld JS. Medication adherence: its importance in cardiovascular outcomes. Circulation. 2009 Jun 16;119(23):3028–35. https://doi.org/10.1161/CIRCULATIONAHA.108.768986. www.ahajournals.org/doi/full/10.1161/circulationaha.108.768986.
2. Brown MT, Bussell JK. Medication adherence: WHO cares? Mayo Clin Proc. 2011;86(4):304–14. https://doi.org/10.4065/mcp.2010.0575.
3. Gast A, Mathes T. Medication adherence influencing factors—an (updated) overview of systematic reviews. Syst Rev. 2019;8:112. https://doi.org/10.1186/s13643-019-1014-8.
4. Jaam M, Ibrahim MIM, Kheir N, et al. Factors associated with medication adherence among patients with diabetes in the Middle East and North Africa region: a systematic mixed studies review. Diabetes Res Clin Pract. 2017 Jul;129:1–15. https://doi.org/10.1016/j.diabres.2017.04.015.

5. Everett Koop C. Drugs don't work in patients who don't take them. (C. Everett Koop, MD, US Surgeon General; 1985).

6. Delamater AM. Improving patient adherence. Clin Diabetes. 2006;24:71–7.

7. Meichenbaum D, Turk DC. Facilitating treatment adherence: a practitioner's guidebook. New York: Plenum Press; 1987.

8. Dobbels F, Van Damme-Lombaert R, Vanhaecke J, et al. Growing pains: non-adherence with the immunosuppressive regimen in adolescent transplant recipients. Pediatr Transplant. 2005;9:381–90.

9. Caetano PA, Lam JM, Morgan SG. Toward a standard definition and measurement of persistence with drug therapy: examples from research on statin and antihypertensive utilization. Clin Ther. 2006;28:1411–24.

10. Cramer JA, Benedict A, Muszbek N, et al. The significance of compliance and persistence in the treatment of diabetes, hypertension and dyslipidaemia: a review. Int J Clin Pract. 2008 Jan;62(1):76–87.

11. Agency for Healthcare Research and Quality. Effective health care program. Available from: www.effectivehealthcare.ahrq.gov/ehc/products/296/1248/EvidenceReport208_CQGMedAdherence_FinalReport_20120905.pdf.

12. Musaus JW and Bahr M. The increasing trend of adherence packaging and the implicaions to manufacturing. Pharm Eng. The Official Magazine of ISPE. 2012;32(5). www.ispe.gr.jp/ISPE/02_katsudou/pdf/201310_en.pdf.

13. Bosworth HB. How can innovative uses of technology be harnessed to improve medication adherence? Medscape; Apr 1, 2012.

14. World Health Organization. Adherence to long-term therapies: evidence for action. Available from: www.who.int/chp/knowledge/publications/adherence_full_report.pdf.

15. Khan R. Socha-Dietrich K. Investing in medication adherence improves health outcomes and health system efficiency: adherence to medicines for diabetes, hypertension, and hyperlipidaemia. In: OECD health working papers. Paris: OECD Publishing; 2018.

16. Omotosho A, Ayegba P. Medication adherence: a review and lessons for developing countries. Int J Online Biomed Eng (iJOE), 2019;15(11). https://online-journals.org/index.php/i-joe/article/view/10647.

17. Reportlinker, 2019. Drug adherence enhancement market: devices and applications, 2018–2030. Available from: www.prnewswire.com/news-releases/drug-adherence-enhancement-market-devices-and-applications-2018-2030-300790788.html.

18. Rubin RR. Adherence to pharmacologic therapy in patients with type 2 diabetes mellitus. Am J Med. 2005;118:27S–34S.

19. Macquart de Terline D, Kane A, Kramoh KE, et al. Factors associated with poor adherence to medication among hypertensive patients in twelve low and middle income Sub-Saharan countries. PLoS ONE. 2019 Jul 10;14(7):e0219266. https://doi.org/10.1371/journal.pone.0219266.

20. CDC. High blood pressure fact sheet. In: DfHDaSP, editor. National Center for Chronic Disease Prevention and Health Promotion. Atlanta, GA: Centers for Disease Control and Prevention; 2015.

21. Burnier M. Managing 'resistance': is adherence a target for treatment? Curr Opin Nephrol Hypertens. 2014 Sep;23(5):439–43.

22. Wofford MR, Minor DS. Hypertension: issues in control and resistance. Curr Hypertens Rep. 2009 Oct;11(5):323–8.

23. Agbor VN, Takah NF, Aminde LN. Prevalence and factors associated with medication adherence among patients with hypertension in sub-Saharan Africa: protocol for a systematic review and meta-analysis. BMJ Open. 2018;8:e020715. https://doi.org/10.1136/bmjopen-2017-020715.

24. De Geest S, Ruppar T, Berben L, et al. Medication non-adherence as a critical factor in the management of presumed resistant hypertension: a narrative review. EuroIntervention. 2014 Jan 22;9(9):1102–9.

25. Jung O, Gechter JL, Wunder C, et al. Resistant hypertension? Assessment of adherence by toxicological urine analysis. J Hypertens. 2013 Apr;31(4):766–74.

26. Kolandaivelu K, Leiden BB, O'Gara PT, et al. Nonadherence to cardiovascular medications. Eur Heart J. 2014 Dec;35(46):3267–76. https://doi.org/10.1093/eurheartj/ehu364.

27. Ho PM, Spertus JA, Masoudi FA, et al. Impact of medication therapy discontinuation on mortality after myocardial infarction. Arch Intern Med. 2006;166:1842–7.

28. Jackevicius CA, Li P, Tu JV. Prevalence, predictors, and outcomes of primary non-adherence after acute myocardial infarction. Circulation. 2008;117:1028–36.

29. Lanouette NM, Folsom DP, Sciolla A, et al. Psychotropic medication nonadherence among United States Latinos: a comprehensive literature review. Psychiatr Serv. 2009;60(2):157–74. https://doi.org/10.1176/appi.ps.60.2.157.

30. Velligan DI, Sajatovic M, Hatch A, et al. Why do psychiatric patients stop antipsychotic medication? A systematic review of reasons for nonadherence to medication in patients with serious mental illness. Patient Prefer Adherence. 2017;11:449–68. https://doi.org/10.2147/PPA.S124658.

31. Lacro JP, Dunn LB, Dolder CR, et al. Prevalence of and risk factors for medication nonadherence in patients with schizophrenia: a comprehensive review of recent literature. J Clin Psychiatry. 2002;63(10):892–909.

32. Sajatovic M, Valenstein M, Blow FC, et al. Treatment adherence with antipsychotic medications in bipolar disorder. Bipolar Disord. 2006;8(3):232–41.

33. Vergouwen ACM, Bakker A, Katon WJ, et al. Improving adherence to antidepressants: a systematic review of interventions. J Clin Psychiatry. 2003;64(12):1415–20.

34. Scott J, Pope M. Nonadherence with mood stabilizers: prevalence and predictors. J Clin Psychiatry. 2002;63(5):384–90.

35. Cochran SD. Preventing medical noncompliance in the outpatient treatment of bipolar affective disorders. J Consult Clin Psychol. 1984;52(5):873–8.

36. Stein MB, Cantrell CR, Sokol MC, et al. Antidepressant adherence and medical resource use among managed care patients with anxiety disorders. Psychiatr Serv. 2006;57(5):673–80.

37. Lanouette NM, Folsom DP, Sciolla A, et al. Psychotropic medication nonadherence among United States Latinos: a comprehensive literature review. Psychiatr Serv. 2009;60(2):157–74. https://doi.org/10.1176/appi.ps.60.2.157.

38. Maher RL, Hanlon J, Hajjar ER. Clinical consequences of polypharmacy in elderly. Expert Opin Drug Saf. 2014;13(1):57–65. https://doi.org/10.1517/14740338.2013.827660.

39. Sabaté E. Adherence to long-term therapies: evidence for action. Geneva: World Health Organization. 2003. Available from: www.who.int/chp/knowledge/publications/adherence_report/en/ (accessed 10 June 2017).

40. DiMatteo MR, Giordani PJ, Lepper HS, et al. Patient adherence and medical treatment outcomes: a meta-analysis. Med Care. 2002;40(9):794–811.

41. Granger BB, Bosworth HB. Medication adherence: emerging use of technology. Curr Opin Cardiol. 2011;26(4):279–87. https://doi.org/10.1097/HCO.0b013e328347c150. www.ncbi.nlm.nih.gov/pmc/articles/PMC3756138/.

42. Anon. Poor medication adherence increases healthcare costs. PharmacoEconomics and Outcomes News. 2005;480:5.

43. International Labour Organization. Economic impact: productivity. Available from: www.social-protection.org/gimi/ShowWiki.action?wiki.wikiId=2523.

44. Osterberg L, Blaschke T. Adherence to medication. N Engl J Med. 2005;353:487–97.

45. Kim J, Combs K, Downs K, et al. Medication adherence: the elephant in the room. US Pharm. 2018;43(1):30–4. www.uspharmacist.com/article/medication-adherence-the-elephant-in-the-room.

46. Zijp TR, Mol PGM, Touw DJ, et al. Smart medication adherence monitoring in clinical drug trials: a prerequisite for personalised medicine? EclinicalMedicine. 2019;15:3–4. https://doi.org/10.1016/j.eclinm.2019.08.013. www.thelancet.com/journals/eclinm/article/PIIS2589-5370(19)30152-X/fulltext.

47. Sinhasane S. Medication adherence panaceas: latest technologies and human intervention. 2019. Available from: https://mobisoftinfotech.com/resources/blog/medication-adherence/.

48. Choudhry NK, Krumme AA, Ercole PM, et al. Effect of reminder devices on medication adherence: the REMIND randomized clinical trial. JAMA Intern Med. 2017 May 1;177(5):624–31. https://doi.org/10.1001/jamainternmed.2016.9627.

49. Bosworth HB, Granger BB, Mendys P, et al. Medication adherence: a call for action. Am Heart J. 2011;162(3):412–24.

50. Cramer JA, Roy A, Burrell A, et al. Medication compliance and persistence: terminology and definitions. Value Health. 2008;11:44–7.

51. McDonough R. MTM: improving positioning and integration. PharmacyToday. 2012;18(2):40. https://doi.org/10.1016/S1042-0991(15)32007-7.

52. Aldeer M, Javanmard M, Martin R. A review of medication adherence monitoring technologies. Appl Syst Innov. 2018;1(2):14. https://doi.org/10.3390/asi1020014.

53. McCormick JB, et al. Medication nonadherence: there's an app for that! Mayo Clin Proc. 2018;93(10):1346–50. https://doi.org/10.1016/j.mayocp.2018.05.029.

54. Arndt RZ. Building trust through technology for medication adherence. 2018. Available from: www.modernhealthcare.com/article/20180526/TRANSFORMATION01/180529960/building-trust-through-technology-for-medication-adherence.

55. Bova CA, Fennie KP, Knafl GJ, et al. Use of electronic monitoring devices to measure antiretroviral adherence: practical considerations. AIDS Behav. 2005;9:103–10.

56. Chaudhry SI, Mattera JA, Curtis JP, et al. Telemonitoring in patients with heart failure. N Engl J Med. 2010;363(24):2301–9.

57. Christensen A, Christrup LL, Fabricius PE, et al. The impact of an electronic monitoring and reminder device on patient compliance with antihypertensive therapy: a randomized controlled trial. J Hypertens. 2010 Jan;28(1):194–200.

58. Gazmararian J, Jacobson KL, Pan Y, et al. Effect of a pharmacy-based health literacy intervention and patient characteristics on medication refill adherence in an urban health system. Ann Pharmacother. 2010 Jan;44(1):80–7.

59. Tamblyn R, Reidel K, Huang A, et al. Increasing the detection and response to adherence problems with cardiovascular medication in primary care through computerized drug management systems: a randomized controlled trial. Med Decis Making. 2010;30(2):176–88.

60. Park JYE, Li J, Howren A, et al. Mobile phone apps targeting medication adherence: quality assessment and content analysis of user reviews. JMIR Mhealth Uhealth. 2019;7(1):e11919. https://doi.org/10.2196/11919.

61. Armitage LC, Kassavou A, Sutton S. Do mobile device apps designed to support medication adherence demonstrate efficacy? A systematic review of randomised controlled trials, with meta-analysis. BMJ Open. 2020;10:e032045. https://doi.org/10.1136/bmjopen-2019-032045.

62. Xu J. Tech-based medication adherence: closing the gaps. Omada. 2021. Available from: www.omadahealth.com/news/tech-based-medication-adherence-solutions-closing-the-gaps.

63. Ingerski LM, Hente EA, Modi AC, et al. Electronic measurement of medication adherence in pediatric chronic illness: a review of measures. J Pediatr. 2011;159(4):528–34. https://doi.org/10.1016/j.jpeds.2011.05.018.

6 Automation in Hospital Settings

Mohammed Alshennawi and Ahmed Al-Jedai

CONTENTS

BACKGROUND

Nowadays, automation and informatics solutions in most medical and nonmedical fields have become a mandatory requirement in many countries throughout the developed and developing world. We need to know that the pharmacy profession is growing rapidly and all available pharmacy automation solutions in the market are getting smarter year after year. As a common target for all of us as pharmacists, administrators, healthcare providers, and patients, we are looking for technology with a mixture of higher quality, cost-effectiveness, and efficiency. Implementing successful pharmaceutical technology in any hospital or organization will bring pharmaceutical care into the next era and will enhance the pharmacist's role in that hospital or organization.

In this chapter, we concentrate on the following points:

1. Providing historical data and examples on implementing some pharmacy technologies
2. Discussing how to evaluate, select, monitor, and build pharmacy automation systems
3. Discussing different pharmacy automation solutions available currently on the market
4. Building a pharmacy automation team of specialists that will ensure efficient utilization of the pharmacy automation solution
5. Building a continuous strategy to ensure having a stable momentum in generating reports and enhancements for any implemented pharmacy automation solution

HISTORICAL BACKGROUND

Since the 1960s, pharmacies have started to implement pharmacy automation equipment/solutions. However, the most extensive and rapid spreading of pharmacy automation solutions started in the late 1980s (like all technological solutions) with simple tablet/capsule counting machines (Figure 6.1).

There is a need for increased pharmaceutical automation, starting with having digital data systems for patients' medications safety. Further, continuous rapid improvement is absolutely necessary to minimize any possible

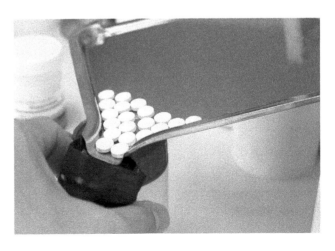

FIGURE 6.1 A pharmacist's pill funnel.

Source: www.shutterstock.com/image-photo/drug-pills-on-counting-tray-pour-1422377612

DOI: 10.1201/9781003002345-7

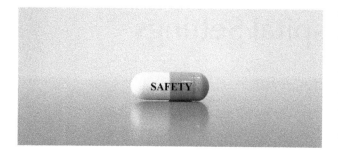

FIGURE 6.2 Medication safety is the pharmacist's top priority.

Source: www.shutterstock.com/image-photo/pharmacovigilance-pv-phv-known-drug-safety-1551448919

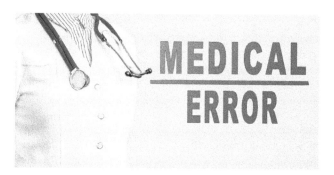

FIGURE 6.3 Continuous improvement of safety protocol is paramount to preventing medical error.

Source: www.shutterstock.com/image-photo/words-medical-error-on-white-background-1873787659

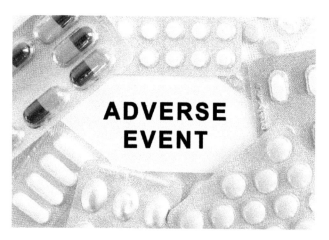

FIGURE 6.4 Adverse medication events must be avoided completely through increased safety protocol.

Source: www.shutterstock.com/image-photo/text-adverse-event-on-white-background-1867148848

human errors and enhance the medication safety, as well as increase the efficacy and speed to prepare correct and proper dispensation of medications to patients (Figures 6.2 & 6.3).

In 1995, JAMA released a statistical study with data for the incidence of adverse drug events (Figure 6.4) and potential adverse drug events (Figure 6.5). Hence, all pharmaceutical automation solutions started to concentrate on these possible medication-dispensing errors and to provide an automated machine to help in minimizing them. The

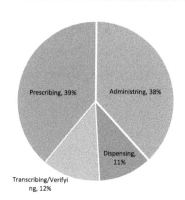

FIGURE 6.5 Incidence of adverse drug events and potential adverse drug events, JAMA 1995.

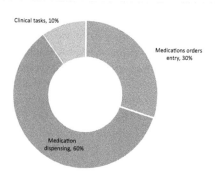

FIGURE 6.6 Pharmacist's daily work distribution.

data for the pharmacist's time also played a significant role in finding solutions that will help pharmacists in playing their original role in providing a medication's clinical information to patients and other healthcare providers instead of having the majority of the pharmacist's time wasted in technical and nonclinical tasks (Figure 6.6).

PHARMACY AUTOMATION BENEFITS

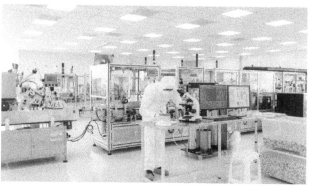

FIGURE 6.7 An example of the sterile environment required for medication formulation.

Source: www.shutterstock.com/image-photo/shot-sterile-pharmaceutical-manufacturing-laboratory-where-1268263639

1. Better security:

   Having medications stored in pharmacy automation solutions provides better medication security and accountability instead of having the medications stored on shelves for the manual dispensing process.

2. Better utilization of medication's shelf life:

   Pharmacy automation solutions provide a better monitoring and stocking process that help pharmacy staff to minimize the possibility of having expired medications on the shelves or dispensing expired medications to patients.

3. Better stock management:

   Planning of the required medications' budget and quantities will be enhanced, and it becomes more accurate by utilizing pharmacy automation solutions integrated directly with the hospital or organization supply chain systems (ERP systems).

4. Greater patient confidentiality:

   Pharmacy automation solutions provide better patient information confidentiality because some patient information may contain sensitive data (e.g., narcotics and other controlled drugs) that necessitates tracking whoever is accessing it.

5. Better accuracy:

   Pharmacy automation solutions provide a better and more accurate medication-dispensing process that tracks the correct and exact quantities leading to enhancing medication safety and minimizing medication errors and adverse drug reactions.

6. Enhancing pharmacists' confidence:

   Pharmacy automation solutions provide pharmacists with all required information, medication history, and supporting clinical decisions; these systems also help pharmacists to become more confident in providing better patient counseling and better drug information.

7. Increasing the speed of the medications-dispensing process:

   Because more demand is now found in the medication-dispensing process, the need to accelerate this process has become a very important task that each hospital and organization should perform accurately.

TYPES OF PHARMACY AUTOMATION

Pharmacy automation solutions have different types. They can be classified in many ways, and classifications can be done based on hospital pharmacy locations (e.g., inpatient, outpatient, sterile preparations). Moreover, they can be classified based on the function that a particular pharmacy automation can perform (e.g., counting, inventory management, clinical supporting systems, secure storage). This chapter covers some of the most famous pharmacy automation types.

AUTOMATED DISPENSING CABINETS (ADCS)

These are the cabinets that are meant to store and dispense the medications to patients on the nursing floors (Figure 6.7.1). They are divided into fully automated cabinets and semi-automated cabinets. The fully automated ones are used to stock almost 80–90% of the nonsterile dosage forms ready to be dispensed directly to patients in nursing units. These cabinets use different storage drawers, and some provide highly secured access to medication (e.g., narcotics and controlled medications). In contrast, the rest can be used to store low-level secure items. These cabinets grant secure access to medications through bio-ID fingerprint access to employees and follow the hospital, organization, and country policies and regulations with medication dispensation (e.g., requirements for witness in any medication process).

Automated dispensing cabinets should be tailored according to the most-used medications in the nursing units (e.g., cardiology, nephrology, neurology, surgery).

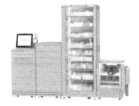
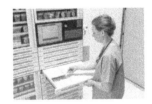
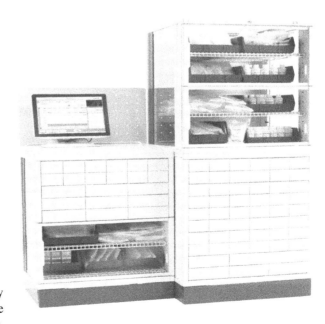

FIGURE 6.7.1 An automated dispensing cabinet.

ANESTHESIA MEDICATION DISPENSING CABINETS (AMDCS)

These are similar to the ADCs; however, they are meant to dispense anesthesia medications to anesthesiologists in operating rooms (Figure 6.7.2). The way of operating these cabinets was designed to provide faster access to medications. One of the differences between ADCs and anesthesia medication dispensing cabinets is that ADCs should perform the medication removal actions electronically before accessing the medication physically, while vice versa in the case of AMDCs.

MEDICATION REPACKING MACHINES

These are the machines that provide packaging for each single medication dosage form (Figure 6.7.3). These machines provide every single dose within a single package with barcode identification for each medication. These machines could be integrated with both ADCs and ERP systems to provide repacking according to the inventory need for each medication.

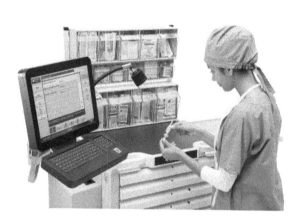
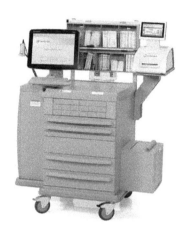

FIGURE 6.7.2   An anesthesia medication dispensing cabinet.

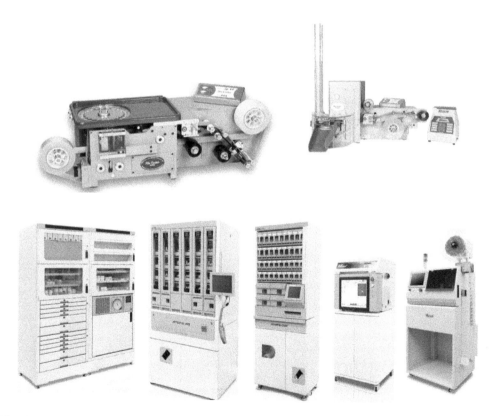

FIGURE 6.7.3   A medication repacking machine.

STERILE PREPARATION MACHINES

These machines are growing nowadays very quickly, and from many providers (Figure 6.7.4). They can be divided into two main types, one for regular sterile products and another for sterile chemotherapy products. The best utilization of such machines can be found for the stock preparations of standardized doses. These machines use either gravimetric or volumetric methods in calculating the amount of the required injected drugs.

PARENTERAL NUTRITION (PN) PREPARATION MACHINES

These machines perform the compounding of macro and micronutrients of parenteral nutrition in bags to be delivered to patients in hospitals or to home patients that require these preparations (Figure 6.7.5). These machines are usually accompanied by operating systems that provide better calculations of the medications and salts added to each bag.

PHARMACY AUTOMATED CAROUSELS

These are the automated pharmacy solutions meant to dispense medications from inpatient pharmacies to patients and ADCs within hospitals and organizations (Figure 6.7.6). These machines are integrated with the hospital's health information systems, ADCs systems, and ERP systems.

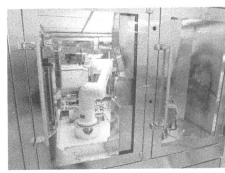
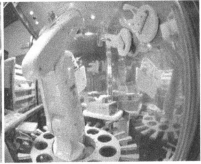

FIGURE 6.7.4   A sterile preparation machine.

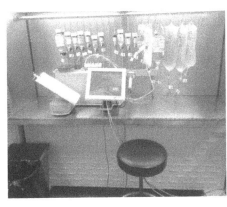
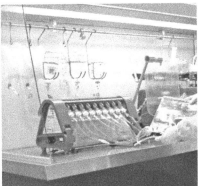

FIGURE 6.7.5   A parenteral nutrition preparation machine.

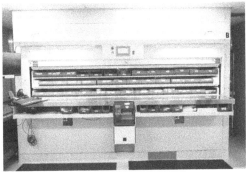
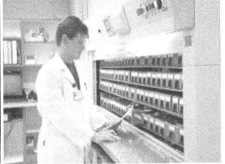

FIGURE 6.7.6   A pharmacy automated carousel.

OUTPATIENT AUTOMATED PHARMACY MACHINES

These can be mainly divided into two types: loose tablet dispensers and medication box dispensers. These machines use the barcode technology to identify the medications, stock them in specific compartments inside the robots, and dispense them according to the need of each patient. The medication is either retrieved by a robotic arm or pushed off the shelf to fall to the dispensary window by gravity (Figure 6.8.1 & Figure 6.8.2).

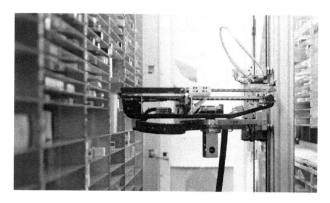

FIGURE 6.8.1   An outpatient pharmacy machine with a robotic arm.

Source: www.shutterstock.com/image-photo/modern-pharmacy-storage-room-two-robot-1568576131

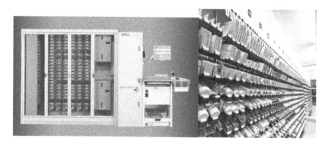

FIGURE 6.8.2

BARCODE MEDICATION ADMINISTRATION MACHINES

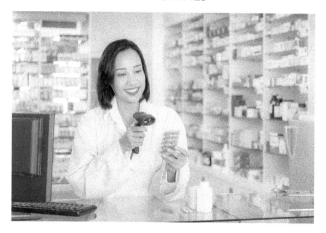

FIGURE 6.9   Pharmacy or other medical staff scan the barcode on medications to verify correct administration.

Source: www.shutterstock.com/image-photo/pharmacist-scanning-barcode-medicine-drug-pharmacy-1900414099

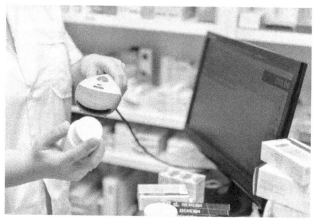

FIGURE 6.10   Barcode administration is an easy way to verify correct medication administration.

Source: www.shutterstock.com/image-photo/pharmacist-scanning-barcode-medicine-drug-pharmacy-1323681521

This technology provides a medication-verification process at the bedside to ensure that the right medication is administered to the right patient through the right route of administration at the correct time (Figure 6.9, 6.10).

PHARMACY AUTOMATION AND ITS IMPACT ON THE PHARMACEUTICAL WORKFORCE

One of the biggest challenges in pharmacy automation is its impact on the pharmaceutical workforce. This challenge increases the resistance from pharmacy staff to work with any automated solution because they feel it is threatening their persistence in work. This challenge was studied extensively by many researchers. They concluded that there is no relationship between implementing any automated pharmacy solution or machine and pharmaceutical manpower. All studies proved that pharmacy automated solutions and machines are meant to improve the pharmaceutical care

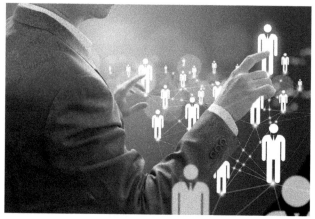

FIGURE 6.11   Pharmacy automation strengthens the links between patients and healthcare providers, including pharmacists.

Source: www.shutterstock.com/image-photo/business-administrator-action-manpower-human-resource-1336612235

manpower clinical abilities and free pharmacists to spend more time with patients and other healthcare members.

WHAT IS NEEDED TO START OR TO IMPLEMENT A PHARMACY AUTOMATION SOLUTION IN YOUR FACILITY?

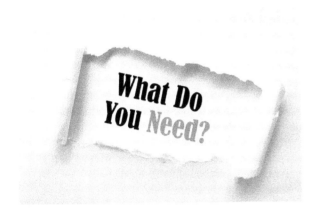

FIGURE 6.12   What do you need?

Source: www.shutterstock.com/image-photo/text-sign-showing-what-do-you-1951901905

1. Study your issues and problems carefully.
2. Make a strategic plan for your pharmacy for the next 5 or 10 years.
3. Identify the weaknesses.
4. Gather and choose the best option (relatively).
5. Implement the best options.
6. Monitor and interfere with problems accordingly.

Keep in mind a very important thing: there is no such best pharmacy automation solution for everyone; the best solution is simply what fulfils your needs and resolves your problems and issues.

TIPS TO MAKE THE PHARMACY AUTOMATION SOLUTION A SUCCESSFUL STORY

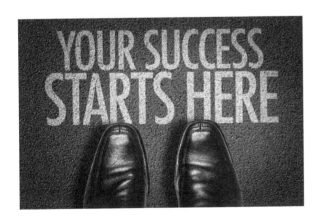

FIGURE 6.13   Success begins with the first step.

Source: www.shutterstock.com/image-photo/top-view-business-shoes-on-floor-347458070

1. Build your implementing team (believers): this is the main cornerstone and the most important step in the transformational journey toward any pharmacy automation solution. The team members' selection should be done very carefully for members who believe in automation in general and the specific solution that they are going to implement. It is very important to choose and select members who have an excellent background and experience in the workflow and process in the pharmacy area in which you will implement the automation solution.
2. Train your team very well: after selecting your team members, you need to invest in them by giving them all the tools to train them adequately, keeping in mind that whatever you will invest in them will be paid back to you during and after the implementation with a smooth and successful launch.
3. Prepare your infrastructure: any required infrastructure like electricity, network, physical space, interface with other systems, etc. must be secured during this phase with cooperation with all pharmacy staff, the solution vendor, hospital information technology, and others.
4. Prepare your users: your end-users should be oriented to the new solution. For example, if the pharmacy automation solution involves inpatient nursing floors (ADCs), all nursing staff should be involved and trained well in how to use the system. Furthermore, if the pharmacy automation solution is outpatient-based, all of your outpatient pharmacists should be aware of and oriented to the solution and its advantages.
5. Test and test and test: create all possible scenarios and do extensive testing on the system in the presence of experts from your pharmacy area of implementation, mark all comments, and try to find solutions for anything unexpected.
6. Prepare a draft of downtime policy and procedure: this is one of the most critical steps because it will guide all users on what to do in case of scheduled or unscheduled downtime with all of its scenarios.
7. Monitor closely: especially after the launching of the pharmacy automation solution (the "go-live" date), this is the period in which the maximum support, follow-ups, and changes must take place.
8. Improve the performance and solve any problems: after launching, and continuously afterward, make sure to create both operational and quality key performance indicators (KPIs) for your pharmacy automation solution, monitor them periodically, and make any necessary changes or interactions as needed.

DURING THE GO-LIVE OR LAUNCHING OF ANY PHARMACY AUTOMATION SOLUTION, YOU MUST ENSURE THE FOLLOWING

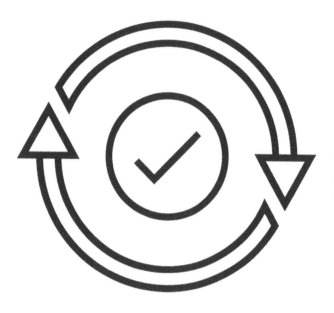

Ensure

FIGURE 6.14   Ensure by reinforcement.

Source: www.shutterstock.com/image-vector/ensure-vector-line-icon-597264665

1. Pharmacy administration must always be on site to give support psychologically and administratively to all end-users and to assure them that all their issues are taken into consideration.
2. Write down all issues and work on resolutions through systematic problem-solving techniques or models, knowing the importance of providing feedback on each issue.
3. Share the knowledge and experience between all end-users about any possible solution(s) using various communication tools (e.g., newsletters, videos, emails, etc.)
4. Confront the resistance. As expected, resistance is one of the most complex problems that you may face in any change, especially when it involves regular daily work.
5. Share the advantages. Always concentrate on the pharmacy automation solution's advantages and the way it will help improve the services and problems that were previously identified. Keep in mind that all pharmacy automation solutions require updates and modifications (similar to any

information technology solutions); these updates and modifications will depend on the feedback from end-users.
6. Improve performance by working collaboratively with all stakeholders to facilitate any issues and resolve all problems.
7. Calculate the ROI. Create a way to calculate the financial return on investment (ROI) and publish it so others can benefit from this data.

POINTS TO REMEMBER

We have to keep in our minds some general concepts that are essential across all pharmacy automation solutions in any hospital or organization.

1. No solution is the best solution for all (Figure 6.15). Available solutions in the market vary in many aspects, specifications, outcomes, and processes. Selecting any pharmacy automation solution should go through extensive evaluation based on each hospital's and organization's needs and requirements. Each hospital and organization should find the best-tailored solution based on good problem-solving and decision-making techniques.
2. The relationship between the hospital or the organization and the selling company should be built on mutual benefits and win-win concepts (Figure 6.16). The hospital or organization will win their needs in providing better pharmaceutical care, minimizing the possibility of medication errors and adverse drug reactions, and enhancing the patients' safety. The selling company should win reputation in the market and cover its expenses for the technology. In the end, the biggest winner for this relationship will be patients who will win safety and pharmaceutical care in an efficient and timely manner.
3. Building a confident and believing pharmacy automation team is the most challenging and successful step in all pharmacy automation solution implementation process (Figure 6.17).
4. The endorsement and support from higher administration of the hospital or health system regarding pharmacy automation solution is an essential step that must be considered.
5. The creation of rules and tasks governing pharmacy automation solutions is mandatory for continuous improvements and enhancements of this technology.
6. Standardizing regular key performance and quality indicators for each pharmacy automation solutions will ensure better monitoring and enhancements of each solution.

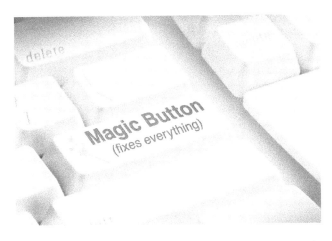

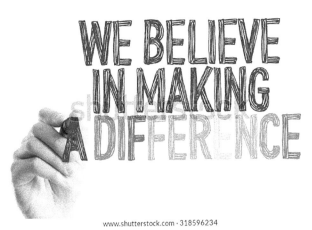

FIGURE 6.15 Pharmacy automation solutions are the magic button that fixes (almost) everything.

Source: www.shutterstock.com/image-photo/closeup-magic-button-on-computer-keyboard-264062756

FIGURE 6.17 Believing in making a difference is the core of problem-solving.

Source: www.shutterstock.com/image-photo/hand-marker-writing-we-believe-making-699167446

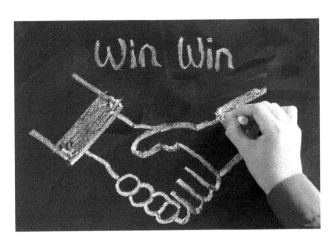

FIGURE 6.16 Pharmacy automation sets up a win-win scenario for all involved.

Source: www.shutterstock.com/image-photo/businessman-draw-handshake-on-chalkboard-win-699167446

Section II

Medical Devices for Clinical Specialties

Monica Zolezzi

CONTENTS

DOI: 10.1201/9781003002345-9

INTRODUCTION

This chapter focuses on the most common medical devices that are used in mental health practice. The chapter is divided into two sections, the first describing devices that are available mostly for inpatient use such as electroconvulsive therapy and point-of-care devices used for monitoring certain psychotropic medications that are mostly accessible at inpatient or outpatient tertiary care settings; and the second for devices that are available for purchase at retail settings accessible to the community in general.

SECTION 1: DEVICES AVAILABLE AT INPATIENT OR OUTPATIENT TERTIARY CARE SETTINGS

1. ELECTROCONVULSIVE THERAPY

a. Background

Electroconvulsive therapy (ECT) is a type of neuromodulation therapy, which is used to treat various serious mental disorders. Neuromodulatory therapies involve stimulating the brain with electricity, magnetic fields, or other forms of energy.[1] In the case of ECT, electricity is applied to the scalp to induce a therapeutic seizure in a patient who is under anesthesia. The person remains under constant medical monitoring by an anesthesiologist and a psychiatrist, as well as nursing staff, throughout the procedure. The decision to use ECT depends on several factors, including the severity and duration of the patient's illness, the likelihood that alternative treatments

would be effective, the side effects of alternative treatments, the patient's preference, and a weighing of the risks and benefits.[2–4] Guidelines stipulate that ECT is typically reserved for use after medications have been tried and were found to be unsuccessful, but it can also be used earlier in the course of illness in severe life-threatening situations such as suicidal ideation, catatonia, and psychotic depression. It works more quickly than medication. ECT has also been used in treatment-resistant schizophrenia, bipolar disorder, and schizoaffective disorder. There is also potential application of ECT in the treatment of severe parkinsonism not responsive to medication

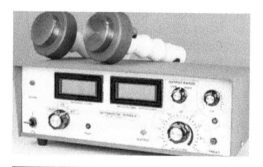

Legend: Image depicts the Ectonustim Series 6+ ECT device. Manufacturer: Ectron, UK

Reference: [Internet]. 2020. [cited 15 March 2020]. Available from: https://www.ectron.co.uk/

FIGURE 7.1 Electroconvulsive therapy machine.

with the on/off phenomenon, and the occasional use of ECT for intractable temporal lobe epilepsy.

b. Device Description

ECT devices were originally placed in the Class III (higher risk) category by the United States Food and Drug Administration (FDA) since 1976. They were reclassified as Class II (moderate risk) devices in 2018. The reclassified uses for ECT devices into Class II are limited to the treatment of catatonia or a severe major depressive episode associated with major depressive disorder or bipolar disorder in patients age 13 years and older who are treatment-resistant or who require a rapid-response treatment due to the severity of their psychiatric or medical condition.

ECT devices machine consists of a brief-pulse, constant-current ECT machine with a wide output range.[5]

Most modern ECT machines transmit electric currents to the brain in brief-timed pulses, which is believed to cause less cognitive impairment than the sine-wave current originally used in ECT. Several modern machines are available from reputable manufacturers, which are usually supplied with electrodes, an electroencephalogram (EEG) monitor, and conducting gel or solution. Examples of ECT machines available include the Thymatron System IV (Somatics, LLC, Lake Bluff, IL, USA), MECTA Spectrum 5000Q (MECTA Corporation, Lake Oswego, OR, USA), and the Ectonustim Series 6 + ECT Apparatus (Ectron Ltd, Bristol, UK). Additional equipment necessary for the administration of ECT includes the following:

- Electrocardiographic monitor with electrodes
- Pulse oximeter to determine oxygen saturation
- Capnograph to measure end-tidal carbon dioxide levels in an intubated patient
- Mouth gag to prevent the patient from accidentally biting his or her tongue

The following should be available in the treatment room and easily accessible to all other ECT areas during treatment sessions:

- A cardiac defibrillator
- A laryngoscope, laryngeal masks, endotracheal tubes, and associated connectors
- Intravenous infusion sets, fluids, stand, and associated sundries
- A stethoscope
- A thermometer
- Ice packs
- An emergency drug box, the contents of which will have been agreed upon by local protocol

c. The ECT Procedure

Informed consent in the part of the patient is usually followed by a pretreatment medical evaluation, as well as a medication review, including an assessment of fitness for general anesthesia, since different classes of medications can influence ECT outcomes. Figure 7.2 provides a summary of medications used during an ECT procedure and the rationale for its use.[6]

In the ECT suite, the patient is given a short-acting anesthetic and a muscle relaxant. The anesthetist will connect monitoring equipment to check the patient's heart rate, blood pressure, oxygen levels, etc. There are two different ways of placing the electrodes, which are illustrated in Figure 7.3 and described here:

- Bilateral ECT: The center of the electrode should be 4 cm above, and perpendicular to, the midpoint of a line between the lateral angle of the eye and the external auditory meatus. Therefore, one electrode is applied to each side of the head. This positioning is referred to as bi-temporal.

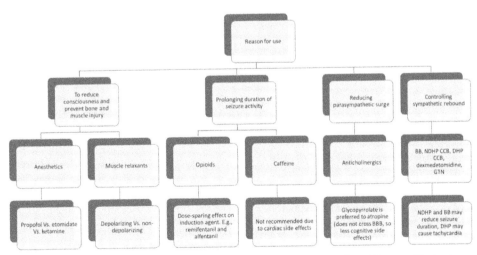

Reference: Zolezzi M. Medication management during electroconvulsant therapy. *Neuropsychiatric Disease and Treatment,* 2016; 12:931–939).

FIGURE 7.2 Medications during ECT procedure.

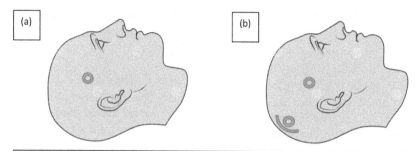

Legend: (a) Bilateral ECT. The electrodes are in each hemisphere (bi-temporally), approximately 4 cm above midpoint the distance between the lateral angle of the eye and the external auditory meatus. (b) Unilateral ECT. The two electrodes are placed in a temporo-parietal positioning, on the head arch, approximately 18 cm from the first electrode position.
Reference: Vishal Uppal, MBBS DA FRCA, Jonathan Dourish, MB ChB MRCPsych, Alan Macfarlane, BSc MBChB MRCP FRCA, Anaesthesia for electroconvulsive therapy, Continuing Education in Anaesthesia Critical Care & Pain, Volume 10, Issue 6, December 2010, Pages 192–196, https://doi.org/10.1093/bjaceaccp/mkq039

FIGURE 7.3   Electrode placement for ECT.

TABLE 7.1

Differences between Bilateral versus Unilateral ECT.

Item	Unilateral ECT	Bilateral ECT
Usage	Less common	More common
Position of electrodes	One on right temporal, one on vertex	Bitemporal or bifrontal
Pulse width and threshold	1.0 ms pulse width at 5–6 x threshold	1.0 ms pulse width at 1.5 x threshold or 0.5 ms pulse width at 1.5–2.5 x threshold
Adverse effect	Less common	More common
Cognitive impairments	Less common (40%)	More common (80%)
Increased seizure threshold		
Efficacy	Less effective than bilateral	More effective than unilateral
	Three times per week is more effective than twice per week	No difference between twice and three times per week admission on efficacy
Speed of response	Six sessions needed to show response	One session needed to show response

- Unilateral ECT: This positioning is usually referred to as the temporoparietal or d'Elia position, in which one electrode is in the same position as in traditional bilateral ECT and the other applied over the parietal surface of the scalp. The exact position on the parietal arc is not crucial. Unilateral ECT is usually applied over the non-dominant hemisphere, which is the right side of the head in most people.

On a worldwide scale, bilateral electrode placement appears to be preferred.[7] Table 7.1 provides a summary on the differences in usage, adverse effects, and efficacy based on electrode placement.

d. Interpretation of Readings

The electrodes deliver an electrical stimulus in excess of an individual's seizure threshold. Selection of the electrical dose (referred to as stimulus dosing) for the individual patient is an important decision at the time of administering ECT. The relative efficacy of each is dependent on the dose relative to the individual's seizure threshold.

- Seizure threshold: This refers to the minimum electrical dose to induce the necessary generalized cerebral seizure activity. The vast majority of patients will have an initial seizure threshold of less than 200 mC, with either electrode placement. It should be noted that the ECT practitioner will occasionally encounter patients with unusually high initial seizure thresholds, for example a bald, dehydrated, elderly man who is prescribed an anti-epileptic drug for mood stabilization and who requires a larger – than-usual dose of induction agent because of severe agitation. The only reliable way to identify patients with a low seizure threshold is to give a low electrical dose initially at the first treatment, to establish whether or not it is sufficient to induce the necessary seizure activity. In the general case, it may be reasonable to start at 50 mC. The exception may be in the management of life-threatening illness.
- Dosing: It is reasonable to start the course with a treatment dose 50% above (i.e., one-and-a-half times) the initial seizure threshold. The exception may be in the emergency treatment of life-threatening illness, when an initial dose 50–100% above the initial seizure threshold would be better. The majority of patients will recover with treatment given at a dose six times the seizure threshold, but at the cost of more pronounced adverse cognitive effects.
- Dose adjustments during the course of treatment: The seizure threshold may, but not inevitably, rise over the course of treatment. Clinical monitoring is the best guide to what, if any, adjustment to the electrical dose is required over a course of treatment;

absent or inadequate clinical improvement indicates a need for a higher electrical dose, while the emergence of significant cognitive adverse effects indicates that a lower electrical dose should be used.

- Missed seizures: In case the electrical stimulus does not generate a seizure, re-stimulation may be necessary while the patient is still unconscious, otherwise the treatment session will have no therapeutic benefit. It is advisable to wait 20 seconds before re-stimulation to miss the latent period. A new seizure threshold may need to be established, in which case stimulation with a dose only slightly higher is indicated (i.e., 25–50 mC). The occurrence of a missed seizure should prompt a review of the anesthetic technique as well as concomitant psychotropic drug treatment, to identify any factors that may be modified to ease the induction of cerebral seizure activity at the next treatment session. Figure 7.4 shows common medications that have been shown to interfere with the ECT seizure response.[6]
- Monitoring seizure activity: The typical seizure is characterized on the EEG by widespread high-frequency spike waves ("polyspike activity") followed by slower spike and wave complexes, typically around 3 cycles per second, or Hertz (Hz). The hallmark of generalized cerebral seizure activity is the tonic-clonic (or grand mal) convulsion. After an initial tonic contraction of the muscles, there is a longer, clonic phase of rhythmic alternating contraction and relaxation of the muscles of the limbs on both sides of the body.
- Seizure duration: If at the first treatment the convulsion lasted less than 15 seconds or the EEG recording showed seizure activity lasting less than

25 seconds, the efficacy of the treatment should be questioned, because it is possible that a generalized cerebral seizure activity did not occur.

The patient should be assessed after each treatment to see if further treatments are necessary because some patients respond dramatically to only few treatments. Some patients may require 12 or more treatments. It is recommended that a set number of treatments should not be prescribed at the start of a course of ECT. If no clinical improvement is seen after 6 properly given bilateral treatments, then the course should be abandoned. There are some patients with depression who do not respond to high-dose right unilateral ECT, but who subsequently respond to bilateral ECT. The ineffective unilateral treatments should be disregarded in the assessment of the need for further bilateral treatments.

Additional methods of monitoring for efficacy and safety include the following:

- The cuff technique: This is a simple technique that minimizes the influence of a muscle relaxant on the assessment of convulsive activity. It involves isolating one forearm or leg by inflating a blood pressure cuff to above systolic pressure as the patient is drifting off to sleep, but before the muscle relaxant is administered. It is recommended when only brief convulsive activity has been seen at the outset of the course of treatment, and where EEG monitoring is not available.
- EEG monitoring: The Special Committee on ECT has decided to recommend that EEG monitoring must be available in all ECT clinics from 1 January 2006. This is useful in two scenarios: to paralyze

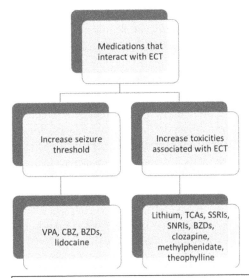

Legend: VPA=Valproic acid; CBZ=Carbamazepine; BZDs=Benzodiazepines; TCAs=Tricyclic antidepressants, SSRIs=Selective serotonin reuptake inhibitors
Reference: Zolezzi M. Medication management during electroconvulsant therapy. Neuropsychiatric Disease and Treatment, 2016:12

FIGURE 7.4 Medications known to interfere with ECT.

the patient completely, and for the detection of prolonged seizures, which might lead to markedly increased cognitive adverse effects without any commensurate therapeutic benefit.

e. Important Safety Issues

ECT is a low-risk procedure with a mortality rate similar to that of anesthesia for minor surgical procedures, estimated to be 1 per 10,000 to 1 per 80,000 treatments.[2,8] The mortality rate may be higher in patients with severe medical disorders. The most commonly reported complications related to ECT include cognitive adverse effects, headaches, muscular aches, drowsiness, weakness, nausea, and anorexia. Headaches after ECT appear to be more common than myalgia, and it usually is mild and tolerable, and subsides within 6 hours. No predictors for post-ECT headache and myalgia have been identified.[9]

The most marked cognitive adverse effects occur immediately postictally, when patients may experience a variable period of disorientation associated with impaired attention, memory, and praxis. These effects resolve over time and are generally short-lived. This form of delirium may be related in part to the ECT procedure or may be secondary to repeated episodes of general anesthesia. ECT can also cause changes in both anterograde and retrograde memory. After ECT, anterograde amnesia resolves rapidly. With retrograde amnesia, deficits are greatest for events closest to the time of treatment and appears to be greater for impersonal than for personal memory. However, it remains unclear how long this may persist. A small proportion of people complain of persisting memory difficulty after treatment and may have persisting loss of memory for events during a period before, during, and after ECT. The ability to learn new information and non-memory cognitive functions (intelligence, judgment, abstraction, etc.) are not affected.[10]

f. Important Features and Special Advantages

One of the most important advantages of ECT is its short onset of action and its effectiveness in the management of more severe forms of major depressive disorder (MDD). Research has shown that 64% to 87% of patients with severe MDD respond to ECT, with response rates as high as 95% for patients with MDD with psychotic features.[11]

Although patients may respond more quickly than with pharmacological treatment, 6 to 12 sessions are typically required to resolve a severe depressive episode.

Studies have also shown that ECT is an effective therapeutic intervention in elderly patients with MDD, especially those with psychosis, suicidality, catatonia, nutritional compromise, and resistance to medications. Response rates have been reported to be as high as 80%. Studies have also shown that compared to the younger adult population, the elderly appear to respond better to ECT as indicated by a relatively lower rate of rehospitalization in geriatric patients treated with ECT with respect to the nongeriatric population. However, the existence of comorbidities and a higher risk for cognitive side effects may be of greater concern in this population.[12]

TABLE 7.2

Information that Should Be Included in a Patient Leaflet about ECT

What is ECT?
When is ECT given?
What happens during ECT treatment?
How do I prepare for ECT?
Will ECT help me?
Is ECT safe?
How often is ECT given?
How many treatments will I need?
Are there any side effects?
What may happen if ECT is not given?
What are the alternatives to ECT?

---

g. Special Tips for Patient Counseling

Despite the substantial evidence behind its efficacy, ECT continues to be one of the most controversial and misunderstood treatments in medicine. Considerable stigma surrounds its use, which undermines public acceptance. Guidelines on the use of ECT vary, but most commonly highlight the need for patient consent that includes full explanation, in a form absent of coercion, and in a suitable language that the patient can understand

- the purpose, method, likely duration, and expected benefit;
- possible pain, discomfort, risks, and associated side effects;
- alternative treatment options; and
- the implications of not having the treatment.[4]

The consent process should conform to all local laws and hospital policies. Several examples of what should be included in a patient information leaflet about ECT are available. Table 7.2 provides an outline of the information that should be included in a patient information leaflet about ECT.

h. Available Evidence on Effectiveness and Safety

Overall, ECT is an effective treatment with a strong evidence base, particularly for the treatment of severe depressive disorders. There are several systematic reviews and some randomized controlled trials that compare the effectiveness and safety of ECT therapy with pharmacological therapy. Several practice guidelines provide the following recommendations based on the evidence resulting from these studies:[2–4,13]

- ECT can be used in MDD that is not responding to medication or psychotherapy.
- Combination of pharmacological treatment with ECT therapy is more effective than the use of some pharmacological agents alone, and it is not inferior to ECT alone.
- Individuals who respond to ECT benefit from continuing of pharmacotherapy.

- ECT is particularly useful in life-threatening conditions (suicidal patients), when rapid response is needed, or when there is resistance to multiple pharmacological agents.
- Cognitive impairment may occur immediately after the ECT session or during the course of treatment. The incidence of this side effect appears to be dose-dependent.
- The cause of harm does not depend on age, but individuals with comorbidities are at higher risk.
- ECT can cause complications during pregnancy but it is preferable to pharmacological therapy due to higher risk of teratogenicity with the use of medications.

i. Economic Evaluation

There is no published evidence regarding the cost-effectiveness of ECT. Several modeling exercises have been used to evaluate the economic implications of ECT compared to other treatments, mostly in MDD and schizophrenia. The modeling exercises undertaken are based on a number of uncertain assumptions, and suggest that—for those with severe depressive illness and treatment-resistant schizophrenia—ECT and pharmacological treatment may be equally cost-effective, with no consistent differences in costs or outcomes.[3,14–18]

j. Implication to the Pharmacy Profession and Pharmacy Practice

Prior to the decision to administer ECT, mental health pharmacists have most likely participated in assessing the patient's medication history at the time of admission and response to treatment throughout the course of hospitalization. The results of this ongoing medication assessment are considered by the treatment team when deciding the need for ECT. Patients who will undergo ECT have similar pharmaceutical care needs as those undergoing any procedure that requires general anesthesia. As a consequence, an important role for the pharmacist is to undertake a thorough pre-ECT medication assessment to identify medication-related issues that may affect the safety and efficacy of ECT. At this time, factors that may place patients at risk are assessed and strategies to reduce this risk are proposed. Recommendations for treating medication-related complications before, during, and after the ECT procedure are provided. Table 7.3 summarizes the management strategies in which pharmacists may be able to participate for pre-existing medical conditions in patients who will undergo ECT.[19]

In addition, pharmacists should be knowledgeable of 1) medications that are used during the ECT procedure and 2) interactions between regularly prescribed medications and medications used during the ECT procedure itself. Figure 7.2 illustrates the medications used during an ECT procedure and the rationale for the use of each, and Figure 7.4 illustrates common medications that have been shown to interfere with the ECT seizure response.[6]

TABLE 7.3

Management Strategies for Pre-Existing Medical Conditions in Patients Undergoing ECT

Condition	Management	Comments
Aortic stenosis	For severity of stenosis, echocardiography should be done before ECT.	Limited data suggest using IV beta blocker to reduce hypertension and tachycardia during ECT. In general, it is safe to use ECT in patient with cardiac issues.
Respiratory disorders	Discontinue theophylline if it's possible. Continue standard treatment.	Theophylline will increase the incidence of status epilepticus after ECT.
Diabetes	Check blood glucose before and after ECT. Withhold oral agents and short-acting insulin until patient can eat. ECT in early morning is preferable.	The effect of ECT on blood glucose is unpredictable.
Hypertension	ECT is applicable if hypertension is well controlled (< 140/90 mmHg). Avoid beta blockers.	Blood pressure will increase during ECT. Beta blockers will increase seizure threshold and reduce efficacy of ECT.
Implantable cardioverter defibrillator (ICD)	Turn off detection mode of ICD during ECT. Perform ECG monitoring during ECT therapy.	In general, it is safe to use ECT in ICD patients.
Long-term warfarin	It is safe to use an anticoagulation agent with INR up to 3.5. It is better to hold ECT in case of high risk of intracranial hemorrhage.	In general, it is safe to use ECT with anticoagulation medications.
Pregnancy	Noninvasive fetal monitoring should be used for pregnant women in second and third trimesters. After 24 weeks, non-stress test should be performed before and after treatment.	In general, it is safe to use ECT during pregnancy. Anesthetic technique modification is needed.

Educating patients and families on ECT and any medication-related issues is also an important role for psychiatric pharmacists. Misconceptions about ECT and the role of medications pre and post procedure should be addressed by pharmacists at this time. Studies have shown that although the majority of patients reported receiving general information about ECT, information about alternative treatments, possible outcomes of ECT, and side effects were not always provided. The importance of detailed discussions with patients and their families, supported by written information in a patient-appropriate form, should be emphasized. Most hospitals have their own educational material about the ECT procedure which can be used by all members of the multidisciplinary team, including pharmacists, as a standardized way to educate patients and families. Table 7.2 provides an outline of the information that should be included when educating patients and families about ECT.[20]

k. Challenges to the Pharmacists and Users

Despite the availability of guidelines, large variations between countries and regions in ECT utilization, rates, and clinical practice are displayed, possibly due to lack of universal consensus about its indications, duration, and frequency of administration.[7] Cognitive side effects of ECT are sometimes underestimated and may last much longer after completed treatment than is usually expected. Cognitive assessment during ECT treatment is usually not comprehensive enough and is limited to bedside assessment. A more proactive approach to careful neuropsychological assessment and consideration of combined maintenance medication treatment after ECT is essential.[21]

l. Recommendations: The Way Forward

Worldwide improvement of ECT utilization and practice is needed, alongside development of an international minimal dataset standard applied in all countries. Continuous and mandatory monitoring and use of ECT health registrar reporting systems would also ultimately reduce knowledge gaps and contribute to more uniform worldwide ECT practice.

ECT research will continue to focus on refining aspects of technique and personalizing ECT type and schedule, as well as further elucidating its mechanisms of action. Technical refinements are aimed at preserving antidepressant efficacy while increasing cognitive tolerability. Techniques to more precisely target particular brain structures or areas for seizure initiation and/or to limit the spread of the seizure are under development.

Further research, including biomarker discovery for response/relapse prediction, should help inform practitioners about how to determine the optimal type and number of acute treatments for a given patient and how to individualize continuation/maintenance ECT schedules.

Stigma remains the biggest impediment to the appropriate use of ECT. The level of knowledge about modern ECT among patients and medical practitioners is low. The portrayal of ECT in the media as a crude and coercive treatment remains problematic, frightening off patients who might benefit from it. Improved education about ECT among healthcare professionals will lead to more favorable perceptions about its use.[7,19,21]

m. Conclusions

ECT has demonstrated to be highly effective and safe in many psychiatric disorders, particularly for patients with life-threatening MDD. The procedure involves application of small electrical currents through the scalp to induce therapeutic seizures, lasting 30 to 90 seconds in duration.

Modern ECT devices deliver continuous currents and are often featured with an EEG for monitoring seizure adequacy. Brief (0.5–2 ms)/ultra-brief (0.2–0.5 ms) pulse widths are the ideal waveforms which are associated with fewer cognitive side effects. To administer ECT, a multidisciplinary team of experts who have knowledge and skills on ECT is needed. Because most patients who require ECT are also on concurrent pharmacotherapy, pharmacists must be knowledgeable on the medications used during an ECT procedure and on the effects of concurrent psychiatric and non-psychiatric medications on the effectiveness and safety of ECT.

n. Lessons Learned

- ECT is a safe and effective treatment for adults and adolescents with certain psychiatric disorders.
- The primary indication for ECT is for the treatment of major depression that is refractory to antidepressant medications, psychotic depression, catatonia, severe suicidality, and other situations in which a rapid antidepressant response is required.
- Adverse cognitive effects associated with ECT include confusion and amnesia. However, objective tests indicate that neuropsychological impairment caused by ECT is generally short lived.
- Pharmacists have an important role addressing medication-related issues in the preparation, administration, and recovery stages of ECT.

REFERENCES

Section 1: Electroconvulsive Therapy

1. Trapp NT, Xiong W, Conway CR. Neurostimulation therapies. Handb Exp Pharmacol. 2019;250:181–224.
2. Rasmussen KG. Principles and practice of electroconvulsive therapy, 1st edn. Washington, DC: American Psychiatric Association Publishing; American Psychiatric Association; 2019.
3. Procopio M. NICE guidelines and maintenance ECT. Br J Psychiatry. 2003;183:263.
4. Weiss A, Hussain S, Ng B, et al. Royal Australian and New Zealand College of Psychiatrists professional practice guidelines for the administration of electroconvulsive therapy. Aust N Z J Psychiatry. 2019;53(7):609–23.
5. United States Food and Drug Administration (FDA). [Internet]. FDA in brief: FDA takes action to ensure regulation of electroconvulsive therapy devices better protects patients, reflects current understanding of safety and effectiveness. FDA, Dec 21, 2018. Available from: www.fda.gov/news-events/fda-brief/fda-brief-fda-takes-action-ensure-regulation-electroconvulsive-therapy-devices-better-protects (accessed 28 Apr 2020).
6. Zolezzi M. Medication management during electroconvulsant therapy. Neuropsychiatr Dis Treat. 2016;12:931–9.
7. Leiknes K, Schweder L, Høie B. Contemporary use and practice of electroconvulsive therapy worldwide. Brain Behav. 2012;2(3):283–344.
8. Benbow SM. The practice of electroconvulsive therapy recommendations for treatment, training and privileging. A Task

Force Report of the American Psychiatric Association. 2nd edn. Washington, DC: American Psychiatric Association; 2001.

9. Haghighi M, Sedighinejad A, Naderi Nabi B, et al. The incidence and predictors of headache and myalgia in patients after electroconvulsive therapy (ECT). Anesth Pain Med. 2016;6(3):e33724.

10. Mankad MV, Beyer JL, Weiner RD, et al. Clinical manual of electroconvulsive therapy, 3rd edn. Washington, DC: American Psychiatric Association; 2010.

11. Husain M, Rush A, Fink M, et al. Speed of response and remission in major depressive disorder with acute electroconvulsive therapy (ECT). J Clin Psychiatry. 2004;65(4):485–91.

12. Rosen B, Kung S, Lapid M. Effect of age on psychiatric rehospitalization rates after electroconvulsive therapy for patients with depression. J ECT. 2016;32(2):93–8.

13. Middleton H, Shaw I, Hull S, et al. NICE guidelines for the management of depression. BMJ. 2005;330(7486):267–8.

14. Oh PI, Iskedjian M, Addis A, et al. Pharmacoeconomic evaluation of clozapine in treatment-resistant schizophrenia: a cost-utility analysis. Can J Clin Pharmacol. 2001;8(4):199–206.

15. Dardennes R, Lafuma A, Fagnani F, et al. Economic assessment of a maintenance treatment strategy in prevention of recurrent depressive disorder. Value Health. 2000;3(1):40–7.

16. Revicki D, Brown R, Palmer W, et al. Modelling the cost effectiveness of antidepressant treatment in primary care. Pharmacoeconomics. 1995;8(6):524–40.

17. Greenhalgh J, Knight C, Hind D, et al. Clinical and cost-effectiveness of electroconvulsive therapy for depressive illness, schizophrenia, catatonia and mania: systematic reviews and economic modelling studies. Health Technol Assess. 2005;9(9):1–156, iii–iv.

18. Ross E, Zivin K, Maixner D. Cost-effectiveness of electroconvulsive therapy vs pharmacotherapy/psychotherapy for treatment-resistant depression in the United States. JAMA Psychiatry. 2018;75(7):713.

19. Kellner C. Overview of electroconvulsive therapy (ECT) for adults. UpToDate. [Internet]. Available from: www.uptodate.com.overview-of-electroconvulsive-therapy-ect-for-adults (accessed 28 Apr 2020).

20. Maguire S, Rea SM, Convery P. Electroconvulsive therapy—what do patients think of their treatment? Ulster Med J. 2016;85(3):182–6.

21. Kolar D. Current status of electroconvulsive therapy for mood disorders: a clinical review. Evid Based Ment Health. 2017 Feb;20(1):12–14.

2. Point-of-Care (POC) Testing for Clozapine

a. Background

Clozapine, a second-generation antipsychotic, has proven to be the most effective medication in the management of treatment-resistant schizophrenia (TRS).[1] Despite its effectiveness, clozapine has been reported to be underutilized mostly due to its associated side effect profile and the blood testing that is required in view of associated agranulocytosis.[2,3] It has been suggested that a potential solution to optimizing clozapine therapy and improving clinical outcomes should include monitoring clozapine levels and hematological parameters using point-of-care (POC) devices.[4] The use of POC devices creates a decentralized method of rapidly obtaining clinical measures using a smaller blood specimen to ultimately provide earlier results or alert clinicians to adjust their plan of action.[5]

b. Device Description

POC devices to measure clozapine concentrations: Saladax Biomedical, a commercial-stage diagnostics company, presented positive data demonstrating the performance of a POC testing device at the 2019 European College of Neuropsychopharmacology (ECNP) Annual Meeting and the International College of Neuropsychopharmacology (CINP) Annual Meeting.[6,7] The device called MyCare™ Insite measures patients' clozapine levels using a single drop of blood from a finger stick. The test takes six minutes which enables healthcare professionals to make immediate decisions in the care of their patients. MyCare™ Insite is the first and, at this point, the only rapid point-of-care test available for determining levels of clozapine.[6] This device uses immunoassay technology to detect clozapine levels. Figure 7.5 illustrates the MyCare™ Insite device available from Saladax Biomedical and the four-step procedure for its use.

4-step procedure

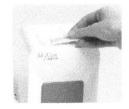 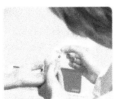 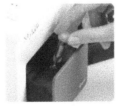 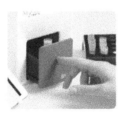

1 | Place the RFID card 2 | Collect the sample 3 | Insert the cartridge 4 | Close the door - done!

Legend: Image depicts the *MyCare™ Insite* POC device manufactured by Saladax Biomedical, Inc. Bethlehem, USA
Reference: [Internet]. 2021. [cited 27 August 2021]. Available from: https://www.sopachem.com/diagnostics/wp-content/uploads/2019/09/MyCare-Insite-User-Manual.pdf

FIGURE 7.5 POC device for measuring clozapine levels.

POC devices to monitor hematologic counts during clozapine treatment: The Hemocue WBC Diff system is designed to provide quantitative measurements of either capillary or venous total white blood cells (WBC) and differential counts (absolute and percentages of neutrophils, monocytes, lymphocytes, basophils, and eosinophils). A single drop of 10 μL blood obtained using a capillary puncture method is needed for the device to provide accurate readings. The device has been designed with a measurement range of 300–30,000/μL and a measuring time of approximately 5 minutes.[8] A strong correlation (r = 0.99) has been reported for WBC count measurements across the reported measurement range.[9] Hemocue is still pending approval by the US FDA; however, it has been approved in Europe, and cleared in the US for WBC count testing only.

Chempaq XBC is another POC device that has been designed to provide quantitative measurement of hemoglobin, WBCs, and a 3-part differential (lymphocytes, monocytes, and granulocytes). Figure 7.6 illustrates the Chempaq XBC device and the sample collection procedure. Chempaq XBC requires a drop of blood sample of 20 μL obtained using the finger prick method. The device has demonstrated acceptable ranges of linearity, reliability, and validity.[10] This device has been approved by the FDA and meets the Clinical Laboratory Improvement Amendments (CLIA) waiver requirements.[11]

Another POC device that is designed for the quantification of WBC counts and neutrophil percentages is Athelas One. This device has been approved by the FDA for use in either venous or capillary blood testing. For the device to produce accurate results, blood samples of 3.5 μL should be taken from patients and collected into a device-specific test strip to be analyzed using computer vision technology. The device needs to be connected to either a smartphone or tablet in order to operate it and displays the results once the procedure is completed. Athelas One has shown linearity on a range of 1–20,000/μL of WBC count measurement. In order to evaluate its performance, a previous study has compared Athelas One with a predicate device (Sysmex 500). Results have shown 0% clinical range error and a correlation of r = 0.99 and 0.97 for WBC counts and neutrophil percentages, respectively between Athelas and Sysmex 500.[12]

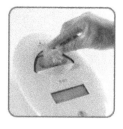

FIGURE 7.6 POC device for monitoring hematological counts during clozapine treatment.

c. Versions/Generations

POC devices are considered in-vitro diagnostics (IVDs) used to perform tests near a site where patient care is practiced. These devices are regulated by FDA and/or by the Centers for Medicare and Medicaid Services (CMS).[13] Validity and reliability of these devices are regulated by quality standards for quality testing established by Clinical Laboratory Improvement Amendments (CLIA).[11] POC devices should pass FDA premarketing and postmarketing regulatory phases in order to have them available in the market. Depending on the indication, intended use, and risk level associated with each device, the FDA classifies them as Class II or Class III devices.[13] In addition, POC devices are also subject to CLIA certification and they get classified as either "waived" or "unwaived" tests (of moderate or high complexity).[11,14]

d. Purposes of Use, Proper Use or Operation, and Operational Requirements

All the aforementioned devices utilize a simple capillary puncture (finger prick) blood collection method to measure the parameters of interest. For this, patients are instructed to relax their hands, perform gentle massage to either the middle or ring fingers, and clean them with alcohol wipes. Disposable lancets are used to puncture the fingertip, wiping off the first three blood drops. The following blood drop is then collected in a device-specific cartridge, microcuvette, or strip and placed in the device. Time to obtain results is approximately 7 minutes for MyCare™ Insite, 5 minutes for Hemocue and Athelas One, and 3 minutes for the Chempaq XBC.

There are some operational instructions specific for each device that need to be followed in order to obtain the most accurate results, as per the user manual instructions.

The MyCare™ Insite device is composed of 6 items: touch screen stand, RFID card, test rack, power cable, power adapter, and analyzer. Before operating the device, the healthcare provider should ensure that all the cables and the touch screen are connected properly. Following this step, the RFID card is placed well on top of the analyzer and a test menu will appear on the screen from which the type of test is selected. When the door opens, the cuvette filled with patient's sample is placed. When the test is completed, the results are displayed on the screen.[15]

For the Hemocue WBC Diff device, the analyzer should be started as described in the "Start-Up" section in the user manual, and the cuvette moving arm should be placed in a loading position. The screen will display the main menu from which the settings may be adjusted. The microcuvette should be taken out from the package and filled with the sample, ensuring that the blood drop is not too large, and that the filling is completed in one continuous process without refilling. Once filled with the sample, the microcuvette is placed appropriately in the device, and the start button is pressed. When the test is completed, the results are displayed on the screen.[16]

The Chempaq XBC system has 3 parts: the Particle Analyzer and Quantifier (PAQ), a small disposable cassette, and a reader. The capillary blood sample is collected in the PAQ and placed directly in the reader. Results are obtained after 3 minutes and displayed on the reader screen. A printout of the results may be obtained if a supplied printer is connected to the device.[17]

For the Athelas One system, a sample is taken from the patient and placed on the test strip directly from the finger or by using a pipette. Once the sample is placed, the test strip stains and forms a monolayer of the sample. Then, the strip is placed in the test strip slot of the device and the analysis takes place. Test results will return after 5 minutes and will be displayed on an application on a smartphone or tablet connected to the device.[18,19]

e. Interpretation of Readings

After the test is completed, readings of the different parameters of interest will be displayed on the device screen for MyCare™ Insite, Hemocue WBC diff, and Chempaq XBC, and on a connected tablet or smartphone for Athelas One.

Clozapine serum levels: The consensus is that 350 ng/mL is the lowest threshold of therapeutic efficacy to define an adequate trial of clozapine.[20] There is still no clearly defined threshold for the upper limit of therapeutic efficacy or toxicity. These values depend on an individual's characteristics such as metabolism, ethnicity, smoking, and concomitant medications or conditions. Clozapine plasma level can be checked after an initial target dose is reached for two weeks before any further dose increase.[20,21] Clinicians are advised to use clinical judgment in order to make informed decision to determine the target level for each patient depending on their individual characteristics.

Absolute neutrophils count (ANC) and WBC: To ensure the safe use of clozapine and avoid clozapine-induced agranulocytosis, patients taking clozapine need to have their ANC and WBC monitored on a regular basis. Monitoring requirements differ around the world and are established by each country's drug regulatory authorities. In the US, the FDA Clozapine Risk Evaluation and Mitigation Strategy (REMS) specifies that clinicians need to be registered and demonstrate that they are competent to prescribe clozapine (i.e., review clozapine-related materials from the Clozapine REMS program website and pass a knowledge test).[21,22] Pharmacies also need to be certified if they dispense clozapine. Patients on clozapine should be monitored weekly during the first 6 months of initiation, every other week for the following 6 months, and every 4 weeks after the first year of initiation.[22] At least levels of 1.5 x 10^9/L are required prior to treatment initiation except for patients with benign ethnic neutropenia (BEN); levels of 1.0 x 10^9/L are acceptable. For patients on clozapine, the neutrophils count should be maintained > 2.0 x 10^9/L. If levels are found to be 1.0–1.49 x 10^9/L clozapine should be maintained but patients need three times weekly monitoring for ANC. If levels are < 1.0 x 10^9/L, clozapine should be stopped and a full blood count test should be performed daily until values normalize.[21,22]

f. Important Safety Issues (Including Cautions and Common Adverse Effects)

The procedure implemented to perform POC is generally well tolerated and minimally invasive. However, pain due to the needle prick might be inconvenient to some patients, especially those who require frequent monitoring. Currently, there are many studies conducted to figure out strategies to minimize lancet needle pain. These strategies include optimizing needle tip shape, enhancing the needle polishing, directing the needle with better angles, and enhancing the skin penetration depth in ways that reduce the pricking pain. As an additional strategy to reduce pain and skin-pricking side effects, patients/clinicians are advised to prick at the side of the fingertip, alternate the test fingers, and perform gentle massage to the fingers prior to the procedure.[23]

In addition to the physical effects surrounding blood sampling, medical errors in the context of POC devices could be present anywhere starting from ordering the device to interpreting test results. Therefore, it is highly important to ensure the quality, accuracy, and precision of the POC devices used in the clinical setting as well as having well-trained personnel capable of performing the procedures correctly.[24]

g. Storage Conditions and Maintenance

MyCare™ Insite: The device should be kept on a dry, clean, level surface that avoids direct sunlight. Temperature of the work space should be 20–28°C, and 10–85% relative humidity.[15]

Hemocue WBC Diff: The microcuvettes should be stored at 15–35°C, < 90% non condensing humidity, and should be allowed to reach 15–35°C before use. They should be used prior to the expiration date that is printed on the package. Regarding the analyzer, it may be stored in temperatures between 0–50°C, < 90 % noncondensing humidity, and should be allowed to reach ambient temperature before use.[16]

Chempaq XBC: The instrument should be stored at 4–30 °C, and 20–85 % noncondensing relative humidity. During the working time, the instrument should be allowed to reach 16–35°C, and 10–70 % noncondensing relative humidity.[17]

Athelas One: The device and the test strips should be placed in an environment with a temperature between 20°C and 25°C.[18]

h. Important Features (Capabilities and Limitations) and Special Advantages

As compared to traditional methods for monitoring clozapine, POC facilitates adherence to and safety and efficacy of clozapine through the implementation of noninvasive techniques that provide real-time, laboratory-quality values for clinicians in a timely manner. This should help healthcare providers to make rapid clinical decisions and encourage patients to demonstrate better adherence patterns to clozapine. This should minimize complications of under-treatment which would, eventually, improve utilization of resources. Moreover, these devices are user-friendly and could be used by any healthcare professional with brief training (not necessarily laboratory personnel).

In addition, most of these devices are either factory-calibrated or perform automatic calibration once started, which saves time and effort as opposed to manual calibration methods. POC devices are also versatile because they are able to perform different tests such as WBC, differentials, and hemoglobin at the same time using a single blood sample. Also, most of them could be used with either venous or capillary blood samples.[5]

As a limitation of the discussed instruments, *Chempaq XBC* can measure WBC and 3-part differential (lymphocytes, monocytes, and granulocytes) only; which limits its use in the context of clozapine monitoring. This is because the most important monitoring parameter associated with clozapine treatment is neutrophils. Since 90% of granulocytes are accounted for by neutrophils, their values could be estimated indirectly; however, it is still less favorable than the direct methods.[25] Additionally, MyCare™ Insite is still not available in the market and pending FDA approval. Therefore, there is no available POC to monitor clozapine concentrations in the clinical practice yet.[5]

Furthermore, inappropriately performed tests or inaccurate results could compromise care delivered to the patients especially if performed by untrained personnel.[26]

i. Special Tips for Patient Counseling if a Device Is Used for Self-Care

POC in the context of clozapine monitoring is only available to be performed by trained clinicians, and are not recommended to be used for self-care. Patients, however, should be educated about the test and its benefits in order to encourage them to adhere to their course of treatment and facilitate the monitoring process. Patients should be advised to report any side effects, medications, or newly discovered medical conditions at the time of the test to avoid any false results. Specific training programs for clinicians should include the following[27]:

- How to start up and use the instrument properly
- How to perform calibration (if needed)
- How to report and interpret results
- How to ensure quality control of the instrument
- What to do in case of problems/errors with the instrument

j. Available Evidence on Effectiveness and Safety

Clozapine is considered the most effective option in patients with schizophrenia and failed prior treatment attempts. Despite the drug effectiveness, it remains underutilized by many patients due to many factors; most importantly the frequent monitoring that the drug mandates. POC devices that utilize capillary puncture for sample collection are considered a good alternative. Available data derived from studies which assessed the safety and efficacy of POC devices for clozapine monitoring show a favorable trend towards their use, although the sample sizes of these studies were relatively small.

Bui et al. compared WBC and differentials counts obtained from the Hemocue WBC Diff device (capillary sample) with data obtained from traditional laboratory procedure (venous sample).[9] Results have shown moderate correlation between the two methods r = 0.77 and 0.82 for WBCs and neutrophils, respectively. When venous samples were analyzed by Hemocue and compared to traditional methods, a strong correlation was observed r = 0.95. However, there was a tendency for Hemocue WBC Diff to measure lower WBC counts than the routine laboratory method.

Another randomized controlled cross-over study was conducted to compare the burden of testing using the two methods on patients and clinicians.[28] The majority of participants favored the capillary puncture method applied by Hemocue WBC Diff over the traditional procedure because it was associated with fewer and less severe adverse effects (pain, anxiety, fear), saved time, and provided quicker turnaround for clinicians than using the traditional method.

Nielsen et al. conducted a randomized cross-over trial to assess performance of the Chempax XBC device.[25] Investigators used the 10 cm visual analog scale (VAS) to assess patients' satisfaction with the blood monitoring method in 77 patients taking clozapine. Results showed statistically significant differences in the VAS scores between the two groups, indicating patients favoring capillary puncture over venous sampling since it was less painful and more convenient. In addition, the majority of patients (62.8%) indicated that capillary blood sampling was their choice, and the majority of psychiatric caregivers (87.1%) found the Chempaq XBC blood monitoring to be a more convenient option for their patient.

k. Economic Evaluation

No economic evaluation studies that compare POC devices for clozapine monitoring to conventional testing methods are currently available.

l. Implication to the Pharmacy Profession and Pharmacy Practice

Pharmacists working in inpatient or outpatient psychiatric hospital settings are well positioned to detect issues related to clozapine safety and efficacy during medication therapy management sessions with patients. Since POC devices are able to provide quick and accurate results, data collected can be communicated to the healthcare team by the pharmacist in order to make timely clinical decisions. Pharmacists are also able to provide proper interpretation and education to patients depending on the nature of the results during the same visits. If patients are found to have alerting levels and require therapy modification, they could be referred to their physicians or the prescribing clinician without having to wait for laboratory results. By having pharmacists performing clozapine monitoring tests using POC devices, waiting time will decrease which is more convenient for patients and clinicians and will help save resources for other patients in need. Also, patient adherence to therapy should improve as a result of the thorough education and counseling given by the pharmacists.[29]

m. Challenges to the Pharmacists and Users

Despite the potential effectiveness of POC devices in clozapine monitoring, there is a lack of guidelines informing clinicians about the best instruments to adopt into their practice. This lack of guidelines is possibly influenced by the lack of studies with strong methodologies comparing POC results against traditional laboratory methods, and comparing different POC devices. This represents a challenge to healthcare providers who are seeking faster and more convenient results. The lack of economic evaluation of the available POC devices also raises uncertainties whether or not they are more cost-effective than the traditional testing methods. Furthermore, the lack of proper training to perform these tests could impact the validity and reliability of the results, and consequently, affect the patient care process negatively.

n. Recommendations: The Way Forward

POC research in the psychiatry field will continue to focus on enhancing techniques and developing new instruments that have better performance, involve a wider range of tests, and produce results with fewer potential errors.

By having these tests in place, the concept of individualized medicine will be further reinforced through identification of specific population target levels, respond to their treatment needs, and achieve optimum safety and efficacy outcomes specific to each patient.

o. Conclusions

The use of POC technology for monitoring clozapine therapy has been expanding dramatically to replace routine laboratory procedures resulting in facilitated monitoring and enhanced adherence. A variety of tests are approved and available for use in clinical practice. The procedure involves analyzing blood samples using finger prick methods for which results will be available within a few minutes. These tests are user-friendly and minimally invasive and could be used by any healthcare provider with brief training. Pharmacists play an important role in clozapine monitoring and the use of POC devices can be important and safe tools to enhance their clinical practice. Guidelines informing the use of POC devices for monitoring the safety and efficacy of clozapine and other medications used in the area of psychiatry are warranted.

p. Lessons Learned

- Clozapine is the only antipsychotic medication with evidence for the treatment of TRS. However, the use of the drug is challenged by the frequent monitoring of hematological parameters needed to avoid clozapine-induced neutropenia.
- POC testing for clozapine monitoring is reliable and produces comparable results to standard laboratory procedures.
- There is only one POC device available to detect clozapine concentration in plasma (pending FDA approval) whereas there is a variety of options available to test WBC and ANC counts.
- Performance evaluation and pharmacoeconomic studies are warranted to build a strong evidence base for the use of POC for clozapine monitoring.

REFERENCES

Section 1: Point-of-Care (POC) Testing for Clozapine

1. Kane J, Honigfeld G, Singer J, et al. Clozapine for the treatment-resistant schizophrenic: a double blind comparison with chlorpromazine. Arch Gen Psychiatry. 1988;45:789–96.
2. Warnez S, Alessi-Severini S. Clozapine: a review of clinical practice guidelines and prescribing trends. BMC Psychiatry. 2014;4:102.
3. Curry B, Palmer E, Mounce C, et al. Assessing prescribing practices of clozapine before and after the implementation of an updated risk evaluation and mitigation strategy. Ment Health Clin. 2018;8:63–7.
4. Kelly DL, Ben-Yoav H, Payne GF, et al. Blood draw barriers for treatment with clozapine and development of a point-of-care monitoring device. Clin Schizophr Relat Psychoses. 2018;12:23–30.
5. Kalaria SN, Kelly DL. Development of point-of-care testing devices to improve clozapine prescribing habits and patient outcomes. Neuropsychiatr Dis Treat. 2019;15:2365–70.
6. Business Wire. Studies feature clinical validations of clozapine point of care testing using a single drop of blood to aid psychiatrists in better treatment of patients with schizophrenia. [Internet]. Available from: www.businesswire.com/news/home/20191024005516/en/ (accessed 4 July 2020).
7. Abstracts of the 32nd ECNP Congress, 7–10 Sept 2019, Copenhagen, Denmark. [Internet]. Available from: www.sciencedirect.com/journal/european-neuropsychopharmacology/vol/29/suppl/S6?page=8 (accessed 4 July 2020).
8. Saladax Biomedical, Inc. My Care™ Insite. [Internet]. Available from: https://mycaretests.com/wp-content/uploads/2019/09/lit-psy-004-rev-03-mycare-insite-intro-flyer.pdf (accessed 4 July 2020).
9. Bui HN, Bogers JP, Cohen D, et al. Evaluation of the performance of a point-of-care method for total and differential white blood cell count in clozapine users. Int J Lab Hem. 2016;38:703–9.
10. Rao LV, Ekberg BA, Connor D, et al. Evaluation of a new point of care automated complete blood count (CBC) analyzer in various clinical settings. Clin Chim Acta. 2008;389:120–5.

11. Center for Medicare and Medicaid Services (CMS). Department of Health and Human Services: Clinical Laboratory Improvement Amendments of 1988 (CLIA); 1998.

12. Athelas. Clinical third party accuracy validation of the Athelas device: CBC device compared with venous Sysmex 5000 in POC clinic. [Internet] Available from: https://athelas.com/ a4ab6c781c91ee7290ced2991f4036e9.pdf (accessed 22 July 2020).

13. Van Norma GA. Drugs, devices, and the FDA: part 2: an overview of approval processes: FDA approval of medical devices. JACC Basic Transl Sci. 2016;1:277–87.

14. US Food and Drug Administration (FDA). Guidance for industry and FDA staff. Administrative procedures for CLIA categorization; 2017.

15. MyCare-Insite Quick Reference Guide. [Internet]. Available from: www.sopachem.com/diagnostics/wp-content/uploads/2019/09/MyCare-Insite-Quick-Reference-Guide.pdf (accessed 22 July 2020).

16. HemoCue Quick Reference Guide. [Internet]. Available from: http://policyandorders.cw.bc.ca/resource-gallery/Documents/Lab%20and%20Pathology%20Medicine/HemoCue%20Hb%20201%20Quick%20Reference%20Guide.pdf (accessed 22 July 2020).

17. Scandinavian Evaluation of Laboratory Equipment for Primary Health Care (SKUP). Chempaq XBC eXpress Blood Counter manufactured by Chempaq A/S. [Internet]. Available from: https://skup.org/ (accessed 23 July 2020).

18. United States Food and Drug Administration (US FDA). [Internet]. Available from: www.accessdata.fda.gov/cdrh_docs/pdf18/K181288.pdf (accessed 23 July 2020).

19. Athelas. [Internet]. Available from: https://athelas.com/ (accessed 23 July 2020).

20. Ellison JC, Dufresne RL. A review of the clinical utility of serum clozapine and norclozapine levels. Mental Health Clinician. 2015;5(2):68–73.

21. Freudenreich O, McEvoy J. Guidelines for prescribing clozapine in schizophrenia. UpToDate. [Internet]. Available from: www.uptodate.com/contents/guidelines-for-prescribing-clozapine-in-schizophrenia (accessed 22 July 2020).

22. United States Food and Drug Administration (US FDA). Information on clozapine. [Internet]. Available from: www.fda.gov/drugs/postmarket-drug-safety-information-patients-and-providers/information-clozapine (accessed 31 July 2020).

23. Heinemann L. Finger pricking and pain: a never ending story. J Diabetes Sci Technol. 2008;2(5):919–21.

24. Ehrmeyer SS. Plan for quality to improve patient safety at the point of care. Ann Saudi Med. 2011;31(4):342–6.

25. Nielsen J, Thode D, Stenager E, et al. Hematological clozapine monitoring with a point-of-care device: a randomized cross-over trial. Eur Neuropsychopharmacol. 2012;22(6):401–5.

26. ACBI. Guidelines for safe and effective management and use of point of care testing. [Internet]. Available from: www.acbi.ie/Article.asp?pID=215 (accessed 23 July 2020).

27. Joint Commission International. Point of care testing. [Internet]. Available from: www.jointcommissioninternational.org/standards/hospital-standards-communication-center/point-of-care-testing/ (accessed 23 July 2020).

28. Bogers JP, Bui H, Herruer M, et al. Capillary compared to venous blood sampling in clozapine treatment: patients' and healthcare practitioners' experiences with a point-of-care device. Eur Neuropsychopharmacol. 2015;25:319–24.

29. Ní Dhubhlaing C, Young A, Sahm LJ. Impact of pharmacist counselling on clozapine knowledge. Schizophr Res Treatment. 2017;2017:6120970.

SECTION 2: DEVICES AVAILABLE FOR PURCHASE AT RETAIL SETTINGS

1. POLYSOMNOGRAPHY AND ACTIGRAPHY

a. Background

There are multiple methods for evaluating sleep complaints, including clinical interviews, sleep diaries, polysomnography (laboratory- or home-based), and actigraphy. Polysomnography (PSG) is considered the gold standard method used to assess sleep disorders because it objectively measures not only wake and sleep time, but also sleep architecture.[1] This technique employs surface electrodes to measure physiologic parameters of sleep using electroencephalography (EEG), eye movements, muscle activity, heart physiology, and respiratory function. Time-series data are aggregated, processed, and visually examined or mathematically transformed in order to reveal insights about sleep/wake states and many aspects of physiology.[2] PSG is used to diagnose, or rule out, many types of sleep disorders, including narcolepsy, idiopathic hypersomnia, periodic limb movement disorder (PLMD), rapid eye movement (REM) behavior disorder, parasomnias, and sleep apnea. Although it is not directly useful in diagnosing circadian rhythm sleep disorders, it may be used to rule out other sleep disorders. The use of PSG as a screening test for persons having excessive daytime sleepiness as a sole presenting complaint is controversial.[3] However, PSG is limited by cost and inconvenience because this method typically requires individuals to spend the night in a sleep laboratory (and less often, at home) under the continued supervision of a sleep technician.[2]

When compared to PSG, actigraphy is a low-cost, noninvasive method of capturing body movements that is emerging as a viable alternative to PSG. It was originally developed as a research-based method for estimating sleep parameters across multiple nights in the individual's natural sleep setting (home environment) rather than measuring sleep during a single night in the sleep laboratory environment.[4] Actigraphic devices can be worn on the wrist, ankle, or waist, relatively unobtrusively over a period of days to weeks. For sleep, the devices are typically worn on the wrist or ankle. Clinical guidelines and research suggest that wrist actigraphy is particularly useful in the documentation of sleep patterns prior to a multiple sleep latency test, in the evaluation of circadian rhythm sleep disorders, to evaluate treatment outcomes, and as an adjunct to home monitoring of sleep-disordered breathing.[4,5]

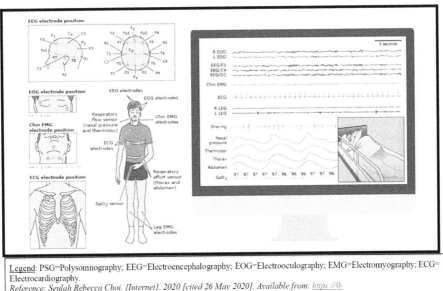

FIGURE 7.7 Placements of PSG derivations and related recordings.

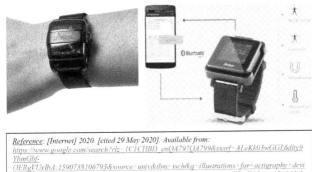

FIGURE 7.8 Classic actigraphy wrist devices.

b. Device Description

A polysomnogram will typically record a minimum of 12 channels requiring a minimum of 22 wire attachments to the patient. These channels vary in every laboratory and may be adapted to meet the doctor's requests. There is a minimum of three channels for the EEG, one or two measure airflow, one or two are for chin muscle tone, one or more for leg movements, two for eye movements (EOG), one or two for heart rate and rhythm, one for oxygen saturation, and one for each of the belts, which measure chest wall movement and upper abdominal wall movement.[6] Polysomnography also uses video and sound recordings. The video recording is added to observe the patient and detect position changes or unusual behavior that may occur during sleep, and the recording of sounds is used to detect snoring patterns, other breathing disorders such as stridor, vocal parasomnias, and vocalizations. Figure 7.7 illustrates placement and recordings of these derivations.

Sleep actigraphs are generally watch-shaped and worn on the wrist of the nondominant arm for adults and usually on the ankle for children. Actigraphs have movement detectors (e.g., accelerometers) and sufficient memory to record for up to several weeks. Movement is sampled several times per second, translated into digital data, and stored for later analysis. In some brands the data are transmitted and analyzed in real time, and some units also measure light exposure.[7] Computer programs are used to derive levels of activity/inactivity, rhythm parameters (such as amplitude or acrophase), and sleep/wake parameters (such as total sleep time, percent of time spent asleep, total wake time, percent of time spent awake, and number of awakenings).[8] Several devices and computer software are available, and assessment can vary depending on the chosen device, procedure, and software program.[9] Most devices use a rechargeable lithium battery that must be charged prior to use.[7] Figure 7.8 illustrates a classical wrist actigraphy device.

c. Various Versions/Generations

The American Academy of Sleep Medicine (AASM) classifies PSG devices into four types, listed here:

- Type I devices are considered the standard laboratory-based PSG.[10]
- Type II devices are portable PSG devices that measure the same parameters at home as those by Type I devices. Home-based PSGs do not use the audio and video recordings.
- Type III devices measure four physiological variables including the heart rate and respiratory function.
- Type IV devices measure only oxygen saturation or airflow.

In addition, there are different protocols that are used in laboratory PSG such as full-night study, split-night study (procedure in which sleep and breathing variables are recorded during the first 2 hours of the sleep period), and daytime study. Full-night PSG is the preferred method since benefit has been well established, whereas for the other methods there is insufficient evidence.[10]

The first actigraphs were developed in the early 1970s. In February of 2008, actigraphy transitioned from a Current Procedural Terminology Category III (emerging technology) to a Category I code (95803), which is a stand-alone code.[4] The AASM "Clinical Practice Guideline on the Use of Actigraphy for the Evaluation of Sleep Disorders and Circadian Rhythm Sleep-Wake Disorders" provides recommendations for the use of actigraphy as described under this code.[4] Over the years, additional types of actigraphs were developed leading to the digital types used today.[8] Despite lack of validation against the gold standard of PSG, consumer sleep technologies (CSTs) are widespread applications and devices purported to measure and even improve sleep. It is the position of the AASM that CST must be FDA-cleared and rigorously tested against current gold standards if it is intended to render a diagnosis and/or treatment. Given the unknown potential of CST to measure sleep or assess for sleep disorders, these tools are not substitutes for medical evaluation. However, CSTs may be utilized to enhance the patient-clinician interaction when presented in the context of an appropriate clinical evaluation.[11]

d. Purposes of Use, Proper Use or Operation, and Operational Requirements

PSG is largely performed in sleep centers or major hospitals which meet the standards of the AASM.[10] The standard procedure usually starts 2 hours before the patient's bedtime. During this time, the patient is introduced to the setting and connected to the devices to monitor heart rate, breathing, and brain activity. The monitoring electrodes are placed on the patient's scalp, temples, chests, and legs to serve as channels of data that are recorded as the patient falls asleep. The room is also connected to cameras and microphones to help the observer in monitoring the patient's movements and breathing sounds (presence or absence of snoring and its volume). The entire study is usually completed by 7 a.m. the next day, unless a Multiple Sleep Latency Test (MSLT) is to be done during the day to test for excessive daytime sleepiness.[12] Most recently, healthcare providers may prescribe home studies to enhance patient comfort and reduce expenses.[13]

Actigraphy devices are relatively easy to use and require very little preparation. As previously mentioned, actigraphs are basically accelerometers that need to be programmed prior to use.[7] Accelerometers function by integrating a filtered acceleration signal over a user-defined time sampling interval, which is commonly referred to as an "epoch." As such, device programing typically involves entering patient information, setting the epoch length, and selecting data collection start and end times.[7] The most validated and commonly used epoch lengths are 30 seconds and 1 minute.[14] At the end of each epoch, the summed value (i.e., activity count) is stored in the monitor memory; this process is repeated until data collection is complete. Patients should be provided with written instructions on use and care of the actigraph, along with an actigraphy log with an explanation on how specific events show up on the actigram (e.g., wake time, bed time, and nap start and end times).[7] It is important that patients understand the importance of completing the log daily for the entire monitoring period.

e. Interpretation of Readings

After the PSG study is completed, a "scorer" analyzes the data by reviewing the study in 30-second "epochs." The score consists of the following information:

- Onset of sleep from time the lights were turned off: This is called "sleep onset latency" and normally is less than 20 minutes. It is important to note that determining "sleep" and "awake" is based solely on the EEG recordings.
- Sleep efficiency: This is the number of minutes of sleep divided by the number of minutes in bed. Normal is approximately 85–90% or higher.
- Sleep stages: These are based on 3 sources of data coming from 7 channels: EEG (usually 4 channels), EOG (2), and chin EMG (1). From this information, each 30-second epoch is scored as "awake" or one of 4 sleep stages: 1, 2, 3, and REM sleep. Stages 1–3 are together called non-REM sleep. Figure 7.9 illustrates a 30-second epoch REM sleep from an overnight PSG.[6]
- Breathing irregularities such as apneas and hypopneas: Apnea is a complete or near-complete cessation of airflow for at least 10 seconds followed by an arousal and/or 3% oxygen desaturation; hypopnea is a 30% or greater decrease in airflow for at least 10 seconds followed by an arousal and/or 4% oxygen desaturation.[6]
- Arousals: These are sudden shifts in brain wave activity. They may be caused by numerous factors, including breathing abnormalities, leg movements, environmental noises, etc. An abnormal number of arousals indicates "interrupted sleep" and may explain a person's daytime symptoms of fatigue and/or sleepiness.
- Cardiac rhythm abnormalities: Although most arrhythmias detected during sleep are benign, they may indicate an underlying disorder in need of investigation and treatment, such as obstructive sleep apnea (OSA). OSA is prevalent among patients with cardiovascular risk factors which predispose them to further cardiovascular events, including arrhythmias, which may be prevented by recognition and treatment of sleep disordered breathing.

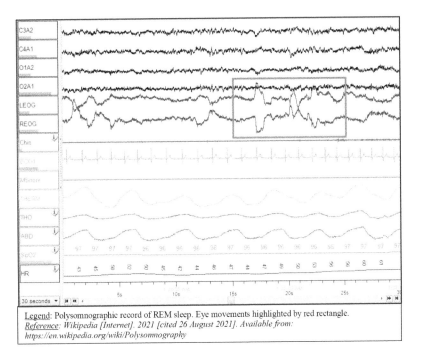

Legend: Polysomnographic record of REM sleep. Eye movements highlighted by red rectangle.
Reference: Wikipedia [Internet]. 2021 [cited 26 August 2021]. Available from:
https://en.wikipedia.org/wiki/Polysomnography

FIGURE 7.9 Example of a 30-second epoch REM sleep from an overnight PSG.

- Leg movements: Abnormal movements during sleep are part of a larger group of nocturnal events that may occur during sleep, wake, or the transitions into or out of sleep. Simple movements during sleep are typically quick, involving only one body area, such as leg cramps which are painful, sustained muscle contractions, most commonly in the calf, foot, or thigh, that may occur at any time during the night. Periodic limb movements of sleep are episodes of repetitive and highly stereotyped limb movements occurring every 5 to 90 seconds, primarily during the first half of the night and during non-REM sleep.
- Body position during sleep: It is known that there is a relationship between body posture and sleep disturbances, particularly for certain sleep disorders such as OSA. For example, it has been observed that the avoidance of the supine position leads to a decrease in the number and severity of obstructive episodes.
- Oxygen saturation during sleep: Oxygen desaturations may be associated with increases in the heart rate. These events may suggest the presence of OSA because it involves periodic pauses in breathing and drops in the oxygen level of the blood that lead to a spike of cortisol (stress hormone) that impacts the heart. In general, it is considered abnormal if the oxygen levels fall below 88% in adults or below 90% in children.

Once scored, the test recording and the scoring data are sent to the sleep medicine physician for interpretation. Ideally, interpretation is done in conjunction with the medical history, a complete list of drugs the patient is taking, and any other relevant information that might impact the study such as napping done before the test.[6]

Actigraphy devices generally come with software that uses a validated algorithm to score the motion data as "sleep" or "wake." The actigraph and log data measure the following variables[7]:

- Average activity counts are measured as an average value over an entire period scored as "wake" by the software algorithm. Average activity counts are provided for each 24-hour period.
- Time in bed is the total amount of time indicated as "rest" according to the sleep log.
- Total sleep time represents the total number of minutes scored as "sleep" within the 24-hour day.
- Sleep onset latency, the time elapsed between the beginning of "rest" as noted on the actigraphy log and the beginning of "sleep" as scored by the software algorithm. Of note, sleep onset latency measured by actigraphy may be less reliable than sleep onset latency measured by in-laboratory PSG.
- Light intensity can also be measured by some actigraphs, which will be useful for determining how light exposure may be contributing to a sleep pattern that is either delayed or advanced.

Qualitative review of the actigram, the aforementioned measured variables and derived information (e.g., sleep efficiency, diurnal variation, number of sleep periods, wake after sleep onset, fragmentation index, and midsleep time) will assist clinicians in the evaluation of circadian sleep-wake rhythm disorders, since each has characteristic

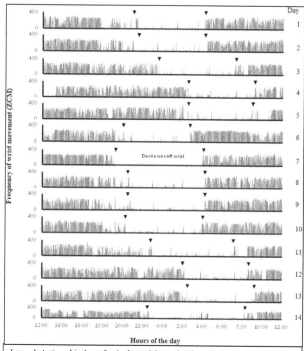

Legend: Actigraphic data of a single participant showing minute-by-minute wrist movement values (activity counts) across 14 days. Downward arrows show 'in bed times' and 'get up times' for each day ascertained based on information from the event marker and sleep diary.
Reference: Fekedulegn D, et al. Actigraphy-based assessment of sleep parameters. Ann Work Expo Health. 2020; 64(4):350–367. Available online: https://doi.org/10.1093/annweh/wxaa007
Published by Oxford University Press on behalf of The British Occupational Hygiene Society 2020. This work is written by (a) US Government employee(s) and is in the public domain in the US.

FIGURE 7.10 Example of actigraphy-based sleep parameters.

findings on actigraphy, and also will provide clinicians with an objective way to measure treatment response. Figure 7.10 illustrates a typical actigraph.

f. Important Features and Special Advantages

As stated earlier, PSG is considered as the gold standard to objectively assess sleep behavior and sleep physiology. Because PSG studies are usually conducted in a sleep laboratory or clinic, PSG is expensive. Although PSG studies are possible to be conducted at home, the procedure is still considered too invasive to be used in clinical studies in which the primary focus is quantification of sleep time, wake time, or both. Consequently, actigraphy has been suggested as an alternative assessment method to PSG. Based on differences in movements associated with wakefulness and sleep, actigraphy provides an estimate of sleep/wake schedules. Being independent of patients' ratings and personal judgments of their sleep, actigraphy may offer a less time-consuming and less expensive alternative to PSG. However, its accuracy is approximately 90% for total sleep time and only around 55% for determining the correct sleep stage when compared to PSG.[14] Total sleep time and sleep efficiency tend to be overestimated by actigraphy, primarily because the delineation of sleep onset is difficult. This leads

TABLE 7.4
Main Differences between PSG and Sleep Actigraphy

Characteristic features	PSG	Actigraphy
Cost	Expensive	Less expensive than PSG
Objective information	Records activity during sleep only	Records both daily variability and sleep quality
Patient burden	High (needs multiple connection wires)	Low (wireless, easy to remove device)
Preparation time	Long time preparation	Less time preparation
Indications	Gold standard for assessing sleep disorders	More beneficial in specific conditions: paradoxical insomnia, cardiometabolic syndrome
Duration	One-night study (maximum of two nights)	Can be used for multiple days and nights (benefit in insomnia condition)
Data type	At least three types of data (EEG, EOG, EMG)	One-dimensional data

Legend: **EEG: Electroencephalography; EOG: Electrooculography; EMG: Electromyography**.

to overestimation of sleep time in situations in which patients lie in bed relatively motionless (e.g., patients with insomnia, those who lie in bed watching television, older adults in a nursing home environment).[7] In contrast, actigraphy may underestimate sleep in patients with a movement disorder. Table 7.1 provides a summary of the differential features of PSG and actigraphy, including the advantages and disadvantages of each. Data from consumer wearable devices that assess sleep (also known as CSTs) should be interpreted with caution. CSTs rely on indirect measures of sleep and have data loss problems, and some devices are more accurate than others. Most CSTs are not validated to be a screening tool for sleep disorders.[7,11]

g. Special Tips for Patient Counseling if a Device Is Used for Self-Care

On the **PSG** study day, it is important to advise the patients of the following:

- Avoid napping.
- Shower and avoid using hair products like gel or hairspray that may interfere with the recording.
- Follow regular routine as much as possible.
- Avoid alcohol and caffeinated beverages.
- Avoid taking any sedative medications.
- Take medications for other conditions as prescribed.
- Bring anything that makes patient comfortable during the night.

As outlined in Section d, prior to the start of sleep study using actigraphy, patients should be provided with written instructions on use and care of the actigraph and be advised to do the following[7]:

- Continue with their days as normal for the entire duration of the study.
- Take regular medications as prescribed.
- Complete the log daily for the entire monitoring period.
- If removed, place the actigraphy device back on the same wrist.
- Water resistance should be noted and addressed appropriately with the patient.
- If a light sensor is being used, patients must ensure that clothing does not cover the sensor.

h. Available Evidence on Effectiveness and Safety

PSG is considered a safe and gold-standard method for diagnosing different sleep disorders. There are no absolute contraindications to PSG when indications are clearly established. However, risk-benefit ratios should be assessed if medically unstable inpatients are to be transferred from the clinical setting to a sleep laboratory for overnight polysomnography.[15] Some precautions and complications related to PSG include the following:

- Skin irritation may occur as a result of the adhesive used to attach electrodes to the patient or from the use of adhesive remover at the end of the study period.
- Collodion-based adhesives and acetone-based adhesive removers should not be used, or used with caution due to their flammability, particularly in patients who require oxygen. If used, they should be applied in well-ventilated areas.
- The integrity of polysomnographic equipment's electrical isolation must be certified by engineering or biomedical personnel qualified to make such an assessment.

There are no clinically significant and undesirable outcomes associated with actigraphy.[4] Therefore, if actigraphy is used as described in Section a, the risk of harm is minimized and the probability of clinical benefits increases.[4] Rarely, patients may develop local skin irritation or hypersensitivity to materials in the device.[7] In addition, care should be taken when wearing the device near magnetic resonance imaging (MRI) machines, since MRI compatibility is not well established.[7,14]

i. Economic Evaluation

Most economic evaluations have assessed differences in costs between laboratory PSG and home-based PSG, particularly for the diagnosis of OSA. The results of a non-inferiority cost-effectiveness study showed that the home-based PSG was not only lower in cost, but also resulted in overall cost savings of €292.70–€571.10.[16] However, other studies suggest that although home-based PSG is the least expensive diagnostic tests, over time laboratory PSG is more cost effective, mostly due to higher rates of false-positive diagnoses with the use of home-based PSG.[10,17,18] Actigraphy is more costly than sleep logs in terms of the technical and professional components of the service. However, these costs are relatively low and compare favorably to the technical and professional costs associated with PSG. Guidelines suggest that actigraphy may be more cost effective if an objective measurement of sleep is needed.[4] However, economic analyses comparing the cost-effectiveness of these devices for the assessment of insomnia or the evaluation of treatment response have not been conducted.

j. Implication to the Pharmacy Profession and Pharmacy Practice

Pharmacists are often involved in assisting individuals with sleeping disorders by initiating conversation, assessing medication history, screening for sleep disorders using self-reported questionnaires and sleep logs (particularly insomnia), monitoring treatment outcomes, and providing medication counseling and sleep hygiene education. The use of actigraphy in particular has been reported as an objective measure to monitor and follow –up with individuals in community pharmacy settings to assist them in the management of sleeping disorders.[19] Furthermore, as health professionals, community pharmacists in particular are at an ideal position to provide information on CSTs in view of the increased commercial availability of these devices. Having a basic understanding of how these devices work is imperative for pharmacists. As patients engage with CST, opportunities will arise to have a dialogue with them about their expectations of the CST as well as their underlying sleep concerns.

k. Challenges to the Pharmacists and Users

The detection of sleep disorders is important to facilitate earlier diagnosis and delivery of treatment. Community pharmacies are often the first point of entry into the healthcare system for individuals experiencing symptoms of sleep disorders, and pharmacists are well placed to check medication profiles that may be suggestive of sleep disorders. However, most studies are limited to the use of self-reported sleep questionnaires.[19] Increasing knowledge about actigraphy may provide pharmacists with the opportunity to more objectively assess sleep disturbances that enable them to refer patients to sleep specialists. In addition, in view of the increased commercial availability of CSTs, there is increased need for consumers to seek the opinion of health professionals about these devices, including pharmacists. The AASM's position statement on CSTs outlined guiding principles for these encounters[11]:

- Clinicians should have a general awareness of CST and be ready to discuss CST with patients.

- Clinicians should understand the general framework of devices and applications available and have a basic knowledge of available evidence or lack thereof.
- Most CSTs are not FDA-cleared or validated clinical devices/applications, but widespread accessibility and use by patients (and potential patients) may augment patient engagement.
- Data can be utilized as a tool for opening discussions with patients.
- Clinicians should recognize the patient's use of CST as a commitment to focus on sleep wellness.

l. Recommendations: The Way Forward

There has been inadequate evidence on the effectiveness of models in specific primary healthcare settings for detecting sleep disorders. Guided by health professionals, actigraphy is a method/device which can be used by patients in the community not only to identify undiagnosed poor sleep, but also to monitor the efficacy of treatments used by patients with sleep disturbances. The community pharmacy is a feasible setting for screening and intervention services which has not been sufficiently explored. Studies exploring the use of actigraphy in the pharmacy setting for screening and improving sleep health management in the community are needed, including patients' and community pharmacists' opinions about the feasibility and cost of such services.

m. Conclusions

PSG is the gold standard method used to assess sleep disorders because it objectively measures not only wake and sleep time, but also sleep architecture. However, it is complex and requires, in most instances, attending a sleep laboratory or clinic. In contrast, wrist actigraphy is less invasive and less expensive than PSG, and particularly appropriate in the study of treatment effects because it can identify changes over time. There is also increased availability of wearable CSTs, although data derived from these should be interpreted with caution since most have not been validated. Actigraphy offers opportunities for pharmacists to become more involved in the management of sleeping disorders. Community pharmacists in particular are at an ideal position to provide information on CSTs in view of their increased commercial availability.

n. Lessons Learned

- PSG is the gold standard method used to assess sleep disorders. This technique employs surface electrodes to measure physiologic parameters of sleep using EEG and measuring eye movements, muscle activity, heart physiology, and respiratory function.
- Actigraphy is basically the use of accelerometers that capture body movements. Actigraphic devices can be worn on the wrist, ankle, or waist, relatively unobtrusively.

- Whereas PSG is often performed in a clinic or laboratory setting to record various physiological characteristics over a limited period of time, actigraphy is a noninvasive method that can be used over longer periods of time in the natural sleep setting of the patient.
- Pharmacists may increase their role in the screening and management of sleep disorders by becoming more knowledgeable, particularly in regards to actigraphy and CSTs.

REFERENCES

SECTION 2: POLYSOMNOGRAPHY AND ACTIGRAPHY

1. McCall C, McCall WV. Comparison of actigraphy with polysomnography and sleep logs in depressed insomniacs. J Sleep Res. 2012;21(1):122–7.
2. Marino M, Li Y, Rueschman MN, et al. Measuring sleep: accuracy, sensitivity, and specificity of wrist actigraphy compared to polysomnography. Sleep. 2013;36(11):1747–55.
3. Lerman SE, Eskin E, Flower DJ, et al. Fatigue risk management in the workplace. J Occup Environ Med. 2012 Feb 1;54(2):231–58.
4. Smith MT, McCrae CS, Cheung J, et al. Use of actigraphy for the evaluation of sleep disorders and circadian rhythm sleep-wake disorders: an American Academy of Sleep Medicine clinical practice guideline. J Clin Sleep Med. 2018;14(7):1231–7.
5. Martin JL, Hakim AD. Wrist actigraphy. Chest. 2011;139 (6):1514–27.
6. Kushida CA, Littner MR, Morgenthaler T, et al. Practice parameters for the indications for polysomnography and related procedures: an update for 2005. Sleep. 2005 Apr 1;28(4):499–523.
7. Thomas SJ, Gamble K, Harding SM, et al. Actigraphy in the evaluation of sleep disorders. UpToDate; Jan 17, 2020. [Internet]. Available from: https://0-www.uptodate.com.mylibrary. qu.edu.qa/contents/actigraphy-in-the-evaluation-of-sleep-disorders?search=sleep%20actigraphy&sectionRank= 1&usage_type=default&anchor=H2666349229&source= machineLearning&selectedTitle=1~150&display_rank=1# H1757092177 (accessed 15 May 2020).
8. Ancoli-Israel S, Cole R, Alessi C, et al. The role of actigraphy in the study of sleep and circadian rhythms. Sleep. 2003;26(3):342–92.
9. Sadeh A, Acebo C. The role of actigraphy in sleep medicine. Sleep Med Rev. 2002;6(2):113–24.
10. Kapur VK, Auckley DH, Chowdhuri S, et al. Clinical practice guideline for diagnostic testing for adult obstructive sleep apnea: an American Academy of Sleep Medicine clinical practice guideline. J Clin Sleep Med. 2017 Mar 15;13(3):479–504.
11. Khosla S, Deak MC, Gault D, et al. Consumer sleep technology: an American Academy of Sleep Medicine position statement. J Clin Sleep Med. 2018;14(5):877–80.
12. Prihodova I, Paclt I, Kemlink D, et al. Sleep disorders and daytime sleepiness in children with attention-deficit/hyperactivity disorder: a two-night polysomnographic study with a multiple sleep latency test. Sleep Med. 2010 Oct 1;11(9):922–8.

13. Bruyneela M, Liberta W, Ameyeb L, et al. Comparison between home and hospital set-up for unattended home-based polysomnography: a prospective randomized study. Sleep Med. 2015;16(1):1434–8.

14. Ancoli-Israel S, Martin JL, Blackwell T, et al. The SBSM guide to actigraphy monitoring: clinical and research applications. Behav Sleep Med. 2015 Jul 17;13(Sup 1):S4–38.

15. AARC-APT (American Association of Respiratory Care-Association of Polysomnography Technologists) clinical practice guideline. Polysomnography. Respir Care. 1995;40(12):1336–43.

16. Corral J, Sánchez-Quiroga MÁ, Carmona-Bernal C, et al. Conventional polysomnography is not necessary for the management of most patients with suspected obstructive sleep apnea. Noninferiority, randomized controlled trial. Am J Resp Crit Care Med. 2017;196(9):1181–90.

17. Pietzsch JB, Garner A, Cipriano LE, et al. An integrated health-economic analysis of diagnostic and therapeutic strategies in the treatment of moderate-to-severe obstructive sleep apnea. Sleep. 2011;34(6):695–709.

18. Pack AI. Does laboratory polysomnography yield better outcomes than home sleep testing? Chest. 2015;148(2):306.

19. Noor ZM, Smith AJ, Smith SS, et al. A feasibility study: use of actigraph to monitor and follow-up sleep/wake patterns in individuals attending community pharmacy with sleeping disorders. J Pharm Bioallied Sci. 2016;8(3):173–80.

2. Bright Light Therapy

a. Background

Bright light therapy (BLT) is a nonpharmacological treatment recommended primarily for major depressive disorder with seasonal pattern, also known as seasonal affective disorder (SAD).[1] The concept of using BLT to address mood disorders associated with changes in the circadian rhythm due to increased number of hours of darkness during winter months started in the early 1980s. Since then, BLT has also been used in the management of sleep/wake disorders (e.g., jet lag, shift work), bulimia nervosa, and adult attention-deficit/hyperactivity disorder (adult ADHD).[2] It has been demonstrated that light affects mood in several ways, particularly by modulating serotonin activity and other monoaminergic pathways in several regions of the brain, enhancing alertness, and regulating sleep homeostasis.[1] These effects of light therapy on mood depend on several factors such as light intensity, wavelength spectrum, illumination duration, time of the day, and individual circadian rhythms.[3]

b. Device Description

BLT is classically delivered through a light box containing fluorescent lamp tubes, a reflector, and a diffusing screen. Light boxes have filters that remove ultraviolet (UV) light to reduce risk of eye or skin damage. White light is recommended. Some lamps claim to provide "full-spectrum light"; however, there is no known advantage to their use. They also produce different intensities of light. The intensity of light is measured in units known as "lux." Ideally, the device for bright light therapy should provide light of 10,000 lux intensity.

c. Various Versions/Generations

Different models are available with varying shapes, sizes, and light intensities. Larger-sized lamps are recommended because as the apparatus becomes smaller, the field of illumination narrows, and even small changes in head position can substantially reduce the intensity of light that reaches the eyes. This problem is a liability of recently marketed miniature lighting devices.[3]

BLT may also be administered through light glasses or visors and dawn simulators. Light visors (or helmets) are portable head-mounted light sources whereas dawn simulators offer natural dawn conditions. However, these have not been as well studied and are not recommended at this time. Figure 7.11 illustrates a few models of light boxes available on the market.

d. Purposes of Use, Proper Use or Operation, and Operational Requirements

The person sits in front of the light box with his/her eyes open. Depending on the treating condition, the person will sit at a specified distance and for a specified duration. It should be noted that the light intensity specified for the lamp (e.g., 10,000 lux) is at a particular distance as specified by the manufacturer. If the person using the lamp sits at a distance greater than that specified by the manufacturer,

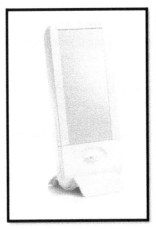
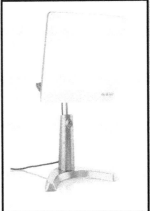
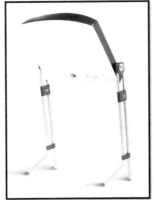
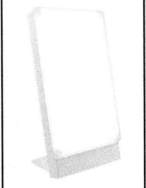

FIGURE 7.11 Light therapy devices.

the intensity of the light received will be less. Only a few devices can provide 10,000 lux at 18 inches or more. Other devices require the person's face to be only 12 inches from the device in order to receive the full 10,000 lux intensity of light.

e. Interpretation of Readings

Table 7.5 summarizes the guidelines for BLT in the management of different mood disorders. BLT treatment for SAD may begin with exposition duration of 30 min, using a light intensity of 10,000 lux. Early morning administration offers greater chances for remission.[1] Measured at eye level, a therapeutic distance of 60–80 cm from the light box can be seen as standard requirements. Lower intensities also appear to be effective, but need longer exposure durations: 2,500 lux for 2 hrs/day, 5,000 lux for 1 hr/day. Significant effects appear only at 2–3 weeks of treatment. Treatment is usually continued until the time of usual spontaneous remission in the spring or summer.

f. Important Safety Issues

BLT is well tolerated, although some people report experiencing headache, eyestrain, nausea, and agitation. These usually subside after several days of treatment. If persistent, they can be reduced or eliminated with dose decreases. Some people have reported the emergence of sleep disturbances, which may indicate a need for adjustment of treatment timing: if evening light is scheduled too late, one often sees initial insomnia and hyperactivation. If morning light is timed too early, one often sees premature awakening with the inability to resume sleep.[3] Rarely have patients discontinued treatment due to side effects. It is contraindicated in case of ophthalmic disorders (cataract, macular degeneration, glaucoma, and retinitis pigmentosa) and disorders affecting the retina (retinopathy, diabetes, herpes, etc.). It is recommended that individuals at risk should have pretreatment ophthalmological examinations.[3] Use of photosensitizing drugs (e.g., hydrochlorothiazide, lithium, tetracycline, or tricyclic antidepressants) should be avoided.[4]

g. Important Features and Special Advantages

Advantages:

a. The main advantage of using BLT is that it is low-cost, home-based, easy to use, and it has a lower side effect profile when compared to pharmacotherapy.

b. Unlike pharmacological agents, it is fast acting in the acute phase of depression (within 1–3 weeks) which will help to improve adherence of patients to the treatment. The results of a meta-analysis on 419 patients with bipolar or major depression showed significant improvement of symptoms within the first week of treatment when they received light therapy as an add-on therapy.[5]

TABLE 7.5

Guidelines for Bright Light Therapy in the Management of Mood Disorders

Features	Recommendations
Recommended treatment	• Seasonal: First line of treatment as monotherapy or as adjuvant to pharmacotherapy
	• Nonseasonal: As adjuvant to pharmacotherapy (antidepressant)
	• Bipolar depression: As adjuvant to pharmacotherapy (mood stabilizer)
Light box	• Fluorescent light box using light intensities from 2,500 to 10,000 lux is the preferred device for light therapy
	• Full spectrum visible light with ultraviolet light filter
Lamp position	• At eye level, at a distance of 60–80 cm (depending on the light box used; check manufacturer's recommendations)
	• No need to stare into the light
Dose and frequency	• Seasonal and nonseasonal depression: First line 10,000 lux for 30 min/day or 2,500 lux for 2 hrs/day
	• Bipolar depression: Initiate slowly (2,500–5,000 lux for 2/1 hr/day, respectively), monitor for manic switch
Time of day	• As early as possible (e.g., before/during breakfast) because morning light is more effective than evening light
	• Bipolar depression: Midday (especially if there is a history of manic switch)
Onset of action	• Usually 1 week, although some patients may respond as early as 3 days
Treatment duration	• Seasonal depression: Until spontaneous symptom remission (usually spring or summer)
	• Nonseasonal depression: 2–5 weeks
	• Bipolar depression: Until reduction of depressive symptoms
Duration of therapeutic effect	• Symptom recurrence shortly after stopping therapy
Non-response	• Ensure patient adherence to treatment
	• If there is insufficient response after two treatment weeks, the dose should be doubled to 30 min in the morning plus 30 min in the evening
	• Consider adjuvant pharmacological treatment if patients continue non-responsive
Side effect	• Mild: headache, eyestrain, nausea, insomnia, agitation
	• Manic switch in seasonal and bipolar depression
Contraindication	• Ophthalmic disorder

Adapted from: Maruani J., et al. *Front Psychiatry*. 2019; 10:85 and Pail G., et al. *Neuropsychobiology*. 2011; 64:152–162.

c. This treatment modality may be advantageous for certain populations who may not be suitable candidates for depression pharmacotherapy, such as prenatal and geriatric patients. The efficacy of light therapy in perinatal depression has been reported in only five published studies, which have produced mixed results.[6] The sample size of these studies was small, and compliance of patients was questionable. Results of a systematic review on the use of light therapy in the geriatric population showed significant improvement of depression when compared to other treatment alternatives.[7]

Disadvantages:

The main limitation of light therapy is the high rate of relapse by discontinuation of treatment. Because of this, in the management of mood disorders in particular, it is recommended to combine this method with pharmacotherapy.[4]

h. Special Tips for Patient Counseling if a Device Is Used for Self-Care

Instructions for the use of BLT vary depending on the condition for which it will be used, and also on the specific manufacturer's recommendations. Several examples of what should be included in a patient information leaflet about BLT are available in the internet. The following information should be covered when counseling a patient about BLT:

- What is BLT?
- How does BLT work?
- What light box should be used?
- How should a light box be used?
- How long will BLT take to work?
- What are the side effects of BLT?
- What are the contraindications for BLT?
- For how long should BLT be used?

i. Available Evidence on Effectiveness and Safety

Various randomized controlled trials (RCTs) on BLT use in SAD and nonseasonal depression suggest it is efficacious, with effect sizes equivalent to those in most antidepressant pharmacotherapy trials. However, many of these reports were not based on rigorous study designs (e.g., adequate group sizes, randomized assignment, defining parameters of active versus placebo conditions), which are necessary to evaluate light therapy for mood disorders. Nevertheless, BLT is now widely considered as first-line treatment of SAD. Specifically, two meta-analyses of eight randomized blinded and controlled studies (n = 703 total) were consistent in demonstrating that BLT showed efficacy in treatment of SAD when compared to a control condition.[8,9]

Several studies have been conducted on the effectiveness of BLT in treating nonseasonal depression. In the most recent meta-analysis, nine trials demonstrated that use of BLT led to a significant reduction of nonseasonal depressive symptoms (standard mean difference = −0.62, 95% CI −0.88 to −0.35, p < 0.001).[10] Studies comparing the effect of antidepressants alone to antidepressants plus BLT treatment in nonseasonal depression have reported similar positive results.[11,12]

Several studies and case reports have evaluated the use of BLT for bipolar depression. Overall, evidence suggests that it is effective and well tolerated, and enhances the remission rate as an adjunct treatment for bipolar depression. However, the number of participants in these studies is small, and there is no uniformity of methodology or patient selection.[13] A meta-analysis of nine studies of the efficacy of BLT in the treatment of bipolar depression showed a reduction in disease severity in patients treated with either BLT monotherapy or in combination with other treatments (effect size = −0.69, 95% CI −0.90 to −0.48, p < 0.001).[14] A 2018 systematic review conducted to find out about the rate of switching to manic phase in bipolar patients who used BLT as adjuvant reported a relatively small switch rate of 4.2%, compared to a switch rate of 15–40% reported with antidepressant drug treatment.[15]

j. Economic Evaluation

Only one economic study conducted in 2012 is available in which the direct mental healthcare costs of using BLT were compared with the use of fluoxetine in patients with SAD. The result of this study shows that using pharmacological treatment has low mental healthcare direct cost unless the amortized cost of the light box is considered. Further cost-effectiveness studies are needed.[16]

k. Implication to the Pharmacy Profession and Pharmacy Practice

As health professionals, community pharmacists in particular are in an ideal position to provide information on light boxes. Having a basic understanding of how these devices work and how these should be used is important so that they can provide this information to patients. In particular, pharmacists should be aware of the following before educating patients on BLT[17]:

- Light box selection criteria: There are many different types of light boxes available. Light boxes can be purchased at most department stores and online. The price of a light box can range from forty to several hundred dollars. Bigger and more intense light boxes are usually more expensive. When selecting a light box or related BLT treatment apparatus, the Center for Environmental Therapeutics recommends consideration of the following factors: clinical efficacy, ocular and dermatologic safety, and visual comfort.[18] The light box selected should emit full-spectrum white light with UV filter. The newest filters use LED, which is less expensive and more durable. A light box that emits white light is preferable. Many wavelengths of light are used in light boxes. White light has been researched the most. Blue light may also be effective, but there is less research to support using blue light. Also, white light causes fewer eye side effects than blue light.[17]

- Selecting a dose: The dose received is determined by the intensity emitted from the light source, distance from the light box, and duration of exposure. A higher-intensity box will require less time per day. A 10,000 lux light box is recommended. The intensity of light boxes that work best range from 2,500–10,000 lux. A box less than 2,500 lux will not be helpful. A box that has more than 10,000 lux is not more helpful and will still require 30 minutes of daily exposure. Patients need not stare directly into the light source as long as the light is able to meet the eye at an angle of 30° to 60°. The upper limit of midday light is 45 to 60 minutes, beyond which patients are more likely to have difficulty with adherence. For patients who respond to BLT, it is reasonable to continue light therapy for 12 months after remission to prevent relapses, similar to the recommendations for antidepressant therapy.
- Monitoring for adverse effects: Generally, BLT is well tolerated. Adverse effects are rare; the most common ones include headache, eyestrain, nausea, and agitation. Light boxes with larger screens cause fewer eye side effects than do small ones. Adverse effects tend to remit spontaneously or after dose reduction. Evening administration of BLT may increase the incidence of sleep disturbances. Like other biologic treatments for bipolar depression, BLT can precipitate manic/hypomanic and mixed states in susceptible patients, although the light dose can be titrated against emergent symptoms of hypomania.[13]

l. Challenges to the Pharmacists and Users

As explained previously, the beneficial effects of light therapy depend on the intensity, spectral composition, duration, and timing of light exposure. To facilitate or cue light exposure that is correctly timed and of adequate duration, modifications to the daily routine (lifestyle and occupational routine) will often be needed. These are not often considered within BLT protocols, and the most convenient and effective fit or compromise between current life circumstances and optimal light exposure requires personalization. Because BLT is applied over a prolonged period of time (typically 30 minutes or more, daily), compliance with the treatment regimen may be challenging. The associated time, effort, and organization burden can impact treatment adherence as well as quality of life which should not be ignored. It has been suggested that light interventions are similar to dietary interventions, wherein individual baseline consumption should be considered.[19] As such, everyone has a light consumption baseline which will have to be manipulated in a personalized manner. What manipulations are likely to be beneficial as well as tolerable will depend upon baseline light exposure patterns, circadian phase, sleep timing, and other aspects of lifestyle and occupational routines.

Overall, there is also a need for guidelines and evidence-based protocols for the use of BLT in psychiatric disorders, which makes this type of treatment more challenging than pharmacotherapy.

m. Recommendations: The Way Forward

The accumulated data on BLT for SAD and nonseasonal depression support its broad application in clinical practice. Clinicians should consider adjunctive light therapy when the response to antidepressants is delayed or incomplete. At the same time, further research is needed to clarify mechanisms of action that complement circadian rhythm phase shifting to produce the antidepressant effect. The promise of automated treatment delivery during sleep, removing the challenge of behavioral compliance, motivates further investigation of dawn simulation. Furthermore, examining the dynamic light exposure of an individual at baseline might enable more targeted light exposure recommendations.

Measurement and reporting of many indicators of acceptability of BLT is inconsistent or limited and should be explored in future research. Improved measurement and reporting of acceptability and adherence-related factors may help to optimize adherence, reduce burden, and improve user experiences. This may in turn contribute toward improved intervention effectiveness.[19]

Further research is also needed on its effectiveness in other psychiatric disorders and on its use in special populations such as the elderly, children, and pregnant women.

n. Conclusions

BLT represents a nonpharmacological, efficacious, and well-tolerated, treatment primarily for seasonal and nonseasonal mood disorders. BLT in treating mood disorders is characterized by rapid and sustained effects both in mono- and adjunct therapy, combined with antidepressants. The side effect profile is favorable in comparison with medications. In view of the wide variety of light boxes available on the market, pharmacists are in an ideal position to advise patients on how to select and use light boxes, as well as to educate them on their efficacy and safety profile. To maximize adherence to treatment, BLT interventions should be optimized to best fit routines, personal values, and social context.

o. Lessons Learned

- BLT is a noninvasive, low-cost treatment option for the management of seasonal and nonseasonal mood disorders, with a definite biological action comparable with antidepressant medication.
- These effects of light therapy on mood depend on several factors such as light intensity, wavelength spectrum, illumination duration, time of the day, and individual circadian rhythms.
- Different models are available with varying shapes, sizes, and light intensities. Pharmacists are

in an ideal position to help patients select the most suitable light box, as well as provide information on how these devices work and how they should be used.

ACKNOWLEDGEMENTS

The author would like to acknowledge the help of the following individuals who took part in the literature review required to write this chapter. Without their support, this chapter would not have become a reality.

Mahtab M. Noorizadeh, PharmD, Research Assistant, College of Pharmacy, Qatar University

Shimaa A. Aboelbaha, BScPharm, MSc Candidate, Research Assistant, College of Pharmacy, Qatar University

REFERENCES

Section 2: Bright Light Therapy

1. Maruani J, Geoffroy PA. Bright light as a personalized precision treatment of mood disorders. Front Psychiatry. 2019;10:85.
2. Pail G, Huf W, Pjrek E, et al. Bright-light therapy in the treatment of mood disorders. Neuropsychobiology. 2011;64:152–62.
3. Terman M, Terman JS. Light therapy for seasonal and nonseasonal depression: efficacy, protocol, safety, and side effects. CNS Spectr. 2005;10:647–63.
4. Avery D, Roy-Byrne PP, Solomon D. Seasonal affective disorder: treatment. UpToDate; June 28, 2020. [Internet]. Available from: www.uptodate.com/contents/seasonal-affective-disorder-treatment.
5. Al-Karawi D, Jubair L. Bright light therapy for nonseasonal depression: meta-analysis of clinical trials. J Affect Disord. 2016;198:64–71.
6. Crowley SK, Youngstedt SD. Efficacy of light therapy for perinatal depression: a review. J Physiol Anthropol. 2012 Dec;31(1):1–7.
7. Chang CH, Liu CY, Chen SJ, et al. Efficacy of light therapy on nonseasonal depression among elderly adults: a systematic review and meta-analysis. Neuropsychiatric Dis Treat. 2018;14:3091.
8. Golden RN, Gaynes BN, Ekstrom RD, et al. The efficacy of light therapy in the treatment of mood disorders: a review and meta-analysis of the evidence. Am J Psychiatry. 2005;162(4):656–62.
9. Martensson B, Pettersson A, Berglund L, et al. Bright white light therapy in depression: a critical review of the evidence. J Affect Disord. 2015;182:1–7.
10. Al-Karawi D, Jubair L. Bright light therapy for nonseasonal depression: metaanalysis of clinical trials. J Affect Disord. 2016;198:64–71.
11. Guzel Ozdemir P, Boysan M, Smolensky MH, et al. Comparison of venlafaxine alone versus venlafaxine plus bright light therapy combination for severe major depressive disorder. J Clin Psychiatry. 2015;76(5):e645–54.
12. Lam RW, Levitt AJ, Levitan RD, et al. Efficacy of bright light treatment, fluoxetine, and the combination in patients with nonseasonal major depressive disorder: a randomized clinical trial. JAMA Psychiatry. 2016;73(1):56–63.
13. Nasr SJ. Bright light therapy for bipolar depression. Curr Psychiatry. 2018;17(11):28–32.
14. Tseng PT, Chen YW, Tu KY, et al. Light therapy in the treatment of patients with bipolar depression: a meta-analytic study. Eur Neuropsychopharmacol. 2016;26(6):1037–47.
15. Benedetti F. Rate of switch from bipolar depression into mania after morning light therapy: a historical review. Psychiatry Res. 2018;261:351–6.
16. Cheung A, Dewa C, Michalak EE, et al. Direct health care costs of treating seasonal affective disorder: a comparison of light therapy and fluoxetine. Depress Res Treat. 2012;2012:628434. https://doi.org/10.1155/2012/628434.
17. Center for Environmental Therapeutics. [Internet]. Available from: www.cet.org/. Center for Environmental Therapeutics (accessed 30 June 2020).
18. University of Wisconsin. School of Medidine and Public Health. Bright light therapy: a non-drug way to treat depression and sleep problems. [Internet]. Available from: www.fammed.wisc.edu/files/webfm-uploads/documents/outreach/im/handout_light_therapy.pdf (accessed 30 June 2020).
19. Faulknerab SM, Dijkcd DJ, Drakeab RJ, et al. Adherence and acceptability of light therapies to improve sleep in intrinsic circadian rhythm sleep disorders and neuropsychiatric illness: a systematic review. Sleep Health. 12 Mar 2020. Available from: www.sciencedirect.com/science/article/pii/S2352721820300619#bib17 (accessed 30 June 2020).

8 Medical Devices for Neurology

Abderrezzaq Soltani

CONTENTS

DOI: 10.1201/9781003002345-10

GENERAL INTRODUCTION

The industry of medical devices with diagnostic and therapeutic applications including the modulation neurological disorders and brain-machine interfaces with neuroenhancement purposes is a very dynamic field; thousands of medical- and commercial-grade neurosystems are being introduced into the market every year. The dramatic increase in licensed neurodevices is attributed to the ever-increasing demand for improved patient outcomes and quality of life in an aging population with greater predisposition to neurological disorders. It is also propelled by the ground-breaking advances in data processing, machine learning, and modern robotics.

There is general scientific and clinical consensus on the merits of existing pharmacotherapeutic agents in modulating specific aspects of various neurological conditions. However, despite the considerable progress made in designing effective pharmacological interventions, the need for alternative safer approaches which offer more effective symptomatic relief and greater neuroprotective/neurorestorative potential is undeniable. Neurotechnology presents a fascinating and debate-provoking approach which offers exciting avenues to fulfil such unmet needs.

Neurotechnology encompasses a wide array of instruments and methods which provide an interface that directly connects technical elements such as electrodes, intelligent prostheses, and computers to the nervous system. These closed-loop systems can either monitor and record brain signals, translating them for diagnostic and therapeutic applications (*readout* systems), or they can be used to apply electrical or electromagnetic stimuli to modulate/overwrite brain activity (*stimulation* systems). Recording *electrodes* can either be placed directly/via a cap on the surface of the head in a *noninvasive* approach or, if high-resolution electrodes are used, can be part of an implantable neurosystem with greater precision. The latter electrodes have recording and stimulatory capabilities (inhibitory or excitatory) and are placed deep inside the brain in specific regions/nuclei via an *invasive* neurosurgical procedure.

The recording/stimulatory electrodes in implanted devices are wirelessly connected to a computing device for signal processing purposes in order to offer prompt and precise control over the electrical stimulus. Enhancements in biomaterials, modern robotics, and machine learning aim to optimize these implanted neurotechnologies by optimizing their stability and biocompatibility, while also conferring a degree of autonomy to these devices for greater adaptability in interpreting and modulating brain activity.

The evidence for the clinical effectiveness of neurological devices is compelling and well documented; both as complementary approaches to standard pharmaceutical methods, or as viable alternatives when standard care no longer offers sufficient therapeutic control, as discussed in the next sections. The highly complex and intricate neurotechnology-based interferences with brain activity raise inevitable ethical and anthropological questions nonetheless. These stem from a number of issues including unsubstantiated claims over neuroenhancement from licensed consumer-grade neurodevices, the concept of self-mechanization by implanting autonomous artificial intelligence into the brain; or importantly, inadvertent neuropsychiatric and neurocognitive changes secondary to neurostimulation which could, in theory, precipitate transient or irreversible alterations in the patient's character traits and/or behavioral patterns. There is an ongoing ethical debate between proponents and detractors over the impact of such interventions on the patient's personal identity or "personhood." While implicit and explicit personality and character changes are evidenced and recognized, there is tacit assumption that, from philosophical and ethical perspectives, the patient's personal identity is not compromised. Identity is used here as the reference is to a person's self-consciousness, responsibility, integrity, accountability, and privacy. It is therefore of paramount importance that such alterations caused by neurotechnological interventions are investigated for greater clarity by comprehensive psychological and cognitive assessment in order to establish universally accepted ethical standards to govern the marketing of neurosystems.

Compared to pharmacological interventions which have been validated and robust mechanisms to evaluate their cost-effectiveness, the economic evaluations of neurodevices are still under scrutiny. This is especially prudent given that the current regulatory framework of neurotechnologies is still in its infancy compared to established standard pharmaceutical practice. High-level and timely clinical evidence (a prerequisite for a thorough economic evaluation of neurosystems) is hindered by the current regulatory environment which has less-stringent rules compared to standard care. There is also a need to design fit-for-purpose neurotechnology assessment methods and reimbursement strategies which take into account determinants of device effectiveness and aspects of reusability to permit valid and reliable cost analyses.

In the next subsections, we will explore the pathophysiological and therapeutic rationale behind the clinical use of medical devices which employ various neurotechnical methods. The operational aspects of the licensed devices and their clinical and cost-effectiveness will be explored and reviewed and the role of a pharmacist highlighted in maximizing the sought clinical benefit and minimizing the risk of adverse events commonly experienced with these systems.

PART 1: ANALGESIC TRANSCUTANEOUS ELECTRICAL NERVE STIMULATION (TENS) FOR PAIN MODULATION

A) BACKGROUND

Transcutaneous electrical nerve stimulation (TENS) devices provide a cost-effective nonpharmacological treatment pathway for acute and chronic pain conditions. They mediate pain modulation by targeting the A-alpha and A-beta subtypes of the large-diameter primary afferent fibers [peripheral mechanism].[1,2] The stimulation of the afferent input is transmitted to the central nervous system [central activation theory][3,4] leading to the activation of the descending inhibitory pathways (which originate in the midbrain and terminate in the spinal dorsal horn).[5] These TENS-mediated antihyperalgesic effects [central mechanism] are a result of stimulating opioid,[5] cholinergic,[6] adrenergic,[7] GABAergic,[8] and serotoninergic[9] receptors in the rostral ventromedial medulla (RVM), periaqueductal gray (PAG), and the spinal dorsal horn neuron which translate into antinociception.[5,10–12] It has also been shown that high-frequency (HF) TENS leads to increasing the release of β-endorphins and methionine-enkephalins in the cerebrospinal fluid.[13,14] Several lines of experimental evidence have proposed the reduction in the excitability of peripheral nociceptors (by reducing substance P and blockade of peripheral opioid receptors) as possible pathways justifying the analgesic effects of TENS.[15,16]

B) DEVICE DESCRIPTION/IMPORTANT FEATURES

The TENS device is a small portable battery-powered machine which delivers nonpainful low-voltage but

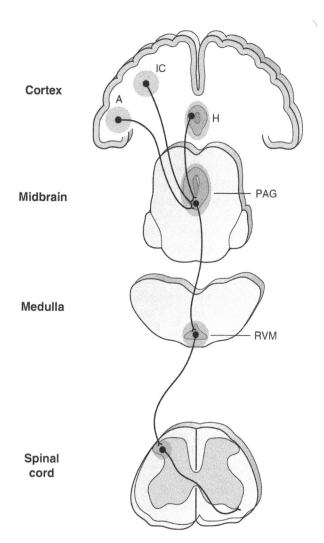

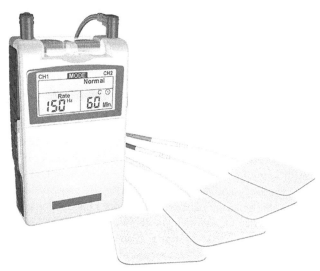

FIGURE 8.2   Med-Fit Dual Channel TENS machine with pads.

Source: Courtesy of tensmachineuk.com; used with permission.

c)   Purpose and Use

The device is designed for self-care during which the user has full control over adjusting the settings. An initial assessment consultation with the doctor is recommended to explore the viability of using the device prior to referral to a pain clinic or physiotherapist. The machine can be used multiple times daily (commonly three times daily) with a session interval between 20 and 45 mins.[17–19] It is always advisable to follow the precise instructions supplied by the manufacturer considering the various types of TENS devices available on the market. The wearable nature of the technological kit makes it easier for the user to either tuck the device into a pocket or clip it onto a belt, depending on the brand. The electrodes are designed as self-adhesive or flexible rubber pads that require applying a thin layer of conductive gel. Pain relief is attained by finetuning the intensity via the TENS dial, the frequency, commonly using preset programs, and duration expressed in number of microseconds that the current enters the skin during each electrical pulse. The intensity of the pulse can be adjusted using the dial on the device and 100 Hz frequency being generally recommended as the starting point prior to increasing the frequency progressively until a tingling sensation is felt (strong but comfortable).[17,18] After a few minutes, the tingling sensation should fade as the pain-relief mechanisms reach full effect. Different brands provide various pre-set programs for specific conditions. However, the optimal settings vary from one patient to another even if they have the same type of pain.

d)   Important Safety Issues (Cautions and Common Adverse Effects)

Several lines of investigation have demonstrated that TENS could play a positive role in reducing pain for women in

FIGURE 8.1   The descending pain control system and sites of antinociception in the rostral ventromedial medulla (RVM), peri-aqueductal gray (PAG), and the spinal dorsal horn neuron.

Source: Used with permission from Rang and Dale's Pharmacology, 8th edition, Rang HP, Ritter JM, Flower RJ, Henderson G, figure 42.4 p513, Copyright Elsevier (2016).

strong-intensity electrical currents via cutaneous electrodes in form of adhesive pads that are positioned in the proximity of the pain-afflicted area(s). TENS machines can deliver high- or low-frequency pulse rates to mediate pulse modulation. High-frequency pulses (90–130 Hz) are the most commonly used therapeutically; they modulate pain via the central activation theory which involves the descending inhibitory pathways.[3,4] Low-frequency pulses (2–5 Hz) on the other hand are thought to exhibit their antinociceptive effects via the release of endorphins.[14] The patient-friendly device is relatively inexpensive with prices ranging from £10 to £200 with no significant difference in pain outcomes between different brands. TENS devices are widely available in primary care, and can be purchased over the counter in retail shops including community pharmacies.

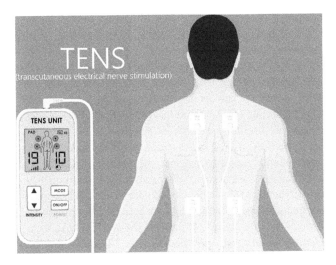

FIGURE 8.3 Example of pad placement for a digital TENS unit and the adjustable modalities to finetune the intensity, frequency, and duration.

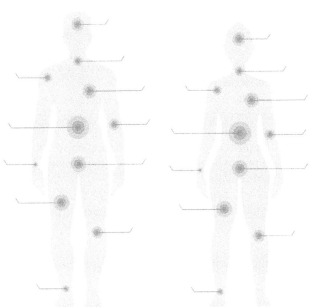

FIGURE 8.4 Site of TENS acupoints to attain optimal antinociceptive effects.

labor.[20] Nonetheless, a consultation with the midwife/obstetrician is warranted prior to considering the use of the device. The electrode pads could cause local skin irritation, for which it is recommended that the site of application is rotated with pads repositioned regularly. Alternatively, a different hypoallergenic pad may be used.[17,18] The pads are not suitable for application in front or the side of the neck, inside the mouth, on the temples, or close to eyes.[18] It is also advisable to avoid using the TENS device in the shower or while operating heavy machinery. The cohort of patient groups who are advised against using TENS machines to relieve pain include patients with pacemakers (or implantable cardioverter defibrillator [ICD]), epilepsy, or arrythmias; pregnant women (especially in the first trimester); patients with undiagnosed pain or pain caused by varicose veins or originating from a site with previous surgery involving metal inserts (e.g., screws, wires, and implants).[17,18,21]

E) STORAGE CONDITIONS AND MAINTENANCE

The "self-adhesive" electrode pads should not be washed with water after use. The device should never be immersed in water. The unit should be stored in a cool and dry place. The average storage life of the electrodes is 2 years but varies depending on the brand. If the device is unlikely to be used for a long period, then it is advisable to remove the batteries from the TENS unit to avoid the potential leakage of corrosive fluid.

F) IMPORTANT FEATURES (CAPABILITIES AND LIMITATIONS) AND SPECIAL ADVANTAGES

TENS devices are portable, noninvasive, easy to use, and side effect free compared to pharmacological interventions

if used according to the manufacturer's supplied instructions. They can be used alone or in combination with pharmacotherapy which could have long-term benefits in reducing the intake of analgesics.[22,23] It is important to note that they are not suitable for all types of pain. They are commonly used to manage musculoskeletal or neuropathic pain such as chronic back pain and knee joint arthritis. Analgesic tolerance to repeated application of the same frequency (HF or LF), same intensity, and pulse duration for chronic pain conditions has been reported.[24] This issue can be circumvented by increasing the pulse intensity to the highest tolerated level,[25,26] modulating between high and low frequencies,[27] or using adjunct pharmacotherapy which inhibits NMDA and glutamate receptors.[28] The positioning of electrodes plays a pivotal role in defining the treatment success. It has been shown that the application of TENS on acupoints is more effective than on nonacupoint sites.[29] This involves the application of electrodes on traditional acupuncture points which is thought to augment the antinociceptive effects of TENS by combining the pain-modulating effects of acupuncture.

G) SPECIAL TIPS FOR PATIENT COUNSELING

- Ensure that the device is switched off prior to placing the electrode pads onto the skin area in proximity to the site of pain.
- The site of application should be clean and dry with no signs of damaged skin including cuts, grazes, ulceration, or lesions reducing pain sensation.

- To test that the device is working appropriately, hold the pads between the fingers, switch the machine on and you should feel a tingling sensation.
- Place the self-adhesive pads on the surface of either side of the affected site (2.5 cm apart) and use a tape to ensure they are fixed on the site if you intend to move around.[18]
- Do not turn the frequency too high because it may cause overstimulation which in turn could aggravate the pain.
- A frequency of 80–100 Hz and duration of 100–200 microseconds are usually recommended as initial settings.
- Once you complete using the device for the day, turn the device off, then carefully remove the pads and clean the application site.

H) EVIDENCE OF EFFECTIVENESS AND SAFETY

Several high-quality studies including randomized clinical trials (RCTs), systematic reviews and meta-analyses have explored the clinical effectiveness of TENS in managing pain associated with several specific conditions including acute pain,[30,31] postoperative pain,[22,32,33] osteoarthritis pain,[34–36] low back pain,[37–39] cancer pain,[40,41] and pain associated with diabetic neuropathy.[42,43] While the accumulated body of evidence points to the excellent safety profile of TENS intervention compared to pharmaceutical measures, the studies are differing and conflicting in drawing conclusions regarding the effectiveness of the approach. Multiple systematic reviews and meta-analyses reported that TENS is ineffective or, at best, results are inconclusive to establish TENS efficacy in pain relief.[34,37,44] Contrastingly, several lines of high-quality clinical evidence have reported significant reduction in pain compared to placebo in multiple conditions including postoperative pain,[22] acute pain,[45,46] lower back pain,[38] and diabetic neuropathy.[42] Bjordal and co-workers also demonstrated that TENS helps in reducing analgesic intake.[22] More recently, emerging evidence is growing in support of use of TENS to alleviate pain associated with fibromyalgia[47] and spinal cord injury.[48]

The lack of consistency in the body of evidence stems from the fundamental differences in the population homogeneity and the adopted dosing regimen (including placement of electrodes, and the frequency, intensity, and duration of TENS application). There is a clear need for further well-designed investigations to provide conclusive results on TENS efficacy.

I) ECONOMIC EVALUATION (COST-EFFECTIVENESS)

There is limited information available on the cost-effectiveness of TENS across the conditions wherein clinical efficacy was demonstrated with varying degrees as discussed previously. One of the instruments used to establish the cost-effectiveness of TENS is the EuroQol-5D (EQ5D). This instrument measures the quality of life in Europe based on 5 dimensions: mobility, self-care, usual activities, pain/discomfort, and anxiety/depression. Using the threshold criteria (EQ5D) adopted by the National Institute for Health and Care Excellence (NICE), the economic evaluation of TENS to manage pain in osteoarthritis of the knee from 88 RCTs including 7,507 patients has shown that TENS is cost-effective at thresholds of £20–30,000 per Quality Adjusted Life Years ($QALY_{EQ5D}$) as described by NICE guidance with an incremental cost-effectiveness ratio (ICER) of £2,690 per QALY against usual care.[49] Paradoxically, a study assessing TENS cost-effectiveness as adjunct to standard primary care management of tennis elbow in a multicenter pragmatic 2-armed RCT involving 241 patients showed that $QALY_{EQ5D}$ outcomes point to adverse effectiveness.[50] Tantalizingly, the same study reported that $QALY_{SF6D}$ outcomes were favorable towards TENS which indicates that not only does the degree of cost-effectiveness depend on the type of pain being managed, but also how economic health outcomes are estimated. The short-form six-dimension (SF6D) health index is based on the 36-item Short Form Health Survey (SF-36), and considered one of the most widely used generic measures of health-related quality of life (HRQoL).[51] This is more significant when considering that SF-6D is more sensitive in detecting differences in a patient's health status, medication use, and degree of disability than EQ5D.[52]

J) IMPLICATION TO THE PHARMACY PROFESSION AND PHARMACY PRACTICE

Considering the compelling evidence demonstrating clinical efficacy, albeit inconclusive, and cost-effectiveness; it is no surprise that TENS is considered an integral part of the recommended nonpharmacological measures to manage pain in an array of clinical conditions as reflected, for example, by the guidance published in the National Institute for Health and Care Excellence (NICE) in the UK and the Agency of Healthcare Research and Quality (AHRQ) in the US.[53,54] Despite the established safety profile of the device, it is paramount for the pharmacist to recognize patient groups for whom the use of TENS machines is not recommended. Providing appropriate advice on the optimal intensity and correct placement of electrodes on acupoints while emphasizing the importance of modulation between HF and LF would ensure that the risk of analgesic tolerance is reduced. Knowledge of the available brands, particularly those approved for use by recognized healthcare bodies (e.g., the National Health Service [NHS] in the UK) would ensure that the patient opts for an effective, affordable, and noninvasive approach to pain relief that is both clinically and cost-effective.

K) CHALLENGES TO PHARMACISTS AND USERS

The patient may need to optimize the settings of the TENS machine prior to attaining the full sought antihyperalgesic effect. Patients with widespread pain could also find it challenging to select the optimal area to place the electrodes.

With the exponential proliferation of TENS manufacturers, and often combining them with other nonpharmacological approaches including neuromuscular stimulation and ultrasound therapy, it is challenging to keep up to date with the underlying mechanisms and safety aspects of multiple brands which are approved by the regulatory bodies. It is therefore fundamental that pharmacists keep up to date with evidence on clinical efficacy and safety of TENS devices.

L) RECOMMENDATIONS AND THE WAY FORWARD

In order to ensure that patients attain the maximum sought antinociceptive benefits of TENS devices, pharmacists should work very closely with general practitioners, physiotherapists, and pain clinics to ensure that patients are assessed appropriately on the merit of using the complementary approach while being counseled thoroughly on using the device correctly. Despite the conflicting nature of evidence supporting TENS clinical efficacy, the current trend points towards a more prominent role of TENS in the realm of nonpharmacological interventions especially when combined with other approaches including ultrasound therapy and acupuncture.

M) CONCLUSIONS

TENS devices provide a nonpharmacological, noninvasive, and patient-friendly approach to alleviating pain. The underlying mechanism involves stimulating the afferent nerve fibers (peripheral) while potentiating the descending inhibitory pathways in the CNS (central). The correct placement of electrodes, using high-intensity pulses and alternating between high and low frequencies are crucial to maximizing the antihyperalgesic effect while reducing the risk of long-term tolerance. TENS machines have an excellent side effect free profile with some evidence of cost-effectiveness. The jury is still out on its clinical efficacy with conflicting reports of established and questionable evidence. Pharmacists could play a pivotal role in optimizing the outcomes from this self-care approach by having a good understanding of its efficacy and safety aspects and working closely with other healthcare professionals.

N) LESSONS LEARNED

- TENS machines are effective against musculoskeletal and neuropathic pain.
- When used concurrently with pharmacological interventions, they help in reducing the intake of analgesic medicines.
- TENS devices are not suitable for pregnant women (especially in the first trimester) and patients with epilepsy, arrythmias, pacemakers, and pain caused by varicose veins; or those with undiagnosed pain.
- Consult the manufacturer's guide and seek the help of a healthcare professional regarding the optimal areas of the body to which to apply the electrodes.

REFERENCES

1. Levin MF, Hui-Chan CW. Conventional and acupuncture-like transcutaneous electrical nerve stimulation excite similar afferent fibers. Arch Phys Med Rehabil [Internet]. 1993 Jan;74(1):54–60 [cited 2020 Jan 7]. Available from: www.ncbi.nlm.nih.gov/pubmed/8420521.

2. Radhakrishnan R, Sluka KA. Deep tissue afferents, but not cutaneous afferents, mediate transcutaneous electrical nerve stimulation-induced antihyperalgesia. J Pain. 2005 Oct;6(10):673–80.

3. Nardone A, Schieppati M. Influences of transcutaneous electrical stimulation of cutaneous and mixed nerves on subcortical and cortical somatosensory evoked potentials. Electroencephalogr Clin Neurophysiol Evoked Potentials. 1989;74(1):24–35.

4. Xiang L, Zhu B, Zhang S. Relationship between electroacupuncture analgesia and descending pain inhibitory mechanism of nucleus raphe magnus. Pain. 1986;24(3):383–96.

5. Kalra A, Urban MO, Sluka KA. Blockade of opioid receptors in rostral ventral medulla prevents antihyperalgesia produced by transcutaneous electrical nerve stimulation (TENS). J Pharmacol Exp Ther. 2001;298(1):257–63.

6. Radhakrishnan R, Sluka KA. Spinal muscarinic receptors are activated during low or high frequency TENS-induced antihyperalgesia in rats. Neuropharmacology. 2003;45(8):1111–19.

7. Li P, Zhuo M. Cholinergic, noradrenergic, and serotonergic inhibition of fast synaptic transmission in spinal lumbar dorsal horn of rat. Brain Res Bull [Internet]. 2001 Apr;54(6):639–47 [cited 2020 Jan 7]. Available from: www.ncbi.nlm.nih.gov/pubmed/11403990.

8. Maeda Y, Lisi TL, Vance CGT, et al. Release of GABA and activation of GABAA in the spinal cord mediates the effects of TENS in rats. Brain Res. 2007 Mar 9;1136(1):43–50.

9. Radhakrishnan R, King EW, Dickman JK, et al. Spinal 5-HT(2) and 5-HT(3) receptors mediate low, but not high, frequency TENS-induced antihyperalgesia in rats. Pain [Internet]. 2003 Sep;105(1–2):205–13 [cited 2020 Jan 7]. Available from: www.ncbi.nlm.nih.gov/pubmed/14499437.

10. Basbaum AI, Fields HL. Endogenous pain control systems: brainstem spinal pathways and endorphin circuitry [Internet]. 1984 [cited 2020 Jan 7]. Available from: www.annualreviews.org.

11. Desantana JM, Da Silva LFS, De Resende MA, et al. Transcutaneous electrical nerve stimulation at both high and low frequencies activates ventrolateral periaqueductal grey to decrease mechanical hyperalgesia in arthritic rats. Neuroscience. 2009;163(4):1233–41.

12. Dailey DL, Rakel BA, Vance CGT, et al. Transcutaneous electrical nerve stimulation reduces pain, fatigue and hyperalgesia while restoring central inhibition in primary fibromyalgia. Pain. 2013;154(11):2554–62.

13. Salar G, Job I, Mingrino S, et al. Effect of transcutaneous electrotherapy on CSF β-endorphin content in patients without pain problems. Pain. 1981;10(2):169–72.

14. Han JS, Chen XH, Sun SL, et al. Effect of low- and high-frequency TENS on Met-enkephalin-Arg-Phe and dynorphin a immunoreactivity in human lumbar CSF. Pain. 1991;47(3):295–8.

15. Rokugo T, Takeuchi T, Ito H. A histochemical study of substance P in the rat spinal cord: effect of transcutaneous

electrical nerve stimulation. J Nippon Med Sch = Nihon Ika Daigaku Zasshi. 2002;69(5):428–33.

16. Sabino GS, Santos CMF, Francischi JN, et al. Release of endogenous opioids following transcutaneous electric nerve stimulation in an experimental model of acute inflammatory pain. J Pain. 2008 Feb;9(2):157–63.

17. Rull G. TENS Machine | How does a TENS machine work? | Patient.info [Internet]. 2018 [cited 2020 Jan 8]. Available from: https://patient.info/treatment-medication/painkillers/tens-machines.

18. NHS. TENS (transcutaneous electrical nerve stimulation)—NHS [Internet]. 2018 [cited 2020 Jan 8]. Available from: www.nhs.uk/conditions/transcutaneous-electrical-nerve-stimulation-tens/.

19. Smith J. How does TENS work? | Tens Machine UK [Internet]. 2019 [cited 2020 Jan 8]. Available from: https://tensmachineuk.com/blog/post/how-does-tens-work-2.

20. Dowswell T, Bedwell C, Lavender T, et al. Transcutaneous electrical nerve stimulation (TENS) for pain management in labour. Cochrane Database Syst Rev [Internet]. 2009 Apr 15 [cited 2020 Jan 8]; Available from: http://doi.wiley.com/10.1002/14651858.CD007214.pub2.

21. GOSH. Pain relief using transcutaneous electrical nerve stimulation (TENS) | Great Ormond Street Hospital [Internet]. 2019 [cited 2020 Jan 8]. Available from: www.gosh.nhs.uk/conditions-and-treatments/procedures-and-treatments/pain-relief-using-transcutaneous-electrical-nerve-stimulation-tens.

22. Bjordal JM, Johnson MI, Ljunggreen AE. Transcutaneous electrical nerve stimulation (TENS) can reduce postoperative analgesic consumption. A meta-analysis with assessment of optimal treatment parameters for postoperative pain [Internet]. 2003 [cited 2020 Jan 9]. Available from: www.EuropeanJournalPain.com.

23. Johnson MI. Transcutaneous electrical nerve stimulation (TENS) as an adjunct for pain management in perioperative settings: a critical review. Expert Rev Neurother. Taylor and Francis Ltd. 2017;17:1013–27.

24. Liebano RE, Rakel B, Vance CGT, et al. An investigation of the development of analgesic tolerance to TENS in humans. Pain. 2011 Feb;152(2):335–42.

25. Sato KL, Sanada LS, Rakel BA, et al. Increasing intensity of TENS prevents analgesic tolerance in rats. J Pain. 2012 Sep;13(9):884–90.

26. Barlas P, Ting SLH, Chesterton LS, et al. Effects of intensity of electroacupuncture upon experimental pain in healthy human volunteers: a randomized, double-blind, placebo-controlled study. Pain. 2006 May;122(1–2):81–9.

27. DeSantana JM, Santana-Filho VJ, Sluka KA. Modulation between high- and low-frequency transcutaneous electric nerve stimulation delays the development of analgesic tolerance in arthritic rats. Arch Phys Med Rehabil. 2008 Apr;89(4):754–60.

28. Hingne PM, Sluka KA. Blockade of NMDA receptors prevents analgesic tolerance to repeated transcutaneous electrical nerve stimulation (TENS) in rats. J Pain. 2008 Mar;9(3):217–25.

29. Cheing GLY, Chan WWY. Influence of choice of electrical stimulation site on peripheral neurophysiological and hypoalgesic effects. J Rehabil Med. 2009 May;41(6):412–17.

30. Walsh DM, Howe TE, Johnson MI, et al. Transcutaneous electrical nerve stimulation for acute pain. In: Walsh DM, editor. Cochrane Database of Systematic Reviews [Internet]. Chichester, UK: John Wiley & Sons, Ltd; 2009 [cited 2020 Jan 9]. Available from: http://doi.wiley.com/10.1002/14651858.CD006142.pub2.

31. Simpson PM, Fouche PF, Thomas RE, et al. Transcutaneous electrical nerve stimulation for relieving acute pain in the prehospital setting. Eur J Emerg Med [Internet]. 2013 Jul [cited 2020 Jan 9]; 1. Available from: http://content.wkhealth.com/linkback/openurl?sid=WKPTLP:landingpage&an=00063110-900000000-99597.

32. Sbruzzi G, Silveira SA, Silva DV, et al. Transcutaneous electrical nerve stimulation after thoracic surgery: systematic review and meta-analysis of 11 randomized trials. Brazilian J Cardiovasc Surg. 2012 Mar;27(1):75–87.

33. Engen DJ, Carns PE, Allen MS, et al. Evaluating efficacy and feasibility of transcutaneous electrical nerve stimulation for postoperative pain after video-assisted thoracoscopic surgery: a randomized pilot trial. Complement Ther Clin Pract. 2016 May 1;23:141–8.

34. Rutjes AW, Nüesch E, Sterchi R, et al. Transcutaneous electrostimulation for osteoarthritis of the knee. Cochrane Database Syst Rev [Internet]. 2009 Oct 7 [cited 2020 Jan 9]; Available from: http://doi.wiley.com/10.1002/14651858.CD002823.pub2.

35. Zeng C, Li H, Yang T, et al. Electrical stimulation for pain relief in knee osteoarthritis: systematic review and network meta-analysis. Osteoarthr Cartil. 2015 Feb 1;23(2):189–202.

36. Osiri M, Welch V, Brosseau L, et al. Transcutaneous electrical nerve stimulation for knee osteoarthritis. In: Cochrane Database of Systematic Reviews. Chichester, UK: John Wiley & Sons, Ltd; 2000.

37. Khadilkar A, Odebiyi DO, Brosseau L, et al. Transcutaneous electrical nerve stimulation (TENS) versus placebo for chronic low-back pain. In: Cochrane Database of Systematic Reviews. Chichester, UK: John Wiley and Sons Ltd; 2008.

38. Machado LAC, Kamper SJ, Herbert RD, et al. Analgesic effects of treatments for non-specific low back pain: a meta-analysis of placebo-controlled randomized trials. Rheumatology. 2009;48(5):520–7.

39. Hazime FA, de Freitas DG, Monteiro RL, et al. Analgesic efficacy of cerebral and peripheral electrical stimulation in chronic nonspecific low back pain: a randomized, double-blind, factorial clinical trial. BMC Musculoskelet Disord [Internet]. 2015 Dec 31;16(1):7 [cited 2020 Jan 9]. Available from: http://bmcmusculoskeletdisord.biomedcentral.com/articles/10.1186/s12891-015-0461-1.

40. Robb KA, Bennett MI, Johnson MI, et al. Transcutaneous electric nerve stimulation (TENS) for cancer pain in adults. In: Robb KA, editor. Cochrane Database of Systematic Reviews [Internet]. Chichester, UK: John Wiley & Sons, Ltd; 2008 [cited 2020 Jan 9]. Available from: http://doi.wiley.com/10.1002/14651858.CD006276.pub2.

41. Hurlow A, Bennett MI, Robb KA, et al. Transcutaneous electric nerve stimulation (TENS) for cancer pain in adults [Internet]. In: Robb KA, editor. Cochrane Database of Systematic Reviews. Chichester, UK: John Wiley & Sons, Ltd. Available from: http://doi.wiley.com/10.1002/14651858.CD006276.pub2.

42. Jin DM, Xu Y, Geng DF, et al. Effect of transcutaneous electrical nerve stimulation on symptomatic diabetic peripheral neuropathy: a meta-analysis of randomized controlled trials. Diabetes Res Clin Pract. 2010 Jul;89(1):10–15.

43. Stein C, Eibel B, Sbruzzi G, et al. Electrical stimulation and electromagnetic field use in patients with diabetic neuropathy: systematic review and meta-analysis. Braz J Phys Ther. 2013;17:93–104.

44. Dubinsky RM, Miyasaki J. Assessment: efficacy of transcutaneous electric nerve stimulation in the treatment of pain in neurologic disorders (an evidence-based review): report of the therapeutics and technology assessment subcommittee of the American academy of neurology. Neurology. 2010;74(2):173–6.

45. Barker R, Lang T, Steinlechner B, et al. Transcutaneous electrical nerve stimulation as prehospital emergency interventional care: treating acute pelvic pain in young women. Neuromodulation Technol Neural Interface [Internet]. 2006 Apr;9(2):136–42 [cited 2020 Jan 9]. Available from: http://doi.wiley.com/10.1111/j.1525-1403.2006.00053.x.

46. Gardner SE, Blodgett NP, Hillis SL, et al. HI-TENS reduces moderate-to-severe pain associated with most wound care procedures: a pilot study. Biol Res Nurs [Internet]. 2014 Jul;16(3):310–19 [cited 2020 Jan 9]. Available from: www.ncbi.nlm.nih.gov/pubmed/23956353.

47. Carbonario F, Matsutani LA, Yuan SLK, et al. Effectiveness of high-frequency transcutaneous electrical nerve stimulation at tender points as adjuvant therapy for patients with fibromyalgia. Eur J Phys Rehabil Med. 2013 Apr;49(2):197–204.

48. Norrbrink C. Transcutaneous electrical nerve stimulation for treatment of spinal cord injury neuropathic pain. J Rehabil Res Dev. 2009;46(1):85–94.

49. Woods B, Manca A, Weatherly H, et al. Cost-effectiveness of adjunct non-pharmacological interventions for osteoarthritis of the knee. PLoS ONE. 2017 Mar 1;12(3).

50. Lewis M, Chesterton LS, Sim J, et al. An economic evaluation of TENS in addition to usual primary care management for the treatment of tennis elbow: results from the TATE randomized controlled trial. 2015 [cited 2020 Jan 9]; Available from: www.icmje.org/.

51. Brazier J, Roberts J, Deverill M. The estimation of a preference-based measure of health from the SF-36. J Health Econ. 2002 Mar 1;21(2):271–92.

52. Petrou S, Hockley C. An investigation into the empirical validity of the EQ-5D and SF-6D based on hypothetical preferences in a general population. Health Econ. 2005 Nov;14(11):1169–89.

53. NICE. Osteoarthritis: care and management Osteoarthritis: care and management clinical guideline [Internet]. 2014 [cited 2020 Jan 9]. Available from: www.nice.org.uk/guidance/cg177.

54. AHRQ. Noninvasive treatments for low back pain [Internet]. 2016 [cited 2020 Jan 9]. Available from: www.effectivehealthcare.ahrq.gov.

PART 2: DEEP BRAIN STIMULATION (DBS) TO MODULATE MOTOR FUNCTIONS AND CONTROL SEIZURES

A) BACKGROUND

Deep brain stimulation (DBS) has emerged as a viable, safe, and effective interventional treatment approach for an array of refractory neurological conditions including Parkinson's disease (PD) and epilepsy. The implantable system-mediated chronic neurostimulation targets the neural circuitry (corticostriatal-thalamocortical loops) of subcortical nuclei (hypothalamic and basal ganglia) and reversibly disrupts their abnormal function.[1,2] This is attained by shifting the oscillatory activity of the stimulated nuclei to a higher frequency in addition to addressing the aberrant electrical activity of neurons in the basal ganglia by altering their firing rate and pattern.[3–5] Therefore, it can be thought of as a brain pacemaker which addresses brain arrhythmias underlying certain neurological disorders by entraining irregular firing patterns. The chronic high-frequency stimulation (typically above 100 Hz with 130 to 160 Hz as the recommended starting point) blocks abnormal signals while also inducing a gradual inactivation of Na^+-mediated action potentials which silences the pathologically hyperactive neurons.[6] Another hypothesis underlying DBS-mediated effects stems from regulating the release of specific neurotransmitters which modulates neuronal network activity involving in these refractory disorders.[7] Ostrem and coworkers also postulated that high-frequency stimulation has a positive influence on neuronal plasticity by inducing long-term synaptic changes in subcortical nuclei.[8] In addition, stimulating neurogenesis and regulating gene expression are thought to also play a role in DBS's modulating effects.[9]

B) DEVICE DESCRIPTION/IMPORTANT FEATURES

DBS devices commit patients to a lifelong implant considering the nature of the neurological conditions they correct. The implanted device warrants subsequent surgical interventions for battery replacements. A standard DBS system encompasses four principal components, namely, the lead, the neurostimulator, extension wire(s), and the programmer. The quadripolar brain lead is implanted surgically into the targeted brain region via stereotactic procedure which is guided by neuroimaging and physiological confirmation techniques such as intraoperative microelectrode recording (MER).[10] The DBS lead target depends on the refractory neurological condition being treated. While modulation the motor function in Parkinson's disease involves targeting the subthalamic nucleus (STN) or the globus pallidus internus (GPi), controlling seizures in refractory epilepsy would preferentially involve the neurostimulation of anterior nuclei of the thalamus (ANT) and hippocampus (HC).[11] The surgical procedure is conducted under general anesthesia. Alternatively, the patient can be kept awake while the DMS lead is implanted under local anesthesia, an approach which is advantageous to prove for DBS-induced adverse effects and optimize the physiological response. The single/dual channel pulse generator (neurostimulator) is implanted subcutaneously in the subclavicular region. The single channel neurostimulators are non-rechargeable (e.g., Soletra®, Medtronics, Inc.) while dual channel models can be designed as rechargeable (e.g., Activa RC®, Medtronics, Inc.). Single channel device batteries tend to last twice as long as dual channel pulse generators with their life span

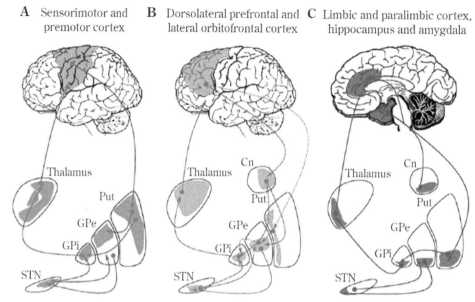

A Sensorimotor and premotor cortex   **B** Dorsolateral prefrontal and lateral orbitofrontal cortex   **C** Limbic and paralimbic cortex, hippocampus and amygdala

Schematic representation of motor (A) associative (B) and limbic circuits (C) of the cortico-striato-pallido-thalamo-cortical loops (CSPTC).
(Reprint with permission from "Lapidus KA, Kopell BH, Ben-Haim S, Rezai AR, Goodman WK : History of psychosurgery : a psychiatrist's perspective. *World Neurosurg* 80 : S27. e21-16, 2013.")

FIGURE 8.5 Schematic representation of motor (A), associative (B), and limbic circuits (C) of the corticostriatal-thalamocortical loops of subcortical nuclei.

Source: Reprint with permission from Lapidus KA, Kopell BH, Ben Haim S, Rezai AR, Goodman WK; History of Psychiatry: a psychiatrist's perspective, World Neurosurg 80: S27. E21–16, 2013—Figure 9 (page S27.E6).

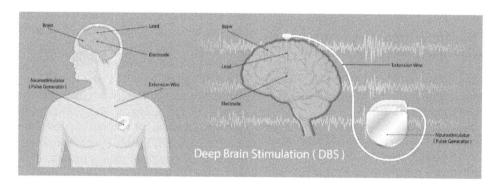

FIGURE 8.6 Site of subcutaneous implantation for the pulse generator (neurostimulator) in the subclavicular region.

being dependent on the clinical indication (on average 6–7 years). The dual channel stimulators offer the advantage of bilateral therapy using a single compact and rechargeable device.

It is noteworthy that dual chamber devices are unsuitable for patients with substantial motor disability or cognitive impairment because the battery needs to be recharged weekly. Instead, the non-rechargeable single channel analogues are better suited because they do not require regular maintenance. The DBS leads and the neurotransmitter are connected by extension wires which are channeled under the skin. Two portable programmers are provided as part of

the supplied DBS device. The clinician programmer controls the lead and the neurostimulator to determine (assign what electrode is active) and configure (electrode polarity) which electrodes of the quadripolar lead are elicited based on adjustable amplitude, duration (width), and pulse rate (frequency) of stimulation. The patient programmer allows the patient to adjust the neurostimulator settings within the clinician's configured range. While the implantation procedure needs to be conducted in a specialized neurosurgical unit, the programming and ongoing monitoring of the prescription-only device is commonly conducted in a regular neurology clinic.

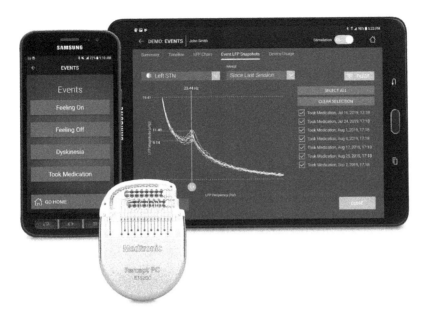

FIGURE 8.7 DBS patient and physician programmers.

Source: [Percept PC Family with Stimulation BrainSense Technology View—Courtesy of Medtronics, Inc; used with permission].

c) Purpose and Use

- Initial programming is performed by the clinician.
- The patient programmer/controller serves as a "remote control" for the patient/caregiver to modulate the neurostimulator.
- The controller can be operated in simple or advanced modes depending on the clinician-patient agreed plan.
- The number of functionalities available depends on the model. Most DBS patient programmers incorporate the following: the device on/off switch, therapy on/off function, battery status check, and a combination of selection/navigation functions for adjustable stimulation parameters (pulse amplitude, width, and rate) accompanied by a number of default group settings (4 group settings in case of Activa®, Medtronics, Inc.).
- Some controllers connect to the neurostimulator wirelessly, while other models feature a connecting antenna and a synchronization function on the controller handset.
- Once the programmer is on, the patient is advised to hold the controller (or the supplied antenna, depending on the brand) over the chest (clavicular region) where the neurostimulator implant is, then, select the synchronization function (it also serves as a check button to ensure that the implanted system is functioning correctly).
- Once synchronized, the therapy screen displays the neurostimulator status (on/off), the battery status, and the therapy parameters.
- The patient can navigate between parameters using the selection/navigation buttons to choose between stimulation parameters and/or group settings.

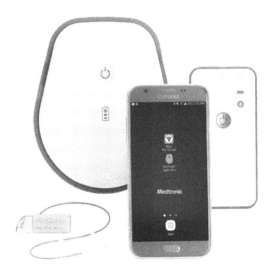

FIGURE 8.8 DBS neurostimulation device and its functionalities.

Source: Interstim Micro with Recharger and Smart programmer—courtesy of Medtronics, Inc; used with permission.

- DBS therapy can be switched on or off at any time by placing the controller over the neurostimulator area and pressing the appropriate function.
- Patients with rechargeable models are advised to maintain a regular schedule of recharging depending on the therapeutic parameters and battery usage.

d) Important Safety Issues (Cautions and Common Adverse Effects)

The long-term safety profile points towards rare adverse effects, barring those linked to unintended stimulation of neighboring nuclei, an undesirable outcome which is reversible upon optimizing the system's parameters.[12] Most DBS-related adverse effects are linked to surgical complications, or they can be hardware-induced or stimulation-related. Reports of intracerebral hemorrhage [3.7%],[13] seizures [7.4%],[14] and stroke/pulmonary embolism have been documented [0.7%].[15] The implanted components could also cause infection and skin damage [4.5%][16]; and reports of neurostimulator-induced pain [10.9%],[17] malfunction, and migration also appear in the literature.[18] The surgical procedure to implant the neurostimulator and DBS leads is contraindicated in patients with severe diabetes or those in need for chronic immunosuppression because both conditions increase the risk of hemorrhagic stroke and device-related infection.[19–21] DBS is also contraindicated for patients in whom preliminary test stimulation was unsuccessful.

Increasing the amplitude by adjusting the voltage or the current corresponds to a positive symptomatic outcome as the field of stimulation spreads further radially to affect a larger neural area. However, excessive stimulation could lead to motor (tonic contractions, dyskinesia, and postural instability) and non-motor complications (heating and brain tissue damage).[19] Heating of the DBS device is a significant safety issue which could lead to irreversible thermal damage.[22,23] Hence, DBS is contraindicated in patients exposed to diathermy because concurrent use could lead to severe tissue injury and fatal electrode heating.[22,24] Magnetic resonance imagining (MRI) procedures involving the use of a full body/head transmit coil extending over the chest are also contraindicated for patients with certain DBS devices because they also cause tissue lesions from component heating.[22,25] Therefore, it is imperative that patients refer to the supplied user manual for comprehensive safety information before they undertake an MRI procedure. They should also exercise caution with equipment which cause strong electromagnetic interference (e.g., theft detectors, security screening devices, electric induction heaters, electric substations, and power generators).[24] Transcranial magnetic stimulation (TMS) is also contraindicated in patients with implanted DBS devices.[24] Patients with other system implants including defibrillators and pacemakers should discuss possible interactions with their respective specialists.

Reports of cognitive and psychiatric adverse events have been documented. These include impaired verbal fluency, transient confusion, anxiety, depression, suicidal thoughts, and psychotic episodes.[26] These complications were closely dependent on the stimulated nuclei and exacerbated by the preexistence of cognitive and psychiatric problems.[27] Management involves reassessing the DPS approach including the placement of lead electrodes in addition to pharmacological interventions.

E)   Storage Conditions and Maintenance

While single channel non-rechargeable DBS devices do not require regular maintenance, the rechargeable dual-chamber models require the neurostimulator battery to be recharged regularly. This commonly involves placing a supplied belt/ shoulder strap with an embedded antenna over the area where

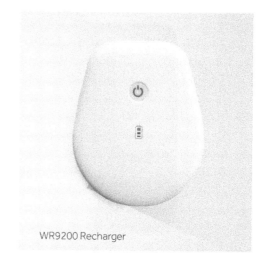

WR9200 Recharger

FIGURE 8.9   DBS wireless charger.

Source: Model WR9200 For Activa RC Devices—courtesy of Medtronics, Inc; used with permission.

the neurostimulator is implanted, then pressing the appropriate button on the supplied charger accordingly. Patients are encouraged to check the battery status regularly in order to avoid the rebound effect of abrupt DBS cessation.[28]

F)   Important Features (Capabilities and Limitations) and Special Advantages

DBS implanted devices are generally safe. With advances in stereotactic and functional neurosurgery and understanding of neural circuitry underlying the pathophysiology of neurological disorders, surgical complications have become uncommon. Compared to ablative surgery, stimulation parameters can be optimized noninvasively with reversibility of stimulation and device adjustability offering a safe and flexible approach to stimulate specific brain centers.

In PD therapy, DBS provides an effective and safer alternative to escalating the number, doses, and frequencies of first-line dopaminergic medication which not only becomes less effective as neurodegeneration becomes more extensive chronically, but might induce motor fluctuations including problematic dyskinesias.[29] The reversibility in DBS therapy provides an opportunity for the patient to address exacerbations of dyskinesia and optimize the dose of levodopa. ANT and HC stimulation has also been shown to reduce seizures by up to 90–95% in drug-resistant cases.[11]

While the DBS device is most effective in alleviating the cardinal features of PD including rigidity, bradykinesia, and tremor; it has proven to be less effective against symptoms of dysphagia, hypomimia, micrographia, postural instability, and frozen gait.[30] The co-presence of non-motor complications (such as cognitive decline and psychiatric symptoms including depression and psychosis) indicative of advanced neurodegeneration affecting other brain regions could also reduce the degree of response to DBS therapy while possibly aggravating the patient's cognitive status.[31]

G) **SPECIAL TIPS FOR PATIENT COUNSELING**

- Patients are advised to always carry their DBS controller with them.
- Patients should be reminded that single-channel devices which are implanted unilaterally provide effects contralaterally (e.g., a right neurostimulator provides effects on the left and vice versa).

- GPi-implanted devices have different stimulation settings compared to STN-implanted systems. The same can be said for ANT and HC stimulations to treat refractory epilepsy.
- Patients are encouraged to keep a record of selected stimulation parameters of the supplied programmer along with the progress of the condition symptoms including the nature and severity of

MY NAME

HOME ADDRESS

EMERGENCY CONTACT · PHONE

PHYSICIAN · PHONE

ALLERGIES/OTHER MEDICAL CONDITIONS

MEDICATIONS THAT MAY BE CONTRAINDICATED IN PARKINSON'S DISEASE

Safe Medications:	Medications to Avoid:
ANTIPSYCHOTICS	
pimavanserin (Nuplazid, FDA approved to treat Parkinson's disease psychosis), quetiapine (Seroquel), clozapine (Clozaril)	avoid all other typical and atypical antipsychotics
PAIN MEDICATION	
most are safe to use, but narcotic medications may cause confusion/psychosis and constipation	if patient is taking MAO-B inhibitor such as selegiline or rasagiline (Azilect), avoid meperidine (Demerol)
ANESTHESIA	
request a consult with the anesthesiologist, surgeon and Parkinson's doctor to determine best anesthesia given your Parkinson's symptoms and medications	if patient is taking MAO-B inhibitor such as selegiline or rasagiline (Azilect), avoid: meperidine (Demerol), tramadol (Rybix, Ryzolt, Ultram), droperidol (Inapsine), methadone (Dolophine, Methadose), propoxyphene (Darvon, PP-Cap), cyclobenzaprine (Amrix, Fexmid, Flexeril), halothane (Fluothane)
NAUSEA/GI DRUGS	
domperidone (Motilium), trimethobenzamide (Tigan), ondansetron (Zofran), dolasetron (Anzemet), granisetron (Kytril)	prochlormethazine (Compazine), metoclopramide (Reglan), promethazine (Phenergan), droperidol (Inapsine)
ANTIDEPRESSANTS	
fluoxetine (Prozac), sertraline (Zoloft), paroxetine (Paxil), citalopram (Celexa), escitalopram (Lexapro), venlafaxine (Effexor)	amoxapine (Asendin)

Share this with your doctor
If you have a deep brain stimulation device (DBS):

MRI Warning
- MRI should not be performed unless the hospital has MRI experience imaging a DBS device safely.
- MRI should never be done if the pacemaker is placed anywhere other than the chest or abdomen.
- Under certain conditions, some DBS devices are safe for full-body MRI and do not need to be turned off.

In other cases, devices should be turned to 0.0 volts and MRI should not be used to image structures of the body lower than the head, because dangerous heating of the lead could occur.
- Always check with your DBS team before having an MRI to make sure the procedure will be safe for you.

EKG and EEG Warning
- Turn off the DBS device before conducting EKG or EEG.
- Diathermy should be avoided.

FIGURE 8.10 Parkinson's medical alert card.

Source: Figure courtesy of Parkinson's Foundation; used with permission.

signs and symptoms of motor fluctuations. Some advanced models have the capability to store patient-specific data (e.g., Activa RC®).

- Patients are advised to use rates above 30 Hz because low programmer rates could exacerbate tremor in PD.[28]
- Stopping DBS abruptly could have a rebound effect in which disease symptoms rerun with greater severity.[28]
- Patients must ensure that they turn the device off if they are scheduled to undertake specific medical tests such as electrocardiography to avoid potential interference.
- Patients should be aware that implanted neurostimulators can potentially be affected by strong magnetic fields in the environment.
- Patients are advised to get a medical alert bracelet which states that they have an implanted DBS system. A medical alert card with details of the system and emergency contact numbers is also warranted.
- Patients should refer to the doctor if they develop new symptoms of depression, suicidal thoughts, or aggravated symptoms of impulse-control disorder.[28]

H) EVIDENCE OF EFFECTIVENESS AND SAFETY

The clinical safety and effectiveness of DBS in managing Parkinson's disease and refractory epilepsy have been extensively investigated. Multiple lines of investigations including RCTs, systematic reviews, and meta-analyses have evaluated the relative efficacy and safety of DBS compared to medication therapy (MT) alone or sham stimulation. The principal outcome measures in PD investigations included impairment/disability [using UPDRS], quality of life (QOL) [evaluated using the Parkinson's Disease Questionnaire (PDQ-39)], levodopa equivalent dose (LED) reduction, and risk/rates of serious adverse events (SAE). The primary outcome measures in epilepsy investigations included changes in the proportion of patients who were seizure-free or experienced a 50% reduction in seizure frequency.[32]

The efficacy of DBS in PD management was superior to MT alone because it led to significant improvements in UPDRS and PDQ-39 scores.[14,33-39] There was also significantly greater reduction in LED scores, both in early-stage and advanced cases of PD.[14,33-36,38,39] Studies have reported that DBS is associated with a reduced risk of complications from therapy [UKPDS-IV] and improvements in mental state, mood, and behavioral problems [UKPDS-I] pointing towards favorable neuropsychiatric and cognitive effects of DBS.[33,35,38] This is conflicting with literature demonstrating negative effects of DBS on some neurocognitive and psychiatric variables.[40,41] Importantly, the risk and severity of SAEs and total number of reported SAEs were significantly greater in DBS groups which highlights glaring limitations in DBS safety profile.[33,42] Indeed, this indicates that

the efficacy outcomes sought from DBS therapy need to be weighed against the higher risk of SAEs.

The use of DBS in managing refractory epilepsy was found to be associated with a statistically significant reduction in seizure frequency compared to sham stimulation.[11,32,43-45] There was a reduction in the proportion of patients who were seizure-free or experienced at least a 50% reduction in seizure frequency but the observed changes were not statistically significant (moderate-quality evidence).[32] Evidence regarding improvements in quality of life as assessed by QOLIE-31 remain inconclusive with conflicting reports on the significance in improvements over baseline.[11,32,46] ATN-DBS therapy was linked to a reduction in epilepsy-associated injuries but caused a significant increase in psychiatric (e.g., depression) and neurocognitive impairments.[32,47] This indicates that the available evidence is inconclusive regarding the efficacy and safety of DBS in managing refractory epilepsy.

I) ECONOMIC EVALUATION (COST-EFFECTIVENESS)

The appraisal of DBS in advanced PD patients based on recent economic evaluation studies on PD management indicated that DBS was more cost-effective than standard and adjunct drug therapies.[48-55] Cost-effectiveness evaluation was either trial-based or model-based, commonly on a Markov model (clinical progression, treatment effect, and cost) in which incremental cost-effectiveness ratios (ICERs) were calculated in terms of costs per QALY. Considering NICE's threshold for determining the cost-effectiveness of PD interventions (US$33,022–US$49,533),[48] and an average of 5-year to lifetime horizon, DBS was found to be more cost-effective with ICERs of US$31,780/QALY,[49] US$28,867/QALY,[50] US$6,700/QALY,[51] and US$23,404/QALY[52] gained. Another study assessing cost-utility analysis (CUA) of DBS therapy demonstrated that it is more cost-effective if implemented in the intermediate stage rather than early (significantly affected by the costs of medical equipment, hospitalization, and maintenance) or late stages of PD.[56] A cost minimization analysis (CMA) following DBS also showed that both GPi and STN approaches result in a significant reduction in medication costs compared to best medical treatment.[57] This was supported by the economic evaluation of McIntosh based on cost-benefit analysis which highlighted the latent cost-saving effect of DBS derived from the long-term reduction of medication use.[58] It is important to note that the reported economic evaluations were sensitive to surgical costs, assumptions in health utilities, and device expenses.

Investigations on the economic evaluation of DBS therapy in refractory epilepsy are very limited. Joglekar et al. used the 5-year data from the SANTE DBS trial[47] to project the treatment response and outcomes over the patients' lifestyle and evaluate DBS cost-effectiveness in managing drug-resistant epilepsy using ICER per QALY.[59] The study demonstrated that DBS was projected to result in an ICER of US$30,492 per QALY gained.

j) IMPLICATION TO THE PHARMACY PROFESSION AND PHARMACY PRACTICE

Pharmacists play a pivotal role in maximizing the benefit sought from pharmacotherapy including neurological conditions. This is notably significant in PD therapy since research has shown that there is a strong correlation between the degree of patient responsiveness to dopaminergic medication, particularly levodopa, and DBS therapy.[60] In addition, adjusting DBS stimulation parameters often warrants changes to PD medication to reduce the risk of motor complications, notably levodopa-induced dyskinesias. Correspondingly, supporting patients in optimizing the parameters of the handheld DBS programmer coupled with knowledge of the Unified Parkinson's Disease Rating Scale (UPDRS) which offers objective assessment of levodopa responsiveness would go a long way towards achieving better disease management and reducing motor deterioration.[61] To achieve this, the pharmacists need to work very closely with other healthcare professionals (neurologists, neurosurgeons, neuropsychiatrists, neurology nurses, physiotherapists, occupational therapists, speech therapists, and nutritionists) in an interdisciplinary approach.

It is also important check the patient's understanding of the reversible nature of therapy; that is, turning off the device would result in the condition reverting to pre-DBS state (medication only-responsive state) and often with greater severity of symptoms (rebound effect). This process can be pivotal in attributing newly developed symptoms to either the device or medication.

k) CHALLENGES TO THE PHARMACISTS AND USERS

The process of progressive degeneration in PD is nonreversible. The cognitive decline in advanced disease states could pose difficulties to achieve optimal DBS outcomes. These include accurately reporting symptoms to optimize DMS parameters and adjust concurrent medication, in addition to practical issues in maintaining the device such recharging the battery-powered machine when needed. Concurrent alteration in PD medication and DBS stimulation settings could be challenging to patients requiring a long process of DBS programming optimizations and frequent follow-ups.

l) RECOMMENDATIONS AND THE WAY FORWARD

The evidence-based clinical and cost-effectiveness of DBS as a therapeutic modality for refractory motor disorders (Parkinson's disease, dystonia, and essential tremor) and epilepsy paved the way for emerging clinical indications which are being investigated in patients with psychiatric disorders,[62,63] cognitive conditions,[64,65] neuropathic chronic pain,[66] cluster headaches,[67] and traumatic brain injury.[68] There is a concerted effort to optimize the clinical use of DBS by shifting from the subjective and trial-and-error empirical approaches to adjusting the stimulation parameters by the patient in the current DBS systems (open loop)

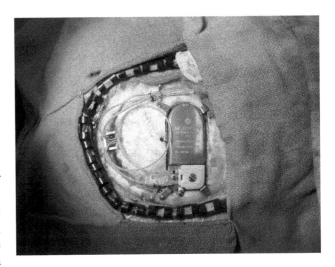

FIGURE 8.11 A brain implant of the RNS system.
Source: Shutterstock.

to implanting a closed-loop "smart" device which records electrical signals and neurochemical concentrations in the proximity of the stimulation site, then modifies stimulation settings accordingly.[69–71] This culminated in the first smart device being approved by the FDA in the US for the treatment of epilepsy (RNS system, NeuroPace®, Mountain View, CA) based on the concept of responsive neurostimulation.[69,72]

m) CONCLUSIONS

DBS provides a safe and reversible intervention to modulate treatment-resistant movement disorders and refractory epilepsy. It involves a stereotaxic surgical procedure to implant electrode leads in specific cortical and subcortical nuclei which are connected to a surgically implanted neurostimulator in the clavicular region. This in turn is controlled by clinical and patient programmers to adjust the stimulation parameters. There is compelling evidence which has established the clinical and cost-effectiveness of the approach to treat advanced PD and epilepsy. The role of DBS in managing other psychiatric, cognitive, and neurological disorders is showing great promise and it continues to evolve with the introduction of adaptive closed-loop smart devices in the responsive neurostimulation strategies.

n) LESSONS LEARNED/POINTS TO REMEMBER

- Ascertaining the patient's understanding of the device capabilities and the procedures involved in the implantation process of components is paramount.
- Managing patient expectations regarding DBS is crucial, particularly regarding the long-term prognosis. DBS does not alter PD disease progression, but it aims to improve motor symptoms and the quality of life.

- The patient may not experience the full positive effects of the DBS device until the concurrent medication and the DBS programmer parameters are optimized to the individual's needs. Hence, record-keeping of DBS programming is crucial, not only to attain optimal parameters but also to avoid duplicating settings which could lead to treatment failure, poor response, or adverse events.
- Adjustments to concurrent medication might be warranted when DBS therapy is initiated.
- DBS therapy is contraindicated in patients exposed to diathermy, TMS, and certain MRI procedures.

REFERENCES

1. Sharma M, Naik V, Deogaonkar M. Emerging applications of deep brain stimulation. J Neurosurg Sci. Edizioni Minerva Medica. 2016;60:242–55.

2. Hammond C, Ammari R, Bioulac B, et al. Latest view on the mechanism of action of deep brain stimulation. Mov Disord [Internet]. 2008 Nov 15;23(15):2111–21. Available from: http://doi.wiley.com/10.1002/mds.22120.

3. Xu W, Russo GS, Hashimoto T, et al. Subthalamic nucleus stimulation modulates thalamic neuronal activity. J Neurosci. 2008 Nov 12;28(46):11916–24.

4. Brown P, Mazzone P, Oliviero A, et al. Effects of stimulation of the subthalamic area on oscillatory pallidal activity in Parkinson's disease. Exp Neurol. 2004 Aug;188(2):480–90.

5. Okun MS. Deep-brain stimulation for Parkinson's disease. New England J Med. Massachussetts Medical Society. 2012;367:1529–38.

6. Magarios-Ascone C, Pazo JH, Macadar O, et al. High-frequency stimulation of the subthalamic nucleus silences subthalamic neurons: a possible cellular mechanism in Parkinson's disease. Neuroscience. 2002 Dec 16;115(4):1109–17.

7. Schiefer TK, Matsumoto JY, Lee KH. Moving forward: advances in the treatment of movement disorders with deep brain stimulation. Front Integr Neurosc. 2011;5:69.

8. Ostrem JL, Marks WJ, Volz MM, et al. Pallidal deep brain stimulation in patients with cranial-cervical dystonia (Meige syndrome). Mov Disord [Internet]. 2007 Oct 15;22(13):1885–91. Available from: http://doi.wiley.com/10.1002/mds.21580.

9. Kalia SK, Sankar T, Lozano AM. Deep brain stimulation for Parkinson's disease and other movement disorders. Curr Opin Neurol [Internet]. 2013 Aug;26(4):374–80. Available from: http://content.wkhealth.com/linkback/openurl?sid=WKPTLP:landingpage&an=00019052-201308000-00008.

10. Ondo WG, Bronte-Stewart H. The North American survey of placement and adjustment strategies for deep brain stimulation. Stereotact Funct Neurosurg. 2005 Dec;83(4):142–7.

11. Li MCH, Cook MJ. Deep brain stimulation for drug-resistant epilepsy. Epilepsia [Internet]. 2018 Feb;59(2):273–90. Available from: http://doi.wiley.com/10.1111/epi.13964.

12. Bhaumik S. Overview of Brain pacemaker. Apollo Med. 2013 Sep;10(3):220–2.

13. Seijo FJ, Alvarez-Vega MA, Gutierrez JC, et al. Complications in subthalamic nucleus stimulation surgery for treatment of Parkinson's disease. Review of 272 procedures. Acta Neurochir (Wien). 2007 Sep;149(9):867–75.

14. Hamani C, Richter E, Schwalb JM, et al. Bilateral subthalamic nucleus stimulation for Parkinson's disease: a systematic review of the clinical literature. Neurosurgery [Internet]. 2005 Jun 1;56(6):1313–24. Available from: https://academic.oup.com/neurosurgery/article/56/6/1313/2744117.

15. Inci S, Erbengi A, Berker M. Pulmonary embolism in neurosurgical patients. Surg Neurol. 1995;43(2):123–9.

16. Oh MY, Abosch A, Kim SH, et al. Long-term hardware-related complications of deep brain stimulation. Neurosurgery [Internet]. 2002 Jun 1;50(6):1268–76. Available from: https://academic.oup.com/neurosurgery/article/50/6/1268/2739846.

17. Sherif C, Dorfer C, Kalteis K, et al. Deep brain pulse-generator and lead-extensions: subjective sensations related to measured parameters. Mov Disord [Internet]. 2008 May 15;23(7):1036–41. Available from: http://doi.wiley.com/10.1002/mds.21973.

18. Lyons KE, Wilkinson SB, Overman J, et al. Surgical and hardware complications of subthalamic stimulation: a series of 160 procedures. Neurology. Lippincott Williams and Wilkins. 2004;63:612–6.

19. Marks WJ. Deep brain stimulation management. In: Deep brain stimulation management. Cambridge: Cambridge University Press; 2015. p. 1–235.

20. Hariz MI. Complications of deep brain stimulation surgery. Mov Disord [Internet]. 2002 Mar;17(S3):S162–6. Available from: http://doi.wiley.com/10.1002/mds.10159.

21. Umemura A, Jaggi JL, Hurtig HI, et al. Deep brain stimulation for movement disorders: morbidity and mortality in 109 patients. J Neurosurg. 2003 Apr 1;98(4):779–84.

22. Rezai AR, Phillips M, Baker KB, et al. Neurostimulation system used for Deep Brain Stimulation (DBS): MR safety issues and implications of failing to follow safety recommendations. Investig Radiol. 2004;39:300–3.

23. Nutt JG, Anderson VC, Peacock JH, et al. DBS and diathermy interaction induces severe CNS damage. Neurology [Internet]. 2001 May 22;56(10):1384–6. Available from: www.ncbi.nlm.nih.gov/pubmed/11376192.

24. Rahimpour S, Kiyani M, Hodges SE, Turner DA. Deep brain stimulation and electromagnetic interference. Clin Neurol Neurosurg. 2021 Apr 1;203:106577.

25. Larson PS, Richardson RM, Starr PA, et al. Magnetic resonance imaging of implanted deep brain stimulators: experience in a large series. Stereotact Funct Neurosurg. 2008 Mar;86(2):92–100.

26. Voon V, Kubu C, Krack P, et al. Deep brain stimulation: neuropsychological and neuropsychiatric issues. Mov Disord [Internet]. 2006 Jun;21(S14):S305–27. Available from: http://doi.wiley.com/10.1002/mds.20963.

27. Okun MS, Fernandez HH, Wu SS, et al. Cognition and mood in Parkinson's disease in subthalamic nucleus versus globus pallidus interna deep brain stimulation: the COMPARE trial. Ann Neurol [Internet]. 2009 May;65(5):586–95. Available from: http://doi.wiley.com/10.1002/ana.21596.

28. Medtronics. Medtronic deep brain stimulation therapy for movement disorders indication-specific information for implantable neurostimulators. 2020. Available from: https://manuals.medtronic.com/content/dam/emanuals/neuro/M927893A106A_view.pdf.

29. Carvalho V, Cunha CV, Massano J. Parkinson's disease: contemporary concepts and clinical management. In: Neurodegenerative diseases: clinical aspects, molecular

genetics and biomarkers. Cham, Switzerland: Springer International Publishing AG; 2018. p. 349–78.

30. Rezai A, Sharma M. Deep brain stimulation (DBS): current and emerging applications. Japanese J Neurosurg [Internet]. 2014;23(8):648–60. Available from: http://jlc.jst.go.jp/DN/JST.JSTAGE/jcns/23.648?lang=en&from=CrossRef&type=abstract.

31. Saint-Cyr JA. Neuropsychological consequences of chronic bilateral stimulation of the subthalamic nucleus in Parkinson's disease. Brain. 2000 Oct 1;123(10):2091–108.

32. Sprengers M, Vonck K, Carrette E, et al. Deep brain and cortical stimulation for epilepsy. Cochrane Database Syst Rev [Internet]. 2017 Jul 18. Available from: http://doi.wiley.com/10.1002/14651858.CD008497.pub3.

33. Bratsos SP, Karponis D, Saleh SN. Efficacy and safety of deep brain stimulation in the treatment of Parkinson's disease: a systematic review and meta-analysis of randomized controlled trials. Cureus. 2018 Oct 22;10(10):e3474.

34. Kleiner-Fisman G, Herzog J, Fisman DN, et al. Subthalamic nucleus deep brain stimulation: summary and meta-analysis of outcomes. Mov Disord. 2006;21.

35. Perestelo-Pérez L, Rivero-Santana A, Pérez-Ramos J, et al. Deep brain stimulation in Parkinson's disease: meta-analysis of randomized controlled trials. J Neurol. Dr. Dietrich Steinkopff Verlag GmbH and Co. KG. 2014;261:2051–60.

36. Weaver F, Follett K, Hur K, et al. Deep brain stimulation in Parkinson disease: a metaanalysis of patient outcomes. J Neurosurg. 2005 Dec;103(6):956–67.

37. Andrade P, Carrillo-Ruiz JD, Jiménez F. A systematic review of the efficacy of globus pallidus stimulation in the treatment of Parkinson's disease. J Clin Neurosci. 2009;16:877–81.

38. Tan ZG, Zhou Q, Huang T, et al. Efficacies of globus pallidus stimulation and subthalamic nucleus stimulation for advanced parkinson's disease: a meta-analysis of randomized controlled trials. Clin Interv Aging. 2016 Jun 21;11:777–86.

39. Xie CL, Shao B, Chen J, et al. Effects of neurostimulation for advanced Parkinson's disease patients on motor symptoms: a multiple-treatments meta-analysas of randomized controlled trials. Sci Rep. 2016 May 4;6.

40. Parsons TD, Rogers SA, Braaten AJ, et al. Cognitive sequelae of subthalamic nucleus deep brain stimulation in Parkinson's disease: a meta-analysis. Lancet Neurol. 2006 Jul;5(7):578–88.

41. Appleby BS, Duggan PS, Regenberg A, et al. Psychiatric and neuropsychiatric adverse events associated with deep brain stimulation: a meta-analysis of ten years' experience. Mov Disord [Internet]. 2007 Sep 15;22(12):1722–8. Available from: http://doi.wiley.com/10.1002/mds.21551.

42. Sharma A, Szeto K, Desilets AR. Efficacy and safety of deep brain stimulation as an adjunct to pharmacotherapy for the treatment of Parkinson disease. Ann Pharmacother [Internet]. 2012 Feb;46(2):248–54. Available from: www.ncbi.nlm.nih.gov/pubmed/22234991.

43. Chambers A, Bowen JM. Electrical stimulation for drug-resistant epilepsy: an evidence-based analysis. Ont Health Technol Assess Ser. 2013;13(18).

44. Larkin M, Meyer RM, Szuflita NS, et al. Post-traumatic, drug-resistant epilepsy and review of seizure control outcomes from blinded, randomized controlled trials of brain stimulation treatments for drug-resistant epilepsy. Cureus. 2016 Aug 22;8(8):e744.

45. Boon P, De Cock E, Mertens A, et al. Neurostimulation for drug-resistant epilepsy: a systematic review of clinical evidence for efficacy, safety, contraindications and predictors for response. Curr Opin Neurol. Lippincott Williams and Wilkins. 2018;31:198–210.

46. Salanova V, Witt T, Worth R, et al. Long-term efficacy and safety of thalamic stimulation for drug-resistant partial epilepsy. Neurology. 2015 Mar 10;84(10):1017–25.

47. Fisher R, Salanova V, Witt T, et al. Electrical stimulation of the anterior nucleus of thalamus for treatment of refractory epilepsy. Epilepsia. 2010 May;51(5):899–908.

48. Afentou N, Jarl J, Gerdtham U, et al. Economic evaluation of interventions in Parkinson's disease: a systematic literature review. Mov Disord Clin Pract [Internet]. 2019 Apr 11;6(4):282–90. Available from: https://onlinelibrary.wiley.com/doi/abs/10.1002/mdc3.12755.

49. Eggington S, Valldeoriola F, Chaudhuri KR, et al. The cost-effectiveness of deep brain stimulation in combination with best medical therapy, versus best medical therapy alone, in advanced Parkinson's disease. J Neurol. 2014 Jan;261(1):106–16.

50. Fundament T, Eldridge PR, Green AL, et al. Deep brain stimulation for Parkinson's disease with early motor complications: a UK cost-effectiveness analysis. PLoS ONE. 2016 Jul 1;11(7).

51. Dams J, Siebert U, Bornschein B, et al. Cost-effectiveness of deep brain stimulation in patients with Parkinson's disease. Mov Disord. 2013 Jun;28(6):763–71.

52. Pietzsch JB, Garner AM, Marks WJ. Cost-effectiveness of deep brain stimulation for advanced Parkinson's disease in the United States. Neuromodulation. 2016 Oct 1;19(7):689–97.

53. Dams J, Balzer-Geldsetzer M, Siebert U, et al. Cost-effectiveness of neurostimulation in Parkinson's disease with early motor complications. Mov Disord. 2016 Aug 1;31(8):1183–91.

54. Becerra JE, Zorro O, Ruiz-Gaviria R, et al. Economic analysis of deep brain stimulation in Parkinson disease: systematic review of the literature. World Neurosurg. 2016 Sep 1;93:44–9.

55. Dang TTH, Rowell D, Connelly LB. Cost-effectiveness of deep brain stimulation with movement disorders: a systematic review. Mov Disord Clin Pract [Internet]. 2019 Jun 17;6(5):348–58. Available from: https://onlinelibrary.wiley.com/doi/abs/10.1002/mdc3.12780.

56. Kawamoto Y, Mouri M, Taira T, et al. Cost-effectiveness analysis of deep brain stimulation in patients with Parkinson's disease in Japan. World Neurosurg. 2016 May 1;89:628–35.e1.

57. Weaver FM, Stroupe KT, Cao L, et al. Parkinson's disease medication use and costs following deep brain stimulation. Mov Disord. 2012 Sep 15;27(11):1398–403.

58. McIntosh ES. Perspective on the economic evaluation of deep brain stimulation. Front Integr Neurosci. 2011;5.

59. Joglekar R, Pietzsch J, Garner A, et al. PD70 cost-effectiveness of deep brain stimulation for epilepsy in Australia. Int J Technol Assess Health Care. 2018;34(S1):155.

60. Charles PD, Van Blercom N, Krack P, et al. Predictors of effective bilateral subthalamic nucleus stimulation for PD. Neurology. 2002 Sep 24;59(6):932–4.

61. Deuschl G, Schade-Brittinger C, Krack P, et al. A randomized trial of deep-brain stimulation for Parkinson's disease. N Engl J Med [Internet]. 2006 Aug 31;355(9):896–908. Available from: www.nejm.org/doi/abs/10.1056/NEJMoa060281.

62. Vicheva P, Butler M, Shotbolt P. Deep brain stimulation for obsessive-compulsive disorder: a systematic review of randomised controlled trials. Neurosci Biobehav Rev [Internet]. 2020 Feb;109:129–38. Available from: https://linkinghub.elsevier.com/retrieve/pii/S0149763419305950.

63. Naesström M, Blomstedt P, Bodlund O. A systematic review of psychiatric indications for deep brain stimulation, with focus on major depressive and obsessive-compulsive disorder. Nord J Psychiatry [Internet]. 2016 Oct 2;70(7):483–91. Available from: www.tandfonline.com/doi/full/10.3109/08039488.2016.1162846.

64. Westwood S, Radua J, Rubia K. Non-invasive brain stimulation as an alternative treatment for ADHD: a systematic review and meta-analysis. Brain Stimul. 2019 Mar;12(2):502.

65. Connors MH, Quinto L, Mckeith I, et al. Non-pharmacological interventions for Lewy body dementia: a systematic review. Psychol Med. Cambridge University Press. 2018;48:1749–58.

66. Frizon LA, Yamamoto EA, Nagel SJ, et al. Deep brain stimulation for pain in the modern era: a systematic review. Neurosurgery [Internet]. 2019 Feb 25. Available from: https://academic.oup.com/neurosurgery/advance-article/doi/10.1093/neuros/nyy552/5364269

67. Neto NNM, Fonoff ET, Dantas SAF, et al. Deep brain stimulation of the posterior hypothalamus for the treatment chronic cluster headache: a systematic review (P4.122). Neurology. 2018;90(15 Supplement).

68. Rezaei Haddad A, Lythe V, Green AL. Deep brain stimulation for recovery of consciousness in minimally conscious patients after traumatic brain injury: a systematic review. Neuromodulation Technol Neural Interface [Internet]. 2019 Jun 13;22(4):373–9. Available from: https://onlinelibrary.wiley.com/doi/abs/10.1111/ner.12944.

69. Morrell MJ. Responsive cortical stimulation for the treatment of medically intractable partial epilepsy. Neurology. 2011 Sep 27;77(13):1295–304.

70. Priori A, Foffani G, Rossi L, et al. Adaptive deep brain stimulation (aDBS) controlled by local field potential oscillations. Exp Neurol. 2013;245:77–86.

71. Rosin B, Slovik M, Mitelman R, et al. Closed-loop deep brain stimulation is superior in ameliorating parkinsonism. Neuron. 2011 Oct 20;72(2):370–84.

72. Epilepsy Foundation. Responsive neurostimulation. RNS System | Epilepsy.com [Internet]. 2018. Available from: www.epilepsy.com/treatment.

PART 3: NONINVASIVE VAGAL NERVE STIMULATION FOR MIGRAINE AND CLUSTER HEADACHES

A) BACKGROUND

Noninvasive vagal nerve stimulation (nVNS) has emerged as an exciting, safe, effective, and patient-friendly alternative approach to managing a range of neurological conditions including migraine and cluster headaches (CHs).[1,2] Exploring the therapeutic potential of nVNS in headache management, both for prophylactic and treatment purposes as a first-line and adjunct option, was driven by the glaring limited treatment options (with off-label use of certain medications such as verapamil for CH and anticonvulsants for migraine) and shortcomings of standard pharmacological interventions. The clinical value of these interventions was limited by the severity of adverse effects and the risk of drug interactions and medication overuse, in addition to the lack of rigorous and compelling evidence to support their clinical use or therapeutic gains from adding or switching between drug treatments.[3–5]

The underlying mechanism of nVNS-mediated neuromodulation in migraine and CH stems from early investigations of the pathophysiological pathways of these neurological disorders identifying the strong cranial parasympathetic activation of the cervical vagal (tenth cranial) nerve during CH attacks.[6] This is also supported by studies illustrating the strong link between VNS antinociceptive properties and blocking vagal afferents to the trigeminal nucleus caudalis (TNC).[7] Indeed, the electrical impulses generated by the nVNS device are transferred transcutaneously to the cervical branch of the vagus nerve to mediate the pain-relieving effects.[1] More recently, experimental evidence demonstrates that nVNS modulates pain by affecting inhibitory neurotransmitter release, predominantly GABA, which decreases TNC glutamate levels.[8]

B) DEVICE DESCRIPTION/IMPORTANT FEATURES

The rechargeable portable device delivers mild electrical signals (1 ms pulses of 5 kHz sine waves repeated at a rate of 25 Hz, 24 Volts and 60 mA output current) to the vagal nerve via the 2 stainless-steel stimulation surfaces (discs) placed in contact with the patient's skin on either side of the neck.[9] Each stimulation lasts for 2 minutes and the device delivers a maximum of 30 stimulations in 24-hour period. The number of remaining doses (stimulations) is indicated

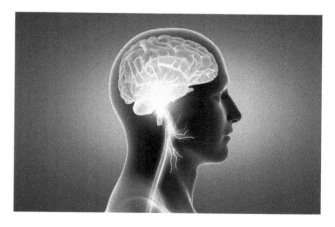

FIGURE 8.12 3D illustration of a strong cranial parasympathetic activation of the cervical vagal (tenth cranial) nerve.

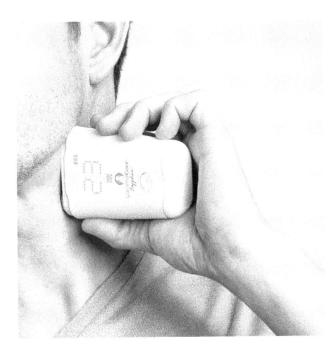

FIGURE 8.13   Site of application of Gammacore device.

Source: Figure courtesy of Electrocore, Inc; used with permission.

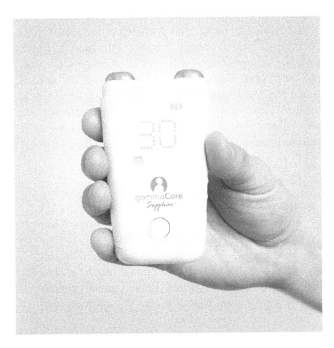

FIGURE 8.14   Gammacore device functions and adjustable intensity.

Source: Figure courtesy of Electrocore, Inc; used with permission.

on the device display screen which also features the battery status and the number of days remaining until the device delivers no further stimulations. The patient has control over the intensity level of the electrical pulses (minimum of 1 to maximum of 40) and mild facial twitching is used as a marker for sufficient vagal nerve stimulation. Considering the legal classification of the system as prescription only,

the device is supplied with a "refill card" which is used to load the system with the days of treatment based on the prescriber's instructions.

c)   PURPOSE AND USE

- Apply a small pea-sized amount of the supplied conductive gel to both stimulation surfaces.
- Locate the treatment site by finding the pulse (vagal nerve) on the side of the neck and ensure that the skin is intact and dry.
- Turn the device on then line up and gently press the stimulation surfaces over the pulse area (treatment location) in front of the large muscle at the side of the neck, just below the lower jaw.
- Maintain the stimulation at the site until it stops automatically after 2 mins (2 short beeps signifying end of treatment dose).
- Remove the device from the application site between successive treatments (the device only counts treatments for stimulations with intensity above 3).
- Adjust the intensity level using the control buttons to the maximum tolerated level.
- To reload the device, turn the power button on, then immediately place the refill card across the device which will display "rd" indicating that the card is being read. The loading is complete once the device beeps twice. If 'bd' is displayed, then this suggests an error and the process needs to be repeated.

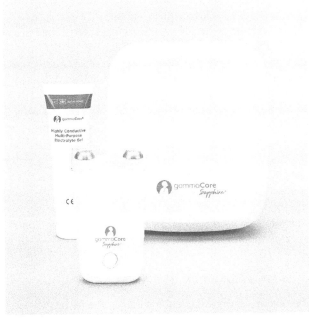

FIGURE 8.15 Contents of an nVNS kit (gammaCore Sapphire™).

D) RECOMMENDED TREATMENT REGIMEN

- The number of stimulations per dose (treatment) and dose frequency depend on the clinical indication. For pain associated with CH, one treatment is defined as "three" consecutive 2-min stimulations. For migraine, one dose (treatment) is defined as "two" 2-min consecutive stimulations.[9]
- For preventive treatment of CHs, the recommended regimen is 2 treatments daily; with the first applied within an hour of waking and the second at least 7–10 hours after the initial dose.[9]
- For acute treatment of episodic CH (eCH), one dose is recommended at onset of attack. If the attack persists, then an additional dose is applied 3 min after the first. The device can be used to treat 4 separate attacks in a day (8 treatments or 24 stimulations in 24 hours).[9]
- For acute treatment of migraine, one treatment is recommended at onset of the migraine attack. If the pain does not resolve, then 2 subsequent treatments are applied with the second after 20 mins and the third after 2 hours of the first dose.

E) IMPORTANT SAFETY ISSUES (CAUTIONS AND COMMON ADVERSE EFFECTS)

Despite the noninvasive nature of nVNS therapy, the approach is associated with some side effects. Application site-linked effects include skin paresthesia/dysesthesia, redness, irritation, and local nociception. Device-induced adverse effects include pain and muscle twitching/contractions in the head/neck area and dizziness. Paradoxically, migraine attacks have also been reported by patients. It is noteworthy that the potential adverse effects associated with chronic use are yet to be evaluated extensively.

The stimulation of the cervical vagal nerve has also been implicated in complications which need further investigations and long-term safety follow-up to in order to be excluded. These include coughing, gastrointestinal discomfort, voice hoarseness, and dyspnea.

The following patient groups are advised against using nVNS systems to manage CHs and migraine: patients with another active implantable medical device, carotid atherosclerosis, history of vagotomy, and/or active/remitting neoplastic disease. It is also not recommended for patients with history of hypertension, congestive heart failure, cardiac arrhythmias, coronary heart disease, history of seizures, aneurysms, or head trauma. In addition, the device is not indicated for children or pregnant women.

F) STORAGE CONDITIONS AND MAINTENANCE

After each use, the stimulation surfaces should be cleaned with a soft, dry cloth to remove the leftover gel. The nVNS device should be stored in a safe place at room temperature in a dry place and away from wireless communication equipment (at least 3.3 m away from wireless devices). The battery life needs to be monitored and charged using the supplied case to maintain an adequate number of treatments. If the device stops functioning, then the patient is advised against replacing the battery if it fails to recharge in the supplied casing. It is recommended that the device is serviced at least once every 3 years.

G) IMPORTANT FEATURES (CAPABILITIES AND LIMITATIONS) AND SPECIAL ADVANTAGES

The portability of gammaCore Sapphire™ device (electroCore, Inc., Basking Ridge, NJ), which is the size of a mobile phone, makes it highly practical and convenient. Importantly, there is well-documented evidence for its safety and tolerability[2] which enhances its accessibility and appeal to patients in light of the unmet medical need by pharmacotherapy. Historically, approved VNS devices warranted surgical implantation for treatment of epilepsy[10,11] and refractory depression.[12,13] On the other hand, nVNS systems circumvent the risks involved with surgical procedures including surgery-related and device-induced serious adverse effects. The flexibility of the approach also permits the patient to administer the transcutaneous stimulation on demand. One significant advantage of using nVNS devices is the potential to reduce the dose and/or number of prescribed medications needed to treat migraine or CH and, importantly, improve the quality of life of patients. It is also noteworthy that most of reported adverse effects resolve immediately after the stimulation is complete which is essential to ensure compliance. The long-term effects associated with the chronic use of nVNS devices have yet to be evaluated and require long follow-ups.

H) SPECIAL TIPS FOR PATIENT COUNSELING

- Ensure that the prescriber and/or the gammaCore customer service team provide the patient adequate training for using the device.
- Nonpainful neck muscle contractions during stimulation are normal and should not be a cause to discontinue treatment. If the patient becomes uncomfortable, then lowering the intensity may alleviate the discomfort.
- Discontinue treatment immediately if the patient experiences chest pain, dizziness, or excessive skin irritation in the treatment area.
- If nVNS treatment does not provide pain relief or if symptoms worsen, then the patient is advised to take the usual prescribed medication and seek medical attention.
- The stimulation surfaces should be capped when not in use. They should not be placed on wet or broken/damaged skin including an open wound, rash, infection, or surgical scar. Jewelry that may come into contact with the treatment area should be removed prior to using the device.

- Patient is advised against using nVNS while driving or operating heavy machinery.
- Do not use nVNS if you have an implanted metallic device. Concurrent use with other electrical devices such as TENS systems should also be avoided.
- Do not use nVNS near microwave or radio frequency instruments, MRI, or computer-aided tomography (CT).
- The nVNS device should not be used if there are signs of defects/damage including cracked casing or stimulation surfaces. If "E7" is indicated on the main display, then this suggests an error.

i) Evidence of Effectiveness and Safety

The licensed clinical indications of nVNS include acute treatment of pain associated with episodic CHs and migraine in addition to prophylactic use in adult patients with CH.[9] The clinical safety and effectiveness of nVNS in acute treatment of CH was derived from two prospective, double-blind, placebo-controlled, randomized clinical trials (ACT1 and ACT2) (150 and 102 patients respectively).[14,15] The RCTs demonstrated that nVNS leads to a significant and sustained improvement of acute pain in patients with eCH but not in chronic CH (cCH) (with primary efficacy end points being reported mild or no pain 15 mins after nVNS treatment and the need for rescue medication within 30–60 mins of treatment).[14,15] Also, nVNS was found to be safe and well tolerated with the majority of adverse effects qualified as mild and reversible upon treatment withdrawal. The transient effects reported in the two studies included application site skin irritation/erythema and burning/stinging sensation. Neuromusculoskeletal side effects were also documented including metallic taste, dysgeusia, and lip/facial drooping/twitching. The investigators also indicated that none of the SAEs were device-induced.

The PREVA study (114 patients), an open-label, controlled, randomized clinical trial, was the first to illustrate the safety and clinical effectiveness of nVNS use for CH prophylaxis.[16] The adjunctive prophylactic use of nVNS (along with standard of care) resulted in significant, rapid, and sustained reductions in the number and frequency of CH attacks and significantly higher response rates compared to control and standard care.[16,17] The nVNS treatment was found to be safe and well-tolerated (reported adverse effects were mild to moderate and included oropharyngeal and neck pain, muscle twitching, and dizziness).

The clinical and safety effectiveness of nVNS in treating acute pain associated with migraine (with or without aura) was established in a prospective, double-blind, placebo-controlled, randomized clinical trial (PRESTO) (243 patients).[2] The abortive efficacy of nVNS (patients becoming pain-free) was significant as early as 30–60 mins after a migraine attack. Similarly to ACT1 and ACT2 studies, the PRESTO study further ascertained the safe and well-tolerated nature of nVNS treatment with similar transient and reversible adverse effects being reported. Other investigations have focused on evaluating the feasibility and safety of nVNS for the prevention of chronic migraine attacks; the most prominent being the EVENT study, a prospective, multicenter, double-blind, placebo-controlled pilot study.[18] Silberstein et al. reported that nVNS was well tolerated and that persistent use may reduce the number of headache days; but larger RCT studies are needed to establish abortive efficacy.

j) Economic Evaluation (Cost-Effectiveness)

The economic evaluation of gammaCore® has shown that it would add costs (£625 for 93 days) to standard care (nasal spray, and subcutaneous preparations of triptans, and high-flow oxygen in the UK).[19] The extra costs, however, are offset by reducing the number and/or doses of prescribed medicines or avoiding the need for more invasive treatment approaches. A pharmacoeconomic model was developed by Morris et al. based on data from the PREVA study to analyze the 1-year economic benefits of nVNS as an add-on to standard care in managing cCH (with the latter typically including verapamil, corticosteroids, lithium, and topiramate).[20] The model estimated that that the adjunctive use of nVNS was more cost-effective than standard care alone as reflected by the reduced yearly costs of managing cCH (from €7511.35 to €7096.69), improved mean $QALY_{EQ5D}$ (from 0.522 to 0.607), and lowered abortive medication costs by 23%.[20] The group also hypothesized that further cost savings could be anticipated in the long term by reducing the number of subsequent clinic visits.

Similar economic gains were shown when nVNS was added to standard care for eCH; with the mean annual costs reduced from US$10,040 to US$9,510) and the mean QALYs improved from 0.74 to 0.83 demonstrating superior cost-effectiveness.[21] A preliminary cost-utility analysis of using nVNS to manage headache in patients with multi-morbidity from the perspective of the NHS further established the improved utility scores and health benefits when nVNS is used. The cost-utility analysis over a 12-month period estimated that adding nVNS to standard care would result in an ICER of £8,310/$QALY_{EQ5D}$ gained, £1,112 net yearly costs saved, and a net health benefit of 0.1 QALYs gained based on a £20,000/QALY threshold.[22]

k) Implication to the Pharmacy Profession and Pharmacy Practice

Considering the prevalence of migraine and CHs and the consistent rise in the use of nVNS devices as alternatives to medicinal interventions, it is crucial for the pharmacist to have a sound understanding of when the approach is considered. Importantly, knowledge of the recommended treatment regimens which are closely dependent on the clinical indication, the common adverse effects, and serious events warranting referral are paramount.

L) CHALLENGES TO THE PHARMACISTS AND USERS

Considering that the assessment of clinical efficacy, safety, and cost-effectiveness research is still in early stages, and that funding for accessing the treatment option in state-based systems (such as NHS in the UK) is closely dependent on individual funding requests (IfRs) which follow interventional procedures guidance (IPG) provided by NICE, it is important that pharmacists ensure that users report all adverse events related to the medical device using the proper channels. The aim is to closely monitor the patient's condition and the tolerability of the device, and establish its long-term safety profile in comparison to standard care. Patient adherence also remains a particular concern when using nVNS as reported previously.[23] Therefore, it is important to emphasize the importance of patient compliance to the treatment regimens; otherwise clinical effectiveness could be limited substantially.

M) RECOMMENDATIONS AND THE WAY FORWARD

The potential clinical benefits offered by nVNS compared to standard pharmacological interventions give us a glimpse of the promising future for neuromodulation devices in managing migraines, trigeminal autonomic cephalgia, and tension-type headaches. It is no surprise then that there is a tremendous concerted effort reflecting the considerable enthusiasm towards investigating the clinical efficacy, safety, tolerability, and economic viability of these systems to cement their place as a standard or adjunct option for patients with most prevalent neurological conditions. Encouraging investigative results extend beyond targeting the vagal nerve to include transcutaneous supraorbital neurostimulation (examples of licensed devices include FDA-approved Cefaly) and transcranial magnetic stimulation (including SpringTMS manufactured by eNeura, Inc.). These innovative devices could provide the perfect alternative to the current unmet clinical needs for patients while offering health authorities a cost-effective approach to managing conditions with a significant economic burden.

N) CONCLUSIONS

Noninvasive vagal nerve stimulation is a noninvasive, safe, and patient-friendly approach for the acute and preventive treatment of headache disorders including eCH and migraines. The portability, ease of –use, and tolerability of the medical device makes it a very attractive approach to patients compared to pharmacological options. The compelling evidence on the clinical efficacy, safety, and economic gains from using nVNS posits a key role of neuromodulation interventions in managing pain associated with these neurological disorders.

O) LESSONS LEARNED

- nVNS devices provide an effective replacement or adjunctive option to standard care in managing acute pain associated with migraine and CHs.

- There is compelling evidence demonstrating the efficacy of nVNS in acute treatment of migraine and eCH. It has also a role to play in the preventive treatment of eCH. The efficacy in managing chronic CH and migraine prophylaxis is yet to be established.
- The patient is advised against exceeding the maximum number of treatments indicated for the clinical indication in 24 hours (no more than 8 per day for acute treatment of CHs and 3 per day for acute treatment of migraine).
- The long-term effects based on the chronic use of the device have yet to be evaluated. The same can be said about the long-term cost benefit considering that most pharmacoeconomic studies are based on short-term savings gains.

REFERENCES

1. Yuan H, Silberstein SD. Vagus nerve stimulation and headache. J Head Face Pain. 2017 Apr 1;57:29–33. Available from: http://doi.wiley.com/10.1111/head.12721.
2. Tassorelli C, Grazzi L, De Tommaso M, et al. Noninvasive vagus nerve stimulation as acute therapy for migraine: the randomized PRESTO study. Neurology. 2018;91(4):e364–73.
3. Nesbitt AD, Goadsby PJ. Cluster headache. BMJ (Online). 2012;344.
4. Francis GJ, Becker WJ, Pringsheim TM. Acute and preventive pharmacologic treatment of cluster headache. Neurology. 2010;75:463–73.
5. Ashkenazi A, Schwedt T. Cluster headache-acute and prophylactic therapy. Headache J Head Face Pain [Internet]. 2011 Feb;51(2):272–86. Available from: http://doi.wiley.com/10.1111/j.1526-4610.2010.01830.x.
6. Goadsby PJ. Pathophysiology of cluster headache: a trigeminal autonomic cephalgia. Lancet Neurol. Lancet Publishing Group. 2002;1:251–7.
7. Bossut DF, Maixner W. Effects of cardiac vagal afferent electrostimulation on the responses of trigeminal and trigeminothalamic neurons to noxious orofacial stimulation. Pain. 1996;65(1):101–9.
8. Oshinsky ML, Murphy AL, Hekierski H, et al. Noninvasive vagus nerve stimulation as treatment for trigeminal allodynia. Pain. 2014;155(5):1037–42.
9. ElectroCore Inc. Instructions for use for gammaCore Sapphire™ (non-invasive vagus nerve stimulator). Basking Ridge, NJ. ElectroCore Inc.; 2018.
10. Schachter SC. Vagus nerve stimulation therapy summary: five years after FDA approval. Neurology. 2002 Sep 24;59(6 Suppl. 4).
11. Ben-Menachem E. Vagus nerve stimulation, side effects, and long-term safety. J Clin Neurophysiol. Lippincott Williams and Wilkins. 2001;18:415–18.
12. Yuan T-F, Li A, Sun X, et al. Vagus nerve stimulation in treating depression: a tale of two stories. Curr Mol Med [Internet]. 2016 Jan 8;16(1):33–9. Available from: www.eurekaselect.com/openurl/content.php?genre=article&issn=1566-5240&volume=16&issue=1&spage=33.
13. Beekwilder JP, Beems T. Overview of the clinical applications of vagus nerve stimulation. J Clin Neurophysiol. 2010;27:130–8.

14. Silberstein SD, Mechtler LL, Kudrow DB, et al. Non—invasive vagus nerve stimulation for the acute treatment of cluster headache: findings from the randomized, double-blind, sham-controlled ACT1 study. Headache. 2016;56(8):1317–32.

15. Goadsby PJ, de Coo IF, Silver N, et al. Non-invasive vagus nerve stimulation for the acute treatment of episodic and chronic cluster headache: a randomized, double-blind, sham-controlled ACT2 study. Cephalalgia. 2018 Apr 1;38(5):959–69.

16. Gaul C, Diener HC, Silver N, et al. Non-invasive vagus nerve stimulation for PREVention and acute treatment of chronic cluster headache (PREVA): a randomised controlled study. Cephalalgia. 2015;36(6):534–46.

17. Gaul C, Magis D, Liebler E, et al. Effects of non-invasive vagus nerve stimulation on attack frequency over time and expanded response rates in patients with chronic cluster headache: a post hoc analysis of the randomised, controlled PREVA study. J Headache Pain. 2017 Dec 1;18(1).

18. Silberstein SD, Calhoun AH, Lipton RB, et al. Chronic migraine headache prevention with noninvasive vagus nerve stimulation: the EVENT study. Neurology. 2016 Aug 2;87(5):529–38.

19. NICE. gammaCore for cluster headache gammaCore for cluster headache. Medtech Innovation Briefing. 2018.

20. Morris J, Straube A, Diener H-C, et al. Cost-effectiveness analysis of non-invasive vagus nerve stimulation for the treatment of chronic cluster headache. J Headache Pain [Internet]. 2016 Dec 22;17(1):43. Available from: https://thejournalofheadacheandpain.biomedcentral.com/articles/10.1186/s10194-016-0633-x.

21. Mwamburi M, Liebler EJ, Tenaglia AT. Cost-effectiveness of gammaCore (non-invasive vagus nerve stimulation) for acute treatment of episodic cluster headache. Am J Manag Care. 2017 Nov 1;23(16):S300–6.

22. Jenks M, Davis S, Amato F, et al. A preliminary cost-utility analysis of non-invasive vagus nerve stimulation therapy in patients suffering with headache and functional disorder multi-morbidity. Value Heal. 2016 Nov;19(7):A698.

23. Paulon E, Nastou D, Jaboli F, et al. Proof of concept: short-term noninvasive cervical vagus nerve stimulation in patients with drugrefractory gastroparesis. Frontline Gastroenterol. 2017 Oct 1;8(4):325–30.

PART 4: EEG PORTABLE DEVICES

A) Background

Electroencephalography (EEG) has emerged as one of the most promising and versatile brain sensing/imaging techniques. EEG has wide and tantalizing clinical, educational, and commercial applications from brain to computer interface (BCI)[1] and to neurofeedback solutions[2,3] to improve meditation and sleep.[4] This neuroimaging technique, which dates back to the 1920s (first human application by the German neurologist Hans Berger[5]), is a crucial and important tool in clinical neurology; both in diagnosing and modulating neurological disorders including epilepsy, sleep disorders, cerebral death, dementia, attention-deficit/hyperactivity disorder (ADHD), autism spectrum disorder (ASD),

and Parkinson's disease. The last decade, in particular, has marked the emergence and proliferation of state-of-the-art portable/mobile EEG devices which allow flexible and real-time recording of electroencephalograms; namely, recordings of electrical activity of the brain using electrodes (small sensors) attached to the scalp reflecting how neural networks in the brain communicate via electrical impulses.

One advantage of EEG over other neuroimaging techniques is its superior high time resolution and sampling rate; thousands of snapshots of electrical activity can be taken from multiple electrodes within a single second. It also offers greater capability to capture the neurophysiological changes underpinning cognitive processes making it a vital tool for neuroscientists to understand the dynamics of cognition and human behavior.[6] The speed at which complex neural patterns are recorded in fractions of seconds is arguably the greatest advantage of EEG.[7]

The principle behind EEG involves directly measuring the generated electrical activity from neurocognitive and affective processes via EEG electrodes attached to the scalp surface. It is these sensors which detect and measure the synchronized activity associated with postsynaptic potentials of pyramidal neurons in cortical brain regions projecting their oscillation patterns towards the scalp surface.[8] Not only does EEG offer key information on processes underlying behavioral responses, but it also helps in monitoring nonbehavioral mental processes including creativity and meditation by taking advantage of the distinct electrical activation patterns. Unlike most physiological recordings which employ a pair of electrodes, EEG devices comprise of a network of electrodes ranging from 10–1000 sensors mounted on elastic caps, mesh platforms, or firm grids which permit faster application and extensive data collection from identical scalp sites.[9]

B) Device Description/Important Features

Mobile EEG devices are marketed in "commercial/consumer" or "medical" grades; the latter is subject to rigorous legal requirements demonstrating their safety and efficacy to cater to specific patient needs. While subtle functional and mechanistic differences exist in hardware and software

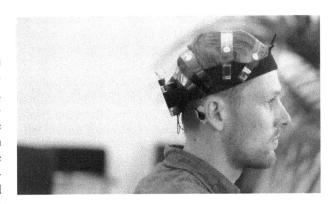

FIGURE 8.16 An electroencephalogram headset.

Source: © iMotions (2019).

designs of marketed portable EEG systems, most encephalographic measurements using these mobile devices employ a recording system which comprises wet/dry electrodes (with or without conductive media) arranged in channels and embedded into the cap/headset (monitoring device). The electrodes acquire and transmit the electrophysiological signals to a control unit which contains amplifiers. The transmission of electrical signals from the scalp to the headcap occurs as a result of the scalp surface, with the attached wet sensors and the electrode gel acting as capacitors.

The electrophysiological signals are then converted from analog to digital EEG data prior to being transmitted wirelessly (Wi-Fi/Bluetooth) to a dedicated host computer with the dedicated software for interpretation. This process is often facilitated by a supplied instrument controller to render the device patient/customer friendly (this software component varies with the marketed device brand and its purpose). The processed data can be analyzed based on frequency bands using spectral methods reflecting various brain waves (delta [0–4 Hz], theta [4–8 Hz], alpha [8–13 Hz], and beta [13–30 Hz]) to measure different neural oscillations reflecting distinct firing patterns associated with certain affective, cognitive, and behavioral states. Medical grade devices are also equipped with a "Packet Loss" alarm systems which are capable of detecting electromagnetic interference; in this event, the patient is advised to stop the recording process.

While medical-grade portable devices are directly controlled by specialized medical personnel to ascertain that the correct recording is attained for diagnostic/therapeutic purposes, consumer-grade systems are stripped to modalities necessary to record specific aspects of brain activity intended for purposes including brain enhancement and cognitive/behavioral wellness.[10] These devices, in contrast to their medical counterparts, offer some degree of flexibility in adjusting the recording settings to fit the customer needs.

c) Purpose and Use

Most common portable EEG devices adopt the 10–20 system, standardized by the International Federation of Electroencephalography and Clinical Neurophysiology, for defining, placing, and naming electrode locations/positions along the scalp.[11] The system defines 21 scalp positions to place the sensors and involves placing the electrodes at 10% and 20% points along lines of longitude and latitude of important reference points: Nasion (Nz), which is the depression between the eyes at the top of the nose; Inion (Iz), which is the bump at the back of the head; and the left and right preauricular points.[7]

Measurements can either be bipolar, quantifying the potential difference between pairs of electrodes, or unipolar measuring the electrode potential compared to a reference electrode.[12] Medical grade devices are used by trained healthcare personnel who facilitate the electrode and device placement on the patient's head with the former directly

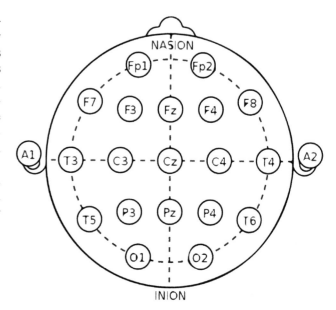

FIGURE 8.17 A top-down map of electrode placement points for EEG according to the 10–20 electrodes system.

Source: © iMotions (2019).

EEG Electrode Placement

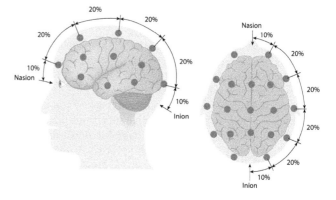

FIGURE 8.18 Lateral and superior views of electrode placement points.

applied to the scalp (preparation phase). This is followed by quality check and recording phase during which the patient is advised to minimize abrupt movements which could affect the signal quality.

d) Important Safety Issues (Cautions and Common Adverse Effects)

It is noteworthy that the headset should be disconnected from the power supply prior to turning the device on. In addition to impacting the quality of generated data, selecting the incorrect conductive paste for the electrode metal could result in its corrosion which in turn would increase the risk of skin irritation.[9] It is also important that the headcap is used on healthy unbroken skin. Reported adverse effects include skin itching, tingling, headache, and burning sensation.[13]

Portable EEG systems should not be used concurrently with the following devices: pacemakers, implanted defibrillators, intracranial devices, implantable neurostimulators, and deep brain stimulators.[12] It is also advised that portable EEG devices are not used in MRI rooms, nor in the proximity of CT instruments, diathermy or electromagnetic detectors, or RF emitters due to interference.

E) STORAGE CONDITIONS AND MAINTENANCE

- The device set should be protected against excessive moisture and immersion in liquid.
- The control unit can be cleaned regularly using a dry paper towel while the headcap should be cleaned (rinsed with water then dried) and disinfected thoroughly after each use.
- It is advised that the electrode quality is checked regularly. If it turns from dull to metallic and shiny, this signifies its deterioration (as it loses ions) and should be replaced.
- The regular maintenance of electrodes depends on the type provided by the marketed brand (standard Ag/AgCl electrodes with conductive gel, dry electrodes, sponge stimulation electrodes with saline, or electrodes with solid gel technology such as Geltrode). Hence, it is recommended to check the instructions supplied with the instrument's manual. It is noteworthy that conductive gel could accelerate the degradation of standard electrodes. Therefore, users are advised to completely remove the gel after each use.

F) IMPORTANT FEATURES (CAPABILITIES AND LIMITATIONS) AND SPECIAL ADVANTAGES

Mobile EEGs are noninvasive, relatively inexpensive (with prices starting from $99),[14] portable, and lightweight, offering a high degree of flexibility in passively collecting/recording data in real-world environments. The high time resolution offers a significant degree of precision in monitoring the time course of cognitive and emotional changes. The price of the device is driven by the number and quality of electrodes, the quality of digitization, and quality and sampling rate of the amplifier.[9]

Adjusting mobile EEG device frequencies gives insight into distinct clinical states. Monitoring EEGs in different frequencies justifies the wide clinical, research, and educational applications of mobile EEG devices including to following: sleep disorders on delta waves;[15] memory recall, mental workload, and spatial navigation on theta waves;[16] meditation, biofeedback, and attention on alpha waves;[17] and motor control on beta waves.[18]

The quality of the generated signal is limited by the nature of the electrode; silver sensors tend to deteriorate over time leading to interference and noisy signals.[9]

G) SPECIAL TIPS FOR PATIENT COUNSELING

- Application of saline-based conductive gel (or paste/cream depending on the brand) is essential for mobile EEG devices that employ wet electrodes to ensure consistent collection of electric potentials from the sensors.
- It is essential to ensure that the headcap is both charged and connected wirelessly to the instrument controller.
- Careful inspection of the scalp under the application site before and after the recording session is warranted in order to screen for any potential adverse effects to the skin.
- The patient/customer is also advised to minimize sudden movements during the quality check phase. They should also avoid touching the headset components during the recording phase to maximize the signal quality and ascertain consistent data collection.
- While results are being analyzed by a specialist for medical-grade devices, patients are advised against self-medication based on the results obtained.
- Electrodes should be cleaned and disinfected with alcohol between sessions.

H) EVIDENCE OF EFFECTIVENESS AND SAFETY

The use of medical-grade wearable EEG devices for ambulatory monitoring and therapeutic yield (change of management) of neurological disorders is established and well documented as illustrated in multiple high-quality clinical studies.[19] This includes their use in detecting and differentiating seizures,[20,21] quantifying the cardinal motor hallmarks of Parkinson's disease and medication-induced adverse effects,[19,22–24] as well as monitoring upper extremity activity and walking capacity in stroke patients.[19,25] The merit of the neuroimaging technique to monitor a wider array of cognitive and psychiatric disorders has also been reported in several lines of investigation including sleep disorders, Alzheimer's, depression, and post-traumatic stress disorder.[26–30] It has to be conceded that a significant limitation of most studies reported is the small dataset adopted involving the wearable sensors, the reported lack of confidence in technology by patients, and ambiguity on the optimal number of sensors to use to record patients' activities accurately and reliably.

The comparative assessment of wearable EEG devices to traditional inpatient analogous systems has demonstrated promising and comparable diagnostic and therapeutic performances to conventional EEG systems.[31,32]

Consumer-grade EEG devices, on the other hand, are still under scrutiny by clinicians, neuroscientists, and regulators with claims of the effectiveness of neurofeedback and cognitive enhancement being called into question. Critics point to the modest to little placebo effect when evidence is evaluated on performance enhancement.[10,33–36] Proponents for using these devices to improve the customer's well-being point to the non-invasive nature of the device with no overt safety concerns, while detractors express concerns over the evidence base for their effectiveness, and importantly the ethical and legal issues with such claims. Indeed, these issues warrant greater attention considering regulators have recently taken action against a number of neurotechnology firms marketing brain enhancement products for unsubstantiated claims linked to clinical indications.[37,38] Beyond the ethical dilemma, there are fundamental differences between consumer EEG devices and medical-grade systems; differences which bring into question the validity and reliability of the recorded brain signals.[33,39]

I) Economic Evaluation (Cost-Effectiveness)

Historically, portable EEG devices were either used as biomarker tools for diagnostic purposes to inform clinical decision-making in managing neurological disorders (including epilepsy, sleep disorders, brain death, and Parkinson's), or merely relegated to research labs for medical and educational purposes aiming to understand cognition and affect. The marketing of consumer-grade versions has only seen a surge in the last decade or so, which explains the scarcity of pharmacoeconomic studies evaluating the economic value added by these interventional systems in improving patient outcomes and quality of life compared to standard care.

Several lines of investigation have highlighted the cost-effectiveness of medical-grade EEG devices compared to traditional onsite EEG systems.[32,40,41] This is partly due to the reduced healthcare costs including hospital stays when comparing the two modalities. Evidence of the cost-effectiveness of these devices remains limited. There are calls for integrating outcome measures to complement the existing collection methods and provide a more accurate picture of their economic value. Examples include a *digital outcome measure* which overcomes the limitations of standard methods that are provider-collected and patient-reported, opening the window for bias.[42]

J) Implication to the Pharmacy Profession and Pharmacy Practice

Pharmacists have a pivotal role to play in assessing and evaluating the safe and effective use of medicines. This role also extends to the effective use of medical devices including portable EEG devices intended for diagnosis and monitoring (medical-grade systems).

The market for direct-to-consumer wearable devices including portable EEG systems for neuromonitoring, neurocognitive training, and stimulation are projected to exceed $3 billion by the end of 2020.[43] Considering their noninvasive nature, the compelling marketing claims (thought control, brain enhancement, and cognitive wellness), and their affordability, it is expected that the next few years will mark a dramatic increase in their use. Taking into account this growing industry of EEG devices used for interventional purposes and the glaring gap of knowledge in the financial realities associated with this new technology, pharmacists are perfectly placed to conduct health technology assessments and economic evaluation of these devices and help patients attain optimal outcomes similarly to assessing pharmacological interventions.

K) Conclusions

The use of wearable EEG devices is on a significant rise. Medical-grade systems provide a reliable and equally effective alternative to conventional onsite EEG instruments as robust diagnostic tools for monitoring purposes. The portability, safety profile, affordability, wireless connectivity, and high signal resolution are examples of the advantages which make these systems superior to the traditional approach with a potential for better therapeutic yields besides the cost-effectiveness of the procedure.

The booming neurotechnology market has seen a proliferation of direct-to-consumer EEG devices with various explicit and implicit cognitive, behavioral, and wellness marketing claims. This calls for greater emphasis on the regulatory, ethical, and legal aspects associated with these claims. Pharmacists could play a pivotal role in providing a clinical, economic, and technological appraisal for these neuroimaging devices by assessing patient outcomes benchmarked to standard interventions.

L) Lessons Learned

- Portable EEG devices are reliable, patient-friendly, affordable, and noninvasive neuroimaging techniques with wide medical applications in differential diagnosis and monitoring of neurological disorders including epilepsy, Parkinson's, stroke, and consciousness disturbances in addition to affective disorders.
- More recently, their applications have extended to providing personalized health data for neurofeedback in an attempt to support patients to self-regulate their brainwaves and alter their behavior.
- There has been a marked shift from promoting thought control to cognitive enhancement and brain wellness, claims which require greater technical, regulatory and medical scrutiny.
- Pharmacists can play a pivotal role in utilizing the best of commercial and medical grades of wearable EEG devices, while providing an invaluable contribution in appraising the health technology and benchmarking the sought outcomes.

REFERENCES

1. Guger C, Edlinger G, Harkam W, et al. How many people are able to operate an EEG-based brain-computer interface (BCI)? IEEE Trans Neural Syst Rehabil Eng. 2003 Jun;11(2):145–7.

2. Ramirez R, Palencia-Lefler M, Giraldo S, et al. Musical neurofeedback for treating depression in elderly people. Front Neurosci [Internet]. 2015 Oct 2;9(Oct):354. Available from: http://journal.frontiersin.org/Article/10.3389/fnins.2015.00354/abstract.

3. Thibault RT, Lifshitz M, Birbaumer N, et al. Neurofeedback, self-regulation, and brain imaging: clinical science and fad in the service of mental disorders. Psychother Psychosom [Internet]. 2015 Jun 15;84(4):193–207. Available from: www.karger.com/Article/FullText/371714.

4. Ülker B, Tabakcioğlu MB, Çizmeci H, et al. Relations of attention and meditation level with learning in engineering education. In: Proceedings of the 9th International Conference on Electronics, Computers and Artificial Intelligence, ECAI 2017. Institute of Electrical and Electronics Engineers Inc.; 2017. p. 1–4.

5. Jung R, Berger W. Fuenfzig jahre eeg. Hans bergers entdeckung des elektrenkephalogramms und seine ersten befunde 1924–1931; cinquante annees d'eeg. Decouverte de l'electroencephalogramme par hans berger et ses premieres constatations, 1924–1931. Arch Psychiatr Nervenkr. 1979;227:279–300.

6. Cohen MX. It's about time [Internet]. Front Human Neurosc. Frontiers Media S. A. 2011;5:1–16. Available from: www.frontiersin.org.

7. Teplan M. Fundamentals of EEG measurement. Measur Sci Rev. 2002;2.

8. Buzsáki G, Anastassiou CA, Koch C. The origin of extracellular fields and currents-EEG, ECoG, LFP and spikes [Internet]. Nat Rev Neurosci. Nature Publishing Group. 2012;13:407–20. Available from: www.nature.com/reviews/neuro.

9. Farnsworth B. EEG (Electroencephalography): the complete pocket guide—iMotions [Internet]. iMotions. 2019. Available from: https://imotions.com/blog/eeg/.

10. Thibault RT, Lifshitz M, Raz A. The climate of neurofeedback: scientific rigour and the perils of ideology. Brain [Internet]. 2017 Dec 6;141(2):e11. https://doi.org/10.1093/brain/awx330.

11. Jasper HH. The ten-twenty electrode system of the international federation. Electroencephalogr Clin Neurophysiol [Internet]. 1958;10:370–5. Available from: https://ci.nii.ac.jp/naid/10017996828.

12. Neuroelectrics. Neuroelectrics user manual enobio [Internet]. 2020. Available from: www.neuroelectrics.com.

13. Neuroelectrics. Neuroelectrics user manual-P2. Electrodes. 2020.

14. Farnsworth bryn. EEG headset prices—an overview of 15+ EEG devices—iMotions [Internet]. iMotions. 2019. Available from: https://imotions.com/blog/eeg-headset-prices/.

15. Krystal AD, Edinger JD, Wohlgemuth WK, et al. NREM sleep EEG frequency spectral correlates of sleep complaints in primary insomnia subtypes. Sleep [Internet]. 2002 Sep 1;25(6):626–36. https://doi.org/10.1093/sleep/25.6.626.

16. Schmidt-Hieber C, Häusser M. Cellular mechanisms of spatial navigation in the medial entorhinal cortex. Nat Neurosci [Internet]. 2013 Mar 10;16(3):325–31. Available from: www.nature.com/articles/nn.3340.

17. Shaw JC. The brain's alpha rhythms and the mind: a review of classical and modern studies of the alpha rhythm component of the electroencephalogram with commentaries on associated neuroscience and neuropsychology. Amsterdam, Boston: Elsevier, 2003.

18. Zaepffel M, Trachel R, Kilavik BE, et al. Modulations of EEG beta power during planning and execution of grasping movements. Di Russo F, editor. PLoS ONE [Internet]. 2013 Mar 21;8(3):e60060. Available from: https://dx.plos.org/10.1371/journal.pone.0060060.

19. Johansson D, Malmgren K, Murphy A. Wearable sensors for clinical applications in epilepsy, Parkinson's disease, and stroke: a mixed-methods systematic review. J Neurol [Internet]. 2018;265:1740–52. https://doi.org/10.1007/s00415-018-8786-y.

20. Rukasha T, Woolley S, Kyriacou T, et al. Evaluation of wearable electronics for epilepsy: a systematic review. Electronics [Internet]. 2020 Jun 10;9(6):968. Available from: www.mdpi.com/2079-9292/9/6/968.

21. Kurada AV, Srinivasan T, Hammond S, et al. Seizure detection devices for use in antiseizure medication clinical trials: a systematic review. Seizure. W.B. Saunders Ltd. 2019;66:61–9.

22. Rovini E, Maremmani C, Cavallo F. How wearable sensors can support parkinson's disease diagnosis and treatment: a systematic review [Internet]. Front Neurosci. Frontiers Media S.A. 2017;11:555. Available from: www.frontiersin.org.

23. Rovini E, Maremmani C, Cavallo F. Automated systems based on wearable sensors for the management of Parkinson's disease at home: a systematic review. Telemed e-Health [Internet]. 2019 Mar 1;25(3):167–83. Available from: www.liebertpub.com/doi/10.1089/tmj.2018.0035.

24. Pasluosta CF, Gassner H, Winkler J, et al. An emerging era in the management of Parkinson's disease: wearable technologies and the internet of things. IEEE J Biomed Heal Informatics. 2015 Nov 1;19(6):1873–81.

25. Dobkin BH, Martinez C. Wearable sensors to monitor, enable feedback, and measure outcomes of activity and practice [Internet]. Curr Neurol Neurosci Rep. Current Medicine Group LLC. 2018;18:1–8. Available from: https://link.springer.com/article/10.1007/s11910-018-0896-5

26. Rohani DA, Faurholt-Jepsen M, Kessing LV, et al. Correlations between objective behavioral features collected from mobile and wearable devices and depressive mood symptoms in patients with affective disorders: systematic review. JMIR Mhealth Uhealth [Internet]. 2018 Aug 13;6(8):e165. Available from: www.ncbi.nlm.nih.gov/pubmed/30104184.

27. Guillodo E, Lemey C, Simonnet M, et al. Clinical applications of mobile health wearable-based sleep monitoring: systematic review. JMIR Mhealth Uhealth [Internet]. 2020 Apr 1;8(4):e10733. Available from: www.ncbi.nlm.nih.gov/pubmed/32234707.

28. Cassani R, Estarellas M, San-Martin R, et al. Systematic review on resting-state EEG for Alzheimer's disease diagnosis and progression assessment. Malaguarnera M, editor. Dis Markers [Internet]. 2018;2018:5174815. https://doi.org/10.1155/2018/5174815.

29. Lobo I, Portugal LC, Figueira I, et al. EEG correlates of the severity of posttraumatic stress symptoms: a systematic

review of the dimensional PTSD literature. J Affect Dis. Elsevier B.V. 2015;183:210–20.

30. Scott H, Lack L, Lovato N. A systematic review of the accuracy of sleep wearable devices for estimating sleep onset. Sleep Med Rev. W.B. Saunders Ltd. 2020;49:101227.

31. Neumann T, Baum AK, Baum U, et al. Assessment of the technical usability and efficacy of a new portable dry-electrode EEG recorder: first results of the HOMEONE study. Clin Neurophysiol. 2019 Nov 1;130(11):2076–87.

32. Neumann T, Baum AK, Baum U, et al. Diagnostic and therapeutic yield of a patient-controlled portable EEG device with dry electrodes for home-monitoring neurological outpatients-rationale and protocol of the HOMEONE pilot study. Pilot Feasibility Stud [Internet]. 2018 Apr 25;4(1):100. Available from: https://pilotfeasibilitystudies. biomedcentral.com/articles/10.1186/s40814-018-0296-2.

33. Wexler A, Thibault R. Mind-reading or misleading? Assessing direct-to-consumer electroencephalography (EEG) devices marketed for wellness and their ethical and regulatory implications. J Cogn Enhanc [Internet]. 2019 Mar 18;3(1):131–7. Available from: https://link.springer. com/article/10.1007/s41465-018-0091-2.

34. Simons DJ, Boot WR, Charness N, et al. Do "brain-training" programs work? Psychol Sci Public Interest [Internet]. 2016 Oct 2;17(3):103–86. Available from: www.ncbi.nlm. nih.gov/pubmed/27697851.

35. Schönenberg M, Wiedemann E, Schneidt A, et al. Neurofeedback, sham neurofeedback, and cognitive-behavioural group therapy in adults with attention-deficit hyperactivity disorder: a triple-blind, randomised, controlled trial. The Lancet Psychiatry. 2017 Sep 1;4(9):673–84.

36. Thibault RT, Raz A. The psychology of neurofeedback: clinical intervention even if applied placebo. Am Psychol [Internet]. 2017 Oct 1;72(7):679–88. Available from: /fulltext/2017-43854-005.html.

37. FTC. Lumosity to pay $2 million to settle FTC deceptive advertising charges for its "brain training" program. Federal Trade Commission [Internet]. 2016. Available from: www. ftc.gov/news-events/press-releases/2016/01/lumosity-pay-2-million-settle-ftc-deceptive-advertising-charges.

38. FTC. Makers of Jungle Rangers computer game for kids settle FTC charges that they deceived consumers with baseless "brain training" claims. Federal Trade Commission [Internet]. 2015. Available from: www.ftc.gov/news-events/ press-releases/2015/01/makers-jungle-rangers-computer-game-kids-settle-ftc-charges-they.

39. Mathewson KE, Harrison TJL, Kizuk SAD. High and dry? Comparing active dry EEG electrodes to active and passive wet electrodes. Psychophysiology [Internet]. 2017 Jan 1;54(1):74–82. Available from: http://doi.wiley.com/10.1111/ psyp.12536.

40. Askamp J, van Putten MJAM. Mobile EEG in epilepsy. Int J Psychophysiol. 2014 Jan 1;91(1):30–5.

41. Dash D, Hernandez-Ronquillo L, Moien-Afshari F, et al. Ambulatory EEG: a cost-effective alternative to inpatient video-EEG in adult patients. Epileptic Disord. 2012 Sep;14(3):290–7.

42. Cohen AB, Mathews SC. The digital outcome measure. Digit Biomark [Internet]. 2018 Sep 21;2(3):94–105. Available from: www.karger.com/Article/FullText/492396.

43. Sharpbrains. Market report on pervasive neurotechnology: a groundbreaking analysis of 10,000+ patent filings transforming medicine, health, entertainment and business. SharpBrains [Internet]. 2018. Available from: https://sharpbrains.com/pervasive-neurotechnology.

PART 5: INTRACRANIAL PRESSURE (ICP) MONITORING DEVICES

A) BACKGROUND

Intracranial pressure (ICP) monitoring is considered a staple diagnostic asset in neurocritical care and a routine clinical surveillance tool for patients with traumatic brain injury (TBI)[1] and chronic neurological diseases.[2]

The pathophysiological rationale behind measuring ICP is underpinned by the Monro-Kellie doctrine which was refined by the American neurosurgeon Harvey Cushing.[3–6] The underlying hypothesis in this model is that the volume of intracranial cavity is constant under physiological conditions, because the skull is solid and brain tissue is incompressible; therefore restricting expansion of the total volume of the intracranial content.[6] The parenchyma of the central nervous system (CNS), cerebrospinal fluid (CS), and arterial/venous blood constitute the intracranial content, the volume of which is constant to maintain a steady ICP.[7] Correspondingly, an increase in the volume of one of these compartments must be compensated for by a reduction in the volume of the other components.[8] In other words, the in- and outflow of fluid components must be balanced to maintain a steady ICP within physiological boundaries to prevent brain injury.[9,10] Physiological boundaries of mean ICP are 7–15 mmHg in adults, 3–7 mmHg in children and 1.5–6 mmHg in infants.[11]

Indeed, it is intracranial pathology (such as intracranial hemorrhage, cerebral edema, or neoplastic mass) which leads to the emergence of an expansive lesion which compromises the compensatory mechanisms. The subsequent brain damage caused by elevated ICP is primarily mediated by cerebral ischemia and brain herniation. Expansive lesions elevating ICP beyond compensation also compromise cerebral perfusion pressure (CPP) and, hence, hamper cerebral blood flow (CBF) to the CNS which could lead to cerebral ischemia.[12] Impaired cerebral blood flow (and energy supply) to the brain represents a major threat to CNS function which justifies the importance of measuring ICP for optimal clinical outcomes.

The other major reason why managing raised ICP is critical for clinical outcomes is the risk of brain herniation. Expansive lesions create pressure gradients between the intracranial cavity and the spinal canal that cause the herniation of the brain tissue.[13] This in turn compromises the blood flow and compresses vital brainstem structures with severely damaging and life-threatening neurological, cardiovascular, and respiratory outcomes including death.[9,14,15]

It is no surprise then, that monitoring ICP in neurointensive care is of paramount importance to guide clinical management and ascertain sufficient blood supply to brain cells.[16] It is the measurement of ICP and ICP-derived

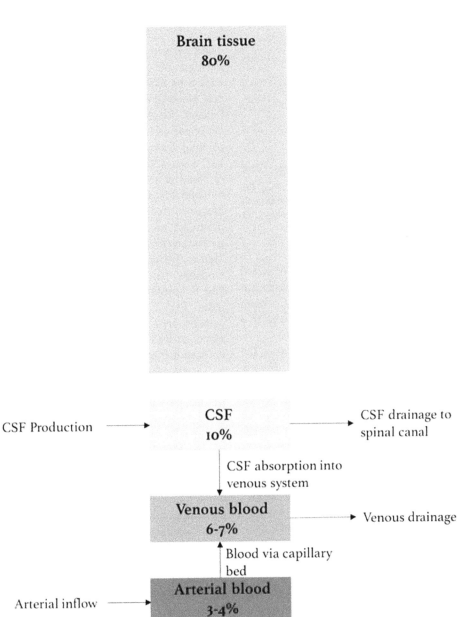

FIGURE 8.19 Schematic representation of the Monroe-Kellie model for the contents of intracranial compartments.

Source: Reproduced with permission from Harary M, Dolmans RGF, Gormley, WB. Intracranial pressure monitoring—Review and avenues for development. Sensors. 2018;18(2): 465.

score (CPP) which is the most widely adopted approach to assess compromised CBF and estimate clinical outcomes.[17] CBF is directly estimated by measuring CPP which can be described using the following relationship: CPP = MAP—ICP in which MAP is the mean arterial pressure.[8]

B) DEVICE DESCRIPTION/IMPORTANT FEATURES

The most common neurological pathologies requiring ICP monitoring include TBI,[15,18] hydrocephalus,[19–21] and subarachnoid hemorrhage (SAH)[22,23] with the modality being used as a surveillance tool for patients being treated

within neurointensive care as a predictor of clinical outcomes including mortality and functional outcomes.[16,24] The most commonly used devices to monitor ICP include fluid-based systems are implantable transducers (invasive ICP devices) and noninvasive ICP devices (nICP) including fluid dynamic systems applying Doppler ultrasonography.

The gold standard method to measure ICP in clinical practice still relies on invasive approaches in which a pressure transducer is implanted surgically; the most widely used fluid-based system involves the insertion of an intraventricular/CNS parenchyma catheter, the therapeutic value of which stems from CSF drainage.[8,16] An alternative, more

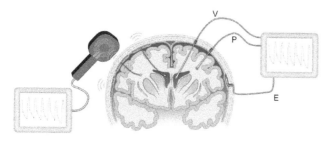

FIGURE 8.20 Overview of wired and wireless methods of ICP.

Source: Reproduced with permission from Evensen KB, Eide PK. Measuring intracranial pressure by invasive, less invasive or non-invasive means: limitations and avenues for improvement. Fluids Barriers CNS. 2020;17(1):34.

technologically advanced approach applying fiber-optic and strain gauge principles,[25,26] involves the invasive placement of a dedicated analog microtransducer system in the brain parenchyma which presents ICP as a numerical value in a connected vital-signs monitor.[27]

Noninvasive approaches to evaluating ICP bypass the need for surgical interventions to measure ICP directly using implanted sensors. Instead, different types of indirect signals are obtained noninvasively; then, a model-based estimation of ICP is processed based on correlating the measured physiological variables with ICP using mechanistic models describing the hydrodynamics of the cerebrovascular system.[28–33] Prominent examples of methods underpinning nICP monitoring include fluid dynamics (e.g., Doppler ultrasonography TCD), ophthalmic (e.g., assessment of the optic nerve sheath diameter (ONSD), otic (e.g., monitoring transcranial acoustic signals (TCA), and electrophysiological approaches.[34] The first method (TCD) will be used as an example in the following section to gain a better understanding of how nICP devices are used.

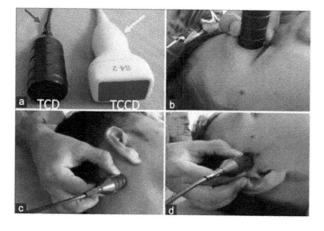

FIGURE 8.21 The use of Doppler ultrasonography in an nICP diagnostic approach.

Source: Reproduced with permission from Patil S, Fadhlillah F. Intracranial pressure monitoring devices. ICU Manag Practice Mindbyte Communications. 2018;48(1).

c) Purpose and Use

The basic principle behind using TCD devices in nICP monitoring is the Doppler effect, in which frequency changes caused by blood movement are used to measure the cerebral blood flow velocity (CBFV) in real time.[35] The relationship between TCD measurements and ICP stems from the impact of raised ICP on blood flow, the cross-section of cerebral vessels, and flow velocity (FV).[33] Indeed, elevated ICP triggers changes in flow dynamics and the geometry of blood vessel walls, leading to an increase of resistance to blood flow and reducing velocity. The change in particle movement within the blood is associated with a scattered ultrasonic wave leading to a Doppler shift, enabling the measurement of blood flow velocity. TCD-derived data are used to provide ICP estimates by applying computational modeling that takes into account CBFV, characteristics of CBFV waveforms, arterial blood pressure, and pulsatility index (PI).[36–39] There is a robust body of evidence which demonstrates a strong correlation between the combined model-derived TCD-ICP estimates and the gold standard invasive ICP measurements.[40]

The Doppler ultrasonic device measures FV in the middle cerebral artery (MCA) indirectly by measuring blood flow parameters in the intra- and extracranial segments of the ophthalmic artery; the intracranial segment reflects ICP in intracranial compartments while the extracranial part is directly impacted by pressure applied externally to the orbit.[34,41]

From a design standpoint, portable versions of TCD-marketed devices typically consist of a headframe to stabilize the probe and a pressure applicator (cuff) to apply pressure externally to the orbit. Some TCD devices feature a cuff with a medium equipped with acoustic transmission capabilities in order to facilitate the propagation of ultrasonic waves between the blood vessels and the ultrasonic transducer. They are also coupled with a pressure sensor to measure the pressure applied by the cuff to the orbit surface. The ultrasonic transducer acts as a transmitter and receiver of ultrasonic waves. Both, the pressure applicator and the ultrasonic transducer are connected to an ultrasonic transorbital Doppler blood flow velocity meter and a data processor. To measure ICP, the pressure applicator is inflated to apply pressure to the eye orbit gradually with ultrasonic waves being picked up and transmitted by the transducer and processed while the meter scans blood flow parameters in the intra- and extracranial segments of the ophthalmic artery. Once these parameters equalize across both sections, this signifies that the external pressure applied via the cuff to the eye orbit is equal to the ICP.[42]

d) Important Safety Issues (Cautions and Common Adverse Effects)

Invasive ICP devices require a high level of surgical expertise, from opening the skull and penetrating the dura to introducing the catheter via the parenchyma and inserting the catheter tip into the lateral ventricles. Considering the complexity of these procedures, it is unsurprising that implanting these invasive devices, particularly fluid-based systems, has an inherent risk of surgical complications including accidental catheter misplacement, intra-cerebral haemorrhage and most notably severe infections.[43–46]

The safety profile of nICP methods, including TCD devices, is vastly superior with attractive affordability of the marketed devices.

E) IMPORTANT FEATURES (CAPABILITIES AND LIMITATIONS) AND SPECIAL ADVANTAGES

The clinical merit of ICP scores has come under scrutiny with several studies demonstrating that ICP devices are not reliable in defining the limits of the brain's compensatory capacity to manage increases in intracranial pressure; a pre-requisite for effective and proactive ICP management.

Beside the surgical complication profile of invasive systems, their use is of very limited benefit in patients with CSF disturbances and shunt failures, since these would affect connectivity to the vital signs monitors and/or impact the accuracy of estimated ICP levels.[8] The external nature of the pressure sensor also presents unavoidable technical difficulties including signal corruption and catheter occlusion, albeit integrated ICP sensors are less prone to obstructions and signal artefacts.[47,48] Having said that, the latter are more prone to baseline drift of the zero-reference pressure level which could give misleading mean ICP levels.[27]

Noninvasive ICP devices, on the other hand, offer unquestionable advantages over invasive analogs including their safety profile, the opportunity to monitor ICP long term without the need for sensor insertion each time, in addition to their portability and usefulness as prescreening tools to decide if invasive ICP monitoring is warranted. Nevertheless, nICP devices have inherent limitations which hinder their application in clinical settings. One is intra- and interobserver variability with results being dependent on the direction from which the orbit and vessels are approached.[8,49] Considering TCD devices give an ICP real-time estimate, this renders it inappropriate for continuous monitoring. Some nICP techniques (e.g., TCD) are also impractical in some patient populations such as the elderly, who demonstrate a lack of TCD windows making their skull impenetrable by ultrasound, limiting the transmission of ultrasound waves.[49,50]

F) SPECIAL TIPS FOR PATIENT COUNSELING

While invasive ICP devices require surgical implantation in specialized neurological units, portable nICP analogs are still restricted to hospital and outpatient settings and the operation can only be performed by a trained operator.

G) EVIDENCE OF EFFECTIVENESS AND SAFETY

A limited number of lines of investigation has evaluated the clinical effectiveness and safety of invasive, and to a significantly lesser extent, noninvasive ICP monitoring in managing various clinical conditions. The strongest evidence comes from an RCT of invasive ICP monitoring in patients with TBI conducted by Chesnut and colleagues.[51–53] The comparative assessment of outcomes in patients whose treatment was guided by invasive ICP monitoring compared to clinical care without ICP monitoring (guided by CT imaging and neurologic examination) demonstrated that 6-month mortality was lower in the ICP group (39% compared to 44% in the non-ICP group).[51,52] Disability (moderate to severe) at 6 months was also lower in the ICP-monitored group (56% compared to 61%). There was no survival benefit seen, however, in ICP-monitored patients in addition to 6% of participants reporting procedure-related complications (focal hemorrhage and local infection). In addition, the general adverse events profile (neurological, cardiovascular, and respiratory events) was comparable between the two groups (45% compared to 46%). The lack of evidence supporting the positive impact of invasive ICP monitoring on survival outcomes was further corroborated by a systematic review of 6 observational studies comparing ICP-monitored patients to those managed with standard care (clinical examination and imaging).[54]

It is clear that there is insufficient Class I evidence for the clinical use of ICP monitoring[8,15] with lines of high-level primary experimental evidence purporting that using ICP levels to guide clinical management resulted in no improved outcomes.[51] Other studies go even further to suggest it could have a negative impact on survival.[55,56] Supporters of ICP monitoring, on the other hand, point to the inherent flaw in the comparative assessment protocol of the studies mentioned where the focal point of the evaluative process is comparing two different treatment modalities rather than the merit of the ICP value itself.[57] The limited standardization and benchmarking of methodologies adopted to estimate ICP could also be a compelling argument which raises questions over drawn conclusions from any comparative assessment aiming to evaluate the effect of ICP monitoring on clinical outcomes.[8,57]

H) ECONOMIC EVALUATION (COST-EFFECTIVENESS)

Similarly to clinical effectiveness and safety, there are limited lines of robust evidence which evaluate the cost-effectiveness of ICP monitoring devices. In a recent cost-benefit analysis study in Mexico, a statistical model was conducted to evaluate the cost-effectiveness of invasive ICP monitoring in pediatric patients with severe TBI.[58] The economic evaluation took into account the severity of TBI lesion (graded by the Glasgow Coma Scale (GCS)), the hospitalization costs, and QALY, the utilities of which were estimated using the Health Utilities Index 2 (HUI-2).[59] The study demonstrated that ICP was cost-effective compared to standard of care reporting an incremental cost in the ICP group of MXN$3,934 (Mexican pesos) with a 0.05 increase in QALY.[58] The incremental cost-effectiveness ratio was MXN$81,062 with an estimated incremental net monetary benefit of MXN$5,358.

I) IMPLICATION TO THE PHARMACY PROFESSION AND PHARMACY PRACTICE

The use of invasive ICP monitoring devices is currently limited to trained personnel in neurological centers and neurointensive units. Noninvasive devices, on the other hand, have wider accessibility considering their price, ease of use, and portability. The current guidance dictates that they are used by trained operators. With the projected breakthroughs in noninvasive neuromonitoring technology, pharmacists in primary and secondary care settings could play a pivotal role in optimizing the use of these systems. This includes the provision of screening services for patients at high risk of elevated ICP, particularly in situations wherein invasive interventions cannot be accessed promptly.

Pharmacists could also play a key role in integrating the wealth of knowledge available from clinical ICP systems and the generated algorithms which would not only guide treatment options effectively, but would also help in foreseeing clinical events and improving short- and long-term clinical outcomes.

J) CONCLUSIONS

The gold standard approach to measure ICP still relies on invasive devices. However, considering the shortcomings and adverse effects of these systems, and considering the questions raised over the reliability of indirect estimation of ICP using noninvasive devices, there is a shift of attention towards more pragmatic approaches by developing digital semi-invasive systems which use implantable telemetric ICP sensors.[60,61] While these miniature devices are less invasive, they maintain a high level of reliability in measuring ICP compared to traditional cable-bound invasive analogs without the need for multiple surgical interventions, reducing the risk of infections. The assessment of ICP from an external receiver, wirelessly connected to the implanted sensor, could be vital for patients in whom the use of classical devices is impractical including patients with suspected shunt failure.[8] Another advantage is that implantable systems offer the chance to measure ICP post-hospitalization on a long-term basis which allows optimal rehabilitation and prompt intervention through early detection of warning signs of intracranial expansion.

Some aspects of ICP monitoring are a subject of ongoing debate with the jury still out on the clinical utility of ICP metrics in predicting outcomes of common ICP clinical indications and treatment protocols. There is still a lack of consensus over the clinical indications of ICP monitoring and its impact on treatment policies with an element of controversy over its merit in reducing mortality and improving survival.[51,55,56,62] Nevertheless, ICP monitoring remains a cornerstone in surveillance and diagnostics areas. It is also essential to appreciate the complexity of pathophysiological cascades which warrant a multimodality monitoring approach extending beyond ICP estimation to include CBF disturbances, brain tissue oxygenation, cerebral metabolism, and cerebral blood flow.[63,64] A recent advent of such a multiparametric tool which adopts the advances in semi-invasive telemetric ICP sensors is the Neurovent-PTO (Raumedic), which is a multimodal integrated catheter with capability to measure ICP, temperature, and brain tissue oxygen simultaneously.[65] The next step in the near future is to eliminate the need for surgical interventions to retrieve the implanted device by using biodegradable pressure sensors; promising emerging studies show the approach is feasible and could present the answer for the optimal ICP monitoring device.[66-68]

K) LESSONS LEARNED

- ICP monitoring is playing an increasingly pivotal role as a surveillance and diagnostic tool in managing traumatic brain injury and chronic neurological disease.

- Invasive ICP measurement is considered the gold standard, of which intraventricular cannulation is the most accurate. The high risk of surgical complications has encouraged exploring noninvasive avenues to estimating ICP, but their clinical application remains very limited with questions raised over the reliability of model-based approach to measuring ICP.

- The clinical merit of ICP measurements remains a topic of debate with the lack of Class I evidence for clinical effectiveness and safety. The emergence of semi-invasive biodegradable and miniature sensors based on telemetric technology, which are monitored wirelessly, presents a compelling argument for a promising future for ICP monitoring devices, particularly when combined with other vital neurological parameters.

REFERENCES

1. Padayachy LC, Figaji AA, Bullock MR, et al. Intracranial pressure monitoring for traumatic brain injury in the modern era. Childs Nerv Syst. 2010;26:441–52.

2. Chawla R, Senthilkumar R, Ramakrishnan N. Intracranial pressure monitoring and management. In: ICU protocols: a step-wise approach, Vol. I [Internet]. Springer Singapore; 2019. p. 327–38. Available from: www.ncbi.nlm.nih.gov/books/NBK326713/

3. Monro A. Observations on the structure and functions of the nervous system. Creech Johnson Edinbourgh, UK [Internet]. 1783; Available from: https://helda.helsinki.fi/handle/10250/2433.

4. Kellie G. Appearance observed in the dissection of two individuals; death from cold and congestion of the brain. Trans Med Chir Soc Edinburgh [Internet]. 1824;1:84. Available from: www.ncbi.nlm.nih.gov/pmc/articles/PMC5405298/.

5. Cushing H. Studies in intracranial physiology & surgery the third circulation, the hypophysics, the gliomas. London: H. Milford, Oxford University Press; 1926.

6. Mokri B. The Monro-Kellie hypothesis: applications in CSF volume depletion [Internet]. Neurology. Lippincott

Williams and Wilkins. 2001;56:1746–8. Available from: https://n.neurology.org/content/56/12/1746.

7. Greenberg M. Handbook of neurosurgery [Internet], 8th edn. New York: Thieme Medical Publishers; 2016. Available from: www.amazon.co.uk/Handbook-Neurosurgery-Mark-Greenberg-M-D/dp/1626232415.

8. Evensen KB, Eide PK. Measuring intracranial pressure by invasive, less invasive or non-invasive means: limitations and avenues for improvement [Internet]. Fluids Barriers CNS. BioMed Central Ltd. 2020;17:1–33. Available from: https://doi.org/10.1186/s12987-020-00195-3

9. Smith M. Monitoring intracranial pressure in traumatic brain injury [Internet]. Anesth Analg. Lippincott Williams and Wilkins. 2008;106:240–8. Available from: https://pubmed.ncbi.nlm.nih.gov/18165584/.

10. Gilland O, Tourtellotte WW, O'Tauma L, et al. Normal cerebrospinal fluid pressure. J Neurosurg [Internet]. 1974;40(5):587–93. Available from: https://pubmed.ncbi.nlm.nih.gov/4817803/.

11. Kukreti V, Mohseni-Bod H, Drake J. Management of raised intracranial pressure in children with traumatic brain injury [Internet]. J Pediatr Neurosci. Medknow Publications. 2014;9:207–15. Available from: /pmc/articles/PMC4302538/?report=abstract.

12. Miller JD, Stanek A, Langfitt TW. Concepts of cerebral perfusion pressure and vascular compression during intracranial hypertension. Prog Brain Res [Internet]. 1972 Jan 1;35(C):411–32. Available from: https://pubmed.ncbi.nlm.nih.gov/5009562/.

13. Sahuquillo J, Poca MA, Arribas M, et al. Interhemispheric supratentorial intracranial pressure gradients in head-injured patients: are they clinically important? J Neurosurg [Internet]. 1999;90(1):16–26. Available from: https://pubmed.ncbi.nlm.nih.gov/10413151/.

14. Treggiari MM, Schutz N, Yanez ND, et al. Role of intracranial pressure values and patterns in predicting outcome in traumatic brain injury: a systematic review [Internet]. Neurocritical Care. Neurocrit Care. 2007;6:104–12. Available from: https://pubmed.ncbi.nlm.nih.gov/17522793/.

15. Carney N, Totten AM, O'Reilly C, et al. Guidelines for the management of severe traumatic brain injury, fourth edition. Neurosurgery [Internet]. 2017 Jan 1;80(1):6–15. Available from: https://pubmed.ncbi.nlm.nih.gov/27654000/.

16. Le Roux P, Menon DK, Citerio G, et al. Consensus summary statement of the international multidisciplinary consensus conference on multimodality monitoring in neurocritical care: a statement for healthcare professionals from the Neurocritical care society and the european society of intensive care medicine. Neurocrit Care [Internet]. 2014 Oct 1;21(2):1–26. Available from: https://link.springer.com/article/10.1007/s12028-014-0041-5.

17. Rosner MJ, Rosner SD, Johnson AH. Cerebral perfusion pressure: management protocol and clinical results. J Neurosurg [Internet]. 1995;83(6):949–62. Available from: https://pubmed.ncbi.nlm.nih.gov/7490638/.

18. Hutchinson PJ, Kolias AG, Czosnyka M, et al. Intracranial pressure monitoring in severe traumatic brain injury [Internet]. BMJ (Online). British Medical Journal Publishing Group. 2013:364. Available from: www.bmj.com/permissionsSubscribe:www.bmj.com/subscribewww.bmj.com/.

19. Frič R, Eide PK. Comparative observational study on the clinical presentation, intracranial volume measurements, and intracranial pressure scores in patients with either Chiari malformation Type I or idiopathic intracranial hypertension. J Neurosurg [Internet]. 2017 Apr 1;126(4):1312–22. Available from: https://thejns.org/view/journals/j-neurosurg/126/4/article-p1312.xml.

20. Eide PK, Sorteberg W. Diagnostic intracranial pressure monitoring and surgical management in idiopathic normal pressure hydrocephalus. Neurosurgery [Internet]. 2010 Jan 1;66(1):80–91. Available from: https://academic.oup.com/neurosurgery/article/66/1/80/2555979.

21. Chari A, Dasgupta D, Smedley A, et al. Intraparenchymal intracranial pressure monitoring for hydrocephalus and cerebrospinal fluid disorders. Acta Neurochir (Wien) [Internet]. 2017 Oct 1;159(10):1967–78. Available from: https://link.springer.com/article/10.1007/s00701-017-3281-2.

22. Heuer GG, Smith MJ, Elliott JP, et al. Relationship between intracranial pressure and other clinical variables in patients with aneurysmal subarachnoid hemorrhage [Internet]. J Neur. American Association of Neurological Surgeons. 2004;101:408–16. Available from: https://thejns.org/view/journals/j-neurosurg/101/3/article-p408.xml.

23. Kumar G, Kalita J, Misra UK. Raised intracranial pressure in acute viral encephalitis. Clin Neurol Neurosurg. Elsevier. 2009;111:399–406.

24. Badri S, Chen J, Barber J, et al. Mortality and long-term functional outcome associated with intracranial pressure after traumatic brain injury. Intensive Care Med [Internet]. 2012 Nov 3;38(11):1800–9. Available from: https://link.springer.com/article/10.1007/s00134-012-2655-4.

25. Gelabert-González M, Ginesta-Galan V, Sernamito-García R, et al. The Camino intracranial pressure device in clinical practice. Assessment in a 1000 cases. Acta Neurochir (Wien) [Internet]. 2006 Apr 27;148(4):435–41. Available from: https://link.springer.com/article/10.1007/s00701-005-0683-3.

26. Koskinen L-OD, Olivecrona M. Clinical experience with the intraparenchymal intracranial pressure monitoring codman microsensor system. Neurosurgery [Internet]. 2005 Apr 1;56(4):693–8. Available from: https://academic.oup.com/neurosurgery/article/56/4/693/2753573.

27. Zhong J, Dujovny M, Park HK, et al. Advances in ICP monitoring techniques. Neurol Res [Internet]. 2003 Jun;25(4):339–50. Available from: www.tandfonline.com/doi/abs/10.1179/016164103101201661.

28. Kashif FM, Verghese GC, Novak V, et al. Model-based non-invasive estimation of intracranial pressure from cerebral blood flow velocity and arterial pressure. Sci Transl Med [Internet]. 2012 Apr 11;4(129):129ra44–129ra44. Available from: https://stm.sciencemag.org/content/4/129/129ra44.

29. Tain RW, Alperin N. Noninvasive intracranial compliance from MRI-based measurements of transcranial blood and CSF flows: indirect versus direct approach. IEEE Trans Biomed Eng. 2009 Mar;56(3):544–51.

30. Ambarki K, Baledent O, Kongolo G, et al. A new lumped-parameter model of cerebrospinal hydrodynamics during the cardiac cycle in healthy volunteers. IEEE Trans Biomed Eng. 2007 Mar;54(3):483–91.

31. Imaduddin SM, Fanelli A, Vonberg FW, et al. Pseudo-bayesian model-based noninvasive intracranial pressure estimation and tracking. IEEE Trans Biomed Eng [Internet].

2020 Jun 1;67(6):1604–15. Available from: https://pubmed.ncbi.nlm.nih.gov/31535978/.

32. Schmidt B, Klingelhöfer J, Schwarze JJ, et al. Noninvasive prediction of intracranial pressure curves using transcranial doppler ultrasonography and blood pressure curves. Stroke [Internet]. 1997 Dec;28(12):2465–72. Available from: www.ahajournals.org/doi/10.1161/01.STR.28.12.2465.

33. Popovic D, Khoo M, Lee S. Noninvasive monitoring of intracranial pressure. Recent Patents Biomed Eng [Internet]. 2009 Nov 1;2(3):165–79. Available from: www.eurekaselect.com/openurl/content.php?genre=article&issn=1874-7647&volume=2&issue=3&spage=165.

34. Zhang X, Medow JE, Iskandar BJ, et al. Invasive and non-invasive means of measuring intracranial pressure: a review [Internet]. Physiol Measur. Institute of Physics Publishing. 2017;38:R143–82. https://doi.org/10.1088/1361-6579/aa7256.

35. Bhatia A, Gupta AK. Neuromonitoring in the intensive care unit. I. Intracranial pressure and cerebral blood flow monitoring [Internet]. Intensive Care Med. Springer. 2007;33:1263–71. Available from: https://link.springer.com/article/10.1007/s00134-007-0678-z.

36. Homburg A-M, Jakobsen M, Enevoldsen E. Transcranial doppler recordings in raised intracranial pressure. Acta Neurol Scand [Internet]. 2009 Jan 29;87(6):488–93. Available from: http://doi.wiley.com/10.1111/j.1600-0404.1993.tb04142.x.

37. Klingelhofer J, Sander D, Holzgraefe M, et al. Cerebral vasospasm evaluated by transcranial Doppler ultrasonography at different intracranial pressures. J Neurosurg [Internet]. 1991 Nov 1;75(5):752–8. Available from: https://thejns.org/view/journals/j-neurosurg/75/5/article-p752.xml.

38. Schmidt B, Klingelhöfer J. Clinical applications of a non-invasive ICP monitoring method. Eur J Ultrasound. 2002 Nov 1;16(1–2):37–45.

39. Heldt T, Zoerle T, Teichmann D, et al. Intracranial pressure and intracranial elastance monitoring in neurocritical care. Annu Rev Biomed Eng [Internet]. 2019 Jun 4;21(1):523–49. Available from: www.annualreviews.org/doi/10.1146/annurev-bioeng-060418-052257.

40. Cardim D, Robba C, Donnelly J, et al. Prospective study on noninvasive assessment of intracranial pressure in traumatic brain-injured patients: comparison of four methods. J Neurotrauma [Internet]. 2016 Apr 15;33(8):792–802. Available from: www.liebertpub.com/doi/10.1089/neu.2015.4134.

41. Horizon Scanning Centre N. Cerepress™ and Vittamed 205™ for non-invasive intracranial pressure measurement technology [Internet]. 2015. Available from: www.hsc.nihr.ac.uk.

42. Bruce BB. Noninvasive assessment of cerebrospinal fluid pressure [Internet]. J Neuro-Ophthalmol. Lippincott Williams and Wilkins. 2014;34:288–94. Available from: /pmc/articles/PMC4284960/?report=abstract.

43. Fried HI, Nathan BR, Rowe AS, et al. The insertion and management of external ventricular drains: an evidence-based consensus statement: a statement for healthcare professionals from the neurocritical care society. Neurocrit Care [Internet]. 2016 Feb 1;24(1):61–81. Available from: https://link.springer.com/article/10.1007/s12028-015-0224-8.

44. Abdoh MG, Bekaert O, Hodel J, et al. Accuracy of external ventricular drainage catheter placement. Acta Neurochir (Wien) [Internet]. 2012 Jan 3;154(1):153–9. Available from: https://link.springer.com/article/10.1007/s00701-011-1136-9.

45. Tavakoli S, Peitz G, Ares W, et al. Complications of invasive intracranial pressure monitoring devices in neurocritical care. Neurosurg Focus [Internet]. 2017 Nov 1;43(5):E6. Available from: https://thejns.org/doi/abs/10.3171/2017.8.FOCUS17450.

46. Eide PK, Sorteberg W. Outcome of surgery for idiopathic normal pressure hydrocephalus: role of preoperative static and pulsatile intracranial pressure. World Neurosurg. 2016 Feb 1;86:186–193.e1.

47. Birch AA, Eynon CA, Schley D. Erroneous intracranial pressure measurements from simultaneous pressure monitoring and ventricular drainage catheters. Neurocrit Care [Internet]. 2006 Aug;5(1):51–4. Available from: https://link.springer.com/article/10.1385/NCC:5:1:51.

48. Eide PK, Holm S, Sorteberg W. Simultaneous monitoring of static and dynamic intracranial pressure parameters from two separate sensors in patients with cerebral bleeds: comparison of findings. Biomed Eng Online [Internet]. 2012 Sep 7;11(1):66. Available from: http://biomedical-engineering-online.biomedcentral.com/articles/10.1186/1475-925X-11-66.

49. Raboel PH, Bartek J, Andresen M, et al. Intracranial pressure monitoring: invasive versus non-invasive methods: a review. Crit Care Res Pract. 2012;2012.

50. Tsivgoulis G, Alexandrov AV, Sloan MA. Advances in transcranial Doppler ultrasonography. Curr Neurol Neurosci Rep [Internet]. 2009 Jan 16;9(1):46–54. Available from: https://link.springer.com/article/10.1007/s11910-009-0008-7.

51. Chesnut RM, Temkin N, Carney N, et al. A trial of intracranial-pressure monitoring in traumatic brain injury. N Engl J Med [Internet]. 2012 Dec 27;367(26):2471–81. Available from: www.nejm.org/doi/abs/10.1056/NEJMoa1207363.

52. Carney N, Lujan S, Dikmen S, et al. Intracranial pressure monitoring in severe traumatic brain injury in Latin America: process and methods for a multi-center randomized controlled trial. J Neurotrauma [Internet]. 2012 Jul 20;29(11):2022–9. Available from: www.liebertpub.com/doi/10.1089/neu.2011.2019.

53. Forsyth RJ, Raper J, Todhunter E. Routine intracranial pressure monitoring in acute coma [Internet]. Cochrane Database Syst Rev. John Wiley and Sons Ltd. 2015;2015. Available from: http://doi.wiley.com/10.1002/14651858.CD002043.pub3.

54. Mendelson AA, Gillis C, Henderson WR, et al. Intracranial pressure monitors in traumatic brain injury: a systematic review. Can J Neurol Sci [Internet]. 2012 Sep 1;39(5):571–6. Available from: www.cambridge.org/core/terms.https://doi.org/10.1017/S0317167100015286Downloadedfromwww.cambridge.org/core.TheUniversity.

55. Shafi S, Diaz-Arrastia R, Madden C, et al. Intracranial pressure monitoring in brain-injured patients is associated with worsening of survival. J Trauma Inj Infect Crit Care [Internet]. 2008 Feb;64(2):335–40. Available from: http://journals.lww.com/00005373-200802000-00012.

56. Farahvar A, Gerber LM, Chiu YL, et al. Increased mortality in patients with severe traumatic brain injury treated without intracranial pressure monitoring. J Neurosurg [Internet]. 2012 Oct 1;117(4):729–34. Available from: http://thejns.org/doi/abs/10.3171/2012.7.JNS111816.

57. Chesnut RM, Bleck TP, Citerio G, et al. A consensus-based interpretation of the benchmark evidence from South American trials: treatment of intracranial pressure trial. J Neurotrauma

[Internet]. 2015 Nov 15;32(22):1722–4. Available from: www.liebertpub.com/doi/abs/10.1089/neu.2015.3976.

58. Zapata-Vázquez RE, Álvarez-Cervera FJ, Alonzo-Vázquez FM, et al. Cost-effectiveness of intracranial pressure monitoring in pediatric patients with severe traumatic brain injury: a simulation modeling approach. Value Heal Reg Issues. 2017 Dec 1;14:96–102.

59. Torrance GW, Feeny DH, Furlong WJ, et al. Multiattribute utility function for a comprehensive health status classification system: health utilities index mark 2. Med Care [Internet]. 1996 Aug 26;34(7):702–22. Available from: www.jstor.org/stable/3766848.

60. Lilja-Cyron A, Kelsen J, Andresen M, et al. Feasibility of telemetric intracranial pressure monitoring in the neuro intensive care unit. J Neurotrauma [Internet]. 2018 Jul 15;35(14):1578–86. Available from: www.liebertpub.com/doi/10.1089/neu.2017.5589.

61. Norager NH, Lilja-Cyron A, Hansen TS, Juhler M. Deciding on appropriate telemetric intracranial pressure monitoring system. World Neurosurg. 2019 Jun 1;126:564–9.

62. Cnossen MC, Huijben JA, van der Jagt M, et al. Variation in monitoring and treatment policies for intracranial hypertension in traumatic brain injury: a survey in 66 neurotrauma centers participating in the CENTER-TBI study. Crit Care [Internet]. 2017 Sep 6;21(1):233. Available from: http://ccforum.biomedcentral.com/articles/10.1186/s13054-017-1816-9.

63. Bouzat P, Sala N, Payen JF, et al. Beyond intracranial pressure: optimization of cerebral blood flow, oxygen, and substrate delivery after traumatic brain injury [Internet]. Ann Intensive Care. Springer Verlag. 2013;3:1–9. Available from: http://annalsofintensivecare.springeropen.com/articles/10.1186/2110-5820-3-23.

64. Roh D, Park S. Brain multimodality monitoring: updated perspectives [Internet]. Curr Neurol Neurosci Rep. Current Medicine Group LLC 1. 2016;16:1–10. Available from: https://link.springer.com/article/10.1007/s11910-016-0659-0.

65. Purins K, Lewen A, Hillered L, et al. Brain tissue oxygenation and cerebral metabolic patterns in focal and diffuse traumatic brain injury. Front Neurol [Internet]. 2014 May 1;5:64. Available from: http://journal.frontiersin.org/article/10.3389/fneur.2014.00064/abstract.

66. Yu L, Kim B, Meng E. Chronically implanted pressure sensors: challenges and state of the field. Sensors [Internet]. 2014 Oct 31;14(11):20620–44. Available from: www.mdpi.com/1424-8220/14/11/20620.

67. Kang SK, Murphy RKJ, Hwang SW, et al. Bioresorbable silicon electronic sensors for the brain. Nature [Internet]. 2016 Feb 4;530(7588):71–6. Available from: www.nature.com/articles/nature16492.

68. Jiang G. Design challenges of implantable pressure monitoring system. Front Neurosci [Internet]. 2010;4(Feb). Available from: https://pubmed.ncbi.nlm.nih.gov/20582269/.

PART 6: SLEEP DISORDER DEVICES

A) BACKGROUND

Insufficient sleep (sleep deprivation) is one of the most pervasive problems of modern society with significant adverse physical and mental morbidities. This in turn makes it a public health pandemic considering its prevalence across all age groups with at least 30% of the general population reporting sleep disturbances lasting several nights per month.[1,2] According to the International Classification of Sleep Disorders (ICSD), insufficient sleep is defined as a restricted sleep pattern that has persisted for at least three months for most days of the week.[3,4] ICSD also classifies sleep disorders into eight major categories: insomnia, sleep-related breathing disorders, central disorders of hypersomnolence, circadian rhythm disorders, parasomnias, sleep-related movement disorders, isolated symptoms, and other sleep disorders.[4]

Insomnia is the most prevalent sleep disorder among adults with an estimated prevalence of approximately 30–43% with 15% reporting chronic insomnia symptoms.[5–11] It is defined as a sleep disorder which occurs despite the patient's having adequate opportunity to sleep, and must be accompanied by mood symptoms (e.g., irritability and anxiety) or impaired daytime functioning (inattention, poor concentration and performance).[3,4,12] Clinical features include difficulty falling asleep/returning to sleep, frequent nighttime awakening, awakening earlier than desirable, and, importantly, dissatisfaction with sleep quality/quantity.[4,13]

There is no universally accepted model to describe the pathophysiology of insomnia. Several paradigms have been proposed to justify the manifested clinical features. One is based on the abnormalities in the neurobiological processes at cellular, molecular, and neurocircuitry levels. Indeed, a strong link has been demonstrated between impaired sleep regulation, circadian rhythmicity, and dysregulation of sleep-promoting (e.g., g-aminobutyric acid [GABA], melatonin, and serotonin) and wake-promoting endogenous molecules (e.g., calcium, catecholamines, and histamine).[9,14–20] It is thought that these sleep-wake regulation molecules are produced in specific brain regions which are characterized by localized Fas activation during sleep.[21] Several lines of experimental evidence have shown that impaired slow wave activity and smaller reduction in brain activity in specific neural circuitries (e.g., anterior ventral and dorsomedial thalamus, raphe nucleus, paramedial preoptic area, and temporal cortices) justify the changes in sleep patterns of patients with insomnia.[22–25] The role of electrophysiological changes in insomnia has been well documented with characteristic EEG indicators being reported including increased β and g activity, diminished d activity, and raised REM EEG arousals indicating REM sleep instability.[26–28]

The difficulty of proposing a once-size-fits-all model becomes more elusive when considering complex clinical presentations of different types of insomnia which could either be primary (idiopathic, pathophysiologic, and paradoxical) or comorbid (secondary to a psychiatric illness, neurological condition, or somatoform disorder; or pharmacologically triggered).[7] Tantalizingly, what seems to be an overarching theme linking these cascades is the premise that insomnia is a disorder of hyperarousal (increased somatic, physiological, and cortical activation:

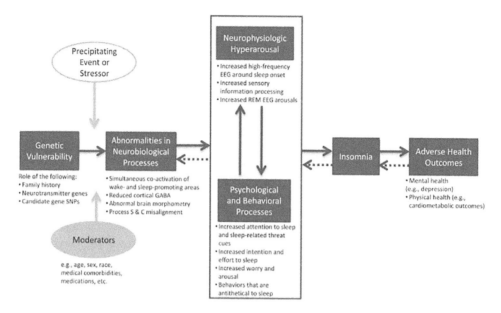

FIGURE 8.22   The pathophysiology of insomnia.

Source: Reproduced with permission from Levenson JC, Kay DB, Buysse DJ. The pathophysiology of insomnia. Chest. (2015);147(4):1179–1192.

neurophysiological hyperarousal) combined with altered behavioral and emotional processes (cognitive and affective hyperarousal).[29–31]

A considerable body of evidence points to the direct and salient role of insomnia in precipitating negative outcomes including the increase in incidence, prevalence, and exacerbation of psychiatric problems (depression, anxiety), impaired cognitive function, cardiovascular morbidity, endocrine disorders (diabetes, obesity), heightened pain perception, and premature mortality.[32–41] The high economic costs are also undeniable with impaired functioning, daytime sleepiness, increased absenteeism, decreased healthcare utilization, poor occupational performance, and vehicular accidents, making it a major multidimensional public health concern.[42–47] Despite this, it remains one of the most poorly managed conditions.[48] Sleep hygiene education, pharmacotherapy (hypnotic medication), and cognitive behavioral therapy remain the mainstay treatment of insomnia.[49] Despite their established efficacy, pharmacological interventions are associated with clinically significant adverse effects, dependence concerns, and long-term tolerance leading to treatment failure with time.[50] CBT is a viable alternative approach with comparable efficacy to hypnotics and treatment gains persistent over time even after active treatment is discontinued.[51,52]

Despite the significant advancements in managing insomnia, there are undeniable concerns over rates of treatment failure coupled with a growing challenge to the preexisting healthcare systems to meet the unmet needs of the ever-increasing population. Policy makers continue to navigate a system with increasing demand for improved quality of care while striving for significant productivity savings. This justifies the calls for designing new innovative

approaches to enhance accessibility and add value without increasing costs.

In the context of technological advances to manage sleep disorders including insomnia, the need for value-based innovation has stimulated the remarkable growth of direct-to-consumer (DTC) neurodevice industry with technologies purporting to improve sleep quality and the overall medical and health state of patients with sleep disorders, which will be the focus of the next segment.

B)   Device Description/Important Features

The new chapter of neurotechnology marketed to the general public to address sleep disorders, including insomnia, is inspired by early research systems recording brain activity with the underpinning rationale closely linked to our understanding of the pathophysiology of insomnia, particularly the electrophysiology of hyperarousal. As such, these neurodevices use EEG (seldom combined with audio-based neurofeedback and binaural beat systems) and pulsed electromagnetic fields (PEMF) to monitor or stimulate the self-regulation and synchronicity of brainwave patterns (both intensity and frequency) and restore the circadian rhythmicity.

Principles governing portable EEG devices and their main features have already been covered extensively in these sections. The rationale behind using these systems in the context of sleep disorders is based on parceling EEG data into prespecified bandwidths (including β, γ, and δ; frequencies which play a prominent role in sleep regulation) then applying learning algorithms to provide key information about the diverging states of sleep and wakefulness. In other words, they can be deemed as a sleep tracking device to analyze brain data taking advantage of the correlation between specific bandwidths and degree of alertness/mental state; namely neurofeedback practice.[53] Some recent marketed technologies even claim that the devices possess the capability to improve sleep quality by directly controlling the brain rate.[54,55] This is attained by combining EEG brainwave monitoring with a binaural beam system of two specific tone frequencies that are capable of controlling the brain rate.[55,56]

Low-frequency PEMF therapy, on the other hand, involves delivering oscillating time-varying (non-static) amplitude-modulated microcurrents from remote electromagnetic coils to stimulate targeted tissue sites at frequencies in the range of 5–300 Hz.[57,58] It is the penetrability of the pulsating current across various biological tissues (from the dermis to the bone) which facilitates PEMF-induced physiological bioeffects at the molecular and cellular levels.[59] The frequency, amplitude, and waveform of the EM field can be adjusted to stimulate specific biological responses, considering that each tissue is characterized by a unique EM signature (which incidentally helps in mapping body organs using EM-based imaging techniques). PEMF bioactivity is owed to the applied alternating current forcing the vibration of ions with significant physiological roles (e.g., calcium, sodium, and chloride), which in turn impacts ion membrane permeability, mitochondrial function, and natural energy production.[60,61] The underlying mechanism of PEMF's effects on sleep could be attributed to modulating calcium release from neuronal cells,[62] modifying the release of GABA,[63] and the concentration of benzodiazepine receptors in the brain.[64] It has also been postulated that low-frequency EM fields could alter melatonin release.[65] This can be accounted for by the direct stimulant effect of specific microcurrents on the magnetosensitive pineal gland leading to reduced sleep latency and increased duration of certain sleep stages.[66] EM-induced EEG changes in the brain and neuro-entrainment (synchronization/tuning of the frequency of applied microcurrents with brainwaves) promoting relaxation and sleep have also been proposed as an alternative hypothesis.[67]

PEMF therapy devices consist of a signal generator and coil applicators which are embedded in the main unit. PEMF's mode of delivery is closely dependent on the marketed design with a high degree of versatility in how the EM signals are emitted. One classical approach involves a control unit to send microcurrents via wired PEMF coil applicators which are secured in the treatment area around the head (e.g., Flexpulse®).[68] Another involves the pulse generator and all other hardware components embedded in a wearable headband which is connected to a mobile device (e.g., Bellabee® and NeoRhythm®).[69,70] The nature of connectivity varies with the brand and can be either wireless (Bluetooth) or via a supplied cable connecting to the earphone jack of a mobile device. Alternatively, the main unit is designed as a miniature handheld device, which is either placed in the palm of the patient's hand (e.g., Bioboosti®),[71] or secured in the treatment area using supplied adhesive patches (e.g., SomniResonance I®).[72]

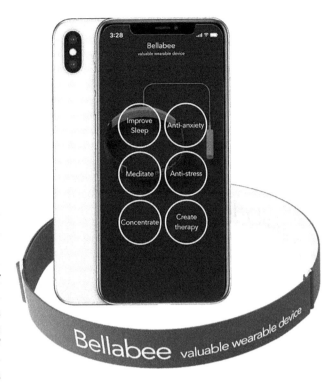

FIGURE 8.23 A PEMF therapy wearable device and the accompanying smartphone app (Bellabee®).

c) How to Use the Device

Despite the fundamental differences in the design features between the marketed DTC PEMF devices as described in the previous section, they all share the attractive feature of user-friendly software platforms (control unit or mobile application) with prerecorded programs. This gives the patient the flexibility to select programs with different settings (pulse rate, frequency, amplitude, intensity, and treatment duration) to cater to their needs. Some are also supplied with a magnetic field detector to ascertain the proximity of the signal generator to the treatment site (e.g., Flexpulse®).[68] Other devices are also equipped with a "test tube" accessory to assess the frequency and strength of the selected programs (e.g., NeoRhythm®).[70]

The initial setup can be as quick as downloading the mobile application, connecting the headband to the mobile device via the earphone jack, then selecting the most appropriate program from the list on the mobile app (e.g., Bellabee®)[69] or the control unit (e.g., Flexpulse®)[68] once the coil applicators are secured in place. Other brands adopting Bluetooth connectivity rely on tapping the device (headband) to pair the headset to the mobile device once the pairing process is initiated from the mobile application (e.g., NeoRhythm®). The tapping mechanism is also adopted to confirm starting and terminating selected programs from the pre-set list. The duration of the treatment session varies with the selected program and the design of the PEMF device ranging from 8 to 60 minutes.

d) Important Safety Issues (Cautions and Common Adverse Effects)

PEMF is a noninvasive and safe approach to treating sleep disorders with no postmarketing safety alerts warranting withdrawal being issued for licensed DTC devices. The frequency range of marketed devices reflects the range of natural brainwave frequencies.[57] Most reported side effects are mild and temporary ranging from discomfort, nausea/vomiting, headache, palpitations, and itching or prickling sensation at the application site; and they tend to disappear after few sessions or when mitigated by finetuning the selected program.[73]

Caution should be exercised with elderly patients or those on antihypertensives because PEMF therapy could reduce blood pressure and slow the heart rate as a result of increased blood flow.[70]

Similarly to other electrical/electromagnetic-based therapies, PEMF therapy is contraindicated for patients with a history of epilepsy, cranial nerve dysfunction, or those with another implantable device such as defibrillators, pacemakers, mechanical heart valves, or electrical stimulators. Manufacturers also advise against using them in the presence of strong EM fields or during pregnancy and breastfeeding, considering the lack of supportive evidence corroborating their safety in such circumstances. The use of PEMF devices is restricted to individuals aged 18 years or older.

e) Storage Conditions and Maintenance

PEMF devices are battery-powered systems (integrated headband/control unit). As with all devices, it is important to follow the manufacturer's instructions carefully to ensure the device is charged correctly. Contact with water should be avoided at all times. Other than storing the system at room temperature in a dry space, PEMF devices warrant minimal regular maintenance (e.g., wiping down the headset with a damp cloth). Users are advised against stretching or bending the headset because this might damage the embedded coils.

f) Important Features (Capabilities and Limitations) and Special Advantages

Perhaps the greatest advantage of PEMF over other brain stimulation therapies is its ability to trigger biological processes that support and heal impaired tissues which extends its beneficial effect beyond regulating brainwaves and aiding sleep to stimulating cellular regeneration in other parts of the body.[57,61] Intriguingly, while other EM modalities attribute their effects theoretically to either electric or magnetic fields, only PEMF is designed specifically to direct precise microcurrents through the tissues to trigger healing mechanisms at molecular and cellular levels.[60,61,74]

Compared to other mechanisms of magnetotherapy (deep brain stimulation, transcranial magnetic stimulation

[TMS]), PEMF devices are undeniably smaller, lighter, and easier to use (with no need for implantation like DBS systems, or attachments/electrodes to the treatment site like TMS), and they are marketed as nonintrusive DTC systems unlike the former which are mostly restricted to hospital use.

g) Special Tips for Patient Counseling

- Depending on the PEMF device brand, it is important not to exceed the maximum number of recommended sessions in 24 hours.
- If the patient is using a headband PEMF design, it is important to ensure that the EM pulse generator is resting against the back of the head (just above the neck, against the cerebellum).
- The headband positioning angle is also critical because the designed coils are embedded in specific stimulation zones pertinent to the chosen program and therapeutic indication.[75]
- Once the mobile app is downloaded and the device is connected via the earphone jack, it is essential that mobile device volume setting is turned to maximum. Then, the desired app can be selected (e.g., Bellabee®).

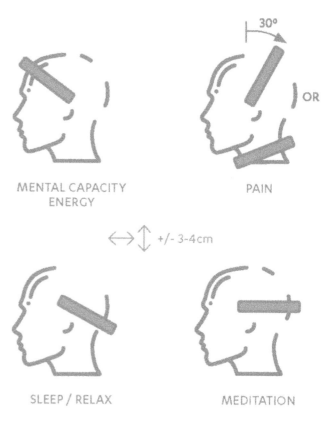

FIGURE 8.24 Illustrations of PEMF headband placement according to specific needs.

Source: Figure courtesy of OmniPEMF, Inc; used with permission.

- Considering that the device is designed to be non-intrusive (no light, sound, or vibration during operating time), to ensure that the device is activated, the user should refer to the mobile interface and check that the time has elapsed once the desired program is launched (e.g., Bellabee®).
- In case the patient experiences any of the anticipated side effects, it is advisable that they shorten the duration or reduce the intensity of the programmed sessions. Persistent side effects suggest hypersensitivity to EM waves and would warrant terminating the treatment modality.
- Patients are also advised against using PEMF devices while driving or operating machinery.

H) EVIDENCE OF EFFECTIVENESS AND SAFETY

There is a modest body of evidence which substantiates using PEMF therapy in managing sleep disorders including insomnia. The experimental lines of evidence date back to over two decades ago, when a double-blind, placebo-controlled study demonstrated that low energy emission therapy (LEET) (a similar low energy EM treatment approach with a different waveform) administered over 20 mins three times a week over 4 weeks increased total sleep time (TST) and reduced sleep latency (SL) in chronic insomnia compared to standard therapy as assessed by polysomnography (PSG) and sleep rating forms.[76] The study also showed that the treatment was safe and well tolerated. In a double-blind cross-over study led by the same group, it was shown that low levels of amplitude-modulated EM fields resulted in EEG changes consistent with reduced SL, longer sleep duration, and deeper sleep in healthy subjects.[66] These findings were also corroborated by the concerted effort of Reite and colleagues in a double-blind cross-over study which illustrated that LEET led to a significant decrease in SL and an increase in total duration of stage B2 of sleep.[77]

Similar positive effects were reported with PEMF therapy more recently. In a double-blind, placebo-controlled study (Class I evidence), a significant improvement in insomnia symptoms (SL, sleeping after rising, daytime sleepiness, difficulty with concentration, and daytime headache) was observed in the active treatment group with no reported adverse effects.[78] The most recent piece of evidence comes from a small prospective pilot study on Bioboosti® in which the miniature PEMF device was effective and well tolerated for the treatment of insomnia based on subjective sleep measures (Pittsburgh Sleep Quality Inventory (PSQI), Insomnia Severity Index (ISI), Epworth Sleepiness Scale (ESS), and Karolinska Sleepiness Scale (KSS).[79]

I) ECONOMIC EVALUATION (COST-EFFECTIVENESS)

While the clinical effectiveness and safety claims are supported to a certain degree, the evidence backing PEMF cost-effectiveness in managing sleep disorders is currently in its infancy; particularly in the absence of economic evaluations with detailed healthcare costs, cost-effectiveness, and cost-utility analyses comparing PEMF value to standard of care (pharmacotherapy, cognitive-behavioral therapy for insomnia CBT-I). It can be speculated that this modality offers an affordable, effective, and safer approach which provides a plausible and attractive alternative when standard of care fails to produce adequate clinical outcomes.[80] What is certain, however, is that the increasing demand for improved quality of care in managing sleep disorders and the growing challenge to policy makers of unmet patient needs by standard therapy could accelerate the implementation of affordable innovative approaches (including PEMF therapy) which in turn would provide more detailed and reliable information to forecast its economic feasibility.

J) IMPLICATION TO THE PHARMACY PROFESSION AND PHARMACY PRACTICE

There is a growing demand for pharmacy professionals to transition from their classical roles in primary and secondary settings to embracing innovative ways in delivering healthcare. Community pharmacists, in particular, could be a key stakeholder and "innovation champion" in the coming years; both in supplying DTC devices (including PEMF systems) and ascertaining if the optimal sought outcomes from these modalities are fulfilled. Importantly, they could be key enablers to champion the delivery of these treatment modalities, facilitate their smooth and rapid uptake and implementation, and align them with standard care. Their knowledge and expertise on the safe and effective use of these devices would make them the preferred reference and consultation point by patients exploring these treatment options. Pharmacists could also take advantage of their wealth of pharmacotherapeutic knowledge to contribute to health policies by assisting in appraising these innovative tools and exploring avenues of synergism between pharmacological agents and licensed DTC devices for a better integration of complementary and alternative therapies to standard care.

K) CONCLUSIONS

Insufficient sleep is a major public health concern with significant physical and mental implications and healthcare costs. Insomnia, in particular, is an undertreated and underestimated issue with an estimated prevalence of 1 in 3 adults. The current state of affairs points to an increasing pressure on existing health systems to meet the ever-growing and complex patient needs. Technological advances which are based on our understanding of the electropathophysiology of sleep disorders and the beneficial biological effects of magnetotherapy could provide the answer for a value-based and sustainable addition to the existing health systems without increasing costs.

While skepticism over the clinical and cost-effectiveness of EEG and PEMF systems is understandable, the prevailing feeling in the scientific community is that of excitement and enthusiasm as the clinical evidence continues to mount, driven by the noninvasive nature of these devices and their affordability coupled with a justified demand for safer and more effective therapeutic options. It is the belief of the author that the future of EEG and PEMF therapy in managing sleep disorders is promising given the recent findings of research; and this opens an exciting avenue for pharmacists to expand their healthcare expertise beyond standard pharmacotherapy.

L)   LESSONS LEARNED

- Sleep disorders including insomnia are a major public health concern for modern society.
- The rapidly expanding value-based neurodevices could be the answer to the concerns raised over standard of care with pervading claims of superior safety, effectiveness, and affordability fueled by increasing demand for improved quality of care.
- EEG and PEMF devices are noninvasive, user-friendly, affordable systems with claims of safety and clinical effectiveness in managing sleep disorders based on our understanding of the electrophysiology of sleep.
- While DTC EEG devices have come under scrutiny with the evidence supporting biofeedback practice being considered inadequate and shaky at best; the safety and clinical effectiveness of PEMF therapy seem to be evidenced by stronger well-designed studies with valid outcome measures.
- This supports the author's prediction that PEMF will be an important modality to complement or provide a viable and attractive alternative to standard treatment approaches.
- Pharmacists could and should play a crucial role as key stakeholders and innovation champions to accelerate the rapid uptake and diffusion of magnetotherapy while achieving alignment with pre-existing health systems.

REFERENCES

1. Chattu V, Manzar M, Kumary S, et al. The global problem of insufficient sleep and its serious public health implications. Healthcare [Internet]. 2018 Dec 20;7(1):1. Available from: /pmc/articles/PMC6473877/?report=abstract.
2. Thorpy MJ. Approach to the patient with a sleep complaint [Internet]. Sem Neurol. Copyright © 2004 by Thieme Medical Publishers, Inc., 333 Seventh Avenue, New York, NY 10001, USA. 2004;24:225–35. Available from: www.thieme-connect.de/DOI/DOI?10.1055/s-2004-835070
3. Thorpy MJ. Classification of sleep disorders. Neurotherapeutics [Internet]. 2012 Oct 14;9(4):687–701. Available from: http://link.springer.com/10.1007/s13311-012-0145-6.
4. Sateia MJ. International classification of sleep disorders-third edition highlights and modifications. Chest [Internet]. 2014 Nov 1;146(5):1387–94. Available from: http://journal.chestnet.org/article/S0012369215524070/fulltext.
5. LeBlanc M, Beaulieu-Bonneau S, Mérette C, et al. Psychological and health-related quality of life factors associated with insomnia in a population-based sample. J Psychosom Res [Internet]. 2007;63(2):157–66. Available from: https://pubmed.ncbi.nlm.nih.gov/17662752/.
6. Yazdi Z, Sadeghniiat-Haghighi K, Loukzadeh Z, et al. Prevalence of sleep disorders and their impacts on occupational performance: a comparison between shift workers and nonshift workers. Sleep Disord [Internet]. 2014;2014:1–5. Available from: /pmc/articles/PMC4055012/?report=abstract.
7. Panossian LA, Avidan AY. Review of sleep disorders. Med Clin N Am. Elsevier. 2009;93:407–25.
8. Ohayon MM. Epidemiology of insomnia: what we know and what we still need to learn. Sleep Med Rev. W.B. Saunders Ltd. 2002;6:97–111.
9. Levenson JC, Kay DB, Buysse DJ. The pathophysiology of insomnia. Chest. 2015 Apr 1;147(4):1179–92.
10. Ohayon MM, Reynolds CF. Epidemiological and clinical relevance of insomnia diagnosis algorithms according to the DSM-IV and the International Classification of Sleep Disorders (ICSD). Sleep Med. 2009 Oct 1;10(9):952–60.
11. Morin CM, Jarrin DC. Epidemiology of insomnia: prevalence, course, risk factors, and public health burden [Internet]. Sleep Med Clin. Elsevier. 2013;8:281–97. Available from: www.sleep.theclinics.com/article/S1556407X13000544/fulltext.
12. National Institutes of Health State of the Science Conference. National Institutes of Health State of the Science Conference statement on Manifestations and Management of Chronic Insomnia in Adults. Sleep [Internet]. 2005;28:1049–57. Available from: https://ci.nii.ac.jp/naid/20001002786.
13. American Psychological Association (APA). Diagnostic and statistical manual of mental disorders: depressive disorders [Internet]. Diagnostic and Statistical Manual of Mental Disorders. American Psychiatric Publishing, Inc.; 2013. p. 1–48. Available from: http://dsm.psychiatryonline.org//content.aspx?bookid=556&sectionid=41101760.
14. Clinton JM, Davis CJ, Zielinski MR, et al. Biochemical regulation of sleep and sleep biomarkers. J Clin Sleep Med [Internet]. 2011 Oct 15;7(5 Suppl). Available from: http://jcsm.aasm.org/doi/10.5664/JCSM.1360.
15. Winkelman JW, Buxton OM, Jensen JE, et al. Reduced brain GABA in primary insomnia: preliminary data from 4T proton magnetic resonance spectroscopy (1H-MRS). Sleep [Internet]. 2008 Nov 1;31(11):1499–506. Available from: https://academic.oup.com/sleep/article/31/11/1499/2454111.
16. Morgan PT, Pace-Schott EF, Mason GF, et al. Cortical GABA levels in primary insomnia. Sleep [Internet]. 2012 Jun 1;35(6):807–14. Available from: https://academic.oup.com/sleep/article-lookup/doi/10.5665/sleep.1880.
17. Riemann D, Klein T, Rodenbeck A, et al. Nocturnal cortisol and melatonin secretion in primary insomnia. Psychiatry Res. 2002 Dec 15;113(1–2):17–27.
18. Backhaus J, Junghanns K, Hohagen F. Sleep disturbances are correlated with decreased morning awakening salivary cortisol. Psychoneuroendocrinology. 2004 Oct 1;29(9):1184–91.
19. Zhang J, Lam SP, Li SX, et al. A community-based study on the association between insomnia and hypothalamic-pituitary-adrenal axis: sex and pubertal influences. J Clin Endocrinol Metab [Internet]. 2014 Jun 1;99(6):2277–87. Available

from: https://academic.oup.com/jcem/article/99/6/2277/2538067.

20. Ban H-J, Kim SC, Seo J, et al. Genetic and metabolic characterization of insomnia. Gaetano C, editor. PLoS One [Internet]. 2011 Apr 6;6(4):e18455. Available from: https://dx.plos.org/10.1371/journal.pone.0018455.

21. Cano G, Mochizuki T, Saper CB. Neural circuitry of stress-induced insomnia in rats. J Neurosci [Internet]. 2008 Oct 1;28(40):10167–84. Available from: www.jneurosci.org/content/28/40/10167.

22. Sallanon M, Denoyer M, Kitahama K, et al. Long-lasting insomnia induced by preoptic neuron lesions and its transient reversal by muscimol injection into the posterior hypothalamus in the cat. Neuroscience. 1989 Jan 1;32(3):669–83.

23. Koenigs M, Holliday J, Solomon J, et al. Left dorsomedial frontal brain damage is associated with insomnia. J Neurosci [Internet]. 2010 Nov 24;30(47):16041–3. Available from: www.jneurosci.org/content/30/47/16041.

24. Altena E, Vrenken H, Van Der Werf YD, et al. Reduced orbitofrontal and parietal gray matter in chronic insomnia: a voxel-based morphometry study. Biol Psychiatry. 2010 Jan 15;67(2):182–5.

25. Joo EY, Noh HJ, Kim J-S, et al. Brain gray matter deficits in patients with chronic primary insomnia. Sleep [Internet]. 2013 Jul 1;36(7):999–1007. Available from: https://academic.oup.com/sleep/article/36/7/999/2453939.

26. Krystal AD, Edinger JD, Wohlgemuth WK, et al. NREM sleep EEG frequency spectral correlates of sleep complaints in primary insomnia subtypes. Sleep [Internet]. 2002 Sep 1;25(6):626–36. https://doi.org/10.1093/sleep/25.6.626.

27. Perlis ML, Smith MT, Andrews PJ, et al. Beta/Gamma EEG activity in patients with primary and secondary insomnia and good sleeper controls. Sleep [Internet]. 2001 Feb 1;24(1):110–17. Available from: https://academic.oup.com/sleep/article/24/1/110/2749965.

28. Riemann D, Spiegelhalder C, Nissen V, et al. REM sleep instability: a new pathway for insomnia? Pharmacopsychiatry [Internet]. 2012;45:1–10.

29. Bonnet MH, Arand DL. Hyperarousal and insomnia: state of the science. Sleep Med Rev. W.B. Saunders. 2010;14:9–15.

30. Riemann D, Spiegelhalder K, Feige B, et al. The hyperarousal model of insomnia: a review of the concept and its evidence. Sleep Med Rev. W.B. Saunders. 2010;14:19–31.

31. Perlis ML, Giles DE, Mendelson WB, et al. Psychophysiological insomnia: the behavioural model and a neurocognitive perspective [Internet]. J Sleep Res. Blackwell Publishing Ltd. 1997;6:179–88. Available from: https://onlinelibrary.wiley.com/doi/full/10.1046/j.1365-2869.1997.00045.x.

32. Silva-Costa A, Griep RH, Rotenberg L. Associations of a short sleep duration, insufficient sleep, and insomnia with self-rated health among nurses. PLoS ONE [Internet]. 2015 May 11;10(5). Available from: https://pubmed.ncbi.nlm.nih.gov/25961874/.

33. Bertisch SM, Pollock BD, Mittleman MA, et al. Insomnia with objective short sleep duration and risk of incident cardiovascular disease and all-cause mortality: Sleep Heart Health Study. Sleep [Internet]. 2018 Jun 1;41(6). Available from: https://pubmed.ncbi.nlm.nih.gov/29522193/.

34. Maric A, Montvai E, Werth E, et al. Insufficient sleep: enhanced risk-seeking relates to low local sleep intensity. Ann Neurol [Internet]. 2017 Sep 1;82(3):409–18. Available from: https://pubmed.ncbi.nlm.nih.gov/28833531/.

35. Lee YJ, Cho SJ, Cho IH, et al. Insufficient sleep and suicidality in adolescents. Sleep [Internet]. 2012 Apr 1;35(4):455–60. Available from: https://pubmed.ncbi.nlm.nih.gov/22467982/.

36. Ayas NT, White DP, Manson JAE, et al. A prospective study of sleep duration and coronary heart disease in women. Arch Intern Med [Internet]. 2003 Jan 27;163(2):205–9. Available from: https://pubmed.ncbi.nlm.nih.gov/12546611/.

37. Janszky I, Ljung R. Shifts to and from daylight saving time and incidence of myocardial infarction [Internet]. New Engl J Med. Massachussetts Medical Society. 2008;359:1966–8. Available from: https://pubmed.ncbi.nlm.nih.gov/18971502/.

38. Copinschi G. Metabolic and endocrine effects of sleep deprivation. [Internet]. Essential Psychopharmacol. 2005;6:341–7. Available from: https://europepmc.org/article/med/16459757.

39. Smith MT, Klick B, Kozachik S, Edwards RE, et al. Sleep onset insomnia symptoms during hospitalization for major burn injury predict chronic pain. Pain. 2008 Sep 15;138(3):497–506.

40. Stiefel F, Stagno D. Management of insomnia in patients with chronic pain conditions [Internet]. CNS Drugs. Springer. 2004;18:285–96. Available from: https://link.springer.com/article/10.2165/00023210-200418050-00002

41. Phillips B, Mannino DM. Do insomnia complaints cause hypertension or cardiovascular disease? J Clin Sleep Med [Internet]. 2007 Aug 15;03(05):489–94. Available from: http://jcsm.aasm.org/doi/10.5664/jcsm.26913.

42. Vishnu A, Shankar A, Kalidindi S. Examination of the association between insufficient sleep and cardiovascular disease and diabetes by race/ethnicity. Int J Endocrinol [Internet]. 2011;2011. Available from: https://pubmed.ncbi.nlm.nih.gov/21754929/.

43. Curcio G, Ferrara M, De Gennaro L. Sleep loss, learning capacity and academic performance [Internet]. Sleep Med Rev. 2006;10:323–37. Available from: https://pubmed.ncbi.nlm.nih.gov/16564189/.

44. De Mello MT, Narciso FV, Tufik S, et al. Sleep disorders as a cause of motor vehicle collisions [Internet]. Int J Prev Med. 2013;4:246–57. Available from: https://pubmed.ncbi.nlm.nih.gov/23626880/.

45. Drake CL, Roehrs T, Breslau N, et al. The 10-year risk of verified motor vehicle crashes in relation to physiologic sleepiness. Sleep [Internet]. 2010 Jun 1;33(6):745–52. Available from: https://pubmed.ncbi.nlm.nih.gov/20550014/.

46. Lockley SW, Barger LK, Ayas NT, et al. Effects of health care provider work hours and sleep deprivation on safety and performance. Jt Comm J Qual Patient Saf. 2007 Nov 1;33(11 Suppl.):7–18.

47. Sallinen M, Holm A, Hiltunen J, et al. Recovery of cognitive performance from sleep debt: do a short rest pause and a single recovery night help? In: Chronobiology international [Internet]. Taylor & Francis; 2008. p. 279–96. Available from: www.tandfonline.com/doi/abs/10.1080/07420520802107106.

48. Edwards J, Goldie I, Elliott I, et al. Fundamental facts about mental health. London: Mental Health Foundation; 2016.

49. NICE. Insomnia [Internet]. Clinical Knowledge Summaries CKS. 2020. Available from: https://cks.nice.org.uk/topics/insomnia/#!management.

50. Kripke DF. Hypnotic drug risks of mortality, infection, depression, and cancer: but lack of benefit [version 3; referees: 2 approved]. F1000Research. F1000 Research Ltd. 2018;5.

51. Morgenthaler T, Kramer M, Alessi C, et al. Practice parameters for the psychological and behavioral treatment of insomnia: an update. Am Acad Sleep Med Rep [Internet]. Sleep. American Academy of Sleep Medicine. 2006;29:1415–9. Available from: https://europepmc.org/article/med/17162987

52. Morin CM, Bootzin RR, Buysse DJ, et al. Psychological and behavioral treatment of insomnia: update of the recent evidence (1998–2004) [Internet]. Sleep. American Academy of Sleep Medicine. 2006;29:1398–414. Available from: https://pubmed.ncbi.nlm.nih.gov/17162986/.

53. Thibault RT, Raz A. The psychology of neurofeedback: clinical intervention even if applied placebo. Am Psychol [Internet]. 2017 Oct 1;72(7):679–88. Available from: /fulltext/2017-43854-005.html.

54. Coates McCall I, Lau C, Minielly N, et al. Owning ethical innovation: claims about commercial wearable brain technologies. Neuron. Cell Press. 2019;102:728–31.

55. Sleep Shepherd. Sleep improvement—sleep shepherd [Internet]. 2016. Available from: https://sleepshepherd.com/sleep-improvement/.

56. Lane JD, Kasian SJ, Owens JE, et al. Binaural auditory beats affect vigilance performance and mood. Physiol Behav. 1998;63.

57. Holden K. Biological eEffects of Pulsed Electromagnetic Field (PEMF) therapy [Internet]. Anti-aging Medical News. 2012. Available from: www.ondamed.net/images/publications/articles/Holden-A4M_Artikel-Biological_Effects_of_pulsed_electromagnetic_Field_Therapie.pdf.

58. Weintraub MI. Magnetotherapy: historical background with a stimulating future [Internet]. Crit Rev Phys Rehabil Med. Begel House Inc. 2004;16:95–108. Available from: www.dl.begellhouse.com/journals/757fcb0219d89390,56be219748b36bea,613213db73532354.html.

59. Vadalà M, Vallelunga A, Palmieri L, et al. Mechanisms and therapeutic applications of electromagnetic therapy in Parkinson's disease [Internet]. Behav Brain Funct. BioMed Central Ltd. 2015;11:26. Available from: /pmc/articles/PMC4562205/?report=abstract.

60. Panagopoulos DJ, Karabarbounis A, Margaritis LH. Mechanism for action of electromagnetic fields on cells. Biochem Biophys Res Commun. 2002 Oct 18;298(1):95–102.

61. Wade B. A Review of Pulsed Electromagnetic Field (PEMF) mechanisms at a cellular level: a rationale for clinical use. Am J Heal Res [Internet]. 2013 Jan 1;1(3):51. Available from: www.sciencepublishinggroup.com/journal/paperinfo.aspx?journalid=656&doi=10.11648/j.ajhr.20130103.13.

62. Blackman C. Calcium release from nervous tissue: experimental results and possible mechanisms. In: Norden B, Ramel C, editors. Interaction mechanisms of low-level electromagnetic fields in living systems. Oxford: Oxford University Press; 1992. p. 107–29.

63. Kaczmarek LK, Adey WR. The efflux of 45Ca2+ and [3H] γ-aminobutyric acid from cat cerebral cortex. Brain Res. 1973 Dec 7;63(C):331–42.

64. Lai H, Carino MA, Horita A, et al. Single vs. Repeated microwave exposure: effects on benzodiazepine receptors in the brain of the rat. Bioelectromagnetics [Internet]. 1992 Jan 1;13(1):57–66. Available from: http://doi.wiley.com/10.1002/bem.2250130107.

65. Reiter RJ. Electromagnetic fields and melatonin production. Biomed Pharmacother. 1993 Jan 1;47(10):439–44.

66. Lebet JP, Barbault A, Rossel C, et al. Electroencephalographic changes following low energy emission therapy. Ann Biomed Eng [Internet]. 1996;24(3):424–9. Available from: https://link.springer.com/article/10.1007/BF02660891.

67. Higgs L, Reite M, Barbault A, et al. Subjective and objective relaxation effects of low energy emission therapy. Stress Med [Internet]. 1994 Jan 1;10(1):5–13. Available from: http://doi.wiley.com/10.1002/smi.2460100103.

68. Flexpulse. Flexpulse PEMF device [Internet]. Flexpulse.com. Available from: https://flexpulse.com/flexpulse-pemf-device/.

69. Bellabee.us. Bellabee—Empower your mind [Internet]. Available from: https://bellabee.us/.

70. Improve your life quality with NeoRhythm [Internet]. Omnipemf. Available from: https://omnipemf.com/.

71. Biomobie. Bioboosti R7—biomobie bioelectric technology—biomobie life core [Internet]. Available from: http://106.14.44.159:9090/r7/.

72. SomniResonance. Placement of the SR1 sleep device—SomniResonance® SR1 [Internet]. SomniResonance—Sleep Naturally. Available from: www.deltasleeper.com/placement/.

73. Bellabee.us. Safety & set-up information—Bellabee [Internet]. Available from: https://bellabee.us/safety-set-up-information/.

74. Ganesan K, Gengadharan AC, Balachandran C, et al. Low frequency pulsed electromagnetic field—a viable alternative therapy for arthritis. Indian J Exp Biol. 2009 Dec;47(12):939–48.

75. Omnipemf. NeoRythm—headband positions section—support—Omnipemf [Internet]. Available from: https://omnipemf.com/support/.

76. Pasche B, Erman M, Hayduk R, et al. Effects of low energy emission therapy in chronic psychophysiological insomnia. Sleep [Internet]. 1996 Jun 1;19(4):327–36. Available from: https://academic.oup.com/sleep/article/19/4/327/2749847.

77. Reite M, Higgs L, Lebet J-P, et al. Sleep inducing effect of low energy emission therapy. Bioelectromagnetics [Internet]. 1994 Jan 1;15(1):67–75. Available from: http://doi.wiley.com/10.1002/bem.2250150110.

78. Pelka RB, Jaenicke C, Gruenwald J. Impulse magnetic-field therapy for insomnia: a double-blind, placebo-controlled study. Adv Ther [Internet]. 2001;18(4):174–80. Available from: https://link.springer.com/article/10.1007/BF02850111.

79. Pavlova M, Matthew P, Veronique L, Puri N. 0391 Gr8 expectations: the efficacy of Bioboosti 8 minute electromagnetic cycles for the treatment of insomnia. Sleep [Internet]. 2018 Apr 27;41(suppl_1):A149—A149. Available from: https://academic.oup.com/sleep/article/41/suppl_1/A149/4988428.

80. Markov MS. Pulsed electromagnetic field therapy history, state of the art and future. Environmentalist [Internet]. 2007 Dec 6;27(4):465–75. Available from: www.curatronic.com.

9 Medical Devices for Pediatrics

Binaya Sapkota and Sunil Shrestha

CONTENTS

DOI: 10.1201/9781003002345-11

GENERAL BACKGROUND

There are various types of pediatric devices available on the market, depending on the pediatric problem. These devices provide no medicinal alternatives to relieve the associated pain and problems. Various lightweight materials, along with a blend of environmentally friendly materials, are currently being emphasized by manufacturers. Nevertheless, the designs of devices, like medicines, are also being improved based on experiences and clinical trials. In this chapter, we will discuss breast pumps, pediatric

thermometers, liquid medicine measuring devices, infant feeding bottles, pediatric inhalation devices, child diapers (disposable napkins), child blood pressure monitors, and child face masks, since these are widely implicated from the pharmacy and pharmacists' point of view. The devices within each category may be of different types depending on their shape, size, or purpose of use. Physicians, pharmacists and other concerned health professionals should select the appropriate device for the patients' conditions and counsel them on their appropriate application or use.

Children are not small adults; they have a different physiological and pharmacokinetic response to diseases and pharmacotherapy, including medicines and medical devices. Breastfeeding is the recommended mode of infant feeding until the first year because it provides nutrition and supports the growth and development of infants. If breastfeeding cannot fulfill the requirements of the child, a breast pump can be used to enhance the amount of milk expression by creating vacuum pressure on the breasts. Fever, along with other clinical complaints, is one of the most familiar symptoms among the pediatric population, for which various types of thermometers, such as digital, ear, forehead, glass, and mercury thermometers, are in clinical practice. Many liquid medications are supplied with measuring devices, such as dosing spoons, calibrated spoons, droppers, dosing cups, and oral syringes, to help parents administer medications to children.

Enteral feeding with bottles and tubes may be necessary for newborn infants if they cannot breastfeed. Respiratory diseases are one of the most typical causes of hospitalizations and emergency department visits among children worldwide. Child diapers are used for the infant and babies during the day or at night; they urinate and defecate within the diaper. High blood pressure in children and adolescents is a global health problem, with primary hypertension as the most common type in these age categories. Children are more susceptible to the risks associated with air pollution, such as chronic respiratory diseases. Masks and respirators protect against air pollutants to some extent.

CHAPTER OBJECTIVES

At the end of the chapter, the readers will be able to understand the details of the following devices:

1. Breast pumps
2. Pediatric thermometers
3. Liquid medicine measuring devices
4. Infant feeding bottles
5. Pediatric inhalation devices
6. Child/baby diapers (disposable napkins)
7. Child blood pressure monitors
8. Child face masks

DEVICE 1: BREAST PUMPS

A) BACKGROUND

Breastfeeding is the recommended mode of feeding for all infants until the first year.[1,2] The World Health Organization (WHO), the American Academy of Pediatrics, and the American College of Obstetricians and Gynecologists recommend exclusive breastfeeding until the age of 6 months, with continued breastfeeding and complementary food items from then onward.[1,3,4] Infants achieve resistance to infectious diseases (i.e., immunity) such as otitis media, gastrointestinal tract infections, respiratory tract infections,

and others, from breast milk. Breastfeeding also reduces sudden infant death syndrome (SIDS) and other causes of childhood mortality and hospitalizations.[1,2] Breast milk also fulfills the requirements for nutrition, growth, and development of infants.[2] Milk expression requires steady production (i.e., galactopoiesis) and secretion of milk from the breast.[5,6] Stimulation of the areola and nipple creates a milk secretion reflex and releases prolactin into the blood from the adeno-pituitary gland,[5] whereas less nipple stimulation reduces prolactin secretion and milk protein synthesis.[6] Milk expression should begin within 2 hours of infant birth. Breastfeeding releases oxytocin, which reduces uterine bleeding and helps in returning the uterus to its normal size more quickly. Breastfeeding also helps reduce body weight, since it consumes 500 calories a day. Hence, breastfeeding is beneficial not only for newborn babies but also for mothers.

Breast pumps are medical devices that are useful for nursing mothers who need to remain separated from their infants for work, school, or other tasks, as well as mothers who face challenges in milk supply.[7,8] The pump is used to enhance the amount of milk expression by creating vacuum pressure on the breasts.[6] Alekseev et al. (1998) found that the blood prolactin level increases by 1.3–1.5 times with breast pump use.[5] A mother with a sick or premature infant in the neonatal intensive care unit (NICU) needs to use a breast pump for uninterrupted milk supply.[3] Mothers who return to work find breast pumps useful to collect and supply their milk while they are away from their baby.[3,6]

B) DEVICE DESCRIPTION/IMPORTANT FEATURES

Normal functioning of the breast pump is based on the principle of milk secretion from the breasts within approximately 1.5 minutes of applying vacuum and compression stimuli to the nipple and areola.

Types of Breast Pumps[6]

Manual or electric breast pumps are available on the market. Before the 1920s, manual expression was the most standard method to extract breast milk, whereas the use of an electric pump began in the 1920s with increased hospital childbirths. Mothers can set the vacuum pressure according to their requirement in almost all pumps—both manual and electric.

i. Manual Pumps

Manual pumps generate a vacuum by repetitive pushing or squeezing of the device with the hands or feet. They do not require electricity or a battery and are convenient to use. They are less costly and noisy and more portable than electric pumps.

ii. Electric Pumps

These pumps are electricity- or battery-operated to generate a vacuum, and they can be personal-use or multiuser pumps. Mothers can set the vacuum pressure according to

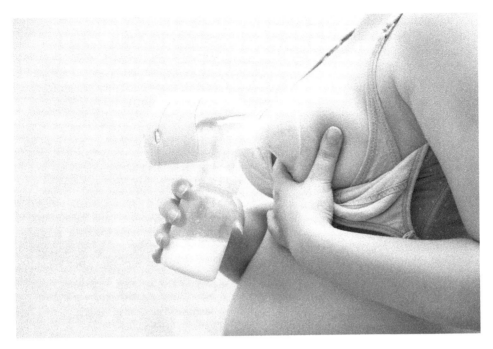

FIGURE 9.1   A breast pump in use; pumped milk is stored in a baby bottle for convenient transition to feeding later.

Source: www.shutterstock.com/image-photo/young-mother-pumped-breast-milk-pump-1049152367

their requirement in almost all pumps—both manual and electric.

A.   PERSONAL-USE PUMPS

Most electric pumps are personal-use types that are not designed for more than one person because filters and non-replaceable parts may be contaminated, causing transmission of infection from one user to another.

B.   MULTIUSER PUMPS (HOSPITAL-GRADE PUMPS)

Mothers generally use these in hospital settings, and their design prevents cross-contamination among different users.

However, these pumps are more expensive than personal-use types.

The breast pump consists of the following parts[5,9]:

i.   Control panel with compressor
ii.   Remote cap consisting of a solid body and an elastic conical tube
iii.   Pneumatic chambers to compress the areola
iv.   Vacuum pusher
v.   Milk collector placed in the holder connected to the body of the cap
vi.   Vacuum conductor of the vacuum and pressure stimuli

C)   PURPOSE AND HOW TO USE

- Relax to allow the release of oxytocin, which stimulates the let-down reflex. Discomfort and distractions can hamper the hormone secretion process.

Therefore, choose a private and comfortable location for breast pumping and ensure that your arms and back are well supported while pumping.

- Place the assembled breast shield on the center of your breast over the nipple. Begin pumping for a few minutes to allow the milk to flow.[9]
- Set a vacuum pressure amplitude of 15–20 kPa at the breast pump. When the maximum vacuum has been achieved, excess pressure is transmitted into the vacuum chambers. Then, compression of the elastic conical tube and the part of the areola within the pneumochamber occurs.
- Control the compression with the regulator on the control panel. After the vacuum inside the elastic conical tube reaches the maximum level, all the stimuli from the pump ceases, and the cycle is repeated.[5]
- The pumping rate can be adjusted to make it similar to a baby's sucking motions once the milk is released.
- Switch breasts every 5 minutes, ensuring that each breast receives 15 minutes of total stimulation. Do not worry if one breast secrets more milk than the other because this is a normal physiological phenomenon.
- Remove the breast shield when you finish pumping. Then, unscrew the bottle and place a cap on it.
- Wash the parts of the manual breast pump that touched the breast or milk in warm soapy water and allow them to air dry.
- You can safely keep the expressed breast milk at room temperature for 4–6 hours or refrigerate it for up to 5 days.[9]

- Always wash your hands before and after using the breast pump and clean the pump parts after use. Additionally, the pump parts should be sanitized at least once daily after cleaning.
- Store the pump set in a clear bag or container after each use and cleaning.

D) IMPORTANT SAFETY ISSUES (CAUTIONS AND COMMON ADVERSE EFFECTS)

- Risks associated with manual breast pumps are breast tissue damage and infection.[7]
- A manual pump is not ideal for mothers with time constraints.[6]
- Adverse events from electric breast pumps include pain, soreness or discomfort, need for medical intervention, and breast tissue damage.
- Serious adverse events include device-related injury, malfunctions, and deaths.[7]
- Bacterial contamination of breast milk may occur with a breast pump.[6,10]
- Breast pumps can cause damage to the nipple and breast tissue.
- Breast pump use can reduce the milk supply, and freezing breast milk depletes the nutritional content.

E) STORAGE CONDITIONS AND MAINTENANCE

- Read the manufacturer's instructions for using and cleaning the pump. Always clean the breast pump parts before each use to avoid contamination of the colostrum (breast milk) with pathogens.[6,9,11,12]
- The mother can store small volumes of breast milk (such as 30–60 mL) in the freezer after the third week postpartum or before returning to work. Expressed milk is safe at room temperature (generally 26°C) for 4 to 6 hours. Milk should be refrigerated within 4 hours at temperatures over 26°C.
- Breast milk refrigerated immediately after expression is safe for approximately 72 hours. Expressed breast milk in the freezer is safe for 6 to 12 months (temperature of −17°C). If milk is expressed under aseptic conditions, it may be safe from bacterial contamination until 5 to 8 days.[6,13]
- Wash breast pump milk collection kits (BPKs) with detergent or sodium hypochlorite followed by a thorough rinsing and drying after each use.[10,12]
- Do not reuse the kits unless they are properly sterilized.[12]

F) IMPORTANT FEATURES (CAPABILITIES AND LIMITATIONS) AND SPECIAL ADVANTAGES

- Breast pumps are useful in human milk banks.[10]
- Breast pumps are beneficial for mothers with breastfeeding problems such as slow infant weight gain or rapid weight loss, or mothers who must return to work early.[3]
- Breast pumps can relieve the breasts from becoming engorged and prevent mastitis.
- Breast pumps can help maintain an adequate milk supply to the baby.

G) SPECIAL TIPS FOR PATIENT COUNSELING

- Fit the breast pump properly to optimize the breast milk supply and prevent injury.
- Express milk in a private location, where you feel less stressed, every 3 to 4 hours for 15 to 30 minutes to maintain milk supply. Wash your hands and pump collection equipment before expressing milk.
- Never use a microwave for reheating the breast milk.[6]
- Never buy a used breast pump or share a pump because previously used pumps may transmit pathogens; however, hospital-grade pumps can be rented and reused.
- If you get injured and suffer from pain or hemorrhage with a breast pump, immediately contact a gynecologist.
- Use the breast pump in the morning because, during this period, you tend to get the most milk secretion.
- Stick to a fixed breast pumping schedule each day because this helps your body produce more milk.
- Remove the pump after 25 to 30 minutes, because both breasts will become entirely empty within this period.

H) EVIDENCE OF EFFECTIVENESS AND SAFETY

Some employers purchase multiuser pumps to promote employee lactation in the office.[6] Informative parameters of breast pump efficacy are the time to milk ejection, amount of milk secreted, and rate of milk secretion.[14]

I) ECONOMIC EVALUATION

Manual breast pumps usually cost between US$40 and $60, whereas electric pumps usually cost between US$175 and $320. Hence, electric breast pumps may not be affordable for many low-income women, but these women can use manual pumps.[3] Retail stores and pharmacies also offer rental options for the pumps.[6] Approximately US$13 billion can be saved on costs associated with premature death and illness with breast pump use every year.[1]

J) IMPLICATIONS FOR THE PHARMACY PROFESSION AND PHARMACY PRACTICE

Breast pumps that work for some women may not work or may cause injury to other women.[7] Nevertheless, breastfeeding and feeding an infant with the breast pump are not equivalent. Infants fed with the pump may gain more weight within one year of age than infants who are breastfed.[15] Health professionals, including pharmacists, should know the details about breast pumps and relevant techniques to help mothers express their milk as needed.[6] They should also counsel women on how early they may use a breast pump.[16]

K) CHALLENGES TO PHARMACISTS AND USERS

Although breastfeeding improves maternal and child health, multiple hurdles prevent some nursing mothers from adopting exclusive breastfeeding. Breast pumps may serve as an alternative for breastfeeding in such a scenario.[15] Manual expression may be needed during times of pump failure, emergencies, and loss of electricity; a mother can manually express first and then use the pump.[6]

L) RECOMMENDATIONS: THE WAY FORWARD

- Health professionals, including pharmacists, should counsel mothers about breast pumping techniques to help them express their milk.
- Pharmacists should instruct mothers to not buy a used breast pump or share a pump, to control the transmission of pathogens.
- Mothers should wash the breast pump milk collection kits with detergent and allow drying after each use.

M) CONCLUSIONS

Breastfeeding is the recommended mode of infant feeding for the first year because it provides nutrition and supports the growth and development of infants. Breast pumps are useful devices for nursing mothers who need to remain separated from their infants due to work-related issues and thus, find difficulty maintaining a timely milk supply. Normal functioning of the pump is based on the principle of milk secretion from the breasts within 1.5 minutes of application of vacuum and compression stimuli to the nipple and areola. Breast pumps that work for some women may not work or may even cause injury to other women.

N) LESSONS LEARNED

- Manual or electric breast pumps are available on the market, and health professionals can choose the pump that fits the mother's need and budget.
- Breast pumps may be useful in human milk banks.
- Bacterial contamination of breast milk may occur with a breast pump. Therefore, necessary care should be taken while using the pump.
- Breast pump efficacy can be evaluated based on the time to milk ejection, amount of milk secreted, and rate of milk secretion.

DEVICE 2: PEDIATRIC THERMOMETERS

A) BACKGROUND

Fever, along with other clinical complaints, is one of the most common symptoms among the pediatric population (e.g., infants and young children), and it is a predictor of occult bacteremia.[17–20] The World Health Organization Expert Study Group recommends axillary temperature ≥ 37.50°C as the threshold for fever, irrespective of the measurement device used, anatomic site chosen for measurement, age, or environmental conditions.[17,18] Fever is responsible for up to 20% of emergency room (ER) visits among pediatric patients.[17–21] Parents and health professionals frequently rely on temperatures measured by parents at home to determine the febrile condition in the child.[22] Therefore, accurate body temperature monitoring of critically ill children is vital,[17–19] and the thermometer is the device used to measure body temperature. The term "thermometer" was derived from the Greek terms *thermē* ("heat") and *metron* measurement).

Oral and rectal temperatures are the most reliable indicators of core temperature; rectal measurement is regarded as the clinical standard. Core temperature closely reflects the temperature in the blood circulation.[18] The temperature of children younger than 4 years is measured with a rectal thermometer in hospital emergency departments because it gives accurate temperature readings in almost all cases; however, it is a physically and psychologically invasive way to measure temperature. An oral electronic thermometer is the most accurate noninvasive method of temperature measurement among adults, but it is not suitable for children younger than 4 years because it demands good patient cooperation.[23]

A mercury rectal thermometer was the only available tool to assess fever for many decades. However, potential heavy metal toxicity due to the direct contact of mercury with the skin and mucosa has limited its use in most countries worldwide.[17,18,21,24,25]

B) DEVICE DESCRIPTION/IMPORTANT FEATURES

Types of Pediatric Thermometers

The most commonly used clinical thermometers are as follows:

i. Digital thermometers (axillary digital thermometers [ADTs], axillary artery thermometer)
ii. Electronic ear thermometers (auricular thermometer, infrared ear thermometers, tympanic membrane thermometers, infrared tympanic thermometer [ITT])
iii. Forehead thermometers (temporal artery thermometers, forehead noncontact thermometers)
iv. Glass and mercury thermometers (doctor's thermometers, rectal glass mercury thermometer)
v. Galinstan thermometers

i. Digital Thermometers

Digital thermometers are the fastest tool for temperature measurement. Readings are taken from the sublingual region, rectum, or armpit (i.e., axillary region). However, axillary temperature reading is the most reliable, appropriate, and accurate method in the pediatric population because minimal patient cooperation is necessary for this route of temperature measurement.[18] These thermometers can easily be purchased in local pharmacies and can be used at home or in the hospital.

ii. Electronic Ear Thermometers

These thermometers were launched onto the market in the 1980s[25]; they use infrared technology for temperature readings. If there is too much wax in the ear, it gives an incorrect reading. These thermometers are expensive but are more comfortable to use in the pediatric population, since they take less time for temperature measurement than digital thermometers.

iii. Forehead Thermometers

These also use infrared technology and measure the heat radiating from the skin on the forehead as the sensor head is moved across the forehead.[23] The forehead is the ideal site for temperature reading because it is innervated by the temporal artery, which receives high blood flow from the carotid artery.[18] These thermometers are painless, noninvasive devices that provide readings within only a few seconds.[26] However, these thermometers are less reliable than digital thermometers.

iv. Glass and Mercury Thermometers

These thermometers were considered the standard for temperature measurement until the 1970s[19,25]; they are the old versions of current thermometers. The thermometer is placed sublingually, and the rise in the mercury tube is observed. Once the mercury stops rising, it indicates the body temperature. These are gradually becoming obsolete due to the potential heavy metal toxicity of mercury.

v. Galinstan Thermometers

Galinstan is a nontoxic eutectic alloy of gallium, indium, and tin; it is liquid at room temperature and even below the freezing point of water. These thermometers provide mercury-free alternatives for temperature measurement.[21] Several companies now replaced mercury thermometers with these thermometers to eliminate the risk of mercury toxicity. Nevertheless, these factors pose potential injury hazards associated with glass encasement.[24]

Of the aforementioned thermometers, axillary digital thermometers (ADTs) and noncontact (infrared) forehead thermometers (NCIFTs) are the most commonly used types

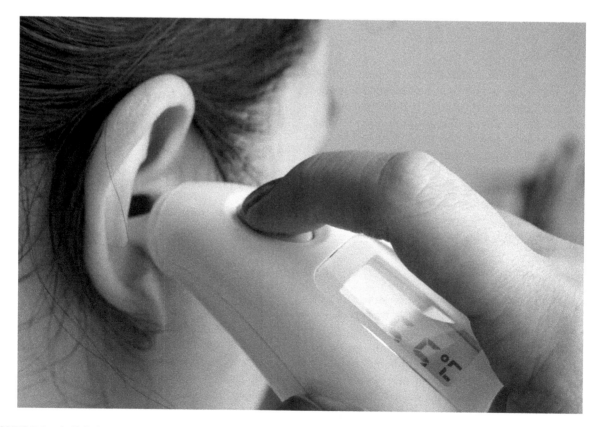

FIGURE 9.2　A digital ear thermometer in use.

Source: www.shutterstock.com/image-photo/woman-checks-temperature-ear-herself-by-1348485365

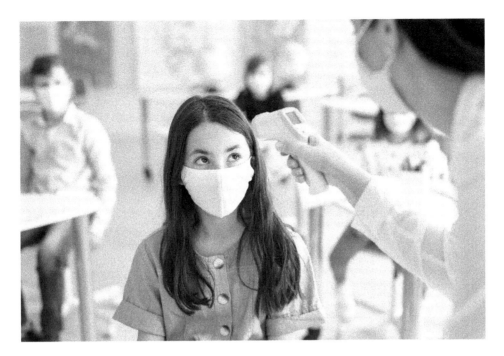

FIGURE 9.3 Noncontact forehead thermometers are often used in schools.

Source: www.shutterstock.com/image-photo/teacher-children-face-mask-school-after-1746069596

in pediatric settings where incorrect temperature measurement may delay treatments or lead to incorrect diagnoses and therapies.[26]

Thermometer Selection

- Consider the following temperature ranges when choosing a particular thermometer for temperature measurement[27]:

Temperature reading	Temperature range
Rectal	36.6°C to 38°C
Ear	35.8°C to 38°C
Oral	35.5°C to 37.5°C
Axillary	34.7°C to 37.3°C

Additionally, consider the following brief guidance for selecting an appropriate temperature reading method based on the age of the child:

Age of the child	Temperature reading technique
Birth to 2 years	Rectal (for a definitive reading); Axillary (for screening purposes)
2 to 5 years	Rectal; Tympanic; Axillary
Age > 5 years	Oral; Tympanic; Axillary

c) PURPOSE AND HOW TO USE

A digital thermometer can be used in the following ways:

- A digital thermometer used for axillary temperature measurement should be calibrated at three-month intervals.[17]
- Turn on the thermometer and ensure that number zero appears on display. This can be ensured by shaking the thermometer down so that it reads below the body temperature.[20]
- Keep the thermometer tip under the armpit or insert it into the anus to measure the child's temperature. If the rectal route is used, lay the child on his or her back to insert only the metallic part of the thermometer into the anus.
- Wait a few seconds until you hear the thermometer alarm.
- Remove the thermometer and check the temperature reading on the screen.
- Clean the metallic tip with cotton and disinfectant or an alcohol swab.

An infrared ear thermometer can be used in the following manner:

- Place the thermometer tip inside the ear, pointing towards the nose.
- Press the power button on the thermometer until you hear a signal.
- Read the temperature measurement, which appears instantly.
- Remove the thermometer from the ear and clean the tip with cotton and disinfectant or an alcohol swab.

A temporal artery thermometer can be used in the following ways:

- Calibrate the thermometer at room temperature at the beginning of each monitoring day.[17]
- Turn the thermometer on.
- Sweep the thermometer gently across the forehead so that the infrared scanner measures the temperature of the temporal artery.
- Record the temperature and time.

D) IMPORTANT SAFETY ISSUES (CAUTIONS AND COMMON ADVERSE EFFECTS)

- Rectal thermometers are painful for infants (i.e., may cause traumatic rectal injury) and time-consuming, and they require good practice for a proper reading. Therefore, these are not the optimal choice for infants, health professionals, or parents.[18,19,23]
- Rectal temperature measurement may disseminate fecal pathogens and is contraindicated in critically ill patients due to immune compromise or coagulopathy.[19]
- Tympanic and forehead thermometers are also not always appropriate because febrile children are generally agitated and do not cooperate with the caregiver.[17]
- Axillary temperature reading with a digital thermometer is time-consuming.
- A noncontact infrared thermometer must be used cautiously due to its high potential for bias.[18]

E) STORAGE CONDITIONS AND MAINTENANCE

- Use an alcohol swab or cotton swab soaked with 70% isopropyl alcohol to clean the thermometer case and the measuring probe, ensuring that no liquid droplets enter the interior of the thermometer.
- Never use an abrasive cleaning agent, such as benzene, for cleaning.
- Never expose the thermometer to water or other liquids.
- You can store the thermometer in a room where the temperature is between $-20°C$ and $+50°C$ and relative humidity is between 15–95%, but its operational temperature is between $16°C$ and $40°C$.

F) IMPORTANT FEATURES (CAPABILITIES AND LIMITATIONS) AND SPECIAL ADVANTAGES

- Thermometers can detect body temperature quickly and with high accuracy.
- They are handy, easy to use, and portable.
- They are usually inexpensive.

G) SPECIAL TIPS FOR PATIENT COUNSELING

- Do not measure oral and rectal temperatures of children younger 5 years due to the invasiveness of the temperature reading procedures.[26]
- Take care not to not scratch the thermometer display by replacing the protective cap after use.
- Take care while reading the temperature on display by keeping the thermometer at your eye level.

H) EVIDENCE OF EFFECTIVENESS AND SAFETY

Tympanic thermometers are fast and easy to handle and minimize the risk of nosocomial infection.[22] A noncontact, accurate, and inexpensive method of temperature measurement is appropriate for the pediatric population.[17] The Canadian Pediatric Society (CPS) still recommends the use of rectal thermometers in children < 5 years of age.[27,28]

I) ECONOMIC EVALUATION

Different thermometers have various cost ranges. Tympanic thermometers can be purchased at the cost of approximately US$50 and can be used at home.[22] Similarly, mercury and glass thermometers usually cost US$3–5, digital thermometers between US$8 and $15, and forehead thermometers between US$2 and $5.

J) IMPLICATION TO THE PHARMACY PROFESSION AND PHARMACY PRACTICE

Large differences in the temperature readings at axillary and rectal sites make the interpretation of the reading difficult in clinical practice.[23] Measuring fever orally or rectally is difficult because it is painful for infants and time-consuming for the health professional; this approach demands good practice.[17,18,21,24,25]

K) CHALLENGES TO PHARMACISTS AND USERS

Tympanic and forehead thermometers are frequently used in clinical practice, but these are not accurate.[17] Frequently encountered problems in temperature measurement are variations in temperature with activity level, meal consumption, measurement timing, time of the day, environmental conditions, improper positioning of thermometer, and hurried readings. Eliminations of these factors is usually not possible. Therefore, reliance on the use of a single temperature reading is not reasonable.[18]

L) RECOMMENDATIONS: THE WAY FORWARD

- Physicians and pharmacists should select appropriate thermometers, from among the many available models or types, for pediatric patients.
- Health professionals should counsel patients that noncontact, accurate, and inexpensive methods of

temperature measurement are appropriate for the pediatric population.

- Mercury thermometers should not be used, since they can lead to heavy metal toxicity and have been banned in many countries.

M) CONCLUSIONS

Fever is one of the most familiar symptoms among the pediatric population and is responsible for up to 20% of emergency department visits among this group. Thermometers can reliably and quickly read body temperature. Oral and rectal temperatures are the most reliable indicators of core temperature, among which rectal measurement is regarded as the clinical standard. Mercury thermometers were previously used in clinical practice, but these are becoming obsolete due to cases of accidental mercury poisoning.

N) LESSONS LEARNED

- Digital, ear thermometers, forehead thermometers, and glass and mercury thermometers are widely used in clinical practice.
- Rectal thermometers are painful for infants and time-consuming for health professionals, and they require good practice for proper reading. Therefore, these are not the optimal choice for infants, health professionals, or parents.
- A noncontact infrared thermometer must be used cautiously due to its high potential for bias.
- Reliance on the use of a single temperature reading is not reasonable. Therefore, repeated temperature readings at various times is necessary to confirm the temperature reading.

DEVICE 3: LIQUID MEDICINE MEASURING DEVICES

A) BACKGROUND

Most of the medications administered to children are oral liquid formulations (such as syrups, solutions, suspensions, and elixirs) to help them swallow the medication easily and prevent the risk of inhalation.[29–31] Liquid medications also facilitate individualized dosages. Pharmacies dispense many liquid medications (e.g., antibiotics, digestive, cold and respiratory medicines, and antipyretics) over the counter (OTC) or on a prescription basis.[30,32] Previously, parents used a household teaspoon (with a capacity of 1.5 mL to 9 mL) to administer liquid medications to their children. Such a wide range in volumes may lead to dosing errors.[32,33] Many of these liquid medications are supplied with the relevant measuring devices, such as dosing spoons, calibrated spoons, droppers, dosing cups, and oral syringes, to help the parents administer medications to their ill children.[32,33,34] Accuracy and precision of dosing can be improved when the dropper is held at a 45° angle.[34] Dosing errors are exceptionally common among children

because pediatric doses mainly depend on age, weight, and body surface area (BSA).[32,33,35] Various studies found that 62–80% of parents routinely administer paracetamol solution to their children at a subtherapeutic (< 10 mg/kg) level.[32,33]

B) DEVICE DESCRIPTION AND IMPORTANT FEATURES

The use of more accurate measuring devices may enhance the probability of obtaining the correct dose.[32] Calibration values of the medication measuring devices should be within ±5% of the indicated value to be accurate.[30]

The following are widely used measuring devices[30]:

i. **Calibration dosing cup:** Dosing cup with calibration marks for every 1 mL to allow dosing up to 20 mL.
ii. **Spoon with a bottle adapter:** Medication measuring device with a spoon-like end and calibration marks for every 0.5 mL, allowing dosing up to 10 mL.
iii. **Oral syringe:** Measures liquid on the same principle as a syringe. The smallest dosing calibration mark is 1.25 mL, and calibration marks are printed for every 0.25 mL, allowing dosing up to 5 mL.
iv. **Dosing spoon:** Calibration marks are present for every 1 mL inside the spoon, and a 2.5 mL dosing line is present in the middle. This allows dosing up to 5 mL.
v. **Dispensing bottle:** Calibration marks for every 1 mL and 2.5 mL are present on both sides; dosing up to 12 mL is possible.

C) PURPOSE AND HOW TO USE[36]

The dosing cup can be appropriately used in the following ways:

- Measure at eye level on a flat stationary surface (not held in hand).

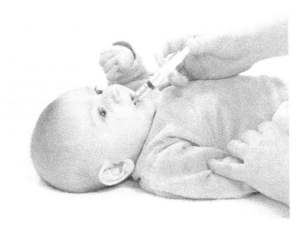

FIGURE 9.4 An oral syringe.

Source: www.shutterstock.com/image-photo/cute-baby-gets-medicine-syringe-his-260735732

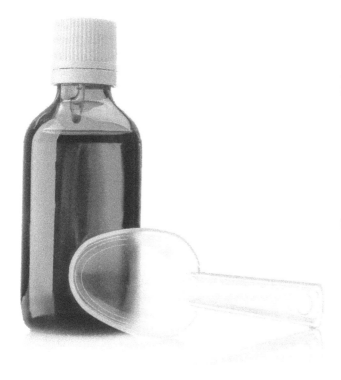

FIGURE 9.5   A dosing spoon.

Source: www.shutterstock.com/image-photo/bottle-cough-syrup-measuring-spoon-on-648426184

- Fill the cup up to the correct dose line.
- If the liquid is thick or sticky, you may add a little water and swirl the cup.
- Close the bottle tightly when you finish giving the medication to the child.

Dosing spoons can be used appropriately in the following manner:

- Measure at eye level and hold the spoon upright.
- Fill the dosing spoon up to the correct dose line.
- If the liquid is thick or sticky, you may add a little water and swirl the spoon.
- Close the bottle tightly when you finish giving the medication to the child.

Droppers or oral syringes can be used accurately in the following ways:

- Carefully draw the medication into the syringe up to the correct dose line.
- Tap out air bubbles, if any.
- Ensure that there is no outward leakage from the dropper or oral syringe.
- Allow a small amount of the medication from the dropper or oral syringe to come out into the space between the tongue and cheek. Keep necessary time gaps to allow the child to swallow.

- Close the bottle tightly once you finish giving the medication to the child.

Follow these simple metrics when measuring a liquid medication:

- 1 teaspoon (tsp) = 5 mL
- 1/2 tsp = 2.5 mL
- 3 tsp = 1 tablespoon (Tbsp)
- 1 Tbsp = 15 mL
- 1/2 Tbsp = 7.5 mL

D)   IMPORTANT SAFETY ISSUES (CAUTIONS AND COMMON ADVERSE EFFECTS)

- Under- or overdosing caused by a measuring inaccuracy can have serious health effects in narrow therapeutic index medicines such as carbamazepine, phenytoin, and digoxin.[30,33]
- Doses measured with medicine droppers can be smaller than those measured using a measuring spoon.[29]

E)   STORAGE CONDITIONS AND MAINTENANCE

- Store the liquid measuring devices in a dirt-free environment at room temperature.
- Wash the device with clean water and allow to dry every time it is used to measure a liquid formulation. Otherwise, microbial growth or colonization may occur in the device.

F)   IMPORTANT FEATURES (CAPABILITIES AND LIMITATIONS) AND SPECIAL ADVANTAGES

- The liquid medication measuring device helps measure liquid dosage forms to obtain an exact amount.
- These devices help gain optimum results for liquid medications.

G)   SPECIAL TIPS FOR PATIENT COUNSELING

- Dosing errors can be clinically significant, especially for infants and the elderly. Underdosing can result in subtherapeutic levels, whereas overdosing can result in supratherapeutic levels.[30]
- Always use the proper measuring device that comes with the medication. If it is not provided, ask the pharmacist to select the best device.
- Do not use the measuring devices that come with one product to measure other medications unless your pharmacist suggests you do so.
- If you lost the measuring device that came with a specific medication, ask the pharmacist for advice.
- Do not mix two or more different liquid medications in a measuring device at the same time.

- Discard any excess medication if you overfill the measuring device but do not return that portion to the bottle because it may contaminate the whole bottle.
- Always wash the measuring device properly after use. Dry it carefully before the next use, because any water droplet may adulterate the next dose.
- Never use hypodermic syringes and only use syringes made for oral use.[36]
- Always use the dosing device that comes with the medicine. Ask your pharmacist for help if a dosing device does not come with the medicine.
- Never use household measuring devices to measure and give liquid medicines because they may be inaccurate and may deliver more or less than required.
- Always observe the measuring device at eye level while measuring the liquid medicine. For dosing cups, measure on a flat surface and not in the hand.
- Never measure liquid medicine in a dim room or when you are distracted.
- Always wash the dosing device after administering the medicine. Otherwise, bacteria can colonize and contaminate any future use. If you wash a dosing device immediately before administration, ensure that it is dry because any liquid droplets or residue on the device can interfere with dosing accuracy.
- If you overfill a cup or dosing syringe while measuring the medicine, discard the excess down the sink. Do not try to pour any excess or unused medicine back into the container because this may contaminate the medicine in the container.
- Do not combine more than one liquid medicine simultaneously in a dosing device to ensure accurate dosing and to minimize potential incompatibility.
- Do not use a hypodermic syringe with a transparent cap, baking or kitchen spoons, or measuring cup with both tablespoon and teaspoon markings to measure liquid medicine. Instead, use dosing cups, oral syringes with colored caps, medicine droppers, dosing spoons, and oral dosing syringes for infants.

H) Evidence of Effectiveness and Safety

Ryu and Lee (2012) reported that pharmacists in South Korea attach a label or write necessary information about the drug name, dosage, indications, and frequency on the container when they dispense liquid medications. They highlight the calibration markings on the medication measuring devices, which helps the parents reduce dosing errors while administering medicine to their children. They reported the percentage dosing errors occurring with dosing spoons (50%), regular dosing cups (47%), calibrated dosing cups (31%), dispensing bottles (7%), spoons with a bottle adapter (4%), and oral syringes (0%).[30] Beckett et al. (2012) also found that oral syringes may be used when administering narrow therapeutic index medications. Parental education on the correct use of the oral syringe can improve dosing accuracy from 37% to 100%.[33] Hence, proper selection and use with educational intervention can prevent liquid dose measurement errors.[35]

I) Economic Evaluation

Economical measuring devices used to administer liquid medications include household teaspoons, dosing cups, droppers, cylindrical spoons, and oral syringes.[37]

J) Implication to the Pharmacy Profession and Pharmacy Practice

Provision of thorough education and counseling and demonstration of medication administration can reduce dosing errors made by parents during the administration of liquid medications. However, more viscous medications (e.g., nystatin) are difficult to measure with a dropper, regardless of the patient education.[34] Community pharmacists are better positioned to educate parents on the selection and use of appropriate measuring devices to improve the accuracy of medication administration in households.[30,32,33] Pharmacists should verify whether the administered volumes of liquid medications are appropriate or not.[29] Health professionals should ensure that an appropriate dosing device has been used to deliver the recommended dose of liquid medicine. Pharmacists should counsel parents to hold the dropper in a vertical position and to see the medicine at eye level to obtain accurate readings.[31]

K) Challenges to Pharmacists and Users

Most cases of overdose among children are caused by the caregiver's failure to use an appropriate preparation (e.g., use of a more concentrated preparation) or the use of an incorrect measuring device.[32] Pharmacists may not even know whether the patients received detailed information on correctly measuring and administering liquid medications. Many patients may have problems reading the calibration markings on the measuring devices.[30] Limited parental education on dosing instructions may lead to dosing inaccuracy and the risk of child morbidity and mortality.[29,33,35]

L) Recommendations: The Way Forward

- Caregivers should routinely measure and administer liquid medication using an appropriate measuring device such as a calibrated spoon or oral syringe.
- Pharmacists should counsel the patients and ensure that they obtain detailed information on correctly measuring and administering liquid medications.

- Pharmacists should verify whether the administered volumes of liquid medications are appropriate by reviewing the usage patterns of the caregivers.

M) CONCLUSIONS

Oral liquid formulations (such as syrups, solutions, suspensions, and elixirs) are usually administered to children to help them swallow medication easily and prevent the risk of inhalation. Household teaspoons, dosing cups, droppers, cylindrical spoons, and oral syringes are economical measuring devices used to administer such medications. The device used to measure liquid medicine should be washed with clean water and allowed to air dry after every use to avoid microbial growth or colonization in the device.

N) LESSONS LEARNED

- The use of more accurate measuring devices may enhance the probability of obtaining the correct dose.
- Calibration values of the medication measuring devices should be within ±5% of the indicated value to be accurate.
- Only the dosing device that comes with the medicine should be used to measure the liquid medicines, and if one is not available, consultation with the pharmacist is necessary.
- The measuring devices that come with a product should not be used to measure other medications unless your pharmacist suggests you do so.

DEVICE 4: INFANT FEEDING BOTTLES

A) BACKGROUND

Breast milk provides infants with a well-balanced mixture of amino acids, sugars, and fats.[38] Breast-milk fat contains long-chain polyunsaturated fatty acids (PUFAs) (docosahexaenoic acid or DHA and arachidonic acid or ARA) that are not present in other milk. These fatty acids are essential for the neurological development of a child.[39] Vitamins, minerals, enzymes, and prebiotics found in breast milk help with digestion. Breast milk also contains cholesterol to support brain growth, hormone development, vitamin D synthesis, and bile production.[38]

Antibodies present in breast milk help develop the infant's immune system and reduce infections such as pneumonia, otitis media, lower respiratory tract infections (LRTIs), and gastrointestinal tract (GIT) infections.[38] Breast milk provides adequate nutrition for newborn babies, and breastfeeding is an excellent way to provide them with breast milk. However, breastfeeding may not always be possible due to medical or physiological conditions, namely, sickness or preterm birth, which may require supplemental feeding. Infants are provided with supplemental feeding in a variety

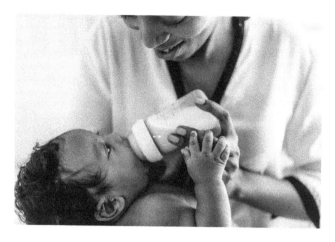

FIGURE 9.6   An infant being bottle-fed.

Source: www.shutterstock.com/image-photo/portrait-enjoy-happy-love-family-african-1715365066

of ways. Traditionally, bottles and nasogastric tubes have been used, and cup feeding is currently popular.[40] Enteral feeding with bottles and tubes may be necessary for the newborn infant if he/she cannot breastfeed.[41] However, partially breastfed babies between the ages of 2 and 6 months may suffer from more regurgitation problems than exclusively breastfed babies.[42] Direct breastfeeding may increase diaphragmatic force, stimulating lung growth, and so may protect the child from respiratory problems. Breastfed infants have lower levels of *Escherichia coli*, *Clostridium difficile*, *Bacteroides*, and *Llactobacilli* and higher counts of *Bbifidobacteria*, whereas formula-fed infants may have a higher bioburden of the former.[43] Considerations during bottle feeding include how bottles deliver milk to infants, how the infant obtains the milk being delivered, and how bottle feeding affects parent-infant intimacy.[44]

B) DEVICE DESCRIPTION AND IMPORTANT FEATURES

Currently, infant feeding bottles are marketed in a variety of appearances and designs because the design may impact the intake of milk by the infants and subsequently their growth or risk of infection.[45] Bottle-feeding device design has advanced due to the introduction of novel materials and extensive studies on research into infants' bottle-feeding patterns.[44]

Infant feeding bottles are available in the following types:

i. Glass bottles: These are durable but also heavy and more expensive, and can shatter (i.e., break) easily.
ii. Plastic bottles: These bottles are made of polypropylene material, i.e., rigid plastic material, but are lightweight and unbreakable. The United Stated Food and Drug Administration (US FDA)

made a rule that plastic bottles be free of a chemical called bisphenol A (BPA).

iii. Stainless steel bottles: These bottles are long lasting and insulated to deliver milk according to the baby's preferred temperature. These are costlier than plastic or glass bottles.

iv. Silicone bottles: Food-grade silicone is available for both bottles and nipples. These are also expensive.

In terms of size, the infant feeding bottles are available in three types, whether they are the glass or plastic type:

i. Small bottles: These have approximately a 60 mL capacity.

ii. Medium bottles: These usually have a 120–150 mL capacity. These are used mainly for the newborns who eat less.

iii. Large bottles: These usually have a 240–300 mL capacity. These are used mainly for older babies who eat more.

Infant feeding bottles are generally available with nipples for feeding infants. These nipples have the following types:

i. Slow flow type (Level 1): useful for newborns to infants < 3 months of age

ii. Medium flow type (Level 2): useful for infants aged 3+ months

iii. Fast flow type (Level 3): useful for infants aged 6+ months

iv. Variable flow type (Level 4): useful for infants aged 9+ months to feed significantly thicker liquids

Flow from the nipple is controlled by the size of the hole of the nipple.

The nipples of the feeding bottles are made of latex and silicone.

i. Latex nipple: It is a soft material but needs to be frequently replaced because it gets easily damaged. Some babies may show allergic reactions to it.

ii. Silicone nipple: Food-grade silicone nipples are firmer and more durable than latex nipples. They should be replaced every few months, less frequently than the latex nipple.

c) Purpose and How to Use[46]

i. Hold baby to be fed in your lap in a semi-upright position, supporting the head and neck.

ii. Touch the baby's lip, so he opens his mouth wide.

iii. Insert the nipple into the baby's mouth.

iv. Let the baby suck for 20–30 seconds for 3–5 continuous swallows.

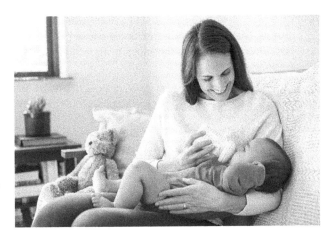

FIGURE 9.7 An infant being bottle-fed.

Source: www.shutterstock.com/image-photo/mother-holding-feeding-baby-milk-bottle-788807785

v. Maintain a short interval after 3–5 continuous swallows.

vi. After a few seconds, let the baby suck again.

vii. Continue feeding at the interval in step (iv) until the baby shows fullness signs.

d) Important Safety Issues (Cautions and Common Adverse Effects)

- Cup feeding may enhance the risk of aspiration pneumonia when an improper technique is used. Other risks may be physiological instability (e.g., bradycardia, apnea, low oxygen saturation) and poor weight gain, which can result in hospitalizations and financial burden.[40]

- Kotowski et al. (2020) reported that bottle-fed infants might have more arrhythmic sucking (AS) patterns than breastfed infants.[44]

- Bottle feeding may impair the infant's ability to learn to breastfeed.[39]

- Expression of breast milk may introduce skin microorganisms into the expressed milk, and storage conditions may increase the bacterial load.[43]

- Formula milk is not as nutritious as breast milk and may put the baby at risk of obesity in early childhood.[47]

- Preparing milk for bottle feeding may be time-consuming, unlike breastfeeding.

- Regular and prolonged bottle feeding may compromise the baby's immune system, putting the baby at risk of bacterial contamination leading to chest, ear, and urine infections or diarrhea because powdered infant formula (PIF) is not a sterile product and provides an ideal growth medium for pathogenic bacteria, resulting in spoilage.[48,49]

- Bottle feeding may lead to transmission of enterobacterial strains, *Bacillus spp.*, *Clostridium spp.*,

Listeria monocytogenes, and *Staphylococcus aureus*, since these strains are prevalent in PIF.[48]
- Bottle feeding is less convenient during nighttime feedings.

E) STORAGE CONDITIONS AND MAINTENANCE

- You may use techniques of boiling, chemical sterilization, electric steam sterilization, or microwave sterilization to clean or sterilize the infant feeding equipment.[49]
- Thoroughly clean and sterilize bottles, lids, and nipples before use to remove the bacterial burden[50]:
  i. Wash your hands with soap water and dry using a clean cloth.
  ii. Wash the equipment (i.e., bottle, lid, and nipple) thoroughly in hot soapy water and use a clean bottle.

The equipment can be sterilized using a sterilizer or a pan and boiling water[50]:

  i. Fill a large pan with water.
  ii. Place the cleaned equipment into the water and cover it entirely with water. Ensure that no air bubbles are present.
  iii. Cover the pan with a lid and boil the water making sure the pan does not boil dry.

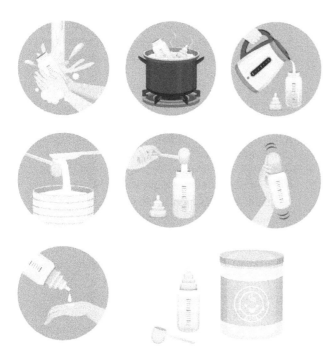

FIGURE 9.8 Sterilization steps for preparing baby bottle-feeding equipment.

Source: www.shutterstock.com/image-vector/icons-set-steps-preparing-baby-bottle-1090897487

Wash and dry your hands with a clean cloth before handling the sterilized equipment. It is better to handle the sterilized equipment with sterilized forceps and to have 3 to 4 bottles for alternative and uninterrupted use while washing or sterilizing the used bottle.

F) IMPORTANT FEATURES (CAPABILITIES AND LIMITATIONS) AND SPECIAL ADVANTAGES

- Anyone can feed the baby with the help of the bottle, even in public places.
- The feeding bottle makes it easy to keep track of the baby's intake.
- Bottle feeding is helpful for babies with lactose intolerance.
- You can measure exactly how much food your baby is getting per bottle feeding.

G) SPECIAL TIPS FOR PATIENT COUNSELING

- Infants may refuse to breastfeed and become addicted to the bottle if they are not breastfed for a prolonged period.[40]
- Freezing and reheating of expressed milk may break down the milk's constituents. Bacterial counts may increase in milk after 48 hours of storage in the refrigerator.[43]
- Proper cleaning and sterilization of infant feeding equipment minimizes risks to the baby and yield better clinical and cost benefits.[49]

H) EVIDENCE OF EFFECTIVENESS AND SAFETY

Formula feeding has intrinsic nutritional and immunological deficiencies compared to breastfeeding. They also include preventable risks, including manufacturing errors, contamination during storage and transport, reconstitution errors at home, and improper cleaning and sterilization of the equipment.[49] The safety and effectiveness of infant feeding bottles may be enhanced by tackling these problems.

I) ECONOMIC EVALUATION

Expressed breast milk provides economically beneficial alternatives if direct breastfeeding is not feasible.[51]

J) IMPLICATION TO THE PHARMACY PROFESSION AND PHARMACY PRACTICE

Supplementing breastfeeding with bottles or cups may increase the extent and duration of breastfeeding. Cups and feeding utensils are easier to clean than bottles and are widely used in low- and middle-income countries.[52] Feeding bottles must not contain toxic substances such as lead, phthalate, polyvinyl chloride (PVC), or bisphenol A (BPA).

K) CHALLENGES TO PHARMACISTS AND USERS

Women who want to breastfeed their infant may not always be able to do so. In such cases, expressed breast milk is usually given by using feeding bottles, but prolonged use of bottles may interfere with breastfeeding.[52]

L) RECOMMENDATIONS: THE WAY FORWARD

- Exclusive breastfeeding should be performed unless not recommended by the concerned healthcare providers; if bottle feeding is necessary, it should be considered supplemental to breastfeeding.
- Infant feeding bottles must not contain toxic substances such as lead, phthalate, polyvinyl chloride (PVC), or bisphenol A (BPA).
- The feeding bottle must be properly cleaned and sterilized to prevent risks of microbial contamination to the baby.

M) CONCLUSIONS

Breast milk provides infants with a well-balanced mixture of amino acids, sugars, and fats. However, breastfeeding may not always be possible due to medical or physiological conditions, which may require supplemental feeding. Traditionally, bottles and nasogastric tubes have been used, and cup feeding is currently popular. Supplementing breastfeeding with bottles and cups may increase the duration of breastfeeding. Expressed breast milk may be given to the baby by using feeding bottles, but their prolonged use may interfere with breastfeeding.

N) LESSONS LEARNED

- Breast milk provides adequate nutrition for newborn babies, and breastfeeding is an excellent way to provide them with breast milk.
- Factors such as patterns of milk delivery to infants via the bottle, the infant's ability to get milk, and the impact of bottle feeding on parent-infant intimacy should be considered.
- Infants may refuse to breastfeed and become addicted to the bottle or cup if they are not breastfed for a prolonged period.
- Feeding bottles and their lids and nipples should be washed thoroughly in hot soapy water after each feeding.

DEVICE 5: PEDIATRIC INHALATION DEVICES

A) BACKGROUND

Respiratory diseases are one of the most common causes of hospitalizations and emergency department visits among children worldwide.[53] Asthma is one such respiratory disease and is characterized by persistent, recurrent bronchial hyperresponsiveness.[54] Asthma affects more than 25 million people worldwide every year.[55] Inhalation therapy is the mainstay therapy for asthma and wheezing acute episodes and maintenance therapy[53] because it exhibits a rapid onset of drug action, requiring minimal doses, and minimizes systemic effects compared with other routes of administration.[56] However, many children with asthma do not correctly use their inhalers and consequently achieve little or no effect from the therapy. Therefore, inhalation therapy should focus on the most comfortable design for use by children and the necessary training for proper administration techniques.[57]

B) DEVICE DESCRIPTION AND IMPORTANT FEATURES

Inhalation therapy in children with asthma can be classified into the following types[53,57–60]:

   i. Nebulizers: Conventional inhalers
  ii. Pressurized metered-dose inhalers (pMDI)
 iii. pMDI with a spacer attached
 iv. Dry powder inhalers (DPIs)

These inhaler systems differ in terms of design, aerosol generation, and optimal inhalation techniques.[57]

i. Nebulizers

These are conventional devices that generate aerosols from solutions and suspensions by vibrations; however, heat is also generated along with aerosols, which may denature drugs (especially proteinaceous drugs).[53,61] Conventional nebulizers are generally less effective and have been modified to enhance the extent of deposition of aerosolized drug particles in the lungs. These novel nebulizers generally have an aerosolized output rate of 0.2 to 0.6 mL/minute. These devices are quiet and portable and can be operated with batteries; however, they are expensive.[53]

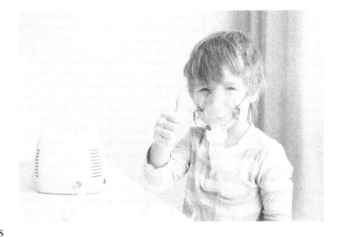

FIGURE 9.9 A pediatric nebulizer in use.

Source: www.shutterstock.com/image-photo/little-boy-making-inhalation-nebulizer-home-1018943911

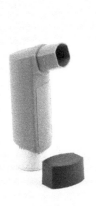

FIGURE 9.10   A pressurized metered-dose inhaler.

Source: www.shutterstock.com/image-photo/metered-dose-inhaler-458352340

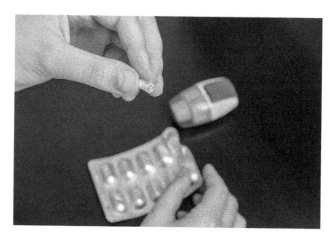

FIGURE 9.11   A capsule of a dry-powder inhaler medication.

Source: www.shutterstock.com/image-photo/drypowder-inhaler-dpi-device-that-delivers-1536801734

ii.   Pressurized Metered-Dose Inhalers (pMDI)

These devices are the most commonly used inhalation devices worldwide. The pMDI is a safe and portable device that can administer multiple doses of the drug and be operated without a power connection. It consists of a reservoir for the drug solution or suspension with surfactants, lubricants, and propellants. Conventionally, chlorofluorocarbons (CFCs) are used as propellants in metered-dose inhalers (MDIs), but hydrofluoroalkanes (HFAs) are currently replacing CFCs due to the ozone layer depletion effects of CFCs.[53]

iii.   pMDI-Spacer Combinations

Holding chambers (spacers) may be attached to the mouthpiece of a pMDI to allow complete evaporation and deposition of the propellants in the device before inhalation. Spacers make the use of pMDIs easier, and these can also be used to deliver bronchodilators during acute bronchoconstriction.[57] Spacers may vary in volume (110 to 750 mL), shape (cylinder, cone, pear-shaped, sphere), and material (plastic, metal).[53,57] Low-volume spacers are more comfortable for use by young children.[57] Spacers connected to the mouthpiece of a pMDI slow the velocity of the aerosolized particles and reduce oropharyngeal deposition of the drug. Furthermore, these are child-friendly.[56,62] Spacers should be connected to a face mask in children younger than 4 years of age because they find it difficult to fit their lips around the mouthpiece tightly; additionally, this inhalation technique is the only possible technique for children in this age category.[53,57] The mouthpiece should be used in older children.[53]

iv.   Dry Powder Inhalers (DPI)

These are propellant-free devices in which a drug is provided as a fine powder in reservoirs, blisters, or gelatin capsules and is fractionated and micronized to generate respirable particles.[53,57] Each blister or capsule contains only a single dose of the drug, necessitating its replacement

before each therapy. Active drug molecules are mixed with carrier molecules (e.g., lactose or micronized glucose) in capsules.[57] The dose deposited in the lungs varies from 15% to 40%. These devices are preferable for children older than 8 years of age to provide maintenance therapy.[53]

c)   PURPOSE AND HOW TO USE

- Press down the canister into the actuator to actuate or generate the aerosol or the metered volume of drug, propellants, and surfactant through the actuator into the air.[57]

How to Use pMDIs[61]

- Shake 4 or 5 times for resuspension and take the cap off.
- Place the inhaler in an upright position.
- Exhale slowly to empty the lungs and place the inhaler immediately in the mouth between the teeth and seal the lips properly.
- Inhale slowly through the mouth and press the canister to actuate a dose at the same time.
- Continue slow and deep inhalation through the mouth for approximately 4–5 seconds until the lungs are full of air.
- Take the inhaler out of the mouth and close the lips when the inhalation is finished.
- Hold the breath at least 10 seconds before breathing normally.
- Repeat the same steps if another dose is to be taken.

How to Use the pMDI-Spacer Combination[61]

- Shake 4 or 5 times for resuspension and take the cap off.
- Insert the mouthpiece of the pMDI into the spacer, ensuring a tight fit.
- Actuate one dose into the spacer chamber.

- Patients should inhale and exhale normally at least 10 times when using the pMDI-spacer combination.
- Rinse mouth if inhaled corticosteroids are used.
- Repeat the same steps if another dose is to be taken.

How to Use DPIs[61]

- Take the cap off and follow the instructions mentioned in the patient information leaflet (PIL).
- Do not point the mouthpiece downwards to prevent dose loss once a dose is prepared for inhalation.
- Exhale slowly to empty the lungs, but do not exhale into the DPI to avoid dispersion of the powder.
- Inhale forcefully through the mouth from the very start (but not gradually) until the lungs are full.
- Take the inhaler out of the mouth and close the lips at the end of inhalation and hold the breath for up to 10 seconds before breathing normally.
- Repeat the same steps if another dose is to be taken.

D) IMPORTANT SAFETY ISSUES (CAUTIONS AND COMMON ADVERSE EFFECTS)

- Talking during administration decreases the delivery of aerosols to the airways.[57]
- Spacers are bulky and inconvenient and require maintenance.[57,61]
- Particles from DPIs are too large to reach the lungs. Therefore, a larger fraction of the inhaled dose is deposited in the oropharyngeal tract after inhalation from a DPI.[57]

E) STORAGE CONDITIONS AND MAINTENANCE

- Spacers should be washed with detergent at least once a month or more frequently. Valves should be replaced at least once a year or more frequently.[57]
- Hydrofluoroalkane (HFA) pMDIs should be stored at a temperature between −20°C and 20°C to gain continuous dose delivery. Outdoor use of pMDIs in freezing weather may decrease aerosol delivery.
- Clean the plastic container of pMDIs at least once a week.
- Periodically clean the spacer with pMDI before use based on the manufacturer's instructions.
- Wipe the mouthpiece of the DPI with a clean, dry cloth. Do not submerge DPIs in water and keep them dry because moisture may decrease drug delivery.
- Periodically clean and disinfect the nebulizers at least once or twice a week and replace the nebulizer to minimize contamination. Additionally, discard all solutions after disinfection.
- Use sterile water (not distilled or bottled) for the final rinse; sterile water can be made simply by boiling tap water for five minutes.
- Thoroughly dry the nebulizers and store them in a clean, dry place between uses because bacteria grow in wet, moist places.[63]

F) IMPORTANT FEATURES (CAPABILITIES AND LIMITATIONS) AND SPECIAL ADVANTAGES

- Nebulizers are usually available with face masks, which makes these more appropriate for patients aged < 2 years as well as the elderly.[61]
- pMDIs are efficacious, and patient acceptance is high with these devices.
- Spacers decrease oropharyngeal deposition of the drug from 80% to 30% (i.e., by 50%). Therefore, a higher dose is delivered to the airways than that from pMDI without the spacer.[57]
- pMDI-spacer combinations decrease side effects associated with inhaled corticosteroid (ICS) therapy (e.g., irritation in the oropharynx, dysphonia, and candidiasis).[53]
- DPIs reduce the inhalation problems or difficulties experienced with pMDIs. They are equally convenient as a pMDI to use.[57]

G) SPECIAL TIPS FOR PATIENT COUNSELING

- Shake the canister for resuspension of the aerosols before inhalation to ensure proper filling of the chamber with the contents.
- Deliver beclomethasone dipropionate, triamcinolone, and other inhaled corticosteroids (ICS) using a spacer to minimize the risk of oropharyngeal deposition.
- Provide necessary training, demonstrations, and assistance to young children to ensure that the inhalation technique is acceptable.[57]
- Actuate only a single dose into the spacer before each inhalation, since multiple inhalations may enhance drug loss within the spacer.[61]

H) EVIDENCE OF EFFECTIVENESS AND SAFETY

Nebulizers help relieve patients with asthma and COPD from severe exacerbations.[61] pMDIs with spacers are equally effective as nebulizers for day-to-day inhalation and acute episodes of wheezing. These are more useful for children ≤ 5 years, since they are convenient and cost-effective, they require less maintenance, and they assure good lung deposition of the drug particles.[53,57] pMDI-spacer combinations are used in maintenance therapy with inhaled corticosteroids because these are more efficient and convenient than conventional nebulizers. DPIs are preferred for children older than 8 years who can exercise high inspiratory flow rates.[53] Data from adult studies may not be directly extrapolated to children because drug delivery to children may vary with their advancing age and disease.[56]

TABLE 9.3

First and Second Recommendations of Inhalation Therapy per Age Group

Age (year)	First choice	Second choice
0–3	pMDI + spacer	Nebulizer
3–6	pMDI + spacer	Nebulizer
6–12 (β2-agonist)	pMDI + spacer; DPI	
6–12 (CS)	pMDI + spacer	DPI
>12 (β2-agonist)	DPI	
>12 (CS)	pMDI + spacer	DPI
Acute asthma	pMDI + spacer	Nebulizer

CS: corticosteroids; DPI: dry powder inhaler; pMDI: pressurized metered-dose inhaler

The effectiveness of therapy should be reassessed when switching from a pMDI-spacer combination to a DPI.[56,61]

Choice of Inhalation Therapy

All inhalation devices may not be appropriate for all patients.[61] Benedictis and Selvaggio (2003) mentioned that inhalation therapy could be chosen according to the following criteria[56]:

I) ECONOMIC EVALUATION

Self-administration of bronchodilators with pMDI-spacer combinations saved US$253,487 per year in the USA. These are more economically beneficial than nebulizers.[53] Generally, pMDI-spacer combinations are the most economical of all the available inhalation therapy modalities.[61]

J) IMPLICATION TO THE PHARMACY PROFESSION AND PHARMACY PRACTICE

Pediatric patients are different from adult patients; they are not capable of following instructions exactly and usually reject inhalation therapy. Clinicians must bear this fact in mind while instructing the children and their caretakers.[58] Selecting an appropriate inhaler, from among > 100 different inhalers, for the treatment of asthma in each patient is a complex issue even for clinicians, because all clinicians may not have sufficient time to obtain experience with each inhaler. Therefore, clinicians should gain in-depth experience with a few inhalers. Training, demonstrations, and consistent follow-ups are helpful to promote correct inhaler use in children who have asthma. Pedersen et al. (2010) reported that children receiving repeated in-depth inhalation instructions on proper inhalation techniques at the pharmacy or in clinical trial settings followed proper inhalation techniques compared to those receiving only a single demonstration.[57]

Most inhaled therapies are not approved for young children, and clinicians may not have good ideas or information about accurate dose prescriptions. Moreover, dose-response measures developed for adults cannot be extrapolated for children due to differences in pharmacodynamic and pharmacokinetic profiles between infants, children, and adults. Therefore, despite being optimized according to height, weight, or body surface area (BSA), a similar respiratory dose in children does not exhibit similar treatment efficacy or risk to these other age categories.[64] Healthcare providers should empower patients to use their inhalers effectively by using training, demonstrations, and follow-up evaluations.[61]

K) CHALLENGES TO PHARMACISTS AND USERS

It is generally challenging to train a child using DPIs to not exhale through the device before inhalation, since this may blow out the dose and increase the humidity within the device. DPIs are single-dose inhalers and are less convenient because they should be loaded before each inhalation, and some children find it challenging to do so. Pedersen et al. (2010) reported that the majority of children younger than 5 years could not consistently use DPI correctly, even after repeated training. Therefore, DPIs should only be used for children older than 5 years, and they should be told to demonstrate the inhalation technique to verify whether there is congruency between what they understood and followed.[57] Some patients do not use spacers due to their size and requirements for cleaning and maintenance.[53] Pharmacists should consult the patients face to face while switching from one inhaler to another to minimize inhalation mistakes, since there may be some technical differences among the various devices.[65]

L) RECOMMENDATIONS: THE WAY FORWARD

- Health professionals, including pharmacists, should remember that children are different from adult patients and may not rigorously adhere to inhalation therapy.
- Dry powder inhalers (DPIs) should only be used for children older than 5 years.
- Pharmacists should consult the patients face to face while switching from one inhaler to another to minimize inhalation mistakes.
- Healthcare providers should instruct patients to use their inhalers via training, demonstrations and follow-up evaluations.

M) CONCLUSIONS

Many children with asthma may not properly use their inhalers and consequently achieve little or no optimum effect from the therapy. Therefore, inhalation therapy should be made child-friendly via necessary training for proper administration techniques. Nebulizers are available with face masks, which are useful for patients aged younger than 2 years as well as the elderly. It is sometimes difficult to train a child using dry powder inhalers to not exhale through the device before inhalation.

N) Lessons Learned

- Various inhalation therapies, such as nebulizers, pressurized metered-dose inhalers (pMDI), pMDI with a spacer attached, and dry powder inhalers (DPIs), are commonly used for pediatric asthmatic patients.
- pMDIs are the most commonly used inhalation devices worldwide, since they are safe and portable and can be operated without power connections.
- Spacers connected to the mouthpiece of a pMDI reduce the velocity of the aerosol and reduce oropharyngeal drug deposition.
- Spacers should be washed with detergent at least once a month.

DEVICE 6: CHILD/BABY DIAPERS (DISPOSABLE NAPKINS)

A) Background

Child diapers are used for infants and babies during the day or at night, allowing them to urinate and defecate within the diaper. This reduces the burden on the parents. However, diapered skin is exposed to friction, overhydration, high pH (> 7), contact with urine and feces, and bacterial colonization, which irritate the skin. Normal microbiota favors acidic pH levels, and increased skin pH in the diaper area facilitates and promotes the growth of pathogenic microorganisms, including *Candida albicans* and *Staphylococcus aureus*, which cause diaper dermatitis (DD).[51,66–69] DD (also known as nappy or diaper rash, napkin dermatitis) is any skin inflammation in the diaper area, and has a prevalence of 25–50% depending on the age of the child and method of diaper application.[66,69,70] Generally, DD peaks between the ages of 9 and 12 months.[70,71] Fecal bacteria increase the activity of fecal proteases, lipases, and ureases, all of which irritate the skin. Fecal ureases catalyze the breakdown of urea to ammonia, which increases the skin pH in the diaper area. DD was observed to be high in babies with diarrhea in the previous 48 hours.[51,66,67,72,73] DD is an acute, episodic inflammatory reaction characterized by erythema, papules, and pustules in the diapered area. DD is common but rarely severe in terms of therapeutics, and it is self-limiting within 3–4 days in many cases. However, it causes discomfort for infants and anxiety for parents and caregivers.[51,66,72,74,75] DD can be managed by ABCDE measures: air (i.e., diaper-free moment), barriers (e.g., zinc oxide, petrolatum), cleansing with a wet cloth or baby wipes, diapers, and education.[71]

B) Device Description and Important Features

Various types of diapers are available on the market:

- i. Reusable (cloth) diapers
- ii. Disposable (single-use) diapers
- iii. Pant diapers
- iv. Pocket diapers

i. Reusable Diapers

Reusable diapers are economical and are currently popular. These are cloth diapers that can be washed and reused, and they are available in a variety of colors and prints to attract the baby.

ii. Disposable Diapers

Disposable diapers are made of inert fiber polymers found in cloth, food containers, and paper products. The pH of disposable diapers is similar to that of normal skin.[75] These are the most widely used diapers, accounting for approximately 95% of the world market.[76] These tend to leak less than the cloth diapers.[77]

iii. Pant Diapers

Pant diapers are preferred by most babies and even mothers, since they are easy to wear and remain in place all day without any discomfort. Children can even run and crawl comfortably with the diapers on.

iv. Pocket Diapers

Pocket diapers are a different style of cloth diaper and are convenient to apply. These are lightweight, and the child finds them comfortable to wear the whole day.

Size of Diapers

Diaper size can vary with the age and weight of the baby as follows:

- Small: 4–8 kgs
- Medium: 7–12 kgs
- Large: 9–14 kgs
- Extra-large: 12–17 kgs

C) Purpose and How to Use[78]

- Wash and dry your hands or use hand sanitizer or a baby wipe.
- Set up a warm, clean area to change your baby's diaper. You may use a changing table or lay a blanket, towel, or mat on the floor or bed to change the baby's diaper.
- Have a clean diaper and plenty of wipes or wet cloths available. Use lukewarm water and gauze for babies with sensitive skin.

Diaper change

- Open up a new clean diaper and place the back half under your baby.
- Fold the dirty diaper in half under your baby, clean side up.
- Clean your baby's front with a damp wipe, cloth, or gauze from the front to the back (never wipe from back to front to prevent the spread of bacteria that can cause urinary tract infections).

- Clean the creases of your baby's thighs and buttocks too.
- Let your baby's skin air dry or dry with a clean cloth.
- Remove the dirty diaper and set it aside. Fold up the dirty diaper and fasten it closed with its tabs, then dispose of it in the trash.
- Wash your hands or use hand sanitizer to prevent the spread of germs.

D) IMPORTANT SAFETY ISSUES (CAUTIONS AND COMMON ADVERSE EFFECTS)

- Persistent DD for longer than a month may be associated with food allergies in infants and children while being fed nonmaternal food. Common allergenic foods in early childhood are cow's milk, eggs, peanuts, and sesame, whereas peanuts and seafood allergies are common in older children.[79]
- DD usually starts from 3 to 12 weeks and reaches a peak level from 9 to 12 months of age; sometimes it may appear in children aged > 24 months of age.[51,67,69,79,80]
- Diarrhea and oral antibiotics also contribute to DD.[79]
- DD has a global prevalence of 7% to 50%.[66,67,69,80]

E) STORAGE CONDITIONS AND MAINTENANCE

- You may rinse the diaper before washing it or spray it with water and baking soda for odor control.
- Wash the diaper separately from other laundry, using mild hypoallergenic detergent, but do not use soap.
- Do not use fabric softener because it can cause rashes on babies' sensitive skin. Fabric softeners can also build a waxy layer on the diapers, making them water-repellent instead of absorbent.
- Use hot water and double rinse each wash.
- Do not use chlorine bleach because it shortens diaper life. Instead, use chlorine-free bleach or washing soda to remove stains.[77]
- Although diapers may not have an expiration date mentioned in the packets, they show better absorbency within 2 years of their purchase.

F) IMPORTANT FEATURES (CAPABILITIES AND LIMITATIONS) AND SPECIAL ADVANTAGES

- Disposable diapers are easy to put on and remove and take less time to wear and change.
- Disposable diapers reduce the need for constant laundering.
- Disposable pant diapers are useful for crawling toddlers during the day as well as at night, as they have higher absorbency and ventilation, protecting against leakage.
- Disposable diapers are easy to use and change within a few minutes.

G) SPECIAL TIPS FOR PATIENT COUNSELING

- Disposable, superabsorbent, and breathable diapers cause less DD than cloth diapers. The diaper area should be gently cleaned with warm water (37–40°C) and a small amount of mild nonirritating cleanser with slightly acidic to neutral pH.[66,68] Traditional soaps are too harsh and have an alkaline pH, which increases the skin pH and decreases the epidermal fat content.[66,68]
- Put on a fresh diaper after each urination or defecation (usually 6–8 times a day).[66,68,69] You may place your child in a highly absorbent diaper meant for 10–12 hours of wear at nighttime.
- Apply antifungals such as nystatin, clotrimazole, miconazole, and ketoconazole to the diaper area during every diaper change. Topical or oral antibiotics are helpful if a secondary bacterial infection is suspected. Topical mupirocin twice a day for 5–7 days is usually sufficient for a staphylococcal infection or a mild local bacterial infection.[66,67]
- Avoid rubbing or friction during diaper changes, and gently cleanse and rinse the diaper area.[66]
- Change diapers regularly to avoid diaper rash.
- Keep extra plastic or biodegradable bags with you to put dirty diapers outside your home if there is no facility to dispose of them.
- Rinse the diaper area with water and a soft cloth or disposable diaper wipes. Use fragrance-free wipes with no alcohol for babies with sensitive skin.[75]

H) EVIDENCE OF EFFECTIVENESS AND SAFETY

In terms of design, the capillary action and surfactants in disposable diapers draw fluids through the top layer of the diaper and prevent rewetting with the hydrophilic qualities of the material.[71] The performance of the baby diaper can be evaluated in terms of retention (i.e., capacity) and rewet (a measure of dryness) values. Currently, disposable diapers are lightweight, compact, very absorbent, leakage proof, and easy to use. Modern diapers have become the diaper of choice for > 95% of parents in advanced economies. Various absorbency evaluations (e.g., in a cupped, flat, or 45° angle position), measuring how dry the surface remains after fluid is absorbed and summing the overall markers, are widely applied while selecting a diaper. Some disposable diapers may have a wetness indicator on them, which is a line that turns color if the diaper is wet. It alerts the parents when it is time for a diaper change.

I) ECONOMIC EVALUATION

Babies use an average of seven disposable diapers per day, which may decrease with the change in the number of meals taken by the baby and toilet training received by the toddler. There is little or no cost difference in laundering cloth diapers and buying disposable diapers.[77] Diapers usually cost an average of US$18 per week or US$936 per year for a single child. Parents who are unable to afford an adequate supply of diapers may do diaper changes less frequently.[81] In Europe, considering a retail price of €0.20 for a single disposable baby diaper, these products render annual expenses of €4.2 billion.[76] Wallace et al. (2017) reported that the average monthly expenditure on diapers is US$70–80, and it may vary if the diapers are bought more frequently or if they are purchased in smaller packets.[82] Individual cloth diapers usually cost between US$13.79 and $20.99 (approximately US$80 per month). The cost of disposable diapers depends on the brand and the age of the child. Essentially, disposable diapers generally cost approximately US$55 per month, whereas natural and eco-friendly diapers cost approximately US$100–150 per month.

j) Implication to the Pharmacy Profession and Pharmacy Practice

Breastfeeding helps prevent DD because the feces of exclusively breastfed infants have low pH, low protease activity, and low lipase activity, which all facilitate irritation. Therefore, DD is less common in exclusively breastfed children than in those fed processed food or cow's milk.[66,67,79] Removing the causes of DD may suffice for mild cases. Allowing periods of rest without diapers exposes the damaged skin to air and reduces contact between skin, urine, and feces. The latter can also be achieved with barrier creams containing zinc oxide and/or petrolatum, which develop a lipid film on the skin surface.[66]

k) Challenges to Pharmacists and Users

DD may cause behavioral disorders, namely, restlessness, irritability, disturbed sleep, discomfort in children, and anxiety in parents. Herbal therapies such as lanolin, aloe vera, bentonite (clay shampoo), honey, olive oil, and beeswax also have beneficial effects in DD. Drugs have side effects, such as respiratory problems, and some antibiotics may lead to hypersensitivity reactions and drug resistance.[80] Parents generally notice and report problems of persistent crying together with agitation and reduced urination and defecation as a result of pain in the diaper area in their children. The severity of DD can be indicated by the rash features (e.g., eruptions, papules, and vesicles), intensity of the rash, and diapered area affected. Prolonged candidal DD in young children may also be due to type 1 diabetes mellitus, chronic candidiasis, or immune deficiency.[66] Smith et al. (2013) reported that there is a link between diapers and child health and between diapers and parental mental health.[81]

l) Recommendations: The Way Forward

- Dirty diapers should be removed, folded up, fastened with their tabs, and set aside. Then, they should be disposed of in the trash.
- Diapers should be washed separately from other laundry using mild, hypoallergenic detergent; do not wash diapers with soap.
- Extra plastic or biodegradable bags should be kept to put dirty diapers outside the home to avoid haphazard disposal in the environment.

m) Conclusions

Child diapers are used for infants and babies during the day or at night, allowing them to urinate and defecate within the diaper. Babies use an average of seven disposable diapers per day, which may decrease with the change in the number of meals taken by the baby and toilet training. The performance of baby diapers should be evaluated in terms of retention (i.e., capacity) and rewet (a measure for dryness) values.

n) Lessons Learned

- Child diapers may be available in various sizes, such as small, medium, large, and extra-large, depending on the bodyweight of the child.
- Various diapers, such as reusable (cloth), disposable (single-use), pant, or pocket diapers, are available on the market.
- Diaper rash may be seen on diapered skin exposed to friction, overhydration, high pH (> 7), contact with urine and feces, and bacterial colonization.
- The diaper area should be rinsed with water and a soft cloth or disposable diaper wipes.

DEVICE 7: CHILD BLOOD PRESSURE MONITORS

a) Background

High blood pressure in children and adolescents is a global health problem, with primary hypertension being the most ordinary type in these age categories.[83] The prevalence of arterial hypertension in childhood is 4.5%.[84] High blood pressure in childhood may be projected to be associated with the same risk of cardiovascular disease (CVD) as in adulthood. Primary (essential) hypertension in children may be associated with CVDs, such as hyperlipidemia and insulin resistance, whereas secondary hypertension has an identifiable cause that is known cause disorder. Family history of hypertension or CVD, male sex, low birth weight (LBW), and maternal smoking during pregnancy are also risk factors for hypertension in children, whereas breastfed children may have a decreased risk.[83,85] The diagnosis of elevated blood pressure, especially in patients with stage

1 hypertension (i.e., mildly elevated blood pressure), is the first step in the treatment of hypertension in children and adolescents.[86] However, pediatric systemic hypertension (HTN) is usually underdiagnosed and undertreated.[87] Frequent BP monitoring is essential for critically ill neonates and children. Invasive direct arterial BP monitoring should be considered in children younger than 3 years of age.[88] Ambulatory blood pressure monitoring (ABPM) helps to confirm hypertension in children and adolescents.[83]

Hypertension in children is initially managed with lifestyle modifications, including weight loss (if overweight or obese), a healthy diet (with no junk food), and regular exercise. Children with persistent hypertension despite lifestyle changes, symptomatic hypertension (e.g., headaches, cognitive problems), stage 2 or any stage of hypertension associated with chronic kidney disease (CKD) or diabetes require antihypertensive medications. Angiotensin-converting enzyme inhibitors (ACEIs), angiotensin (AT) receptor blockers, calcium channel blockers (CCBs), and thiazide diuretics are safe, effective, and well tolerated, but beta blockers are not considered first-line therapy in children. Children should be started on the lowest recommended dosage of the medications and titrated every 2–4 weeks until the blood pressure goal is achieved. If the goal is not achieved with the maximal dose of a single medication, a second medication with complementary action should be added.[83]

B) DEVICE DESCRIPTION AND IMPORTANT FEATURES

Pediatric blood pressure cuffs are dedicated to BP monitoring for children and are not used to monitor BP in older patients. They are designed with an adjustable size to fit around a child's wrist and can be worn all the time to help the parent or caretaker keep track of the child's blood pressure at all times.

Types of Blood Pressure Monitors[89]
   i.   Mercury sphygmomanometer
   ii. Aneroid blood pressure monitors
   iii. Digital blood pressure monitors

i. Mercury Sphygmomanometer

This is one of the oldest BP monitors and includes an inflatable or deflatable cuff. A mechanical bulb assists in the inflation while deflation is done through a valve.

ii. Aneroid Blood Pressure Monitors

Aneroid BP monitor includes a cuff, mechanical bulb, deflating valve, and a round monitor. This monitor has a round dial covered with glass and a metal spring that gives

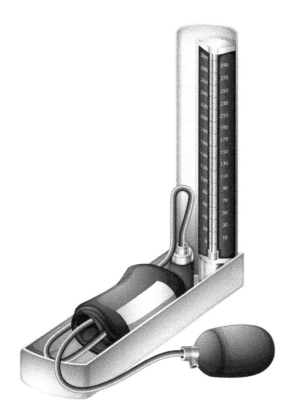

FIGURE 9.12 A mercury sphygmomanometer.

Source: www.shutterstock.com/image-vector/illustration-blood-pressure-measuring-device-on-181541765

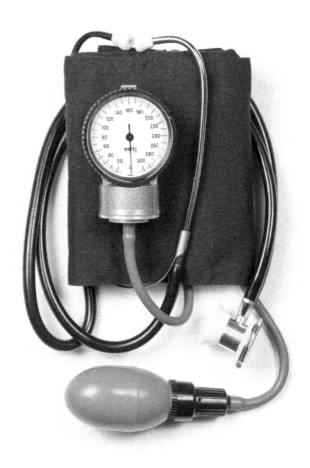

FIGURE 9.13 A classical aneroid blood pressure monitor ("blood pressure cuff").

Source: www.shutterstock.com/image-photo/manual-aneroid-sphygmomanometer-stethoscope-on-white-120709720

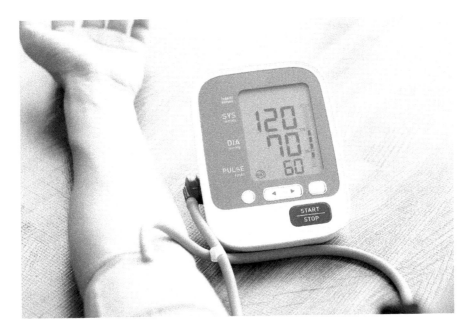

FIGURE 9.14   A digital blood pressure monitor ("automatic blood pressure cuff").

Source: www.shutterstock.com/image-photo/human-check-blood-pressure-monitor-heart-730380310

the reading. Both aneroid and mercury BP apparatuses require a stethoscope for reading the BP.

iii. Digital Blood Pressure Monitors

These devices may be semiautomatic or fully automatic. Semiautomatic models are manually inflated and automatically deflated, whereas fully automatic models are automatically inflated and deflated. Digital BP monitors have a built-in LCD screen to show the readings, so a stethoscope is not required. These models are also used in neonatal ICU.

Cuff Requirements

It is essential to select the right cuff size for measuring BP because a smaller cuff may falsely elevate the BP measurement, whereas a larger cuff may falsely lower the BP measurement.[90] An ideally sized cuff should cover two thirds of the length of the arm and should be 20% wider than the diameter of the limb to which it is fitted. The cuff should encircle at least 75% of the arm.

Choice of BP Monitor

The choice of BP monitor depends on accuracy, ease of use, and cost. Additionally, it is vital to appreciate the limitations of each device and have proper training about using it.

c)   PURPOSE AND HOW TO USE

Before You Check the BP of a Child, You Should[91]

- Wait 30 minutes if the child has been fed something. Tell the child to rest for 3 to 5 minutes without talking.

- Tell the child to sit in a comfortable position, with his/her legs and ankles uncrossed and back supported.
- Tell the child to elevate his/her left arm to the level of his/her heart. Wrap the cuff around the upper part of the child's bare arm. Check the placement of the cuff.

i) Measurement in the Arm[92]

- Place the cuff on your child's right arm, halfway between the shoulder and elbow, around the midline over the brachial artery.
- Measure the pressure in the arm at heart level.
- Place the bell of the stethoscope over the brachial artery below the bottom edge of the cuff.
- Inflate the cuff to approximately 20 mm Hg above the point where the radial pulse disappears and then deflate at 2–3 mm Hg/second.
- The systolic reading is the onset of the Korotkoff sounds or the point when the initial sound is heard.
- In children and adolescents, the diastolic reading is the disappearance of Korotkoff sounds.
- When all sounds have disappeared, the cuff should be deflated entirely and rapidly. An approximately 1–2 minute gap is maintained before further BP monitoring is performed to release blood trapped in the veins.

ii) Measurement in the Thigh[92]

- Tell the child to lie face down and apply the cuff over the posterior of the mid-thigh.

- If the child is unable to lie face down, tell the child to flex the knee to fit the stethoscope and monitor the pressure with the child supine.
- Place the stethoscope over popliteal artery at thigh to obtain the BP reading.

D) IMPORTANT SAFETY ISSUES (CAUTIONS AND COMMON ADVERSE EFFECTS)

- Errors may occur with BP monitoring in the wrist due to movement and incorrect posture.[93]
- Home BP cuffs and wrist monitors are not well validated in children and are not used.[83]
- Cuff size is a critical variable in the accuracy of BP measurement; the width of the cuff should be at least 40% of the mid-arm circumference.

E) STORAGE CONDITIONS AND MAINTENANCE

- Store the BP measurement device with its components in a clean, safe location at a temperature range of −20°C to 60°C within a relative humidity (RH) of 10 to 95%. However, the operating temperature and RH should be maintained at 10°C to 40°C and 15% to 90%, respectively.
- Use a soft and dry cloth and neutral soap to clean the BP measurement device and the arm cuff.
- Do not clean the device using gasoline or similar corrosive agents.
- Do not expose the BP measurement device to moisture or a water source to prevent damage. Additionally, the device and its components should not be washed by immersing in water.
- Do not disassemble the device or its components.
- Do not store the device if it is wet or in locations with extreme temperatures, humidity, direct sunlight, dust or corrosive agents, vibrations, or shocks.

F) IMPORTANT FEATURES (CAPABILITIES AND LIMITATIONS) AND SPECIAL ADVANTAGES

- Pediatric BP cuffs are economical, lightweight and easy to use and read; they have an indicator to show the child's BP.[93]
- Ambulatory blood pressure monitoring (ABPM) helps identify white coat hypertension (i.e., those who present hypertension only in the doctor's office).[86]
- ABPM shows accurate diagnosis and target organ damage (TOD), if present.[85]
- Home BP measurements (HBPM) and ABPM help to confirm hypertension.[94]
- Daily BP readings provide ideas about managing a child's health and hypertension.

G) SPECIAL TIPS FOR PATIENT COUNSELING

- Hold the BP monitor steadily at heart level for an accurate BP reading.[93]
- Use only validated and reliable BP measurement devices.[94]
- Screen your child for elevated BP annually beginning at 3 years of age or at every physician visit if risk factors are present.[83,92]
- Screen your child with hypertension for comorbid CVD, including diabetes mellitus (DM) and hyperlipidemia.[83]
- Use an appropriately sized cuff with an inflatable bladder width that is at least 40% of the arm circumference.
- Monitor BP in the right arm of a relaxed, seated child because coarctation of the aorta may lead to false low readings in the left arm.[83,92]
- Tell your child to watch television, use the computer, or play video games for < 2 hours/day.[95]
- Take BP readings at the same time each day, beginning 2 weeks after a change in treatment and during the week before the next follow-up visit to the physician.
- Take 2 or 3 BP readings with a gap of one minute and record the results. Do not measure BP over clothes.
- Do not depend on the wrist and finger BP monitors because they give less reliable readings.
- Choose a validated monitor, especially for the BP measurement in pregnant women or children.[96]
- Do not use the device on an injured arm that is receiving medical treatment. Do not apply a cuff to an arm receiving an intravenous drip or blood transfusion.
- Do not use the device in a moving vehicle such as a car or airplane.

H) EVIDENCE OF EFFECTIVENESS AND SAFETY

In children and adolescents, ABPM is more accurate than BP measurement in a clinic. ABPM refers to the use of a validated device that assesses BP every 20–30 minutes, around the clock.[83]

I) ECONOMIC EVALUATION

ABPM is cost-effective only if it is used accurately, because it helps diagnose and screen patients who are not hypertensive and who do not require therapy. It is also useful for children requiring long-term therapy for HTN to minimize untoward effects of the therapy. The procedure is also beneficial to monitor patients with borderline HTN and white coat HTN (WC-HTN) and their symptoms.[97] Many of the BP monitors in India are economical, with prices ranging from US$1 to $3.[98] Flynn and Urbina (2012) estimated that initial ABPM would save more than US$2.4 million per 1,000 children in the USA.[99]

J) IMPLICATION TO THE PHARMACY PROFESSION AND PHARMACY PRACTICE

It is essential to confirm the diagnosis of hypertension using ABPM in patients with asymptomatic or mildly elevated BP (stage 1 hypertension).[86] These devices are also used in clinical research in the ICU to test the efficacy of medications. Continual BP measurement is usually performed using an arterial line.[100] Physicians should review any prescription only medications (POM) and over-the-counter (OTC) medications and supplements, performance-enhancing drugs, and illicit drugs that the patient may be using because these can also increase BP. Patients should be evaluated for their family history of hypertension, other CV risk factors, and renal or endocrine disorders.[83] If BP is consistently increased, measure in both arms with the child in a seated position and in a leg with the child in a prone position. BP should be nearly equal in both arms and is usually 10–20 mm Hg higher in the legs. If there is a significant difference in BP between the two arms or the BP in the leg is lower than that in the arms, there may be a heart murmur. Dietary approaches to stop hypertension (DASH) diets may also reduce BP in children and adolescents.[83,101] Children with hypertension should be given a diet enriched with high fresh fruits and vegetables, fiber, and low-fat dairy, and their sodium intake should be reduced.[83]

ABPM should only be used by personnel trained in the application and interpretation of the data in pediatric patients. The device should be programmed to record BP every 20 to 30 minutes during the day and every 30 to 60 minutes during the night. Health professionals, including pharmacists, should instruct the guardians to record the antihypertensive medication administration, activity level, and sleep and wake times of the child in a diary, creating a journal or logbook of daily BP monitoring.[102] Cuff sizes should be standardized and uniformly color-coded for convenience. Selecting an appropriate BP cuff size is vital, because a smaller cuff overestimates the BP reading, and a larger cuff underestimates the reading. This is crucial in the case of children due to their varying arm sizes with age. Therefore, cuffs for children are marketed in various sizes and labeled for neonatal, infant, child and/or pediatric purpose, or thigh BP measurements.[90]

K) CHALLENGES TO PHARMACISTS AND USERS

Wrist devices yield error reporting with the use of cuffs that are too large or too small.[93] Therefore, it is better to use cuffs that are accurately sized for the child's arm.[103] Obtaining an accurate BP reading in children and adolescents can be problematic due to anxiety, caffeine intake, time or timing of BP monitoring, and patient positioning. For accurate reporting, the child should be seated for at least 3–5 minutes with back supported and feet uncrossed and flat on the floor. All children and adolescents with hypertension should be monitored for hyperlipidemia and renal disease with urinalysis and electrolyte, blood urea nitrogen (BUN), and creatinine tests.[83] ABPM should be used by individuals with expertise in using and interpreting it because accurate execution is essential, and only trained staff can ensure this.[103]

L) RECOMMENDATIONS: THE WAY FORWARD

- Ambulatory blood pressure monitoring should only be used by personnel training in using and interpreting the data.
- The child should be in a seated position for at least 3–5 minutes with back supported and feet uncrossed and flat on the floor for accurate blood pressure readings.
- Cuff sizes should be standardized and uniformly color-coded for convenience.

M) CONCLUSIONS

High blood pressure in children and adolescents is a global health problem, with primary hypertension being the most common type. Frequent blood pressure monitoring is essential for critically ill neonates and children. Therefore, guardians or parents should be trained to apply the ambulatory blood pressure monitor and interpret the reading at home. The device should be programmed to record BP every 20 to 30 minutes during the day, and every 30 to 60 minutes during the night.

N) LESSONS LEARNED

- Mercury sphygmomanometers and aneroid and digital blood pressure monitors are the commonly used blood pressure monitors for children.
- ABPM is a cost-effective approach to diagnosing and screening patients who are not hypertensive and do not require therapy.
- Wrist devices yield reporting errors with the use of cuffs that are too large or too small.
- ABPM helps identify white coat hypertension.

DEVICE 8: CHILD FACE MASKS

A) BACKGROUND

Children are more susceptible to the risks associated with air pollution, such as chronic respiratory diseases. Masks and respirators protect against air pollutants to some extent.[104] Masks and respirators are also crucial in newly emerging respiratory disorders such as severe acute respiratory syndrome (SARS) and Middle East respiratory syndrome coronavirus (MERS-CoV).[105] Masks are economical, effective, and easy to use, and they substantially

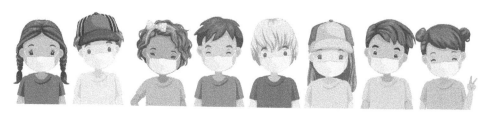

FIGURE 9.15 Illustration of children wearing face masks to protect against airborne and respiratory-droplet-borne pathogens.
Source: www.shutterstock.com/image-vector/kids-mask-set-little-boy-girl-1736243453

reduce the transmission of infectious organisms.[106] Aerosol masks were initially developed for adults and later downsized to fit children.[107]

B) DEVICE DESCRIPTION AND IMPORTANT FEATURES

Masks for aerosol therapy are made of breathable fabric and are available in various shapes and dimensions.[107] Child face masks are comfortable, adjustable with two elastic ear straps, and appealing to users with bright colors and child-friendly prints or patterns. There is a nose wire and a pocket for additional filter inserts. The best material for a homemade face mask is 100% cotton fabric that is tightly woven in multiple layers.

Types of Face Masks[108]
  i. Cloth masks
 ii. Surgical face masks (medical or procedure mask)
iii. N95 respirators (filtering face pieces [FFP])

i. Cloth Masks

Cloth face masks covering the nose and mouth help reduce the transmission of droplets in the community. Homemade or purchased cloth masks can be useful for a child.

ii. Surgical Masks

Surgical masks are loose-fitting and disposable devices that create a physical barrier to control the transmission of contaminants in the environment. These are available in a smaller size for children ≥ 3 years old.

iii. N95 Respirators

N95 respirators are personal protective equipment (PPE) used to protect children from airborne particles and prevent them from transmitting these particles to others. These respirators are available in varying sizes, ranging from extra-small to large. Only immunocompromised children or those at high risk can wear an N95 mask.[109]

C) PURPOSE AND HOW TO USE[110]

When Putting on a Mask
  • Tell the child to wash his/her hands with soapy water before putting on a mask (or you do this for them).

  • Ensure that the mask is clean, not torn or worn, and not dirty or damaged.
  • Adjust the mask to securely cover the mouth, nose, and chin, ensuring that it is comfortable for the child to breathe.

While Wearing a Mask
  • Change the mask if it gets dirty or wet.
  • Ensure that the mask fully covers the mouth and nose of your child.
  • Tell your child not to pull the mask down below the nose or chin or wear it on the head.
  • Do not touch the mask while wearing it, and tell your child the same.

When Taking Off a Mask
  • Wash your hands before and after taking off the mask or tell your child to do so.
  • Tell the child not to touch the front of the mask.
  • Wash fabric masks after each use and store them in a clean bag.
  • Dispose of the medical masks in a closed bin, since these are single-use.

D) IMPORTANT SAFETY ISSUES (CAUTIONS AND COMMON ADVERSE EFFECTS)

  • Cloth masks may reduce hydration and may cause erythema or tissue damage.
  • Use of a worn mask may result in poor perfusion and edema.[111]
  • Children younger than 2 years of age should not wear any type of mask because they would have to struggle to breathe due to their tiny airways.[108]
  • Masks may be uncomfortable to wear, especially for children and in hot and humid environments. This produces poor adherence in these age groups.[112]
  • Self-contamination may occur if nonmedical masks are not changed when wet or soiled due to microbial growth.
  • Overuse of masks may lead to bilateral headache, breathing difficulties, and/or perioral dermatitis with rashes and redness due to the build-up and deposition of saliva, sweat, and moist vapor

between the mask and the skin. This also creates a favorable condition for bacteria to grow or colonize.

- Masks may yield itchy rashes due to contact between the rubber strings and the skin of the nose and ears.[112]
- Masks may give a false sense of security, leading to lower adherence to other critical preventive measures, including physical distancing and hand hygiene, in the case of a pandemic, such as COVID-19.[112,113]
- Wearing face masks may be problematic for children wearing spectacles due to the accumulation of fog.
- Wearing a face mask makes the exhaled air circulate into the eyes, generating an impulse to touch the eyes. This may ultimately lead to an eye infection.[113]

E) STORAGE CONDITIONS AND MAINTENANCE

- Homemade cloth masks should be routinely cleaned and washed in hot water using soap or detergent before they are reused. Then, rinse them well with fresh water and hang to dry.
- Masks can also be disinfected by soaking them in a solution of 2 tablespoons of bleach in a bowl for 5 minutes.
- Wash fabric masks using soap or detergent in hot water (at least 60°C) at least once a day. If they are machine washed, use the appropriate warm setting according to the type of fabric.
- Dry the mask after washing and store it in a clean bag.

F) IMPORTANT FEATURES (CAPABILITIES AND LIMITATIONS) AND SPECIAL ADVANTAGES

- Aerosolized medications can be safely delivered with the use of face masks in the pediatric population.[107]
- Masks or facial coverings prevent the child from generating or receiving droplets during breathing, coughing, sneezing, talking, etc.

G) SPECIAL TIPS FOR PATIENT COUNSELING

- Use a securely fitting mask to minimize leakage of sensitizing agents (e.g., aerosolized antibiotics) into the caregivers' environment.[107]
- Consider the size, fit, fabric, and filters when you choose a child face mask.
- Let your children see others wearing the mask if they refuse to wear it and talk about its benefits.
- Encourage your children to wear masks only if they can remove them without assistance to ensure that there is no suffocation risk.

- Tell your children to not touch their face while wearing masks and tell them to wash their hands immediately after taking masks off.
- Children in good health can wear a nonmedical or fabric mask, whereas those with cystic fibrosis or cancer should wear a medical mask.
- Children should not wear a mask when playing sports or performing rapid movements, including running, jumping, or playing, since these movements may compromise their breathing.[112]
- Do not share masks between children, and disposable masks should be appropriately disposed of when these are removed and not reused.
- Follow instructions on how to put on, take off, and dispose of medical masks with hand hygiene and instruct your child to follow the same instructions.[112]
- Tell your child to maintain frequent handwashing and physical distancing and to wear a face mask correctly and consistently to protect their communities.

H) EVIDENCE OF EFFECTIVENESS AND SAFETY

The effectiveness of masks mainly depends on their correct use to prevent or restrict the spread of microorganisms. Nevertheless, the use of a mask alone may not protect adequately, and other measures should also be adopted.[114] Masks reduce the risk of transmission of droplets from infected persons to others.[112] Although the effectiveness of homemade cloth face coverings is doubtful, surgical masks can prevent inhalation of large droplets and sprays and can prevent transmission of respiratory viruses from the ill.[108,115] Surgical masks should be worn when taking public transportation or when going to or staying in crowded places.[115] However, cloth face coverings can reduce source virus transmission if they are well constructed (e.g., hybrid and multilayer) with optimal material (e.g., high-grade cotton) and used correctly.

However, surgical masks are also poorly effective in filtering submicron-sized airborne particles. Surgical masks and N95 respirators are equivalently effective for the prevention of influenza-like illness (ILI),[108] but N95 respirators are 21.5% effective in protecting against inhalation of nanoparticles, while surgical masks are only 2.4% effective.[109] Children at high risk of infection or who are severely immunocompromised should wear an N95 mask to protect themselves, whereas those at moderate risk may use a surgical or disposable mask for medical use. Similarly, children at low risk may use a disposable mask for medical use, whereas those at very low risk need not wear a mask or can wear nonmedical masks such as cloth masks.

I) ECONOMIC EVALUATION

Face masks are economical and easier to use than most other infection transmission strategies.[109] Mukerji et al.

(2017) reported that N95 respirator use would be cost-effective in the case of a highly pathogenic pandemic.[116]

J) IMPLICATION TO THE PHARMACY PROFESSION AND PHARMACY PRACTICE

Pharmacists should counsel the parents or guardians that children younger than age 2 should not wear masks. Similarly, N95 respirators are not required for the general population (instead, they are required for healthcare personnel) because they achieve a very close facial fit and block 0.3-μm particles, and require an increased effort in breathing, leading to discomfort, tiredness, or headaches after continuous use for a few hours.[108] Use of cloth masks for situations wherein a surgical or N95 mask would not be required or not available is appropriate, but their use may give users a false sense of protection from infectious organisms.[113]

K) CHALLENGES TO PHARMACISTS AND USERS

Face masks may make breathing difficult, particularly if the child is already suffering from respiratory problems. Moreover, a fraction of carbon dioxide previously exhaled is also inhaled at each respiratory cycle, which increases breathing frequency and extent. Users should remove the mask when he/she is sneezing or is in a post-seizure state to facilitate smooth respiration.[106] The issue of mask size and fit is problematic for infants and young children whose faces undergo rapid developmental changes in all dimensions during the first few months/years of life. Therefore, more than one size of mask is needed at the same time during such phases.[107] Adherence and dental side effects of face masks are problematic phenomena.[117] Children of any age with developmental disorders and disabilities should not regularly wear face masks and should be assessed on a case-by-case basis. Similarly, children with severe cognitive or respiratory impairments should not wear masks.[118]

L) RECOMMENDATIONS: THE WAY FORWARD

- Pharmacists should counsel the parents or guardians that children younger than two years should not wear masks.
- Surgical masks should be worn when taking public transportation or when going to or staying in crowded places.
- Children of any age with developmental disorders should not regularly wear face masks and should be assessed on a case-by-case basis.

M) CONCLUSIONS

Children are more prone to the risks associated with air pollution, such as chronic respiratory diseases, for which masks and respirators may play a protective role. Masks are economical, practical, and easy to use, and they reduce the transmission of infectious organisms from one person to another. The effectiveness of masks to restrict the spread of microorganisms mainly depends on their correct use. However, the use of a mask alone may not protect adequately, and other measures should also be adopted.

N) LESSONS LEARNED

- Masks for aerosol therapy are made of breathable fabric and are available in various shapes and dimensions.
- Children in good health can wear a nonmedical or fabric mask, whereas those with cystic fibrosis or cancer should wear a medical mask.
- Only immunocompromised children or those at high risk should wear an N95 mask.
- Masks should not be shared between children and should be appropriately disposed of and not reused after they are removed.

DEVICE 9: OTHER DEVICES USED IN PEDIATRIC PRACTICE

In addition to the aforementioned pediatric devices of importance to pharmacy practice in clinical, hospital, community, or household settings, other pediatric devices are also crucial from the pediatric practitioner's perspective. Some of these devices are:

A) Devices unique to children
- Infant incubators
- Phototherapy light (bili lights) (for treating neonatal jaundice)
- Newborn auditory function screening devices
- Infant caps
- Bilirubinometer

B) Devices developed for children but also used with adults
- Atrial septal defect occluder
- Cerebrospinal fluid shunt

C) Life-saving and life-sustaining medical devices for children
- Mechanical ventilators
- Balloon atrial septostomy (Rashkind procedure)

Since these devices are more applicable to pediatric practitioners than pharmacy practitioners, they are out of the scope of the present chapter. Interested readers are suggested to refer to the relevant literature.

REFERENCES

1. Bream E, Li H, Furman L. The effect of breast pump use on exclusive breastfeeding at 2 months postpartum in an inner-city population. Breastfeed Med. 2017;12(3):1–7. https://doi.org/10.1089/bfm.2016.0160.

2. Clark A, Dellaport J. Development of a WIC single-user electric breast pump protocol. Breastfeed Med. 2011;6(1):37–40. https://doi.org/10.1089/bfm.2010.0012.

3. Chamberlain LB, McMahon M, Philipp BL, et al. Breast pump access in the inner city: a hospital-based initiative to provide breast pumps for low-income women. J Hum Lact. 2006;22(1):94–8. https://doi.org/10.1177/0890334405284226.

4. Slusher T, Slusher IL, Biomdo M, et al. Electric breast pump use increases maternal milk volume in African nurseries. J Tropic Pediatr. 2007;53(2):125–30. https://doi.org/10.1093/tropej/fml066.

5. Alekseev NP, Ilyin VI, Yaroslavski VK, et al. Compression stimuli increase the efficacy of breast pump function. Eur J Obstetr Gynecol Reproduct Biol. 1998;77:131–9.

6. Eglash A, Malloy ML. Breastmilk expression and breast pump technology. Clin Obstetr Gynecol. 2015;58(4):855–67.

7. Brown SL, Bright RA, Dwyer DE, et al. Breast pump adverse events: reports to the food and drug administration. J Hum Lact. 2005;21(2):169–74. https://doi.org/10.1177/0890334405275445.

8. Kapinos KA, Bullinger L, Gurley-Calvez T. The Affordable Care Act, breastfeeding, and breast pump health insurance coverage. JAMA Pediatr. 2018:E1–E2. https://doi.org/10.1001/jamapediatrics.2018.2003.

9. FDA. Breast pumps. US Food and Drug Administration. 2018 Nov 1. Available from: www.fda.gov/medical-devices/breast-pumps/types-breast-pumps (accessed 23 Sept 2020).

10. Flores-Anton B, Martın-Cornejo J, Morante-Santana MA, et al. Comparison of two methods for cleaning breast pump milk. collection kits in human milk banks. J Hospit Infect. 2019;103:217–22. https://doi.org/10.1016/j.jhin.2019.07.007.

11. CDC. How to keep your breast pump kit clean. Center for Disease Control and Prevention, USA. 2018 Aug 20. Available from: www.cdc.gov/healthywater/pdf/hygiene/breast-pump-fact-sheet-p.pdf (accessed 23 Sept 2020).

12. Price E, Weaver G, Hoffman P, et al. Decontamination of breast pump milk collection kits and related items at home and in hospital: guidance from a Joint Working Group of the Healthcare Infection Society and Infection Prevention Society. J Hospit Infect. 2016;92:213–21. https://doi.org/10.1016/j.jhin.2015.08.025.

13. DOHHS. Pumping and storing breastmilk. Office on Women's Health at the U.S. Department of Health and Human Services. 2018 July 9. Available from: www.womenshealth.gov/breastfeeding/pumping-and-storing-breastmilk (accessed 23 Sept 2020).

14. Mitoulas LR, Lai CT, Gurrin LC, et al. Efficacy of breast milk expression using an electric breast pump. J Hum Lact. 2002;18(4):344–52. https://doi.org/10.1177/089033402237907.

15. Crossland N, Thomson G, Morgan H, et al. Breast pumps as an incentive for breastfeeding: a mixed methods study of acceptability. Matern Child Nutr. 2016;12:726–39. https://doi.org/10.1111/mcn.12346.

16. Weisband YL, Keim SA, Keder LM, et al. Early breast milk pumping intentions among postpartum women. Breastfeed Med. 2017;12(1):28–32. https://doi.org/10.1089/bfm.2016.0142.

17. Apa H, Gözmen S, Keskin-Gözmen S, et al. Clinical accuracy of non-contact infrared thermometer from umbilical region in children: a new side. Turk J Pediatr. 2016;58(2):180–6.

18. Apa H, Gozmen S, Bayram N, et al. Clinical accuracy of tympanic thermometer and noncontact infrared skin thermometer in pediatric practice: an alternative for axillary digital thermometer. Pediatr Emer Care. 2013;29(9):992–7.

19. Hebbar K, Fortenberry JD, Rogers K, et al. Comparison of temporal artery thermometer to standard temperature measurements in pediatric intensive care unit patients. Pediatr Crit Care Med. 2005;6(5):557–61. https://doi.org/10.1097/01.PCC.0000163671.69197.16.

20. Porter RS, Wenger FG. Diagnosis and treatment of pediatric fever by caretakers. J Emerg Med. 2000;19(1):1–4.

21. Schreiber S, Minute M, Tornese G, et al. Galinstan thermometer is more accurate than digital for the measurement of body temperature in children. Pediatr Emer Care. 2013;29(2):197–9.

22. Robinson JL, Jou H, Spady DW. Accuracy of parents in measuring body temperature with a tympanic thermometer. BMC Fam Pract. 2005;6:3. https://doi.org/10.1186/1471-2296-6-3.

23. Reynolds M, Bonham L, Gueck M, et al. Are temporal artery temperatures accurate enough to replace rectal temperature measurement in pediatric ED patients? J Emerg Nurs. 2014;40:46–50. https://doi.org/10.1016/j.jen.2012.07.007.

24. Aprahamian N, Lee L, Shannon M, et al. Glass thermometer injuries: it is not just about the mercury. Pediatr Emer Care. 2009;25(10):645–7.

25. Barton SJ, Gaffney R, Chase T, et al. Pediatric temperature measurement and child/parent/nurse preference using three temperature measurement instruments. J Pediatr Nurs. 2003;18(5):314–20. https://doi.org/10.1053/S0882-5963(03)00103-9.

26. Franconi I, Cerra CL, Marucci AR, et al. Digital axillary and non-contact infrared thermometers for children. Clin Nurs Res. 2016:1–11. https://doi.org/10.1177/1054773816676538.

27. Baxter C, Gorodzinsky FP, Leduc D, et al. Temperature measurement in paediatrics [Canadian Paediatric Society (CPS) Statement: CP 2000–01]. Paediatr Child Health. 2000;5(5):273–6.

28. Batra P, Saha A, Faridi MMA. Thermometry in children. J Emerg Trauma Shock. 2012;5(3):246–9. https://doi.org/10.4103/0974-2700.99699.

29. Kairuz TE, Ball PA, Pinnock REK. Variations in small-volume doses of a liquid antibiotic using two paediatric administration devices. Pharm World Sci. 2006;28:96–100. https://doi.org/10.1007/s11096-006-9012-z.

30. Ryu GS, Lee YJ. Analysis of liquid medication dose errors made by patients and caregivers using alternative measuring devices. J Manag Care Pharm. 2012;18(6):439–45.

31. van Riet-Nales DA, Schobben AFAM, Vromans H, et al. Safe and effective pharmacotherapy in infants and preschool children: importance of formulation aspects. Arch Dis Child. 2016;101:662–9. https://doi.org/10.1136/archdischild-2015-308227.

32. Sobhani P, Christopherson J, Ambrose PJ, et al. Accuracy of oral liquid measuring devices: comparison of dosing cup and oral dosing syringe. Ann Pharmacother. 2008;42(1):46–52. https://doi.org/10.1345/aph.1K420.

33. Beckett VL, Tyson LD, Carroll D, et al. Accurately administering oral medication to children isn't child's play. Arch Dis Child. 2012;97:838–41. https://doi.org/10.1136/archdischild-2012-301850.

34. Peacock G, Parnapy S, Raynor S, et al. Accuracy and precision of manufacturer-supplied liquid medication

administration devices before and after patient education. J Am Pharm Assoc. 2010;50(1):84–6. https://doi.org/10.1331/JAPhA.2010.09006.

35. Buddhadev MD, Patel KS, Patel VJ, et al. Perceptions about oral liquid medication dosing devices and dosing errors by caregivers of hospitalised children. J Pharm Res. 2016;10(12):810–13.

36. ASHP Safe Medication. How to use liquid medications. American Society of Health-System Pharmacists. 2014:1–6. Available from: www.safemedication.com/safemed/docs/Liquid-Medications.pdf (accessed 23 Aug 2020).

37. Johnson A, Meyers R. Evaluation of measuring devices packaged with prescription oral liquid medications. J Pediatr Pharmacol Ther. 2016;21(1):75–80.

38. Burca NDL, Gephart SM, Miller C, et al. Promoting breast milk nutrition in infants with cleft lip and/or palate. Adv Neonatal Care. 2016;16(5):337–44. https://doi.org/10.1097/ANC.0000000000000305.

39. WHO. Infant and young child feeding: model chapter for textbooks for medical students and allied health professionals. France: World Health Organization. 2009:1–100.

40. Flint A, New K, Davies MW. Cup feeding versus other forms of supplemental enteral feeding for newborn infants unable to fully breastfeed. Cochrane Database Syst Rev. 2016, Issue 8. Art. No.: CD005092. https://doi.org/10.1002/14651858.CD005092.pub3.

41. Yilmaz G, Caylan N, Karacan CD, et al. Effect of cup feeding and bottle feeding on breastfeeding in late preterm infants: a randomized controlled study. J Hum Lact. 2014;30(2):174–9. https://doi.org/10.1177/0890334413517940.

42. Chen P, Soto-Ramírez N, Zhang H, et al. Association between infant feeding modes and gastroesophageal reflux: a repeated measurement analysis of the infant feeding practices study II. J Hum Lact. 2017:1–11. https://doi.org/10.1177/0890334416664711.

43. Soto-Ramírez N, Karmaus W, Zhang H, et al. Modes of infant feeding and the occurrence of coughing/wheezing in the first year of life. J Hum Lact. 2013;29(1):71–80. https://doi.org/10.1177/0890334412453083.

44. Kotowski J, Fowler C, Hourigan C, et al. Bottle-feeding an infant feeding modality: an integrative literature review. Matern Child Nutr. 2020;e12939. https://doi.org/10.1111/mcn.12939.

45. Fewtrell MS, Kennedy K, Nicholl R, et al. Infant feeding bottle design, growth and behaviour: results from a randomised trial. BMC Res Notes. 2012;5:150. https://doi.org/10.1186/1756-0500-5-150.

46. Minnesota WIC Program. Paced bottle feeding: infant feeding series for breastfed babies that use a bottle and formula fed babies. Available from: www.health.state.mn.us/docs/people/wic/localagency/wedupdate/moyr/2017/topic/1115feeding.pdf (accessed 26 Aug 2020).

47. Ventura AK, Hernandez A. Effects of opaque, weighted bottles on maternal sensitivity and infant intake. Matern Child Nutr. 2019;15:e12737. https://doi.org/10.1111/mcn.12737.

48. Redmond EC, Griffith CJ, Riley S. Contamination of bottles used for feeding reconstituted powdered infant formula and implications for public health. Perspect Publ Health. 2009;129(2):85–94. https://doi.org/10.1177/1757913908101606.

49. Renfrew MJ, McLoughlin M, McFadden A. Cleaning and sterilisation of infant feeding equipment: a systematic review. Publ Health Nutr. 2008;11(11):1188–99. https://doi.org/10.1017/S1368980008001791.

50. WHO. How to prepare formula for bottle-feeding at home. Ireland: World Health Organization; 2007. p. 1–12.

51. Li R, Magadia J, Fein SB, et al. Risk of bottle-feeding for rapid weight gain during the first year of life. Arch Pediatr Adolesc Med. 2012;166(5):431–6.

52. Collins CT, Gillis J, McPhee AJ, et al. Avoidance of bottles during the establishment of breast feeds in preterm infants. Cochrane Database Syst Rev. 2016, Issue 10. Art. No.: CD005252. https://doi.org/10.1002/14651858.CD005252.pub4.

53. Muchão FP, da Silva Filho LV. Advances in inhalation therapy in pediatrics. J Pediatr (Rio J). 2010;86(5):367–76. https://doi.org/10.2223/JPED.2024.

54. Roncada C, Andrade J, Bischoff LC, et al. Comparison of two inhalational techniques for bronchodilator administration in children and adolescents with acute asthma crisis: a meta-analysis. Rev Paul Pediatr. 2018;36(3):364–71. https://doi.org/10.1590/1984-0462.

55. Nalin U, Stout S, Portnoy JM. Single inhaler maintenance and reliever therapy in pediatric asthma. Curr Opin Allergy Clin Immunol. 2019;19:111–17. https://doi.org/10.1097/ACI.0000000000000518.

56. Benedictis FM, Selvaggio D. Use of inhaler devices in pediatric asthma. Pediatr Drugs. 2003;5(9):629–38.

57. Pedersen S, Dubus JC, Crompton G. The ADMIT series—Issues in Inhalation Therapy. 5) Inhaler selection in children with asthma. Primary Care Respir J. 2010;19(3):209–16. https://doi.org/10.4104/pcrj.2010.00043.

58. DiBlasi RM. Clinical controversies in aerosol therapy for infants and children. Respir Care. 2015;60(6):894–916.

59. Murayama N, Murayama K. Comparison of the clinical efficacy of salbutamol with jet and mesh nebulizers in asthmatic children. Pulm Med. 2018, Article ID 1648652:1–6. https://doi.org/10.1155/2018/1648652.

60. Vandewalker M, Hickey L, Small CJ. Efficacy and safety of beclomethasone dipropionate breath-actuated or metered-dose inhaler in pediatric patients with asthma. Allergy Asthma Proc. 2017;38:354–64. https://doi.org/10.2500/aap.2017.38.4078.

61. Laube BL, Janssens HM, Jongh FHC, et al. What the pulmonary specialist should know about the new inhalation therapies. Eur Respir J. 2011;37:1308–31. https://doi.org/10.1183/09031936.00166410.

62. Pedersen S, Mortensen S. Use of different inhalation devices in children. Lung. 1990;Suppl:653–7.

63. Gardenhire DS, Burnett D, Strickland S, et al. A guide to aerosol delivery devices for respiratory therapists, 4th edn. Irving, TX: American Association for Respiratory Care; 2017. p. 1–55.

64. Carrigy NB, Ruzycki CA, Golshahi L, et al. Pediatric in vitro and in silico models of deposition via oral and nasal inhalation. J Aerosol Med Pulm Drug Deliv. 2014;27(3):149–69. https://doi.org/10.1089/jamp.2013.1075.

65. Chrystyn H, Lavorini F. The dry powder inhaler features of the Easyhaler that benefit the management of patients. Expert Rev Respir Med. 2020:1–7. https://doi.org/10.1080/17476348.2020.1721286.

66. Pogacar MS, Maver U, Varda NM, et al. Diagnosis and management of diaper dermatitis in infants with emphasis on skin microbiota in the diaper area. Int J Dermatol. 2018;57:265–75.

67. Shin HT. Diagnosis and management of diaper dermatitis. Pediatr Clin N Am. 2014;61:367–82. https://doi.org/10.1016/j.pcl.2013.11.009.

68. Stamatas GN, Tierney NK. Diaper dermatitis: etiology, manifestations, prevention, and management. Pediatr Dermatol. 2014;31(1):1–7. https://doi.org/10.1111/pde.12245.

69. Sukhneewat C, Chaiyarit J, Techasatian L. Diaper dermatitis: a survey of risk factors in Thai children aged under 24 months. BMC Dermatol. 2019;19:7. https://doi.org/10.1186/s12895-019-0089-1.

70. Blume-Peytavi U, Hauser M, Lunnemann L, et al. Prevention of diaper dermatitis in infants—a literature review. Pediatr Dermatol. 2014;31(4):413–29. https://doi.org/10.1111/pde.12348.

71. Klunk C, Domingues E, Wiss K. An update on diaper dermatitis. Clin Dermatol. 2014;32:477–87. https://doi.org/10.1016/j.clindermatol.2014.02.003.

72. Carr AN, DeWitt T, Cork MJ, et al. Diaper dermatitis prevalence and severity: global perspective on the impact of caregiver behavior. Pediatr Dermatol. 2020;37:130–6. https://doi.org/10.1111/pde.14047.

73. Prasad HRY, Srivastava P, Verma KK. Diaper dermatitis: an overview. Indian J Pedlatr. 2003;70(8):635–7.

74. Cohen B. Differential diagnosis of diaper dermatitis. Clin Pediatr. 2017;56(5S):16S–22S. https://doi.org/10.1177/0009922817706982.

75. Shah K. Myths on chemical burns in the diaper area. Clin Pediatr. 2017;56(5S):13S–15S. https://doi.org/10.1177/0009922817706976.

76. Mendoza JMF, D'Aponte F, Gualtieri D, et al. Disposable baby diapers: life cycle costs, eco-efficiency and circular economy. J Clean Product. 2019;211:455–67.

77. Hayhoe CR, Hsu C. Planning for baby: diaper choices and comfort. Virginia Cooperative Extension: Virginia State University, USA. Available from: https://vtechworks.lib.vt.edu/bitstream/handle/10919/49760/2910-7038.pdf?sequence=1&isAllowed=y (accessed 7 Sept 2020).

78. CDC. Safe and healthy diapering in the home. Center for Disease Control and Prevention National Center for Emerging and Zoonotic Infectious Diseases, USA. Available from: www.cdc.gov/healthywater/pdf/hygiene/diapering-in-home-H.pdf (accessed 7 Sept 2020).

79. Celiksoy MH, Topal E, Okmen ZH, et al. Characteristics of persistent diaper dermatitis in children with food allergy. Pediatr Dermatol. 2019;36:602–6. https://doi.org/10.1111/pde.13733.

80. Sharifi-Heris Z, Farahani LA, Haghani H, et al. Comparison the effects of topical application of olive and calendula ointments on Children's diaper dermatitis: a triple-blind randomized clinical trial. Dermatol Ther. 2018;e12731. https://doi.org/10.1111/dth.12731.

81. Smith MV, Kruse A, Weir A, et al. Diaper need and its impact on child health. Pediatrics. 2013;132;253. https://doi.org/10.1542/peds.2013-0597.

82. Wallace LR, Weir AM, Smith MV. Policy impact of research findings on the association of diaper need and mental health. Women's Health Issues. 2017;27–S1:S14–S21. https://doi.org/10.1016/j.whi.2017.09.003.

83. Riley M, Hernandez AK, Kuznia AL. High blood pressure in children and adolescents. Am Fam Physician. 2018;98(8):486–94.

84. Narogan MV, Narogan MI, Syutkina EV. Validation of A&D UA-778 blood pressure monitor in children. Blood Press Monit. 2009;14:228–31. https://doi.org/10.1097/MBP.0b013e328330ceb2.

85. Yip GW, So H, Li AM, et al. Validation of A&D TM-2430 upper-arm blood pressure monitor for ambulatory blood pressure monitoring in children and adolescents, according to the British Hypertension Society protocol. Blood Press Monit. 2012;17:76–9. https://doi.org/10.1097/MBP.0b013e328351d4a4.

86. Garin EH, Araya CE. Treatment of systemic hypertension in children and adolescents. Curr Opin Pediatr. 2009;21:600–4. https://doi.org/10.1097/MOP.0b013e32832ff3a7.

87. Kaplinski M, Griffis H, Liu F, et al. Clinical innovation: a multidisciplinary program for the diagnosis and treatment of systemic hypertension in children and adolescents. Clin Pediatr. 2019:1–8. https://doi.org/10.1177/0009922819898180.

88. Lang SM, Giuliano JS, Carroll CL, et al. Neonatal/infant validation study of the CAS model 740 noninvasive blood pressure monitor with the Orion/MaxIQ NIBP module. Blood Press Monit. 2014;19:180–2. https://doi.org/10.1097/MBP.0000000000000036.

89. Ogedegbe G, Pickering T. Principles and techniques of blood pressure measurement. Cardiol Clin. 2010;28:571–86. https://doi.org/10.1016/j.ccl.2010.07.006.

90. Arafat M, Mattoo TK. Measurement of blood pressure in children: recommendations and perceptions on cuff selection. Pediatrics. 1999;104(3):e30. https://doi.org/10.1542/peds.104.3.e30.

91. AAFP. Blood pressure monitoring at home. American Academy of Family Physicians 2020 Apr 6. Available from: https://familydoctor.org/blood-pressure-monitoring-at-home/ (accessed 25 Sept 2020).

92. USDOHHS. A pocket guide to blood pressure measurement in children. US Department of Health and Human Services, USA. 2007; NIH Publication 07-5268:1–4.

93. Cuckson AC, Moran P, Seed P, et al. Clinical evaluation of an automated oscillometric blood pressure wrist device. Blood Pressure Monit. 2004;9:31–7. https://doi.org/10.1097/01.mbp.0000122238.15497.47.

94. Beime B, Deutsch C, Krüger R, et al. Validation of the custo screen pediatric blood pressure monitor according to the European Society of Hypertension International Protocol revision. 2010. Eur J Pediatr. 2017:1–8. https://doi.org/10.1007/s00431-017-2874-3.

95. AAFP. High blood pressure in children. Am Fam Physician. 2012;85(7):704.

96. AHA. Monitoring your blood pressure at home. American Heart Association. Available from: www.heart.org/en/health-topics/high-blood-pressure/understanding-blood-pressure-readings/monitoring-your-blood-pressure-at-home (accessed 25 Sept 2020).

97. Portmanl RJ, Yetman RJ. Clinical uses of ambulatory blood pressure monitoring. Pediar Nephrol. 1994;8:367–76.

98. Jeyanthi N, Gokulnath BV, Thandeeswaran R. A complete survey on blood pressure monitoring devices and applications. Biomed Res. 2018;29(21):3751–65.

99. Flynn JT, Urbina EM. Pediatric ambulatory blood pressure monitoring: indications and interpretations. J Clin Hypertens (Greenwich). 2012;14(6):372–82. https://doi.org/10.1111/j.1751-7176.2012.00655.x.

100. Wankum PC, Thurman TL, Holt SJ, et al. Validation of a noninvasive blood pressure monitoring device in

normotensive and hypertensive pediatric intensive care patients. J Clin Monit. 2004;18:253–63.

101. Riley M, Bluhm B. High blood pressure in children and adolescents. Am Fam Physician. 2012;85(7):693–700.

102. Flynn JT, Daniels SR, Hayman LL, et al. Update: ambulatory blood pressure monitoring in children and adolescents: a scientific statement from the American Heart Association. Hypertension. 2014;63:1116–35. https://doi.org/10.1161/HYP.0000000000000007.

103. Genovesi S, Corrado C, Salice P. Arterial blood pressure monitoring in children. Ital J Pediatr. 2015;41(Suppl 2):A35. https://doi.org/10.1186/1824-7288-41-S2-A35.

104. Goh DYT, Mun MW, Lee WLJ, et al. A randomised clinical trial to evaluate the safety, fit, comfort of a novel N95 mask in children. Sci Rep. 2019;9:18952. https://doi.org/10.1038/s41598-019-55451-w.

105. Mukerji S, MacIntyre CR, Newall AT. Review of economic evaluations of mask and respirator use for protection against respiratory infection transmission. BMC Infect Dis. 2015;15:413. https://doi.org/10.1186/s12879-015-1167-6.

106. Asadi-Pooya AA, Cross JH. Is wearing a face mask safe for people with epilepsy? Acta Neurol Scand. 2020;00:1–3. https://doi.org/10.1111/ane.13316.

107. Amirav I, Luder AS, Halamish A, et al. Design of aerosol face masks for children using computerized 3D face analysis. J Aerosol Med Pulm Drug Deliv. 2013;26:1–7. https://doi.org/10.1089/jamp.2013.1069.

108. Esposito S, Principi N. To mask or not to mask children to overcome COVID-19. Eur J Pediatr. 2020:1–4. https://doi.org/10.1007/s00431-020-03674-9.

109. Tracht SM, Valle SYD, Edwards BK. Economic analysis of the use of facemasks during pandemic (H1N1) 2009. J Theor Biol. 2012;300:161–72. https://doi.org/10.1016/j.jtbi.2012.01.032.

110. UNICEF. COVID-19 and masks: tips for families. United Nations Children's Fund, New York, USA. 2020 Aug 26. Available from: www.unicef.org/coronavirus/covid-19-and-masks-tips-families (accessed 25 Sept 2020).

111. Visscher MO, White CC, Jones JM, et al. Face masks for noninvasive ventilation: fit, excess skin hydration, and pressure ulcers. Respiratory Care. 2015;60(11):1536–47. https://doi.org/10.4187/respcare.04036.

112. WHO. Interim guidance: advice on the use of masks in the context of COVID-19. Switzerland: World Health Organization. 2020. Developed on 2020 June 5.

113. Spitzer M. Masked education? The benefits and burdens of wearing face masks in schools during the current Corona pandemic. Trends Neurosci Educ. 2020;20:100138. https://doi.org/10.1016/j.tine.2020.100138.

114. Rubio-Romero JCR, Pardo-Ferreira MC, Torrecilla-García JA, et al. Disposable masks: disinfection and sterilization for reuse, and non-certified manufacturing, in the face of shortages during the COVID-19 pandemic. Safety Sci. 2020;129:104830. https://doi.org/10.1016/j.ssci.2020.104830.

115. Feng S, Shen C, Xia N, et al. Rational use of face masks in the COVID-19 pandemic. Lancet. 2020;8:434–6. https://doi.org/10.1016/S2213-2600(20)30134-X.

116. Mukerji S, MacIntyre CR, Seale H, et al. Cost-effectiveness analysis of N95 respirators and medical masks to protect healthcare workers in China from respiratory infections. BMC Infect Dis. 2017;17:464. https://doi.org/10.1186/s12879-017-2564-9.

117. Minase RA, Bhad WA, Doshi UH. Effectiveness of reverse twin block with lip pads-RME and face mask with RME in the early treatment of class III malocclusion. Prog Orthod. 2019;20:14. https://doi.org/10.1186/s40510-019-0266-0.

118. WHO. Q&A: children and masks related to COVID-19. Switzerland: World Health Organization. 2020. Developed on 2020 Aug 21. Available from: www.who.int/news-room/q-a-detail/q-a-children-and-masks-related-to-covid-19 (accessed 25 Sept 2020).

10 Medical Devices for Urology

Subish Palaian and Kadir Alam

CONTENTS

DOI: 10.1201/9781003002345-12

GENERAL BACKGROUND

Urology deals with disease conditions related to both the male and female genitourinary tracts. A urologist is a physician who belongs to this surgical specialty and deals predominantly with the urinary tract. Urology differs from nephrology in the fact that a nephrologist deals with the physiology and diseases of the kidneys and provides medical treatment without surgical interventions. In addition to the urinary tract, the urologist also deals with conditions associated with male reproductive organs such as the penis, testes, scrotum, prostate, etc. This chapter focuses specifically on urology-related medical devices and excludes those used in nephrology. However, there maybe a few devices which may be used in both urology and nephrology related cases and in some cases even by other specialties.

The urinary tract broadly consists of the kidneys, ureters, urinary bladder, urinary sphincter, and urethra (Figure 10.1). Due to the existing differences between the male and female urinary systems, the medical devices used between sexes also occasionally vary. Age is one of the predisposing factors for urinary problems such as urinary incontinence, erectile dysfunction (ED), etc., and hence the use of medical devices varies across age groups. Medical devices used in urology can be divided into the following categories: prostheses, stents, catheters, and miscellaneous devices such as urobags and urine flow meters. The use of these devices is increasing nowadays with newer versions being launched regularly. Hence, a pharmacist is expected to be knowledgeable on these products and should assist urologists in procurement, and educating patients in their proper use. Urinary catheterization and urostomy services can be offered as extended community pharmacy services. They can add to the professional role and offer more business avenues to community pharmacies.

Urinary System

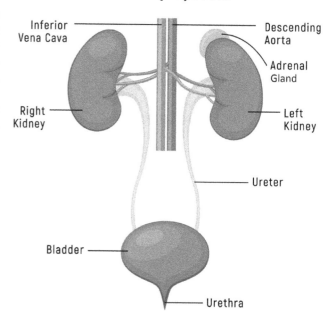

FIGURE 10.1   Diagram of the human urinary system.

Source: www.shutterstock.com/image-vector/urinary-system-anatomy-incontinence-biology-infection-1836780448

eyes, etc. These artificial body parts perform the functions similar to the original body parts and hence are being used commonly these days. In urology, two groups of prostheses are widely used: penile prostheses and vesical sphincter prostheses. The first one is used in males suffering from erectile dysfunction after pharmacological measures fail[1] and the latter are used for people with urinary incontinence.

DEVICE 1: PROSTHESES

A)   BACKGROUND

Prostheses are artificial body parts. Examples for prostheses include artificial heart values, artificial limbs, artificial

B)   DEVICE DESCRIPTION AND IMPORTANT FEATURES

i.   Penile Prostheses

These are mechanical devices implanted inside the bodies of males to provide rigidity of the penile shaft during sexual intercourse. As mentioned earlier, the method is employed only after the failure of already available pharmacological treatments for erectile dysfunction.[2] There are two types: malleable penile prosthesis, and inflatable penile prosthesis. A malleable penile prosthesis is of fixed length and firmness and is inserted through a small incision at penoscrotal junction. The inflatable penile prosthesis makes use of a fluid to achieve rigidity. This fluid moves from a reservoir kept near the urinary bladder to the paired cylinders placed in the erectile bodies of the penis. This device is also inserted through a similar incision to that used for the malleable penile prosthesis. The main advantage of the inflatable penile prosthesis is complete flaccidity and concealment after deflating the device. The surgical procedure for placing the device is performed under anesthesia (epidural or general). More details on penile prostheses are available here.[3]

ii. Vesical Sphincter Prostheses

These are silicone rubber-based devices used in patients with urinary incontinence. The prosthesis is placed through one incision (on the upper part of the scrotum) or two incisions (one in the perineum and another in the groin or abdomen).[5] These are inflatable and adjustable and inflate around the urethra to stop incontinence. The scrotum will include a pump and a tank is kept in the abdomen that keeps the pressure situation intact.[4] Circumference of cuffs lies between 4 and 11 cm and balloon pressure in between 50–80 cm H_2O at 10 cm H_2O increments. At rest, pressure inside the balloon is at equilibrium with the urethral cuff pressure, enabling the urethra to be compressed at the predetermined pressure. The fluid transfers from the cuff to the balloon after squeezing the pump which leads to opening the urethra and permitting voiding or catheterization.[6] More details on vesical sphincter prostheses are available here.[7]

c) Purpose and How to Use

i. Penile Prostheses

These are used to treat severe cases of erectile dysfunction. These may be because of the scarring inside the penis due to conditions such as Peyronie's disease (with painful erections). They are usually indicated for patients with ED resulting in relationship conflict, and patients with uncontrolled diabetes. A video explaining the use of penile prostheses is available here.[8]

ii. Vesical Sphincter Prostheses

These are the most commonly used type of urological implants indicated in incontinent male patients. The device can be operated voluntarily by deflating the cuff in order to create voiding and can stay inflated at other times to raise urethral pressure thus continence.[1,9]

d) Important Safety Issues (Cautions and Common Adverse Effects)

Because these devices require invasive procedures to insert inside the body, their use is associated with surgical site infections. In case of any suspected infections, urgent medical intervention should be made which may require even immediate removal of implant. Other complications include malfunctioning of the device, perforation of urethral mucosa, bleeding after the surgery, scar tissue formation, and erosion of tissue around the implant.[1] These complications often require re-operation and repair.

e) Storage Conditions and Maintenance

i. Penile Prostheses

In malleable prostheses there, is a risk of breakage. However, most people maintain the prosthesis throughout their life. The inflatable one may have to be changed over time.[10]

ii. Vesical Sphincter Prostheses

Since this device remains inside the body once inserted, one must be careful and should inform the physician/surgeon before any other procedures are performed in the urinary tract.

f) Important Features (Capabilities and Limitations) and Special Advantages,[1,11]

Important features of the two different types of penile prosthesis, the inflatable and the semirigid, are reviewed and summarized in this section.

Inflatable implants create a natural and rigid erection. They also provide flaccidity when the device is deflated. This device has a greater number of parts connected and hence has an increased chance of malfunctioning; it also requires a reservoir placed in the abdomen. These are relatively more complicated than semirigid implants and provide less firm erections.

Semirigid rod implants have fewer parts and produce lesser malfunction. Hence, it is also easy to be handled. This device causes a slight rigidity in the penis and puts a constant pressure inside the penis creating a tendency for injury and difficulty in concealing under clothing.

g) Special Tips for Patient Counseling

Since use of these devices requires special care and attention, patients require adequate knowledge prior to and during their use. A few important counseling points for these devices are given here:

i. Penile Prostheses

Just as with any other medical implants, the patient should be screened properly before use of implants and the expectation of outcome should be clarified. The pharmacist should clearly explain that penile implants do not increase sexual desire or sensation, it only helps men to get an erection. The patient should also be informed about the possible risks and complications.[12]

TABLE 10.1

Safety and Effectiveness of Urology Prostheses

Device	Comments
Penile prosthesis	Recent advanced technological developments in design and modern surgery techniques have enabled penile prosthesis implants to be a more natural, durable, and reliable method.[15]
	Safety and efficacy data of Alpha-1 contemporary inflatable devices are much better over inflatable prostheses.[16]
	Nearly all inflatable prosthesis implants (90%-95%) produce erections needed for intercourse. The satisfaction rates of men were found as high as 80–90%.[17]
Vesical sphincter prosthesis	It is an effective option for the treatment of stress urinary incontinence after prostate surgery.[18]

ii. Vesical Sphincter Prostheses

The patient should be advised for prescriptions of antibiotics, pain medication, or stool softeners to prevent constipation (having fewer bowel movements than usual). Post-surgery, the patient can shower after 48 hours and any bandages can be removed while showering. There is no need to put more bandages on the incisions after showering. If the bandages fall off or get dirty in the first 48 hours after surgery, they should be replaced with clean bandages. Sexual intercourse should be avoided during the initial six weeks following the procedure to allow wound healing.[13] In addition, the pharmacist must provide a scrotal support[14] to wear during the first week after surgery. If the scrotal support gets wet, it needs to be replaced.

H) Evidence of Effectiveness and Safety

These devices are being increasingly used since there are studies reporting their safety and effectiveness. A summary of a few studies is listed in Table 10.1.

I) Economic Evaluation of Penile Prostheses

A review of economic evaluations of available ED therapies may not be generalizable to today's ED patients[19] since they do not reflect present-day costs of physicians, pharmaceuticals, and devices, and fail to account for patient comorbidities.

A study suggests sildenafil and vacuum erection device therapy should be considered as first-line strategies for ED. The second-line and third-line choices can include ICI therapy, transurethral alprostadil suppository, and penile prosthesis implant.[20]

J) Implication to the Pharmacy Profession and Pharmacy Practice[21, 22, 23]

Undoubtedly, pharmacists have a big role in assisting urologists in procurement of the devices and also a direct role in patient care during the implantation of these devices. Community pharmacists can also provide extended pharmacy services for patients with erectile dysfunction. Some of the important roles of pharmacists are described here:

1. Penile Prosthesis

Role in Assisting Patients in Choosing a Device

Though these devices are prescribed by specialist doctors after a thorough evaluation, pharmacists can assist patients by providing information that will help them in choosing a device suitable for them. These include people for whom ED fails to respond to initial choice such as oral and extracavernous pharmacological therapies or wherein these therapies are ineffective, contraindicated, or not tolerated. These candidates may be the ones suffering with severe arteriogenic and/or veno-occlusive disease, diabetes, hypertensive arterial syndrome, neurological disorders, and related treatments. Pharmacists can also help select a suitable scrotal support bag for patients using a penile prosthesis.

Prevention and Early Identification of Infections

Risk of infection with post-surgery prosthesis use ranges from 1% to 4 %. Patients with spinal cord injuries, diabetics, and those with long-term corticosteroid use are at a high risk of infection.

Follow-Up

First post-operative follow-up is needed after two weeks to check the wound healing progress, the presence of any infection, and functioning of the device. A 3-month follow-up and further regular annual check-ups are needed to observe the wound, check for the correct functioning of the device, and assess patient-partner satisfaction.

2. Vesical Sphincter Prosthesis

The pharmacist can help with the proper fit and function of incontinence products. There are also treatment options before considering medication or surgery, including bladder control exercises, pelvic floor exercises, sphincter strengthening, catheters, and urethral inserts. Community pharmacists can also help in choosing suitable OTC medications for these patients because many of the medications such as antihistamines and those with anticholinergics may cause further complications in their urinary incontinence.

K) Challenges for Pharmacists and Users

The major challenge for users is the risk of infection associated with the use of devices. Another challenge is the proper usage of the devices. For pharmacists, strengthening product knowledge is the major challenge.

L) Recommendations: The Way Forward

The pharmacists must have good knowledge of these devices. They can suggest these devices for suitable patients after consultation with a urologist. Pharmacists can provide patient care by guiding them on proper usage and precautions to be taken while using the devices. Studies on patient satisfaction with use of the devices and quality of life (QoL) improvements can be conducted by pharmacists. There is also a huge scope for community pharmacists to provide extended services for patients with ED and incontinence, enabling more business opportunities and closer relationships with patients.

m) Conclusions

Urinary tract prostheses (penile and vesical) are unique in improving a patient's QoL. Suitable candidates for these devices should be identified and recommended to use the most suitable for their needs. A pharmacist should counsel the patients on risks related to infection, wound formation, and bleeding due to the invasive nature of these devices. A pharmacist can play an important role in coordination of patients with the urologist.

n) Lessons Learned

- Urology prostheses can largely improve QoL of patients.
- Pharmacists can guide patients in choice of these devices and medications affecting these devices' performance.
- Early identification of device failure and infections is crucial.

DEVICE 2: URINARY STENTS

a) Background

A stent is a tiny tube placed into a hollow structure of the body. The purpose of any stent is to keep the patency and maintaining the flow of fluid in an artery, vein, ureter etc.[24, 25] In urology, three types of stents are commonly used and their purpose is to allow urine to flow freely. They include urethral, ureteric, and prostatic stents. The obstruction to urine flow may be due to renal stones, urinary tract infection (UTI), prostate problems, cancer, etc.

b) Device Description/Important Features

Since the purpose of a stent is to enhance free flow of urine through or beside it, urinary stents are usually hollow in nature. The nature of the stents differs in terms of the place where they are positioned within the urinary tract and the manner in which they are being affixed inside the body and the duration they are kept inside the body. The important features of the urinary stents are described in Table 10.2.

c) Purpose and How to Use

Urethral stent: This is placed to open a blockage or stricture in the urethra. It can be kept for a short or long duration.[29]

TABLE 10.2
Device Descriptions of Urinary Stents

Device	Description
Urethral stent	This stent is placed in urethra and usually made of a metallic alloy, polymer, or a biodegradable material available in multiple designs; rigid enough to maintain the patency of urethra.[26]
Ureteral stent	This stent is flexible in nature and capable enough to be placed in ureter with a length of approximately 10 inches. While placed in ureter, the curl in the top portion sits in the kidney and bottom in the bladder. A string may be present on an end visible outside the body.[25] Commonly called DJ or JJ stent.[27]
Prostatic stent	This stent (both temporary and permanent in nature) is placed into the prostatic urethra through an endoscopic procedure and enhances normal voiding in patients with a functioning detrusor.[28]

Ureteral stent: This is commonly used in treatment of ureteral and renal stones. The details about the use of urethral stents can be viewed in YouTube videos in link given.[30]

Prostate stent: This is used in men unable to empty their bladder and are not fit for surgery. It is alternative to an indwelling catheter in this group of patients. The stent is placed under local anesthesia inserted through the urethra until the tip reaches bladder. The surgeon then confirms the correct positioning of the stent through an ultrasound or a cystoscope.

DJ Stent: This stent is part of ureteroscopic procedures and used to relieve ureteral obstruction.

TABLE 10.3
Safety Issues Associated with Urinary Stents

Device	Safety issues
Urethral stents[31, 32]	UTI, urosepsis, urinary incontinence, stent migration (in approximately 2.5% of cases). Other safety concerns include hematuria (6–14%), perineal pain (2–13%), retrograde ejaculation (0–17%), or painful erections (0–44%).
Ureteral stents	Incontinence, occurs mainly due to the stent being inside the bladder and causing irritation.[33]
Prostatic stents[28]	Migration of stent, painful urination following the procedure, lack of improvement in urine flow, incontinence, stone formation in the stent.
DJ stents	UTI and flank pain may occur due to retrograde urine flow.[34] Other complications occurring in the short-term include infection, hematuria, pain, and sometimes stent syndrome. Long-term complications include encrustations (more common with longer duration of indwelling), renal stones, stent blockades, and hydronephrosis.[35]

d) Important Safety Issues (Cautions and Common Adverse Effects)

Since the stents are placed inside the urinary tract, they can cause irritation in the bladder leading to urine leakage. They also cause discomfort in the groin, bladder, urethra, and genitals.

e) Important Features (Capabilities and Limitations) and Special Advantages

Ureteral Stents

The advantage of ureteral stents is that there is no need of collecting bags associated with stent-related symptoms, and they can be used in coagulopathy or platelet dysfunction. The major limitations are greater X-ray exposure than percutaneous nephrostomy (PCN) insertion and hence need to be used cautiously in pregnant women. There has been mortality reported with forgotten stents.[36]

Prostatic Stents[28, 37]

There are two types of prostatic stents: permanent stents and temporary stents.

i. Permanent stents are placed while the patient is under regional anesthesia and take less than 15 minutes; they possess less bleeding tendency; and the patient need not stay in the hospital even for a single day. The drawbacks and risks are increased urination and incontinence, mild discomfort, and/or dislodgement of the stent leading to incontinence and urinary obstruction. At times it is difficult to remove these stents if deemed necessary, and they do not allow scopes for endoscopic surgical options due to their fixed diameter.

ii. Temporary stents can be also placed quickly like the permanent ones, but are unique in that they can be easily removed like a Foley catheter. The drawback is that they do not provide voiding function in patients without a properly functioning bladder and external sphincter. These stents may also cause urinary frequency in some patients during the first 78 hours, and improper stent selection can lead to incontinence or urinary retention.

f) Special Tips for Patient Counseling[38]

A patient on urinary stents should be recommended to drink at least 1.5 to 2 liters of fluid daily to minimize UTI risk. They can be recommended simple painkillers. The urine may be discolored to slightly pinkish due to irritation from the stent leading to bleeding. If the patient has a stent with a thread coming out of urethra, he or she should be advised not to remove it. The stent should be removed at the appropriate time as suggested by the urologist.

Evidence of Effectiveness and Safety

TABLE 10.4

Evidence of Effectiveness and Safety of Urinary Stents

Device	Evidence of effectiveness and safety
Urethral stents	The use of short-term urethral stenting post-operatively in patients with urethral stones lead to an increase in irritative symptoms, dysuria, hematuria, and longer operative times and a decrease in unplanned hospital readmission.[39]
Ureteral stents	The presence of an extraction string offers a safe and effective method for stent removal. This method gives patients the benefits of reduced pain and shortened stent dwelling time without increasing the risk of UTI.[40]
Prostatic stents	The Spanner stent does not offer any significant advantage over previously designed temporary stents. There is no improvement in peak flow rates (PFR) or international prostate symptom score (IPSS) beyond 1–2 weeks after insertion. The stent causes irritation relieved upon stent removal.[41]
DJ stent	A randomized controlled trial compared covered a metallic ureteral stent and a DJ for malignant ureteral obstruction (MUO), and reported that covered metallic ureteral stent may be effective for MUO.[42]

g) Economic Evaluation

A few studies on economic evaluation of urinary stents are mentioned in Table 10.5.

TABLE 10.5

Economic Evaluation of Urinary Stents

Device	Economic evaluation
Urethral stents	Short segment bulbous urethral strictures with primary reconstruction are less costly than treatment with direct vision internal urethrotomy (DVIU). From a fiscal standpoint it is recommended that urethral reconstruction should be considered over DVIU in the majority of clinical circumstances.[43]
Ureteral stents	Study suggests metal stents are well tolerated and cost effective in contrast to polymer ureteral stents in treating urethral obstruction. In patients with ureteral occlusive disease and who are not fit for surgical intervention, a metal resonance stent is more economic and well tolerated.[44] While managing benign upper urinary tract obstruction, metallic ureteral stents provide effective drainage with significant cost-benefit attributable to shorter exchange interval.[45]
Prostatic stents	In high-risk patients with BPH, prostatic stents are a safe and effective option for symptomatic BPH treatment. They are well suited to treating the frail elderly patient unable to withstand surgery.[46]
DJ stent	DJ stenting compared with ureteral catheterization in standard percutaneous nephrolithotomy (PCNL) is found equally as feasible. A lower cost can be a huge relief to the patients in the third world developing country.[47]

H) IMPLICATION TO THE PHARMACY PROFESSION AND PHARMACY PRACTICE

Since these devices are often used by patients during home care, it is important that pharmacists are knowledgeable on handling these devices, identifying device failures, and educating patients on their proper usage. Any patient having indwelling stents should take special care of their device-related education, including use of OTC medications, early identification of device failure, and device migration.

I) CHALLENGES TO PHARMACISTS AND USERS

Forgotten ureteral stents can lead to multiple complications such as hematuria, stent occlusion, stent migration, fragmentation, encrustation, and stone formation. It can also sometimes cause recurrent UTI, urinary tract obstruction, and kidney failure.[48, 49]

J) RECOMMENDATIONS: THE WAY FORWARD

Often patients receive urinary stents on an outpatient basis and use them in home care, so pharmacists should be able to provide first-hand information to patients and educate them on device failure, infections, and timely removal of the stents. Enhancing product knowledge and offering services to patients with stents are the way forward.

K) CONCLUSIONS

Proper handling of stents by patients and timely removal and device maintenance-related information can be offered by pharmacists to their patients.

L) LESSONS LEARNED

- Urinary stent placement is a common practice used in urology, and the stent remains in the patient's body even after she or he leaves the hospital.
- Improper use of the stents can lead to multiple complications; pharmacists can largely help patients in proper device usage.

DEVICE 3: URINARY CATHETERS

BACKGROUND

Catheters are hollow tubes facilitating drainage of fluid from the body. A urinary catheter collects urine from the bladder. Catheter use is recommended in cases in which urinary drainage and measurement is necessary, such as urinary incontinence, urinary retention, prostate surgery, and many other medical conditions like multiple sclerosis and spinal cord injury.[50] Catheters are used while the patients are admitted in the hospital or at times even while the patients receive home care. Catheters are of different sizes, materials (usually made up of silicone), and types (straight or coudé tip). A Foley catheter (indwelling in nature), named after Frederic Foley, the surgeon who first designed it, is common in medical practice. Broadly there are three types of catheters: intermittent self-catheter, indwelling catheters, and condom catheters.[51] [Figure 10.2]

DEVICE DESCRIPTION/IMPORTANT FEATURES[52, 53]

The nature of catheterization depends upon the patient type and the disease condition. Intermittent catheterization involves catheter insertion at regular intervals for a

Foley Catheter

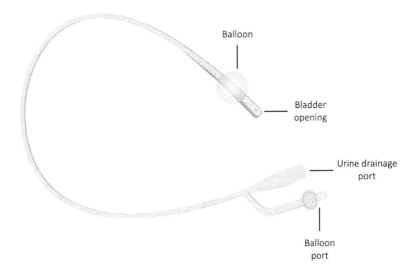

Balloon

Bladder opening

Urine drainage port

Balloon port

FIGURE 10.2   A diagram of a Foley catheter.

Source: www.shutterstock.com/image-vector/foley-catheter-295082864

brief period to empty the bladder. Indwelling catheterization involves catheter insertion in which an inflated balloon places the catheter in the bladder and remains for longer duration. This method is applicable for measuring urine output, incontinence, post-surgery urine output maintenance, and in patients with voiding difficulties due to neurologic disorders.

It is important for a pharmacist to understand the nomenclature of urinary catheters.[54] Catheters are measured in the French scale signifying its girth. For example, 1 "French" or "Fr" is equivalent to 0.33 mm = .013″ = 1/77″ in diameter. The common catheter size in males is 14 Fr (range 14 Fr to 16 Fr) and in females 12 Fr (average 10 Fr to 12 Fr). Catheters are color-coded: black (10 Fr), white (12 Fr), green (14 Fr), orange (16 Fr), and red (18 Fr). The French sizes are not applicable the condom catheters which are measured in mm, depending on the diameter of the condom-shaped receptacle. A description of various types of urinary catheters is provided in Table 10.6.

a) Purpose and How to Use

Catheterization is a common process which involves insertion of the catheter in the urinary tract. The use of specific types of catheters are mentioned in Table 10.7.

b) Important Safety Issues[51,67] (Cautions and Common Adverse Effects)

Though catheterization offers various advantages, they are the leading cause of healthcare-associated UTIs. Other

---

TABLE 10.6
Descriptions of Urinary Catheters

Device	Description
Foley Catheter 2-Way Adult Foley Catheter 2-Way Child Foley Catheter 3-Way Foley Catheter Silicone 2-Way Adult Foley Catheter Silicone 2-Way Child Foley Catheter Silicone 3-Way Adult	Foley catheters are placed in the bladder via the urethra with a balloon at the bladder end, and the catheter tube is connected at the external end to a bag for drain collection, available in many sizes and made up of variety of materials.[55,56] The terms 2-way and 3-way signify the number of lumens present in the catheter. For example, 3-way consists of a lumen for inflating the balloon, a lumen for urine drainage, and another lumen for irrigation. The 2-way has everything except the lumen for irrigation.
Nephrostomy catheter	This is used to relive blockage in urinary system facilitating urine drainage into a bag outside the body directly from the kidney. In some cases, it may also drain into bladder.[57]
Suprapubic catheter	This is a hollow flexible tube used to drain urine directly from the bladder; it is inserted through a cut in the lower abdomen below the navel area under anesthesia.[58]
Cytometry catheter	This is helpful in diagnosing problems related to urine control such as incontinence, difficulty emptying the bladder, overactive bladder, obstructions, or frequent infections.[59]
Condom catheter	Used in men for short-term incontinence, this has a flexible sheath that fits over the penis just like a condom that rolls onto and attachesto the penis by a double-sided adhesive, a jockey-type strap, or a foam strap.[60]

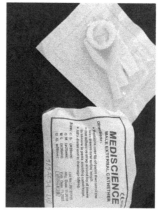

Figure 10.3 A condom catheter and manufacturer instructions.
Source: www.shutterstock.com/image-photo/
melakamalaysia-june-182019-condom-catheter-plastic-1427009801

Nelaton catheter	This has one hole at the side of the tip and a connector at the other end for drainage; used for intermittent catheterization.[61]
Ureteral stent	This is used to drain urine from the kidney to the bladder in occasions such as kidney stone treatment.[62,63,64]

TABLE 10.7
Catheterization Procedures

Foley Catheter 2 Way-Adult Foley Catheter 2 Way-Child Foley Catheter 3-Way Foley Catheter Silicone 2-Way Adult Foley Catheter Silicone 2-Way Child Foley Catheter Silicone 3-Way Adult	The purpose is to drain urine from the bladder. The catheter is inserted into the bladder and left for period of time (indwelling catheter).[55] Catheter lubricated with a water-soluble jelly is inserted through the urethra until it reaches the bladder. Once the catheter is passed, the balloon placed in the bladder is then slowly inflated with about 10 cc of water using a syringe. Inflating the balloon is usually not a painful process.[56,50] More details about Foley catheterization are available here.[65]
Cytometry catheter	These measure the amount of urine that can be held by the bladder. It also measures pressure inside the bladder, and how full it is upon the urge to go.[59]
Condom catheter	A condom catheter is an option as a bladder containment strategy for men who have problems with urinary incontinence. In the case of upper motor neuron deficits, there may be episodes of urinary incontinence that can be managed with this technique. In the case of lower motor neuron deficits, the condom catheter may be part of the long-term strategy to contain urine.[66]

safety concerns are pain and burning in genital area and low back, leaking of urine, latex allergy, renal stones, and physician damage to urinary tract due to catheter insertion.

c) Storage Conditions and Maintenance

Catheters should be protected from direct sunlight. Coated catheters are packaged in opaque packing materials to protect from direct sunlight. The package insert should be read for the expiry dates and any catheters after expiry should not be used. Catheters and drainage bags should be disposed after thorough rinsing with soapy water and placed in a plastic bag for disposal.[68]

d) Special Tips for Patient Counseling

Counseling for a catheterized patient should be focused on catheter replacement and uninterrupted supplies, spotting signs of potential problems, seeking timely medical advice, prevention of infections, etc. Patients should be told to live a relatively normal life with a urinary catheter. The ways of concealing the collection bag under clothes should be discussed, and patients can be encouraged to carry out most everyday activities.[69]

e) Evidence of Effectiveness and Safety

The ESCALE trial does not advocate the regular use of an indwelling catheter because it possesses the challenges of long-term use of urinary catheter in UTIs, which requires further investigation.[70]

f) Economic Evaluation

A probabilistic modeling study in UK hospitals found that catheter prevention offers substantial health-economic gains, but community-oriented interventions are needed to target the large burden imposed by community-onset infection.[71] Another study found hydrophilic-coated catheters are more economical than uncoated ones.[72]

g) Implication to the Pharmacy Profession and Pharmacy Practice

A thorough knowledge of catheterization and urostomy products is needed for pharmacists due to the surge in the number of patients using catheterizations. Community pharmacists should be familiar with individual patients' reasons for catheterization and urostomy, and should possess knowledge of the types of catheterizations, available catheters, and handling of the urostomy bag.[73] There is a substantial opportunity and scope for community pharmacists to offer these services as an extended service.

h) Challenges to Pharmacists and Users

UTI (both upper and lower) is the main challenge associated with catheterizations. The duration a catheter remains in the body influences the risk of infection. A considerable amount of UTI can be minimized through proper catheter insertion, maintenance, and use for the shortest duration possible. At times catheterization is also associated with bladder spasms (similar to stomach cramps), leakages, blockages, and damage to the urethra.[74]

i) Recommendations: The Way Forward

The pharmacists should be knowledgeable of catheter use and should be in a position to explain this knowledge patients. Pharmacists should also possess skills related to catheterization and urostomy.

j) Conclusions

Widespread increase in use of catheters on an outpatient basis gives an opportunity for pharmacists to sell these devices, educate patients, and provide catheter care as a part of extended community pharmacy service. The pharmacy curricula must focus on these aspects and there should be training programs to enhance these skills in the practicing pharmacists.

k) Lessons Learned

- Urinary catheters are of different types and their use is increasing day by day.
- Pharmacists must be proficient in recommending selection of catheters.
- Pharmacists must be knowledgeable about urostomy and should know how to change urobags as an extended community pharmacy service.

DEVICE 4: MISCELLANEOUS

BACKGROUND

In this section authors discuss two urology-related devices, the urine collection bag and urine flow meters. Other urology-related products such as the transurethral resection (TUR) set, transurethral resection of the prostate (TURP) drape, TURP loop, nephrostomy tube, urology guidewires, diamond-tip needle, Chiba needle, fascial dilator set, or disposable trocars are not discussed in detail. Readers are recommended to refer to product manuals for more information on these products.

a. Device Description/Important Features

i. Urine Collection Bag

A urine collection bag, also called night drainage bag, is a specially designed device enabling collection of urine while the patient is in bed, and in a few cases while the person is moving (Figure 10.4). Normally, for adults the bags are of two-liter capacity. They are provided with an efficient non-return valve with top outlet.[75,76] Urine collection bags are available in different sizes (pediatric and adult) and shapes, and are chosen based on patient requirements and preferences. The commonly used urine collection bags are urostomy bags, Malecote drainage sets, urinary drainage bags, leg side urobags, Uro Bag Pant Systems, etc. Uro Bag Pant Systems are specially designed urine collection bags with no external appearance, offering comfort for the patients. A detailed description of the Uro Bag Pant System is available here in this link.[77]

ii. Urine Flow Meter

A urine flow meter is used to measure the flow of urine. It enables tracking of speed of urine flow, urine quantity, and time taken for a specific quantity. This device is used in performing diagnostic tests to assess the urinary tract. The test is recommended by the urologist/physician based on the requirement of individual patients.[78] There are both electronic and manual flow meters available in pharmacies.

b. Purpose/How to Use

i. Urine Collection Bag

Urine collection enable urine collection from the bladder via a catheter or sheath. The collection bag is attached to the external end, enabling the collection of urine from bladder. The bag is connected to the catheter by pushing the tapered end of the collection bag tube firmly into the funnel end of the catheter. The bag volume for adults is normally two liters and once the bag is half to three quarters filled (2 to 3 hours) the patient/patient attendant should empty it. The night bag is suitable for use for about 5–7 days and the urobag pant system about one month.

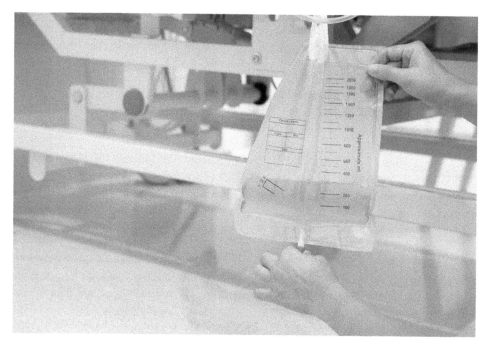

FIGURE 10.4 A urine collection bag as commonly used in hospitals.

Source: www.shutterstock.com/image-photo/hand-holding-urine-pee-catheter-bag-794468998

ii. Urine Flow Meter

As mentioned under the device description, this device is recommended if someone has slow urination, weak urine stream, or difficulty urinating; or to test the urinary sphincter muscle. Measuring the urine flow rates (average versus maximum) can be used to assess the severity of any blockage or obstruction. [79, 80]

More details on urine flowmetry, the recommendations, guidelines on flowmetry, etc., are available here.[81]

c. Special Tips for Patient Counseling

i. Urobag

Since the patients with urobags often received home care, there is a considerable role for the pharmacists to counsel the patients. The counseling is targeted at choosing the right device, using it, and care during use of the device. A brief overview of pharmacists counseling for a patient with Uro Bag Pant System is provided here:

> Step I: The patient should practice proper hand washing techniques while caring for the catheter or collection bag, and should secure the bag properly.
>
> Step II. The leg band should be positioned on the thigh properly as mentioned in the product insert.
>
> Step III: The catheter tubing should be placed over the bag and secured. For every 4 to 6 hours, the bag should be repositioned to prevent pressure from the elastic on leg. This can be done by changing the bag to another leg.
>
> Step IV: The band should be washed as often as needed. Hands should be washed and the leg band dried.[80]

d. Implication to the Pharmacy Profession and Pharmacy Practice

The urine collection bags and urine flow meters are used by patients both in the hospital and in home care. Improper use of the urine collection bags can lead to embarrassment for the patient, urine leakage, and infections. While the nurse handles use of these devices in the hospitals, the pharmacists have a significant responsibility in offering these services as an extended community pharmacy service.

e. Recommendations: The Way Forward

There is a large scope for pharmacists in assisting patients with device choice and caring for them while on home care. Considering the increase in use of urine collection bags, pharmacists must seize the growing opportunity in home care of patients using this device. Pharmacists must be trained in aseptic handling of the urine collection bags and should be offered these skills even in pharmacy education.

e. Conclusions

These devices are largely used by patients on home care and community pharmacists have a significant role to play. Caring for patients with urine collection bags can be a valuable extended service offered by the community pharmacists.

f. Lessons Learned

- Pharmacists can play an important role in serving home care patients with urine collection bags as an extended service.
- Pharmacists can also help patients with urine flowmetry.
- Caring for patients with urine collection bags can enhance patients' quality of life and can bring pharmacists closer to their patients.

ACKNOWLEDGEMENTS

The authors would like to acknowledge Dr. Nirmal Lamichhane, MCh (Urology), Senior Consultant at Department of Surgical Oncology, B.P. Koirala Memorial Cancer Hospital, Bharatpur, Nepal, for reviewing the draft version of the chapter and suggesting modifications. Special thanks to Dr. Gani Alam, Senior Resident, Department of Surgery, Western Regional Hospital, Pokhara Academic Health and Sciences, Pokhara, Nepal, for his views and contribution. Mr. Bimal Lamichhane, the Medicine Retailer and Surgical Goods Supplier at Bimal Pharmacy, Bharatpur, Chitwan, Nepal, is deeply acknowledged for providing the authors with the list of urology devices available on the market.

REFERENCES

1. Mayo Clinic. Penile implants. Available from: www.mayoclinic.org/tests-procedures/penile-implants/about/pac-20384916 (accessed 30 Dec 2020).

2. Department of Urology, University of Washington. Penile prosthesis. Available from: www.washington.edu/urology/penile-prosthesis/ (accessed 30 Dec 2020).

3. What you need to know about penile prosthesis: the penile implant. Available from: www.youtube.com/watch?v=uJOzPNCsp0M.

4. Health Management.org. Available from: https://healthmanagement.org/products/view/vesical-sphincter-prosthesis-for-urinary-incontinence-zsi-375-zephyr-surgical-implants (accessed 30 Dec 2020).

5. Urology Service, University of Utah. Available from: https://healthcare.utah.edu/urology/conditions/incontinence/artificial-urinary-sphincter.php (accessed 30 Dec 2020).

6. González R, Piaggio L. Chapter 59—artificial urinary sphincter. In: Gearhart JP, Rink RC, Mouriquand PDE, editors. Paediatric urology, 2nd edn. W.B. Saunders; 2010. p. 775–82. ISBN 9781416032045. https://doi.org/10.1016/B978-1-4160-3204-5.00059-1.

7. www.medicalexpo.com/prod/ami-agency-medical-innovations/product-110269-952133.html.

8. How penile implants work. Available from: www.youtube.com/watch?v=6JPB2K2wGgg.

9. Brant WO, Martins FE. Artificial urinary sphincter. Transl Androl Urol. 2017;6(4):682–94. https://doi.org/10.21037/tau.2017.07.31.

10. Dr Paulo. FAQ. Available from: www.drpaulo.com.br/en/faq/penile-prosthesis-implantation (accessed 30 Dec 2020).

11. Kuyava CC. Penile prosthesis devices and methods. Available from: https://patents.google.com/patent/US7407482B2/en (accessed 30 Dec 2020).

12. Wintner A, Lentz AC. Inflatable penile prosthesis: considerations in revision surgery. Curr Urol Rep. 2019 Mar 20;20(4):18. https://doi.org/10.1007/s11934-019-0881-9. PMID: 30895471.

13. Drugs.com. Urinary sphincter replacement. Available from: www.drugs.com/cg/urinary-sphincter-replacement-discharge-care.html (accessed 20 Dec 2020).

14. Memorial Sloan Kettering Cancer Center. About your artificial urinary sphincter. Available from: www.mskcc.org/cancer-care/patient-education/artificial-urinary-sphincter (accessed 30 Dec 2020).

15. Blewniewski M, Ostrowski I, Pottek T, et al. Safety and efficacy outcomes of ZSI 475 penile prosthesis. Urologia. 2017 Apr–Jun;84(2):98–101. https://doi.org/10.5301/uj.5000240. PMID: 28430342; PMCID: PMC6154831.

16. Goldstein I, Newman L, Baum N, et al. Safety and efficacy outcome of mentor alpha-1 inflatable penile prosthesis implantation for impotence treatment. J Urol. 1997 Mar;157(3):833–9. PMID: 9072580.

17. WebMD. Erectile dysfunction: penile prosthesis. Available from: www.webmd.com/erectile-dysfunction/guide/penile-prosthesis#1 (accessed 30 Dec 2020).

18. Tutolo M, Cornu JN, Bauer RM, et al. Efficacy and safety of artificial urinary sphincter (AUS): results of a large multi-institutional cohort of patients with mid-term follow-up. Neurourol Urodyn. 2019 Feb;38(2):710–18. https://doi.org/10.1002/nau.23901. Epub 2018 Dec 21. PMID: 30575997.

19. Rezaee ME, Ward CE, Brandes ER, et al. A review of economic evaluations of erectile dysfunction therapies. Sex Med Rev. 2020 Jul;8(3):497–503. https://doi.org/10.1016/j.sxmr.2019.06.001. Epub 2019 Jul 17. PMID: 31326359.

20. Tan HL. Economic cost of male erectile dysfunction using a decision analytic model: for a hypothetical managed-care plan of 100,000 members. Pharmacoeconomics. 2000 Jan;17(1):77–107. https://doi.org/10.2165/00019053-200017010-00006. PMID: 10747767.

21. Narang GL, Figler BD, Coward RM. Preoperative counseling and expectation management for inflatable penile prosthesis implantation. Transl Androl Urol. 2017 Nov;6(Suppl 5):S869–S880. https://doi.org/10.21037/tau.2017.07.04. PMID: 29238666; PMCID: PMC5715186.

22. PharmaChoice. Urinary incontinence. Available from: www.pharmachoice.com/urinary-incontinence/ (accessed 30 Dec 2020).

23. Bettocchi C, Palumbo F, Spilotros M, et al. Penile prostheses. Ther Adv Urol. 2010 Feb;2(1):35–40. https://doi.org/10.1177/1756287209359174. PMID: 21789081; PMCID: PMC3126066.

24. MedlinePlus. Stent. Available from: https://medlineplus.gov/ency/article/002303.htm#:~:text=A%20stent%20is%20a%20tiny,stent%20holds%20the%20structure%20open (accessed 29 Dec 2020).

25. Urology, San Antonio. Ureteral stents: what you need to know. Available from: www.urologysanantonio.com/ureteral-stents#:~:text=Ureteral%20stents%20are%20

26. Duvdevani M, Chew BH, Denstedt JD. Urethral stents: review of technology and clinical applications. In: Baba S, Ono Y, editors. Interventional management of urological diseases, Recent advances in endourology, Vol. 8. Tokyo: Springer Japan; 2006. p. 191–206.

27. Kidney Stone Clinic. Ureteric stent information double J stent. Available from: www.kidneystoneclinic.com.au/urinary-tract-double-j.html (accessed 29 Dec 2020).

28. Europian Association of Urology. Prostate stent. Available from: https://patients.uroweb.org/treatments/prostate-stent/ (accessed 29 Dec 2020).

29. Drugs.com. Urethral stent placement. Available from: www.drugs.com/cg/urethral-stent-placement.html (accessed 29 Dec 2020).

30. Ureteral stent placement: PreO® patient education & engagement. Available from: www.youtube.com/watch?v=qKCpUf8KKv4.

31. Scotland KB, Lo J, Grgic T, et al. Ureteral stent-associated infection and sepsis: pathogenesis and prevention: a review. Biofouling. 2019 Jan;35(1):117–27. https://doi.org/10.1080/08927014.2018.1562549. Epub 2019 Feb 8. PMID: 30732463.

32. Geavlete P, Mulţescu R, Niţă G et al. Urethral stents. In: Geavlete PA. Endoscopic diagnosis and treatment in urethral pathology. Amsterdam: Academic Press; 2016. p. 65–88. ISBN 9780128024065. https://doi.org/10.1016/B978-0-12-802406-5.00003-3.

33. Turney B. Ureteric stent information for patients. Oxford University Hospitals, NHS Foundation Trust. Available from: www.ouh.nhs.uk/patient-guide/leaflets/files/13562Pureteric.pdf (accessed 29 Dec 2020).

34. Sener TE. Is urethral catheter necessary after ureteroscopy and DJ stent placement? Available from: https://clinicaltrials.gov/ct2/show/NCT03713411 (accessed 29 Dec 2020).

35. El-Faqih SR, Shamsuddin AB, Chakrabarti A, et al. Polyurethane internal ureteral stents in treatment of stone patients: morbidity related to indwelling times. J Urol. 1991;146:1487–91.

36. Arora S, Rajesh A. Urology for nephrologists. In: Jha PK, Kher V, editors. Manual of nephrology. New Delhi: Jaypee Brothers Medical Publishers (P) Ltd; 2016. p. 249–64. Available from: www.jaypeedigital.com/book/9789352501625/chapter/ch11.

37. https://en.wikipedia.org/wiki/Prostatic_stent.

38. Fairview Patient Education. Having ureteral stent. Available from: www.fairview.org/patient-education/83047 (accessed 28 Dec 2020).

39. Reynen E, Picheca L. Ureteral stents: a review of clinical effectiveness and guidelines. Ottawa: CADTH; 2017 Mar. (CADTH rapid response report: summary with critical appraisal).

40. Luo Z, Jiao B, Zhao H, Huang T, Geng L, Zhang G. The efficacy and safety of ureteric stent removal with strings versus no strings: which is better? BioMed Res Int. 2020:10. https://doi.org/10.1155/2020/4081409. Article ID 4081409.

41. McKenzie P, Badlani G. Critical appraisal of the Spanner™ prostatic stent in the treatment of prostatic obstruction. Med Devices (Auckl). 2011;4:27–33. https://doi.org/10.2147/MDER.S7107. Epub 2011 Feb 9. PMID: 22915927; PMCID: PMC3417871.

42. Kim JW, Hong B, Shin JH, et al. A prospective randomized comparison of a covered metallic ureteral stent and a double-J stent for malignant ureteral obstruction. Korean J Radiol. 2018 Jul–Aug;19(4):606–12. https://doi.org/10.3348/kjr.2018.19.4.606.

43. Rourke KF, Jordan GH. Primary urethral reconstruction: the cost minimized approach to the bulbous urethral stricture. J Urol. 2005 Apr;173(4):1206–10. https://doi.org/10.1097/01.ju.0000154971.05286.81. PMID: 15758749.

44. Taylor ER, Benson AD, Schwartz BF. Cost analysis of metallic ureteral stents with 12 months of follow-up. J Endourol. 2012 Jul;26(7):917–21. https://doi.org/10.1089/end.2011.0481. Epub 2012 Apr 17. PMID: 22360415.

45. López-Huertas HL, Polcari AJ, Acosta-Miranda A, et al. Metallic ureteral stents: a cost-effective method of managing benign upper tract obstruction. J Endourol. 2010 Mar;24(3):483–5. https://doi.org/10.1089/end.2009.0192. PMID: 20210650.

46. Lam JS, Volpe MA, Kaplan SA. Use of prostatic stents for the treatment of benign prostatic hyperplasia in high-risk patients. Curr Urol Rep. 2001;2:277–84. https://doi.org/10.1007/s11934-001-0064-2.

47. Joshi R, Sharma AS, Dongol U, et al. Double J stenting compared with ureteral catheterization in percutaneous nephrolithotomy. JKMC [Internet]. 9 Oct 2014 [cited 23 Dec.2020];3(2):63–7. Available from: www.nepjol.info/index.php/JKMC/article/view/11228.

48. El-Faqih SR, Shamsuddin AB, Chakrabarti A, et al. Polyurethane internal ureteral stents in treatment of stone patients: morbidity related to indwelling times. J Urol. 1991;146(6):1487–91.

49. Mohan-Pillai K, Keeley JR FX, Moussa SA, et al. Endourological management of severely encrusted ureteral stents. J Endourol. 1999 Jun;13(5):377–9.

50. MedlinePlus. Urinary catheters. Available from: https://medlineplus.gov/ency/article/003981.htm (accessed 30 Dec 2020).

51. Cafasso J. Urinary catheters. Healthline. 2018 Sept 29. Available from: www.healthline.com/health/urinary-catheters#types (accessed Sept 2020).

52. Herter R, Kazer MW. Best practices in urinary catheter care. Home Healthc Nurse. 2010;28:342–9.

53. Robinson J. Urinary catheterisation: assessing the best options for patients. Nurs Stand. 2009;23:40–5.

54. Compact Cath. Urinary catheter types and sizes. Available from: www.compactcath.com/blog/catheter-types-and-sizes/ (accessed 29 Dec 2020).

55. Veluswamy AT. What is foley catheter used for ? Emedicine. 2020 Aug 10. Available from: www.emedicinehealth.com/foley_catheter/article_em.htm (accessed 29 Dec 2020).

56. Drugs.com. Foley catheter placement and care. Available from: www.drugs.com/cg/foley-catheter-placement-and-care.html (accessed 29 Dec 2020).

57. Memorial Sloan Kettering Cancer Center. About your nephrostomy catheter. Available from: www.mskcc.org/cancer-care/patient-education/caring-your-nephrostomy-catheter (accessed 29 Dec 2020).

58. Bladder and Bowel community. Suprapubic catheter. Available from: www.bladderandbowel.org/surgical-treatment/suprapubic-catheter/ (accessed 29 Dec 2020).

59. Urology care foundation. What is a cystometry/cystometrogram (CGM). Available from: www.urologyhealth.org/urology-a-z/c/cystometry (accessed 29 Dec 2020).

60. Healthtalk.org. Living with a urinary catheter. Available from: https://healthtalk.org/living-urinary-catheter/condom-catheters (accessed 29 Dec 2020).

61. Smart Medical Byers. Urethral and nelaton catheter. Available from: www.smartmedicalbuyer.com/collections/urethral-and-nelaton-catheter (accessed 29 Dec 2020).

62. Shlamovitz GZ. Urethral catheterization in men. Emedicine. 2016 Jan 7. Available from: https://emedicine.medscape.com/article/80716-overview (accessed 29 Dec 2020).

63. Lo J, Lange D, Chew BH. Ureteral stents and foley catheters-associated urinary tract infections: the role of coatings and materials in infection prevention. Antibiotics (Basel). 2014 Mar 10;3(1):87–97. https://doi.org/10.3390/antibiotics3010087. PMID: 27025736; PMCID: PMC4790349.

64. UrologyPlace. Coding for ureteral catheters and stents. Available from: https://community.auanet.org/blogs/policy-brief/2018/06/05/coding-for-ureteral-catheters-and-stents (accessed 29 Dec 2020).

65. Urinary catheterization. Available from: www.youtube.com/watch?v=3yYj2a4DjiA.

66. Alverzo JP, Rosenberg JH, Sorensen CA, et al. Chapter three—nursing care and education for patients with spinal cord injury. In: Sisto SA, Druin E, Sliwinski MM, editors. Spinal cord injuries. Mosby; 2009. p. 37–68. ISBN 9780323006996. https://doi.org/10.1016/B978-032300699-6.10003-6.

67. van den Broek PJ, Wille JC, van Benthem BH, et al. Urethral catheters: can we reduce use?. BMC Urol. 2011;11:10. https://doi.org/10.1186/1471-2490-11-10.

68. Continence Product Adviser. Storage and disposal. Available from: www.continenceproductadvisor.org/storageanddisposal#:~:text=Catheters%20should%20not%20be%20stored,or%20two!)%20for%20disposal (accessed 27 Dec 2020).

69. Everest Pharmacy. Urinary catheterisation. Available from: www.everestpharmacy.co.uk/condition/urinary-catheterisation/ (accessed 27 Dec 2020).

70. Bonfill X, Rigau D, Esteban-Fuertes M, et al. Efficacy and safety of urinary catheters with silver alloy coating in patients with spinal cord injury: a multicentric pragmatic randomized controlled trial. The ESCALE trial. Spine J. 2017 Nov;17(11):1650–7. https://doi.org/10.1016/j.spinee.2017.05.025. Epub 2017 May 31. PMID: 28578163.

71. Smith DRM, Pouwels KB, Hopkins S, et al. Epidemiology and health-economic burden of urinary-catheter-associated infection in English NHS hospitals: a probabilistic modelling study. J Hosp Infect. 2019 Sep;103(1):44–54. https://doi.org/10.1016/j.jhin.2019.04.010. Epub 2019 Apr 30. PMID: 31047934.

72. Rognoni C, Tarricone R. Healthcare resource consumption for intermittent urinary catheterisation: costeffectiveness of hydrophilic catheters and budget impact analyses. BMJ Open. 2017;7:e012360. https://doi.org/10.1136/bmjopen-2016-012360.

73. Fletcher L. Catheterization and urostomy for the community pharmacist. US Pharm. 2013;8(38):27–30. Available from: www.uspharmacist.com/article/catheterization-and-urostomy-for-the-community-pharmacist-42387

74. Pharmacy Care Plus. Cather. Available from: www. pharmacycareplus.co.uk/pages/health_advice_184063-action=condition&condition=urinary-catheterization& article=Introduction.cfm; www.uspharmacist.com/article/catheterization-and-urostomy-for-the-community-pharmacist-42387 (accessed 27 Dec 2020).

75. MedlinePlus. Urine drainage bags. Available from: https://medlineplus.gov/ency/patientinstructions/000142.htm (accessed 27 Dec 2020).

76. Healthklin. Urine collection bag. Available from: www. healthklin.com/Romsons-UroBag-Urine-Collecting-Bag (accessed 27 Dec 2020).

77. Uro Bag Pant System. Available from: www.youtube.com/watch?v=rpWfXBtxZ78.

78. Urology care foundation. What is uroflometry? Available from: www.urologyhealth.org/urology-a-z/u/uroflowmetry #:~:text=Uroflowmetry%20measures%20the%20flow%20 of,or%20have%20a%20slow%20stream (accessed 27 Dec 2020).

79. Healthline. Preparing for a uroflow test. Available from: www.healthline.com/health/uroflowmetry#preparation (accessed 27 Dec 2020).

80. SecuriCare. Changing urostomy pouches. Available from: www.securicaremedical.co.uk/advice-and-support/stoma-care/how-to-change-your-stoma-pouch/changing-urostomy-pouches (accessed 27 Dec 2020).

81. International Continence Society 41st Annual Meeting Glasgow 2011. Available from: www.ics.org/Workshops/HandoutFiles/000169.pdf.

11 Medical Devices for Diabetes and Endocrine Disorders

Amir Babiker and Mohammed Aldubayee

CONTENTS

DOI: 10.1201/9781003002345-13

DIABETES

Diabetes still imposes a massive burden on health, the economy, and patients' quality of life as a leading cause of morbidity, including renal failure, ischemic heart disease, lower-limb amputations, and psychosocial comorbidity. Optimizing glycemic control with insulin, especially in type 1 diabetes, can significantly decrease any related microvascular complications.[1] Currently, millions of patients require insulin therapy to manage their diabetes, including patients with type 2 diabetes. This is expected to rise even more with the increasing prevalence of T2D due to several factors.[2] However, advanced technology in the management of diabetes has influenced the outcome significantly.[3–5] This includes familiarity of patients and/or healthcare provider with the devices that are used in the treatment of diabetes and blood glucose monitoring:

1. Insulin delivery devices
2. Glucose monitoring system

1.0   INSULIN DELIVERY DEVICES

Insulin continues to be the mainstay of treatment in most types of diabetes. Thus, a careful selection of insulin delivery device is essential to ensure patient's and health provider's satisfaction.[2] Manual and automatic devices are used for insulin delivery in patients with T1D, and are now increasingly used in T2D with the guidance of the treating physician, as well as in some subtypes of maturity onset diabetes in the young (MODY).[5,6]

Insulin delivery devices are of two types:

Manual:

1.1 Insulin pen: durable (reusable) and dispensable (prefilled) (Table 11.1).
1.2 Insulin port device.

Automated:

1.3 Continuous subcutaneous insulin infusion in an open-loop system (different types of pumps).
1.4 Closed-loop system (artificial pancreas).

TABLE 11.1
Prefilled, Disposable Insulin Pens

Device	Insulin contained in the device (trade name)	Insulin chemical name, manufacturer	Insulin concentration	Dose delivery and increment	References
FlexTouch®					15–18
	Levemir®	Insulin detemir, Novo Nordisk	Contains 300 units of insulin (100 U/mL)	Delivers 1 to 80 units in 1-unit increments	
	Tresiba®U100	Insulin degludec, Novo Nordisk			
	Ryzodeg®	Insulin degludec/insulin aspart, Novo Nordisk			
	Tresiba® U200	Insulin degludec, Novo Nordisk	Contains 600 units of insulin (200 U/mL)	Delivers 2 to 160 units in 2-unit increments	
FlexPen®					19–24
	NovoRapid®	Insulin aspart, Novo Nordisk	Contains 300 units of insulin (100 U/mL)	Delivers 1 to 60 units in 1-unit increments	
	NovoMix® 30	70% Insulin aspart protamine and 30% insulin aspart, Novo Nordisk			

Device	Insulin contained in the device (trade name)	Insulin chemical name, manufacturer	Insulin concentration	Dose delivery and increment	References
SoloSTAR®					25–27
	Lantus®	Insulin glargine injection, Sanofi US	Contains 300 units of insulin (100 U/mL)	Delivers 1 to 80 units in 1-unit increments	
	Apidra®	Insulin glulisine, Sanofi US			
	Toujeo®	Insulin glargine injection, U-300, Sanofi US	Contains 450 units of insulin (300 U/mL)	Delivers 1–80 units in 1-unit increments	
KwikPen™					28–35
	Humalog®	Insulin lispro injection, Eli Lilly and Company	Contains 300 units of insulin (100 U/mL)	Delivers 1 to 60 units in 1-unit increments	
	Humalog® Mix 50/50™	(50% insulin lispro protamine suspension and 50% insulin lispro injection), Eli Lilly and Company			
	Humalog® Mix 75/25™	(75% insulin lispro protamine suspension and 25% insulin lispro injection), Eli Lilly and Company			
	Humulin® N	Human insulin isophane suspension, Eli Lilly and Company			
	Humulin® 70/30	(70% human insulin isophane suspension 30% human insulin injection), Eli Lilly and Company			
	Basaglar® KwikPen®	Insulin glargine injection	Contains 300 units of insulin (100 U/mL)	Deliver 1 to 80 units in 1-unit increments	
	Humalog® U200	Insulin lispro injection, Eli Lilly and Company	Contains 600 units of insulin (200 U/mL)	Delivers 1 to 60 units in 1-unit increments	
	Humulin R U500	Insulin human injection, Eli Lilly and Company	Contains 1500 units of insulin (500U/mL)	Delivers 5 to 300 units in 5- unit increments	

1.1 INSULIN PENS

Evidence

The insulin pen device is intended to provide a simple and less painful means of insulin administration and is a substitute to the conventional insulin vial/syringe. It is, therefore, associated with greater patient preference that leads to improved glycemic control.[5] However, understanding the different types and advantages of these pens and the pharmacodynamic properties of their insulin content is of great benefit to physicians and helps them to decide on the best option for a given patient's needs.

The conventional insulin vial/syringe is still the preferable method in developing countries with limited resources and also preferred by some patients in the US relative to Europe and Canada; however, diabetes management teams encourage routine use of pens because of their superiority in several aspects.[7,8] Studies have shown that insulin pens are less painful, simpler, and more practical to use, aiming to improve glycemic control by resolving barriers of insulin administration.[7,8] Moreover, increased medication adherence was observed within the users of insulin pens.[9,10] All devices have limitations and disadvantages and of course insulin pens are no exception. Nevertheless, because of its convenience and patient preference, healthcare providers should encourage the use of insulin pens over the traditional vial/syringe technique.

Characteristics of Pens and Patient Use

Although most patients are accustomed to vials and syringes, the potential for error remains high, particularly among elderly patients.[10] Previous investigations on insulin accuracy have found that both types of devices are inaccurate. Patients who use syringes appear to be overdosed, while patients who use pen injectors are consistently underdosed, when measuring minimal doses such as one insulin unit (100 units/mL); however, pens are more precise with larger volumes than syringes.[11–13] Pens come with brochures that save time for patients who have never used insulin before and would like to know about the different devices available. Knowing the proper device for a given patient can make a difference in clinical outcomes. There are syringes of different sizes such as 3/10 cc, ½ cc, and 1 cc syringes, as well as needles in various lengths of 28–31 gauge and these should be tailored to the patient's needs including accuracy of dose calculation.[14] For instance, using a 3/10 cc

syringe for a patient who needs 13 units of insulin ensures more accurate dose measurement of over 60% in the calculation of doses.[14] Pen devices offer patients accuracy and convenience, and because they are less painful and socially acceptable, pen devices also offer flexibility of where to use them. Different pens are available to use and pharmaceutical companies strive to meet patients' needs in producing flexible and effective insulin pens (Table 11.1)(Figure 11.1).

There are different types of pens, such as FlexPens which are used to deliver NovoRapid, a rapid-acting insulin; NovoMix 30, a biphasic (rapid and intermediate-acting) insulin; and Detemir (Levemir), a relatively peakless long-acting insulin.[15–23] Each disposable pen contains 300 units, comes in a 5-pen kit, and uses needles from (Novo or BD) pharmaceutical companies. After first use, these pens can be stored at room temperature for 30–35 days.[15–18]

Insulin glargine (Lantus), by Sanofi, comes in Solostar pens and refillables. The Solostar offers a 5-disposal pen kit, each containing 300 units.[24–27] Each pen lasts for 30 days after being opened, which is ideal for patients that use low doses. Another type is the OptiClik pen, which has a unique cartridge with a built-in plunger screw.[24–27]

Moreover, Eli Lilly produces "Turbo" pen to deliver Humulin N and R, as well as Humalog, Humalog 75/25, and Humalog 50/50.[28–35] Some devices come with additional features to support patients with particular needs such as those who tend to forget and might double the dose. HumaPen Memoir, for instance, is a device that requires a 3 ml Humalog cartridge and features a digital read out that can store the time and date of the last 16 doses.[28–35] HumaPen Luxura requires the same 300 u cartridge and delivers an accurate ½ units of insulin (cartridges come in a set of 5 of 300 u each) for kids who need lower insulin doses. The disposable version is KwikPen, which is also available in Humalog, Humalog 75/25, and Humalog 50/50; and its features have improved over the "Turbo" pen (Table 11.1).[28–35] KwikPen, in packs of 5 pens each containing 300 units, has a short throw distance and is easier to read out. Each KwikPen is good after the first use for at least 30 days without refrigeration.[31–35]

More recently, insulin biosimilars, such as Basaglar, a long-acting insulin equivalent to glargine insulin, have become available, aiming to reduce the cost of production and selling of previously known types of insulin with the same level of efficacy.[28–35]

Pen needles are required in order to use insulin pens and the selection of needles vary as well.[14] BD and Novo are the two most popular brands, but others are also available. BD Ultra-Fine needles are available in three sizes:

- 5 mm and 31 gauge Mini Pen Needle
- 8 mm and 31 gauge Short Pen Needle
- 12.7 mm and 29 gauge Original Pen Needle

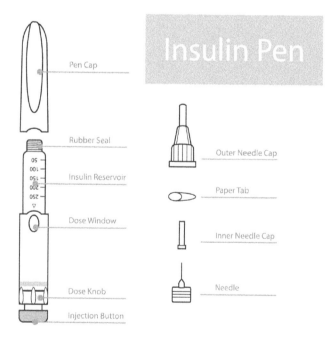

FIGURE 11.1 Parts of durable (reusable) insulin pen.

Source: www.shutterstock.com/image-vector/diabetic-insulin-pen-parts-549081298 www.shutterstock.com/image-vector/insulin-pen-icon-isometric-illustration-vector-742419007

NovoFine Disposable Pen Needles comes in two sizes:

- 31 gauge x6 mm
- 30 gauge x8 mm

The adipose tissue's thickness and density determines the most appropriate needle length and diameter for patients.

1.2 INFUSION PORTS

Patients with diabetes who need insulin injections more than 4–6 times a day often experience discomfort and bruising as a result of frequent sticking. In such patients, an insulin port (I-Port) device is suitable to use (Figure 11.2). I-Port is inserted into the skin every three days and insulin is administered through the port with a pen/syringe.[36] With the help of I-Port, the number of required shots per day is not a source of concern for the patient.

1.3 CONTINUOUS SUBCUTANEOUS INSULIN INFUSION (CSII) OR INSULIN PUMPS

Evidence

Due to different factors that lead to difficulties in interpreting clinical trials of CSII, uncertainties remained about the superiority of the effectiveness of CSII versus multi-dose injections (MDI). These factors include suboptimal use of CSII as per best practice guidelines, differences in baseline control, and psychosocial factors such as lack of motivation and noncompliance.[37] Even most summary metanalyses were not conclusive and can be misleading due to poor trial selection.[37] Hence, both CSII and MDI can be effective in glycemic control in motivated and committed patients. However, CSII is particularly effective in newly diagnosed patients who embark on pump therapy from the beginning, and in those with type 1 diabetes who have not reached the HbA_{1c} target levels without disabling hypoglycemia using best attempts with MDI and for whom MDI is impractical.[37] Future research comparing superiority of CSII versus MDI in terms of efficiency, mortality, and psychosocial impact is required, as well as finding solutions to enhance the adherence and suboptimal glycemic outcomes on CSII.

Characteristics of Pumps and Patient's Use

There is a wide range of pump devices that are currently in use by patients worldwide, with some of these smart pumps,

because of cost-effectiveness, still being used strictly in some parts of the world such as the USA. They have a common feature of a small portable size with a screen and buttons, though they differ in many other detailed features based on their operating systems (Figure 11.3a & 11.3b). We have outlined here the important points from a user guide of one of these pumps, as an example, highlighting some features of this pump and general practical points for effective use of the device Table 11.2). In addition, we give an example of comparing three commonly used smart pumps in the USA to reflect in the variety of advances in technology in serving patients' needs (Table 11.3).

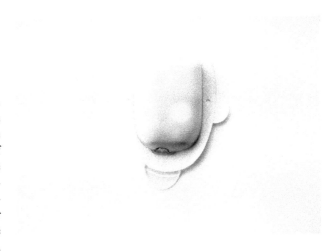

FIGURE 11.3A Different insulin pump devices with variable features.*

*Horizontal and vertical layouts of pumps, and a single unpacked pod for Insulet's Omnipod Insulin Management System.
www.shutterstock.com/image-photo/modern-diabetic-items-diabetes-care-concept-610296500
www.shutterstock.com/image-photo/single-unpacked-pod-insulet-omnipod-insulin-1666973641

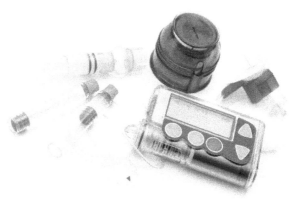

FIGURE 11.3B Pump features, infusion set, reservoir, and infusion of insulin in a patient's body.

Source: www.shutterstock.com/image-photo/education-about-controlling-diabetes-insulin-pump-408502936
www.shutterstock.com/image-vector/insulin-infusion-pump-on-patient-body-725070595

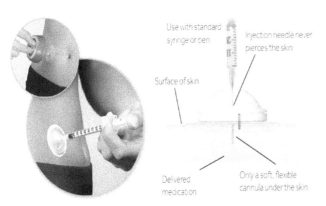

Use with standard syringe or pen

Injection needle never pierces the skin

Surface of skin

Delivered medication

Only a soft, flexible cannula under the skin

FIGURE 11.2 Insulin port.

TABLE 11.2

An Effective User Guide of a Pump (M670 Minimed as an example) with Highlights of the Most Important Practical Points*

User Guide	Contents	Highlights of the most important practical points**
Initial preparations	• Ensure safety: indications, contraindications, and warnings. • Equip with consumables and accessories. • Give clear guidance on insulin starting doses when changed from multidose injections or in insulin-naïve patients	Medical team (dietician, educator, etc.) decide who is appropriate —ready for insulin pump—or not. Some start patients with sensors before transitioning to a pump to understand their background glycemic profile better. Some fix the pump for patients with saline only, but not insulin, to allow the patient to become familiar with settings and wearing a pump. Emphasize how to use pump with hypo and hyper glucose readings. Order supplies early before they finish. Know whom to contact in case it does not work.
First steps	• Introduction to pump • Lock, unlock, and remove pump • Manual and auto modes • Managing batteries	Starting settings should be entered by the educator after discussion with physician and dietician—patients are not encouraged to change them until more experienced. Provide patient/family with extra batteries. No manual mode for patients and parents as yet—this depends on level of education of parents. Pumps get locked within seconds/minutes as a safety measure especially in case of children (parents need to unlock it). Patient or parent can disconnect a pump only for 2 hours for activities.
Basal	• Basal settings: rate and patterns • Viewing information on basal rate • Adding another basal rate and using temporary basal • Canceling temporary basal rate • Stopping insulin delivery and resuming it	It is preferred to set 4–5 basal rates per day. (Some try flat basal initially.) In old pumps, only 3 patterns could be set, but in modern smart pumps, it is feasible to set 7–8 patterns. Temporary basal usually tried inadvanced visits. Also, stopping and resuming insulin delivery is required in old pumps, but it occurs automatically if a sensor is fixed in new smart pumps. Hence, no need for temporary basal rates in these recent pumps. Patients can start using patterns in a second phase of training, if necessary, e.g., during holiday or special events such as Ramadan in Muslim patients and in frequently exercising patients.
Bolus	• Bolus settings: types, delivery, increment, speed, and the "Wizard" • Setting up and turning off the Bolus Wizard • Active insulin • Bolus Wizard warnings • Square Wave bolus • Dual Wave bolus • Preset Bolus: setting up, delivering & stopping	Accuracy of carb (CHO) counting and periodic revision with dietician Reasonable Insulin:Carb (I:CHO) ratios for the patient size In advanced visits: square and dual waves and manual bolus, including overriding suggestions from the pump (used to protect from hypos by some parents in the old pumps with no function of auto suspension) Easy bolus without CHO counting: used for corrections and if still a bit struggling with the dose because of hypos or difficulty in CHO counting in some situations Stopping (canceling) a bolus is a new feature in new pumps (can disconnect if not sure how it works). Old pumps can also do it but stopping the bolus will also stop the basal unlike new pumps.

User Guide	Contents	Highlights of the most important practical points**
Reservoir and infusion set	• The reservoir and infusion set • Disconnecting and reconnecting infusion set	Should change every 3 days Should get rid of bubbles during priming and set the infusion properly Should be changed in case of frequent high BG readings to avoid DKA In new pump resume immediately with reconnection
Meter	• Wireless connection of a meter with the pump • Remote bolus • Deleting a meter	Calibrating the sensor—this particular meter sends results directly to pump; other meters can be used, but are not guaranteed to have this function. Maintained supply of sensors is a real challenge with financial burden. Many diabetes treating teams encourage patients to use sensors in intermittent fashions; i.e., around the times of clinic visits. This could be more cost effective and efficient in supporting decisions about dose adjustment during clinic visits. Can function as a remote for pump and instruct bolus giving + useful in downloads using USB at home
History and events	• History: summary, daily, alarm, glucose sensor, events	Useful in assessment of patient care and assessing existing patterns of events
Reminders	• Reminders: e.g., personal, BG check, calibration, low reservoir, and set change	Good in helping the patients to keep committed for tasks including changing infusion sets, etc. It also gives early warning for a change of reservoir (approximately when 20 units are left)
General settings	• Airplane Mode • Auto Suspend • Block Mode • Display Options • Language • Managing pump settings • Self-Test • Sensor Demo • Time and date	Airplane mode disconnects all parts (pump, sensor, and meter). Auto suspend is a new feature with sensors (with low and high BG in G670 and with low BG only in G640) G670 is available in USA/Canada and other countries; still not available in many other countries. Parents should not try changing settings without referring to supervising treating team.
Setting up continuous glucose monitoring	• Understanding Continuous Glucose Monitoring (CGM) • Technology • Home screen • Understanding glucose settings • High and low settings • Manually resuming basal delivery during a suspend by sensor event • Wireless connection: pump and transmitter using Auto Connect • Wirelessly connecting pump and transmitter using Manual Connect • Deleting the transmitter from pump • Inserting the sensor • Connecting the transmitter to the sensor • Starting the sensor • Calibrating the sensor • When to calibrate • Guidelines for calibrating • Turning off Sensor Settings	Make sure CGM is well connected, calibrated, and merged with the pump. Shortage of supply—may need to be flexible to use CGM that do not match with the pump, such as FreeStyle Libre or Dexcom with G640 or G670 MiniMed. However, the patient should realize that the auto suspension is very important and the peculiar function of these smart pumps are lost during times of using non-CGMS with them or a CGMS that is not connected to the pump. Time of calibration is important to keep accuracy of the sensor (should not be timed with very low or very high BG readings).
Using continuous glucose monitoring	• Identifying sharp changes in sensor glucose • Silencing Alerts	

(Continued)

TABLE 11.2
Continued

User Guide	Contents	Highlights of the most important practical points**
Troubleshooting	• Troubleshooting: sensor, calibration, etc. • What is a Check Settings alarm? • My pump is asking me to rewind. • When a pump is dropped • My pump display times out too quickly.	Rewind with set change—process is clearer and easier to perform in new pumps. When sensor is not well affixed, it gets disconnected and should be changed. Calibration will not and should not be accepted when the time is inappropriate (very low or very high BG, as previous) or if there is a large discrepancy between a pricking test and sensor reading.
Maintenance	• Cleaning and storing: pump and transmitter	Transmitter and sensor should be in room temperature or fridge door—it gets broken in hot whether
Product specifications and safety information	• Product specifications • Alarm and alert escalation • Altitude range • Audio frequency • Backlight • Default, alert, and safety • Characteristics of the pump: weight, dimensions, etc. • Quality of service • Radio frequency communications • Security	For safety issues and suspected occlusion or similar issues, contact the support team, which is available 24.7.

* Adapted from Medtronic information resources of guidance on initial pump settings for diabetes treating teams (Protocol book: from MDI to MM G670).

**These points of practical importance were discussed with experienced diabetes educators in a tertiary center.

TABLE 11.3
Comparison between the Important Features of Three Commonly Used Smart Pumps[38]

Pump	Size (mm)	Weight	Screen	Color	Pros	Cons
  • Tandem t:slim X2 and t:flex	79.5 x 50.8 x 15.2	3.95 oz with full reservoir	Color touch screen	Black, with plastic or leather cases available in multiple colors	• Modern, high-tech appearance: Touch screen • Charges: No disposable batteries • Compact, thin dimensions • Rapid number entry/fastest bolus entry • Full integration with multiple devices, including smartphones and CGMS, e.g., Dexcom G5 • Can calculate boluses up to 50 units • Carb counting calculator • Alert for high temperatures and missed boluses • Secondary basal programs can be linked with secondary bolus formulas • Changing the position of the pump only leads to minimal unintended insulin • Prediction of low, basal suspend and restarts • Updates available free online	• No attached clip • Should be charged every one to two weeks • Unlock procedure required to perform any programming • Difficult handling (small buttons and weak vibration) • Can only be used with the product tubing connections (patient can be stuck if not enough supply) • Might take some time to set since both basal and bolus settings are in the same time slots. • Weak vibrate mechanism • No meter link

Pump	Size (mm)	Weight	Screen	Color	Pros	Cons
• **Medtronic MiniMed 670G with Guardian**	54 x 97 x 25	3.37 oz	Color	Black	• Slim clip with color screen and high resolution • Slim attachable clip • Data from Medtronic CGMS (Guardian connect) can be displayed on the pump screen • Prediction of low and high and automated suspension of basal rate (Hybrid closed loop based on sensor readings and prediction by algorithm) • Remote control for slow or fast bolus delivery • Can set "Presets" for basal and boluses • Can generate statistics of performance, and software (CareLink) can be easily downloaded	• Small screen and text compared to pump size • Basic programming requires many steps • Supplies may not be easily available in some areas • "Airplane Mode" requires additional finger pricking for calibration and safety checks. • Distracting and occasionally distressing system alerts especially when frequently encountered • Insulin-on-board only deducted from correction boluses • Not compatible with other downloading systems (only with CareLink), which can be less convenient for patients and families
• Insulet Omnipod	pod: 61 x 41 x 18 PDM: 66 x 110 x 26	OP: 1.2 oz (full reservoir) PDM: 4.0 oz (w/batteries)	Color	Pod: white Pump: black	• Discrete pump size with large color screen that is ideal for travel • No tubing • No missing insulin because of no connection issues • Fully watertight • Basal and bolus settings can be customized • Freestyle meter can be easily integrated • Can program through clothing from a few feet away • Simple cannula insertion with less risk of lipodystrophy • Personal Diabetes Manager (PDM) data can be displayed on smartphone as well as a "Find My PDM" feature. • The Omnipod VIEW™ app allows up to 12 caregivers to follow the data remotely in their smartphones	• Bulky programmer • Programmer is required every time in order to enter boluses or make settings changes in the pump. • Malfunction of programmer allows the pod to deliver the basal rate. • Pod can result in a residual "bulge" on the site of insertion • Cannula available in only one size • Max reservoir volume 200 u; minimum fill amount 85 u • Pod stops working after 72 hours (plus grace period) • Low-suspend and hybrid closed loop features are not integrated though it has potential to hybrid with Dexcom CGMS • Editing or programming is not possible during bolus delivery • A default in cannula or pod error may require complete pod replacement • Should be suspended during changing basal settings and the limit for temporary basal is only 12 hours • Insulin-to-carb ratios in whole number increments only (DASH PDM will have IC ratio in < 1 g increments)

Initial pump start settings of insulin are by far the standard, so we give an example of one of the postulated models to shed light on this area (Table 11.4). Though, these starting doses should be guided by the diabetes management team; namely, the diabetologist, diabetes educator, and nutritionist. Nevertheless, clinical pharmacists should also be aware of these doses since they deal with this group of patients who get shifted from daily insulin injections to CSII.

2.0 GLUCOSE MONITORING DEVICES

2.1 BLOOD GLUCOSE MONITORING (BGM)

The invention of self-monitoring of blood glucose (SMBG) may be the most notable breakthrough in diabetes management besides the discovery of insulin. SMBG has helped patients to assess glycemic regulation more accurately, allowing for more intelligent adjustment of insulin.

TABLE 11.4
Initial Pump Start Settings**

Patient Name: _____ DOB: _____ Weight: _____ lb/kg

Current Daily Injection Dose: _____ + _____ = _____ units

Pump Model: _____ Pump Serial Number: _____ Date: _____

Calculations for Starting Doses

Pump TDD

Reduced Injection Dose: _____ units/day x 0.75 = _____ units/day
(Daily Injection Dose) (Reduced Dose)

Weight Dose: _____ x 0.23 units = _____ units/day OR _____ x 0.50 units = _____ units/day
(Weight (lbs)) (Weight Dose) (Weight (kgs)) (Weight Dose)

Pump Total Daily Dose: (_____ units/day + _____ units/day) ÷ 2 = _____ units/day
(Reduced Dose) (Weight Dose) (Pump TDD)

Basal Rate

Total Daily Basal Units: _____ units/day x _____ = _____ units/day
(Pump TDD) (% Basal) (Total Daily Basal)

Initial Basal Rate: _____ units ÷ 24 hours = _____ units/hour
(Total Daily Basal) (Initial Basal Rate)

ICR

Total Daily Bolus Units: _____ units/day - _____ units/day = _____ units/day
(Pump TDD) (Total Daily Basal) (Total Daily Bolus)

Insulin-to-Carb Ratio:
_____ grams ÷ _____ units/day =
(Daily Carbs) (Total Daily Bolus)
_____ grams/unit x 1.2
(Pre-pump ICR)
= _____ grams/unit
(Pump ICR)

OR

500 ÷ _____ units/day =
(Pump TDD)
_____ grams/unit
(Insulin-to-Carb Ratio)

ISF

Insulin Sensitivity Factor:
_____ mmol/L/1unit x 1.2
(Pre-pump ISF)
= _____ mmol/L/1unit
(Pump ISF)

OR

100 ÷ _____ units
(Pump TDD)
= _____ mmol/L/1 unit
(Insulin Sensitivity Factor)

Initial Pump Start Settings

Basal Rates		Insulin-to-Carb Ratio	Bolus Wizard™ calculator Settings		
Time	Rate		Insulin Sensitivity Factor	BG Target Ranges	

Basal Rates

	Time	Rate
1)	00:00 @ _____
2)	_____ @ _____
3)	_____ @ _____
4)	_____ @ _____
5)	_____ @ _____

Max Basal Rate: _____ units

Insulin-to-Carb Ratio

	Time	Ratio
1)	00:00	_____
2)	_____	_____
3)	_____	_____

Max Bolus: _____ units

Insulin Sensitivity Factor

_____ mmol/L /unit

Active Insulin Time

_____ hours

*Clinical Considerations**
Adults: 4 – 5 hours
Children: 3 – 4 hours
Pregnancy: 3 – 4 hours

BG Target Ranges

	Day	Night
	__ mmol/L – __ mmol/L	__ mmol/L – __ mmol/L

Clinical Considerations*	Day	Night
Adults and Adolescents (13+ yrs):	5.0 – 5.6 mmol/L	5.6 – 6.1 mmol/L
School Age (6 – 12 yrs):	5.0 – 6.1 mmol/L	5.6 – 6.7 mmol/L
Toddler to Pre-school (0 – 6 yrs):	5.6 – 6.7 mmol/L	6.1 – 7.2 mmol/L
Hypoglycaemia Unawareness:	5.6 – 6.7 mmol/L	6.1 – 7.2 mmol/L
Pregnancy:	4.4 – 5.0 mmol/L	5.0 – 5.0 mmol/L

Make adjustments if BG is outside of these ranges:	Adjustment Instructions for Patients*
Fasting/pre-meal: _____ to _____ mmol/L	• If night, fasting/pre-meal or bedtime BG below target, *decrease* basal 10 – 20%
Post-meal: _____ to _____ mmol/L	• If night, fasting/pre-meal or bedtime BG above target, *increase* basal 10 – 20%
Bedtime: _____ to _____ mmol/L	• If post-meal BG less than 1.7mmol/L above pre-meal BG, *increase* carb ratio by 10 – 20%
Nocturnal: _____ to _____ mmol/L	• If post-meal BG more than 3.3mmol/L above pre-meal BG, *decrease* carb ratio by 10 – 20%
	Elevated BG: Verify trends 2–3 days before adjusting **Low BG:** Consider immediate adjustment

**Adopted with permission from Medtronic information resources of guidance on initial pump settings for diabetes treating teams (Protocol book: from MDI to MM G670, Medtronic).

Temperature and oxygen concentration can influence the results of most meters that use an enzymatic form of glucose calculation (i.e., altitude).[39] Hematocrit, (in)adequacy of peripheral circulation, and contaminated skin surface (with the presence of glucose on the skin surface at the time of testing) are other factors that affect accuracy.[39] Glucose meters have changed considerably since their arrival. The time required for sample analysis has dropped from minutes to seconds as well as the quantity of blood required for analysis, which has declined to around 1/100 of that originally necessary.[40] The meters have also become smaller and easier to operate with larger, easier-to-read displays (Figure 11.4). Early glucose meters used reflectance (optical) technology to estimate glucose levels, but most new meters (still not all) use electrochemical signaling (glucose oxidase) to estimate glucose levels.[41–43]

The American Diabetes Association (ADA) recommends that SMBG should be performed three or more times daily for patients who are using multiple daily doses (MDD) of insulin or CSII.[40] For patients who are on other regimens, such as oral medications or just basal insulin therapy, SMBG may still be useful in achieving adequate glycemic control. However, there are still unmet needs with SMBG from patients' and health practitioners' perspectives:

Patients' perspectives:

- There is a resistance to self-monitoring of blood glucose (SMBG) due to related discomfort, competing priorities, the non-discreet nature of testing, and the fear of repeated failures from the results.
- Many are confused by glucose data and don't know how to read it.

Health practitioners' perspectives:

- Non-optimal decision-making can happen due to limited time of consultation with the patients and lack of overall data.
- Many are frustrated by futile attempts to slow the pace of disease progression and avoid harmful effects.

The American Diabetes Association (ADA) has set a measurement for evaluating meter accuracy, in which 100% of readings should fall within 5% of the reference, such as a laboratory analyzer. Today's finger-prick meters often fail to meet such strict standards.[44–46]

As a result, the need for continuous glucose monitoring (CGM) devices has grown in recent years. They are commercially available, but they are understandably more costly than handled meters, which makes CGM not a feasible option in many countries because of the issue of affordability. These devices have a subcutaneous monitor to measure the glucose level of interstitial fluid (similar to the concentration of blood glucose).[47] However, they are not precise enough to replace the SMBG since they appear to be less accurate than direct

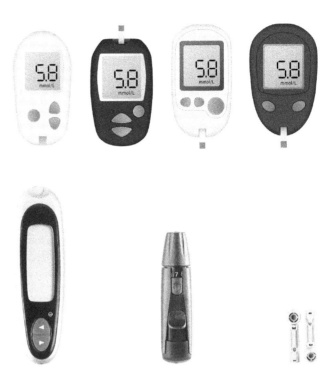

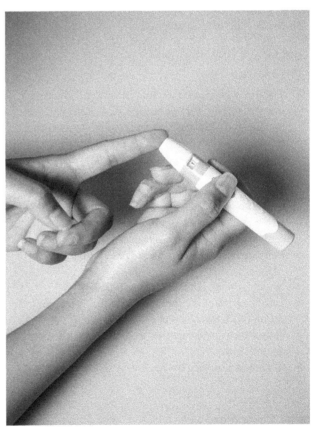

FIGURE 11.4 Different glucose meters used by simple finger-prick method for glucose monitoring.

Source: www.shutterstock.com/image-vector/glucose-meter-icon-set-realistic-vector-1262232721

www.shutterstock.com/image-photo/diabetes-testing-kit-lancing-device-lancets-1846818553

www.shutterstock.com/image-photo/woman-piercing-finger-glucometer-lancing-device-1979914733

measurements at periods of rapid glucose fluctuation and have not yet been proven to enhance overall metabolic glucose regulation and reduce the likelihood of complications.[47,48] Moreover, CGM can be effective in treating patients with type 1 diabetes with respect to adherence to their insulin regimen and may be beneficial in providing stable glucose levels and in indicating hypoglycemia early warning signs in patients who are unaware that they have hypoglycemia[47,49]

2.2 CONTINUOUS GLUCOSE MONITORING SYSTEM (CGMS)

Different pharmaceutical companies try to produce affordable devices for continuous glucose monitoring systems (CGMS) that provide glucose checks that are

- accurate,
- frequent,
- convenient to patients,
- socially acceptable,
- not painful,
- helpful with management decisions (given limited resources), and
- easily explained to patients.

Examples of CGMS Devices

2.2.1 FreeStyle Libre

- The dense glucose data required for a full glycemic image can be easily generated with flash glucose monitoring. This device is remarkable for its speed reading to collect glucose data. The lightweight and fully disposable sensor lasts up to 14 days and needs no calibration or regular finger pricks; it tests, collects, and saves glucose data automatically, which is another main benefit of the flash glucose monitoring device. Fast scanning of the reader over the sensor collects and displays glucose data.
- Fully disposable sensor is intended to be used for 14 days.
- No finger stick calibration is required.
- Sensor operates by standard near-field communication (NFC) wireless protocols.
- Sensor measures, captures, and stores glucose data automatically.
- Color touch-screen reader is easy to use and read.

2.2.2 Dexcom

Sensor Calibration

There are two methods of sensor calibration (Figure 11.8). Factory-calibrated systems are advantageous because they eliminate potential for errors associated with finger-prick calibrations. The FreeStyle Libre System is currently the only factory-calibrated sensor for consumers to use. Accuracy is not dependent on patient compliance and finger-prick results used for calibration.

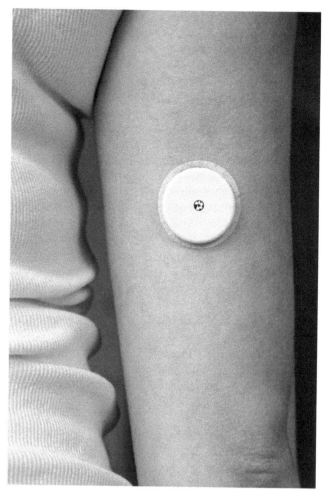

FIGURE 11.5 FreeStyle Libre meter, sensor, and data.

Source: www.shutterstock.com/image-photo/blood-glucose-monitoring-sensor-called-freestyle-1670304901

2.2.3 Guardian Connect***

The Guardian™ Connect Continuous Glucose Monitoring (CGM) system helps patients to manage their diabetes by:

- Tracking their glucose levels day and night.
- Presenting their glucose levels in a convenient and discrete manner using their smartphones.
- Alerting them to glucose events using their smartphones.
- Educating patients on how exercise, diet, and medications can affect their glucose levels.
- Offering patients extra tools such as alerts to help them keep track of their diet, exercise, and insulin in order to avoid excessive and low glucose levels.

System Description

The Guardian Connect system includes the Guardian Connect app, Guardian Connect transmitter, Guardian Sensor (3), charger, tester, one-press inserter, and oval tape.

The Continuous Glucose Monitoring (CGM) system is a device that allows patients to monitor their sensor glucose

The FreeStyle Libre Sensor

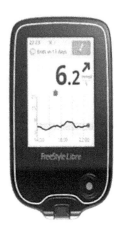

- No lancet

- Compact and lightweight

- Easy to hold, use and carry

- Provides easy to read graphs

- Offers easy-to-understand graphs with a quick summary of glucose history

- Backlit colour touchscreen

- Stores 90 days of glucose data

- Provides a complete glucose picture over 3 months

FreeStyle Libre sensor

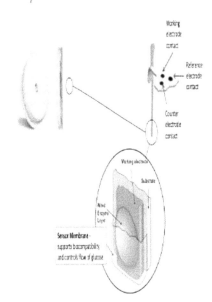

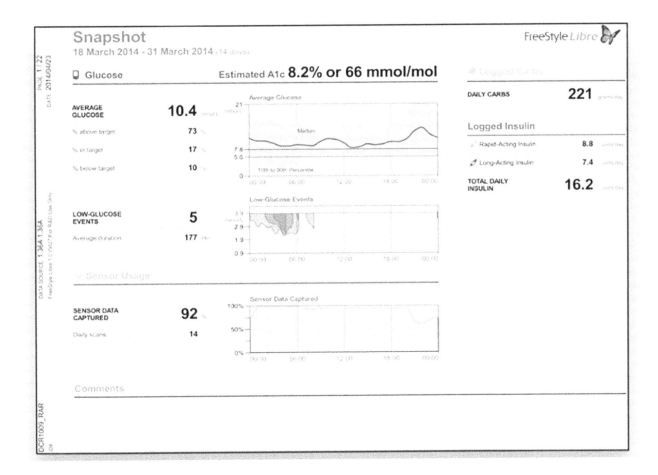

FIGURE 11.6   Dexcom sensor, transmitter, and auto applicator.

Source: www.shutterstock.com/image-photo/sydney-australia-20210130-cgm-continuous-glucose-1943160844
www.shutterstock.com/image-photo/sydney-australia-20210130-cgm-continuous-glucose-1956548359

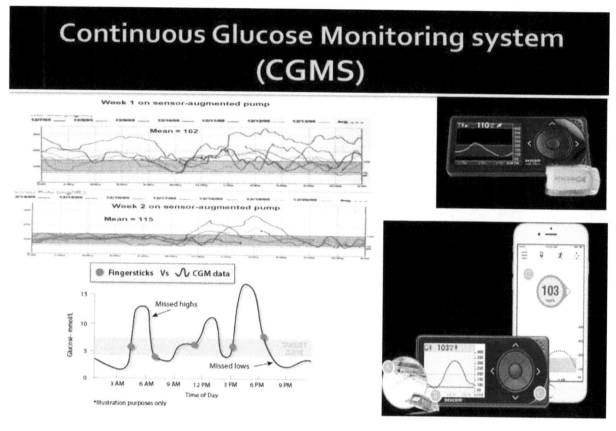

FIGURE 11.7   Dexcom versus finger-stick data.

Two methods for sensor calibration

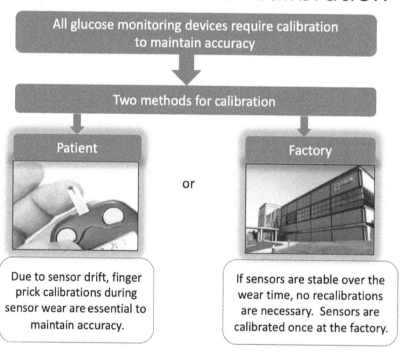

FIGURE 11.8   Patient versus factory calibration of sensor.

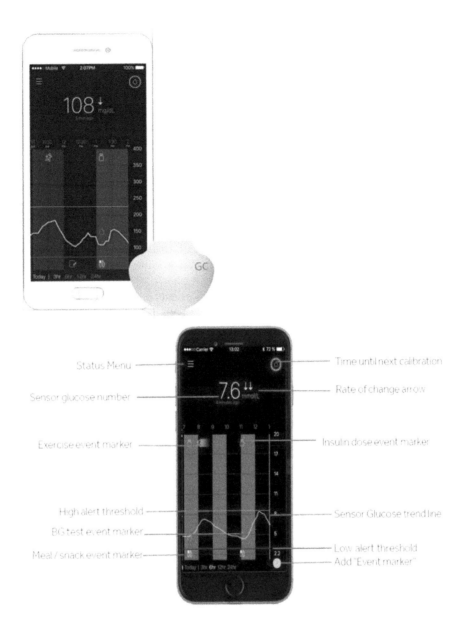

FIGURE 11.9 Guardian Connect.

levels in real time. Guardian Sensor (3) will be placed under the skin to monitors glucose volume in the interstitial fluid. These glucose readings are collected by the Guardian Connect transmitter and converted to sensor glucose values. The glucose values from the sensor are then shown on the Guardian Connect app. The app provides alerts based on glucose levels in the sensor. Only compatible mobile devices should be used for this product.

Indications for Use

- The Guardian Connect system is for regular/irregular monitoring of glucose levels in the interstitial fluid underneath the skin in patients with diabetes mellitus aged 14 to 75. The Guardian Connect system provides real-time glucose values that can be shown on Guardian Connect app in for compatible mobile devices only.
- The application allows users to detect trends and track patterns in glucose concentrations, and will also send alerts if a Guardian Sensor (3) glucose level falls below, rises above, or is predicted to surpass set values. The Guardian Sensor (3) glucose values provide an indication of when a finger-stick test may be required but not to make insulin adjustments.

Guardian Sensor (3)

The Guardian Sensor (3) is a CGMS that uses a Medtronic glucose sensor for up to 7 days of uninterrupted use. It is used as an adjunctive device, but not an alternative, to standard SMBG. Each sensor should be used only once and it needs to be prescribed.

Guardian Connect Transmitter

The transmitter is only compatible with the Guardian Sensor (3). The transmitter powers the glucose sensor, and collects and calculates sensor data before sending it via Bluetooth version 4.0 to the Guardian Connect app installed on a compatible mobile device. It requires a prescription.

Guardian Connect App

Patients should use a compatible mobile device, and should be experienced enough to adjust the mobile audio and notification settings. The app displays the sensor's data, and provides a user interface for sensor calibration, entering data such as exercise and meals, and uploading information to the CareLink Personal website. The app helps patients to detect trends and track patterns of glycemic profile. It provides alerts in case of exceeding certain limits of high or low blood glucose readings, or if predicting to surpass these limits.

2.2.4 Limitations of CGM Systems

A finger-prick test with a blood glucose meter is required when glucose levels shift quickly and CGMS that monitors interstitial fluid glucose levels may not be as accurate in those cases. It also inaccurately detects hypoglycemia or impending hypoglycemia in some occasions, such as in FreeStyle Libre, and should be questioned when the patient's symptoms do not match the CGMS readings.[49–52]

"Too many alarms" and "alarms too often" are among the top reasons for sensor discontinuation.

Certain patients may benefit from sensor-based glucose monitoring system with alarms such as patients[53–54]

- who are diagnosed with hypoglycemia unawareness,
- with nocturnal hypoglycemia, and/or
- with high glucose variability.

However, in order for the alarms to be useful, patients have to wear the sensor, turn on the alarms, and keep the device close to them.

Too many device alarms can create alarm fatigue that may cause important alarms to be missed or turned off completely.[55]

Sensor-based glucose monitoring systems are more effective when utilized through increased wear time.[56] However, there are two issues with regard to utilization:[52]

- Discontinuation: Patients discontinue usage for numbers of reasons.
- Wear time/data capture: Patients may not wear sensors continuously or the receiver may not be within the range of the transmitter.

2.2.5 Potential Risks of Using CGMS Sensors

- Skin irritation or other reactions
- Pain +/– Infection
- Rash
- Residual redness associated with adhesive or tapes or both
- Scarring
- Bleeding and Bruising
- Swelling +/– Allergic reaction
- Fainting secondary to anxiety
- Appearance of a small "freckle-like" dot where needle was inserted, or fear of needle insertion
- Sensor fracture, breakage, or damage
- Minimal blood splatter associated with sensor needle removal

3.0 Closed Loop System (Artificial Pancreas)

Further advances in the field include trying to close an open loop by having insulin pump, continuous glucose monitoring system, and algorithmic device (with individual patient's settings) talking to each other in order to optimize insulin delivery, in what is known as an "artificial/bionic pancreas" (Figure 11.10). The bionic pancreas is one of the recent examples of this basic model and some others will shortly appear on the market. Some smart

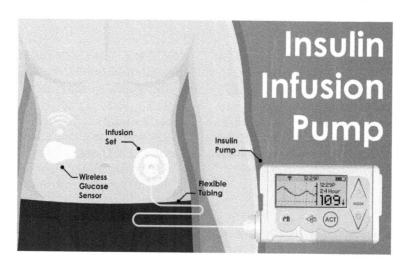

FIGURE 11.10 Closed loop "artificial pancreas" insulin delivery system.

Source: www.shutterstock.com/image-vector/insulin-infusion-pump-on-patient-body-725063101

pumps such as the G670 MiniMed, with the auto-suspension function in hypo- and hyperglycemia are not far from this model.

ESSENTIAL COMPONENTS

- Insulin pump to accurately and precisely deliver variable amounts of insulin
- Continuous glucose sensor to accurately determine ambient glucose levels
- Effective algorithms to vary insulin delivery rates based on
  - real-time glucose sensor outputs

Summary

The injection of insulin combined with intermittent or continuous glycemic control are essential for the management of patients with T1D and some patients with other types of diabetes.[14] The injection technique and dosage of insulin should be consistent, and both should be reviewed by the diabetes care team on a periodic basis.[14] An efficient use of insulin devices should lead to a better metabolic control. This requires an understanding of the various types of insulin, the duration of action, and learning to adjust insulin dosage to achieve individual target goals of blood glucose, which cannot be achieved without an effective use of delivery devices by patients with support from the diabetes care team.

ENDOCRINE DISORDERS

1.0 GROWTH DISORDERS

Pediatric patients with growth disorders can benefit from treatment with recombinant human growth hormone (HGH).[57,58] Patients and families should be educated about how to use the application devices; namely, GH pens (Table 11.5, Figure 11.11) or automated electronic injecting devices (Figure 11.12).[59] Treatment goals should be set and shared with patients/familiesalong with emphasizing the importance of compliance to achieve adequate outcome after using this costly treatment in a narrow window of time; i.e., before completion of puberty.[57]

1.1 MOST COMMON THERAPEUTIC INDICATIONS OF GROWTH HORMONE THERAPY

Children

- Growth hormone deficiency (GHD)
- Intrauterine growth restriction or small for gestational age (SGA), who did not show a catch-up growth by 4 years of age as per practice in the European countries
- Chronic renal disease
- Turner syndrome (TS)

Adults

- Childhood-onset growth hormone deficiency: Children with severe GHD should be retested for GHD upon completion of pubertal growth and before being transferred to adult service.
- Adult-onset growth hormone deficiency: Post traumatic injury. A stimulation test would be required for verification of GHD.

1.2 DOSAGE

Patients' doses should be decided on an individual basis. However, the following are the general guidance based on potentials of response to GH therapy and risks of overdosing. The response depends on how deficient the patient is in GH and how responsive the growth plate would be to GH treatment. There is a direct relationship between GHD, the resistance of the growth plate, and the required effective dose of GH therapy. GHD patients require smaller doses, while growth plate-resistant patients (as in chronic renal disease and TS) require higher doses of GH. SGA patients are in between.

Pediatric population:

- Growth Hormone Deficiency: 0.025–0.035 mg/kg/day or 0.7–1.0 mg/m$_2$/day After growth completion, GH treatment should be continued to achieve full somatic adult development including lean body mass and bone mineral accrual.
- Small for Gestational Age: 0.035 mg/kg/day or 1.0 mg/m$_2$/day
- Chronic renal disease: 0.050 mg/kg/day or 1.4 mg/m$_2$/day
- Turner syndrome: 0.045–0.067 mg/kg/day or 1.3–2.0 mg/m$_2$/day

Adult population:

- Childhood-onset GHD: 0.2–0.5 mg/day with dose adjustment if required, guided by serum IGF-1 level.
- Adult-onset GHD: a low dose 0.1–0.3 mg/day with dose titration as in childhood-onset.
- Women may require higher doses than men, and those on oral estrogen replacement are undertreated while men are overtreated.
- Maintenance dose rarely exceeds 1.0 mg/day.

1.3 METHOD OF ADMINISTRATION

Night injections are preferred and injection sites should be rotated to avoid lipoatrophy.

1.4 CONTRAINDICATIONS

- Hypersensitivity to GH.
- Active intracranial tumors or still on chemo/radiotherapy

TABLE 11.5

Characteristics of Growth Hormone Delivery Devices*

Device type	Device (somatotropin)	Manufacturer	Strength and increment	Use (single or multiple)	Storage	Advantage	Disadvantage
Syringe and needle	MiniQuick (Genotropin®)	Pfizer	Available in dose of 0.2–2.0 mg; Increment in 0.2 mg steps	Single-use disposable syringe	Can be kept outside the refrigerator (maximum 25°C) for up to 6 months before use	Can be kept non-refrigerated for 6 months (useful for holidays, etc.); Prefilled dose in a preloaded cartridge (so no need for dose dialing); Discreet and portable; Optional needle guard; Preservative-free	Reconstitution required (2-chamber cartridge); Only available in 0.2mg increments
Injector pen	Genotropin Pen (Genotropin®)	Pfizer	5.3 mg cartridge (increments of 0.1 mg); 12 mg cartridge (increments of 0.2 mg)	Multi-use pen in two sizes	Cartridge is stored in the pen. The pen is refrigerated.	Clear digital dose display; Optional needle guard; Pen can be personalized (GenoCaps®); Dial back possible; May be stored at room temperature (£ 25°C) for up to one month prior to reconstitution	Cartridge needs to be inserted into the device (not prefilled); Reconstitution required (2-chamber cartridge); Needs to be stored in the refrigerator after reconstitution; Dose cannot be preset
	GoQuick Pen (Genotropin®)	Pfizer	5.3 mg cartridge (increments of 0.05 mg); 12 mg cartridge (increments of 0.15 mg)	Single-dose daily disposable syringe	Can be stored at room temperature (£ 25°C) for up to one month prior to reconstitution	Prefilled with cartridge; The dose can be preset; Optional needle guard; Dial back possible	Reconstitution required (2-chamber cartridge); Needs to be stored in the refrigerator after reconstitution
	HumatroPen™ (Humatrope®)	Lilly	6 mg cartridge (0.025 mg increments); 12 mg cartridge (0.05 mg increments); 24 mg cartridge (0.1 mg increments)	Multi-use pen	Cartridge should be stored refrigerated	Optional needle guard; Dial back possible	Cartridge needs to be inserted into the device (not prefilled); Reconstitution required (the cartridge needs to be reconstituted with the diluent, which is supplied separately, before being inserted into the device); Needs to be stored in the refrigerator before and after reconstitution; Dose cannot be preset
	NordiPen (Norditropin®)	Novo Nordisk	5 mg cartridge (0.05 mg increments); 10 mg cartridge (0.1 mg increments); 15 mg cartridge (0.1 mg increments)	Multi-use pen	After first use, store at room temperature (below 25°C) for up to 3 weeks.	Premixed solution; Storage advantage (as in previous column); NordiPenMate® auto-inject accessory available; Graphic and classic designs available	Cartridge needs to be inserted into the device (not prefilled); If the patient dials above the correct dose, the dose selector needs to be reset; No needle guard on the device; although the NovoFine® Autocover® needle can be used (also, the needle will be hidden if NordiPenMate® is used); Dose cannot be preset

Product	Manufacturer	Concentration/increments	Device	Storage	Features	Notes
NordiFlex (Norditropin®)	Novo Nordisk	Different concentrations (in 1.5 ml): Orange (5mg), Blue (10 mg), Green (15 mg), Purple (30 mg) (increments of 0.025 mg, 0.05 mg, 0.1 mg, 0.1 mg for the 4 pens, respectively)	Multi-use pen	After first use, store at room temperature (below 25°C) for up to 3 weeks.	Prefilled device / Premixed solution / Storage advantage (as in previous column). / NordiFlex PenMate® autoinject accessory available / Dial back possible	No needle guard on the device; although the NovoFine® Autocover® needle can be used (also, the needle will be hidden if Nordi-Flex PenMate® is used) / Dose cannot be preset
NutropinAq Pen (Nutropin®)	Ipsen Genentech	Only 10 mg size available in the UK (0.1 mg increments)	Multi-use pen	Cartridge should be stored in the refrigerator before and after first use	Premixed solution / LCD display / Dial back possible / Optional needle shield	Cartridge needs to be inserted into the device (not prefilled) / Needs to be stored in the refrigerator before and after first use / Dose cannot be preset
SurePal™ Pen (Somatropin®)	Sandoz	5 mg (0.05 mg increments), 10 mg (0.1 mg increments)	Multi-use pen	Cartridge should be stored in the refrigerator before and after first use	Premixed solution (no reconstitution required) / Dose can be preset / Needle is hidden throughout use / No priming is required / Cartridges are dose-specific and will not fit in the incorrect pen	Cartridge needs to be inserted into the device (not prefilled) / Needs to be stored in the refrigerator before and after first use / Dial back not possible; although reset process is simple and will avoid waste
Omnitrope Pen (Somatropin®)	Sandoz	5 mg (0.05 mg increments), 10mg (0.1 mg increments)	Multi-use pen	Cartridge should be stored in the refrigerator before and after first use	Premixed solution (no reconstitution required) / Needle guard	Cartridge needs to be inserted into the device (not prefilled) / Needs to be stored in the refrigerator before and after first use / Dial back not possible (it needs to be reset; otherwise, there will be drug waste) / Dose cannot be preset

(Continued)

TABLE 11.5
Continued

Device type	Device (somatotropin)	Manufacturer	Strength and increment	Use (single or multiple)	Storage	Advantage	Disadvantage
Needle-free injector	ZomaJet VisionX® (Zomacton®)	Ferring	10 mg vial, increments of 0.1 mg	Needle-free device	Reconstituted vial should be stored in the refrigerator	Needle-free / No product waste / Dial back possible / Does not require daily needle change (head needs to be changed every 7 days) / Audible sound with each dose (may be a disadvantage for some) / Automatic locking system after dose given	Vial requires reconstitution using prefilled diluent syringe / The reconstituted vial needs to be stored in the refrigerator / The dose needs to be drawn up from reconstituted vial before each injection / Requires some pressure to be placed on the skin / Dose cannot be preset / May cause skin reactions
Electronic injector	easypod ™ (Saizen®)	Merck Serono	6 mg, 12 mg, and 20 mg liquid cartridges (all 0.01 mg increments)	Electronic auto-injector. Dose programmed.	Cartridge stored within the device. The device is refrigerated.	Automatically injects and delivers dose / Dose is preset by HCP (protected by PIN code) / Records dose history; dose log allows adherence monitoring / Needle hidden throughout use / On-screen instructions for user / Audible and visual signals show when the dose is complete / Can control comfort parameters (e.g., injection depth/time, needle speed) / Device can be personalized (on-screen name; facias) / Dose adjustment function to minimize waste (set by HCP) / Skin sensor to ensure correct placement / Premixed solution	Cartridge needs to be loaded into the device / Batteries need to be replaced approximately once every year / Relatively large device / Needs to be stored in the refrigerator before and after first use / Electronic device—requires care during storage and use

*Reference websites for the devices given in the table are as follows:
- easypod™—growth hormone delivery www.saizenus.com
- Clinicaltrials.gov www.clinicaltrials.gov
- Genotropin® official site www.genotropin.com
- Humatrope www.humatrope.com
- Norditropin® somatropin (rdna origin) injection for growth hormone deficiency www.norditropin-us.com
- NordiTropin—Novo Nordisk A/S www.norditropin.com
- Human growth hormone therapy: nutropin www.nutropin.com
- Merck Serono International SA www.merckserono.net
- justgrowth—Merck Serono's growth hormone disorders website www.justgrowth.com
- Ferring www.ferring.com
- easypod™ www.easypodus.com all cited from [Google Scholar]

- After completion of puberty especially in girls when they have regular cycles
- During acute critical illness, e.g., after major surgery or trauma, respiratory compromise, etc.
- After kidney transplant except for a purpose of catching up in growth

1.5 SPECIAL WARNINGS AND PRECAUTIONS FOR USE

The prescription of GH should be confined to clinicians with expertise and specialization in the field of endocrinology and growth to avoid irrational use of GH, and unnecessary and potentially harmful overdosing GH doses should be guided by IGF-1 level every 6 months and monitoring of thyroid function and A1c level at least once a year. Also, patients with dyslipidemia should have monitoring of their lipid profile during GH therapy.

Children

- GH can lead to impaired glucose tolerance and transient T2DM. It can also result in transient hypothyroidism and transient dyslipidemia. Patients on GH treatment should be monitored for these potential side effects.
- Upper airway obstruction and sudden death were reported in patients with Prader-Willi syndrome following GH therapy and patients with severe obesity.
- SGA children could have other medical diagnoses such as genetic or syndromic etiology, so further workup is warranted before starting GH therapy.
- Dose adjustment is of special importance in patients with TS since they might experience hands and feet overgrowth as well as otitis media with GH therapy.
- Renal function should be monitored during treatment in patient with chronic renal disease.
- Scoliosis can worsen with treatment and should be monitored for, but it is not an absolute contraindication for GH therapy. A collaboration with colleagues in orthopedic and spinal surgery should guide the treatment in a safe way.

Adults

- Growth hormone deficiency in adults is a lifelong disease.

Other risks

- There is no evidence that growth hormone increases the risk for primary neoplasms. However, a slight rise in the incidence of a secondary neoplasm was reported, though most of these could be attributed to commonly used irradiations in treatment and so it is difficult to accuse GH for it. Nevertheless, patients undergoing GH therapy who have had full remission of their malignancy should be carefully watched for a relapse.

- Benign intracranial hypertension (BIH), also known as pseudotumor cerebri, is a rare associated side effect of GH therapy. A funduscopy for papilledema is recommended in case of a serious or frequent headache, vision problems, fatigue, and/or vomiting. GH therapy should be discontinued if BIH is confirmed and can be resumed later when the condition is treated successfully.
- Patients on GH therapy, especially TS, should be monitored for thyroid function and treated for possible associated deficiency as discussed earlier.
- A small percentage of patients can produce antibodies to somatropin, as with all somatropin-containing products. These antibodies have a poor binding capacity and do not affect the growth rate. Any patient who does not respond to the medication should be tested for antibodies to somatropin.

1.6 GROWTH HORMONE DEVICES

1. Pens (Table 11.5 & Figure 11.11)
2. Saizen (Automated Electronic Injection Device) (Figure 11.12)

Motivations for patients undergoing GH therapy can be low because concordance with drug therapy is often poor in chronic non-life-threatening conditions.[60]

Missing GH injections can be due to different reasons[61]:

- Forgetting to take it
- Experiencing side effects
- Inability to pay for it
- Being away from home or traveling
- Forgetting to renew prescription
- Forgetting to order the next refill
- Illness or not feeling well
- Special event
- Requiring a "vacation" from taking medication

Automated Electronic Injection Device[59,61,62]

- Successful GH therapy relies on regular and continued injections. More than one fifth of young patients miss > 2 injections/week on average.
- Missing more than 2 injections a week can impair height velocity outcomes.
- Non adherence with GH ranged 64% to 77% among the 3 age groups.
- The electronic r-hGH auto-injector, easypod™, automatically records the patient's adherence to treatment. Accurate monitoring of adherence enables appropriate intervention if necessary.
- Out of 779 respondents, 720 (92.4%) said that easypod was easy/very easy to use.
- There is no waste of medication due to automatic setting, which balances between daily dose accuracy and no waste in growth hormone cartilage.

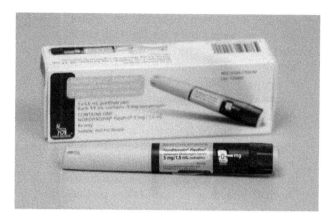

FIGURE 11.11 Norditropin: A commonly used growth hormone (GH) therapy (FlexPro™ 5 mg/1.5 ml pen as an example).

Source: www.google.com/url?sa=i&url=https%3A%2F%2Fwww.shutterstock.com%2Feditorial%2Fimage-editorial%2Fhghgrowing-use-chicago-usa-6231877a&psig=AOvVaw2aiULNcgAoqUVn_vlUtiRG&ust=16237 55552932000&source=images&cd=vfe&ved=0CAIQjRxqFwoTCLDg mIf_lvECFQAAAAAdAAAAABAD

www.shutterstock.com/editorial/image-editorial/hghgrowing-use-chicago-usa-6231877a

- Saizen helps patients to get the most out of their growth hormone.
- In GH patients with poor results, healthcare professionals should distinguish and classify between patients with poor adherences who require further education and low-level respondents who need higher doses of growth hormone.
- Saizen easypod is a free auto-injector device, offered by the company, which provides comprehensive digital history of patient adherence to therapy, enabling the healthcare professional to monitor his/her patient's adherence through Saizen easypod.
- Saizen easypod is easy to use (three steps to inject).
- There is less pain during injection due to comfort-setting options.
- There is less needle phobia since the needle is hidden all the time.
- Poor adherence bears a dual effect: increased therapy cost with decreased efficacy outcome.
- Healthcare professionals must distinguish between the need for an increase in dosage and the need for additional patient education.[63]

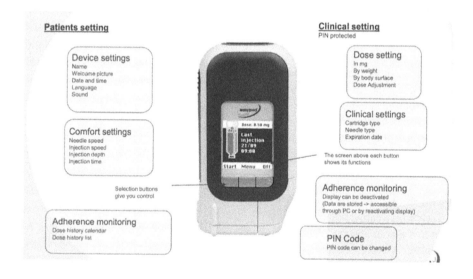

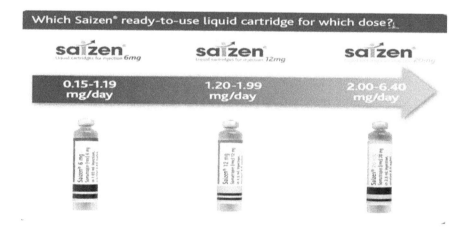

FIGURE 11.12 Easypod™: An automated electronic injection device with cartridge selection guide for appropriate doses.

How Easypod™ Can Help in Identifying Adherence for Better Diagnosis and Better Clinical Outcome

1. Easypod Electronic Injector can **track patient adherence** through a dose calendar screen.
2. Skin sensor ensures that the patient has injected him- or herself; injection will not be performed unless easypod senses skin.
3. In GH patients with poor outcome, for the first time we can **differentiate** between patients with **poor adherences** who need more education and **low responders** who need higher doses of growth hormone.
4. **Personalized comfort settings** ensure less pain during injection, such as flexibility to change injection depth, injection speed, and needle speed.
5. **Pre-set dosing** to be determined by the physician decreasing chance of errors ("No more clicks").
6. Patients endure **less needle phobia** because the needle is hidden all the time.
7. Saizen with easypod is easy to use (three steps to inject).
8. Easypod offers four types of dose-setting (in mg, by weight, by body surface, dose adjustment).

2.0 OTHER ENDOCRINE CONDITIONS

Medical devices are used in variety of endocrine conditions such asthose associated with metabolic syndrome (dyslipidemia, obesity, and T2D), osteoporosis, contraception, and hormonal replacement therapy.

2.1 OBESITY, METABOLIC SYNDROME, AND TYPE 2 DIABETES

2.1.1 Weight Control and Exercise-Monitoring Mobile Apps

Smartphone health applications can be a successful health-improvement plan. Several studies published in peer-reviewed journals have concluded higher health performance for mobile health app users relative to non-users, in comprehensive bibliographic research.[64] Diet, physical activity, health-improving, and overall quality of life were the most common themes. The purpose of these apps includes providing updates on one's health status and tracking individual health status or behavior changes.[64] Mobile health apps are now popular for a number of health-promoting behaviors including physical activity and weight management behaviors within the general population without disease (Figure 11.13).[64]

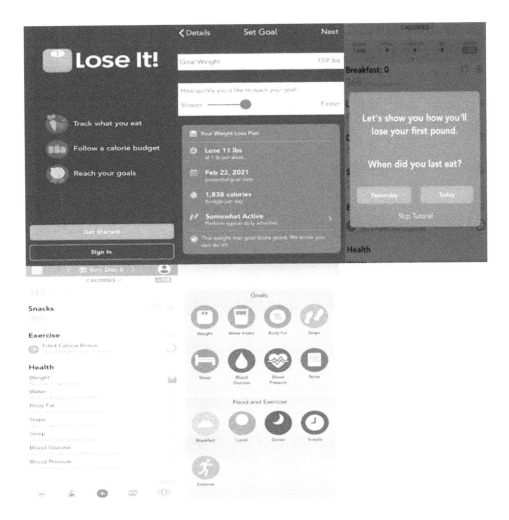

FIGURE 11.13 An example application for exercise-monitoring and weight control.

2.1.2 Liraglutide (Victoza® and Saxenda®) and Semaglutide (Ozempic) Injections

Obesity is a debilitating condition with few treatment options for pediatric patients. Liraglutide can be useful for weight management in adolescents and obese patients with type 2 diabetes. In addition to lifestyle therapy, obese children and young adults who use liraglutide (3.0 mg) can significantly reduce their BMI (Figure 11.14).[65]

During a 56-week clinical trial, one of four trials in the SCALE program, liraglutide 30 mg was found to decrease bodyweight and improve glucose metabolism.[66] Therefore, liraglutide 3.0 mg can have health-promoting benefits by minimizing the risk for diabetes in prediabetic obese people.[66] The three-year assessment of the SCALE Obesity and Prediabetes trial has a limitation—the withdrawing participants were not followed up on after they discontinued participating. More recently, once weekly semaglutide (Ozempic) have been approved for the treatment of type 2 diabetes and obesity in adults (Figure 11.14).[67]

2.2.0 Dyslipidemia

2.2.1 Evolocumab (PCSK9 Inhibitor) Pen

Proprotein convertase subtilisin/kexin type 9 (PCSK9) decreases the expression of LDL receptors on hepatic cells; hence, it boosts the plasma low-density lipoprotein cholesterol (LDL-C).[68] Evolocumab is a human monoclonal immunoglobulin G2 that binds specifically to human PCSK9, exhibiting nonlinear kinetics as a result, to reduce LDL-C within 11 to 17 days of effective half-life.[68] Evolocumab also reduces lipoprotein (a).[68] Evolocumab comes in two doses of 140 and 420 mg (Figure 11.15). The peak reduction of LDL-C takes place around 1 week after a subcutaneous dose of 140 mg every 2 weeks, and around 2 weeks after a dose of 420 mg once monthly, and it gradually returns to baseline over the doses' interval.[68] No dose adjustment is required and in a previous study no meaningful clinical differences were observed when using evolocumab alone or with other lipid-reducing agents such as statins.[68] Although, according to a systematic review and meta-analysis, PCSK9 inhibitors added to moderate-intensity to high-intensity statin therapy

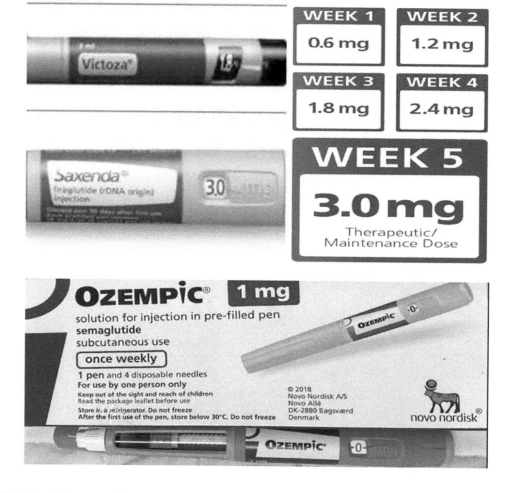

FIGURE 11.14   Liraglutide (Victoza® and Saxenda®) and semaglutide (Ozempic) injections.

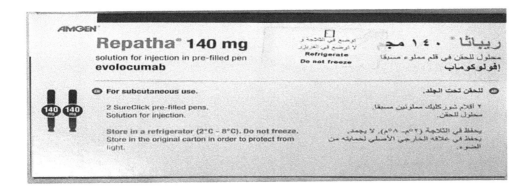

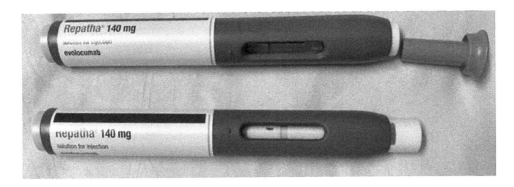

FIGURE 11.15 Evolocumab (PCSK9 inhibitor) pen.*

*When the orange cap is off, the pen is ready to be used for injection. When the yellow safety guard is pushed down and the yellow window appears, this means all the medicine (clear fluid) has been injected (injection is complete).

greatly decreases LDL-C in patients requiring further reduction in LDL-C and evolocumab has shown superiority over alirocumab.[69]

2.2.2 LDL Apheresis

Low-density lipoproteins (LDL) adsorption has many other antiatherosclerotic effects besides LDL elimination (Figure 11.16).[70] Lipoprotein apheresis inhibits the development of atherosclerosis in multiple ways and can improves atherogenic lipoprotein metabolism.[70] Selective LDL adsorption therapy could also eliminate cell adhesion molecules including intracellular adhesion molecule-1, vascular cell adhesion molecules, and coagulation factors including fibrinogen and thrombosis, and plasminogen activator inhibitor-1 as well as inflammatory cytokines.[71–75]

LDL adsorption removes the oxidized LDL in peripheral artery patients, which results in better and longer walking distance.[76] Lipoprotein apheresis was also found to remove vitronectin, micro (VLDL), heavy LDL, and apolipoprotein C-III, each of these have significant atherogenic effects in patients with familial hypercholesterolemia (FH); apolipoprotein C-III is the endogenous lipoprotein that facilitates the progression of atherosclerosis, and vitronectin is removed by apheresis independent from lipoproteins.[77–79] PCSK9, which acts as a key player in lipid metabolism in the liver, could also be removed

with LDL adsorption therapy.[80–83] Lipoprotein apheresis is quite effective at lowering Lp (a) concentrations, and when conducted weekly or biweekly, the mean interval concentrations are significantly reduced by 25%–40%.[70,84] Lipoprotein apheresis has been the most effective way to reduce LDL-C and prevent cardiovascular events in patients with severe FH. The latest lowering drug will now better control LDL-C levels than ever before.[70] Therefore, time will come to determine whether to avoid or decrease the frequency of LDL apheresis, particularly in patients with severe FH.

In 2019, The European Society of Cardiology (ESC) and European Atherosclerosis Society (EAS) released an updated guideline for managing dyslipidemias that target lipid-lowering in accordance with recent validated findings from large outcome trials.[85] The guideline recommended integrating different therapeutic models such as statin with ezetimibe and/or a PCSK9 inhibitor to achieve these new treatment targets.[85] They stated, "If needed, lipid apheresis can complement the medical armamentarium. Moreover, lipid apheresis remains the only approved treatment modality for lowering lipoprotein (a), however medical treatments are under current investigation."[85] Despite the advances in diabetes and kidney disease therapies, LDL apheresis can be useful in patients with diabetes mellitus, severe proteinuria, and dyslipidemia who have low renal prognosis.[86]

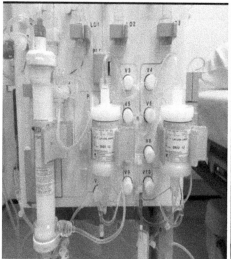
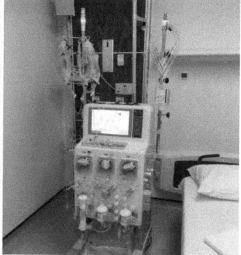

FIGURE 11.16   LDL apheresis machine.

2.3.0   Osteoporosis

2.3.1   Parathyroid Hormone (Teriparatide) Pen

Teriparatide is an accessible and widely used agent for increasing new bone formation repairing architectural flaws in the skeleton of osteoporotic patients (Figure 11.17).[87] Teriparatide greatly lowers the risk of vertebral and non-vertebral fractures in patients with osteoporosis.[88] Teriparatide promotes bone formation more than bone resorption, as shown by biochemical and histological studies.[87] It functions in two distinct ways: by stimulating bone formation on active remodeling sites (remodeling-based bone formation) and previously inactive bone surfaces (modeling-based bone formation).[87] The second is by an increase in the initiation of new remodeling sites. The two methods help to increase overall bone density and this is usually confirmed by bone density DEXA scan. Evidence shows that completing the whole 24-month continuous therapy of teriparatide results in better skeletal health compared to the shorter time span in osteoporosis patients who are at high risk of fractures.[87]

2.4.0   Contraception

2.4.1   Implanted Contraceptive Devices

Unintended pregnancies (UIP) have negative consequences for both women and the economy. The long-acting reversible contraceptives like intrauterine devices (IUDs) and subcutaneous implants are efficient ways in preventing UIPs (Figure 11.18a & 11.18b). Etonogestrel subdermal implants (ESI), levonorgestrel intrauterine system (LNG-IUS), copper intrauterine device (Cu-IUD), and depot medroxyprogesterone

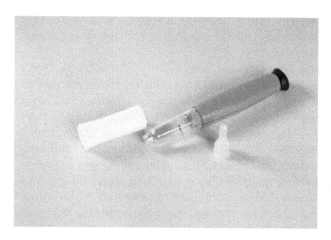

FIGURE 11.17A   Parathyroid hormone (teriparatide) pen

Source: www.shutterstock.com/image-photo/osteoporosis-injection-treatment-pen-injector-used-1205866246

www.shutterstock.com/image-photo/modern-syringe-needle-treatment-home-1595380495

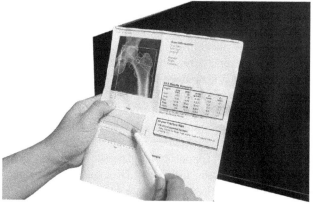

FIGURE 11.17B   Management plan to prevent fractures in a patient with osteoporosis (Reduced bone mass density of the femur and pelvic bone).

Source: www.shutterstock.com/image-photo/bmd-dexa-densitometry-hip-scan-osteopenia-1733642126

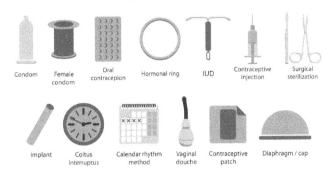

FIGURE 11.18A Different methods of contraception (mostly hormone-based).

Source: www.shutterstock.com/image-vector/pregnancy-icons-set-family-parenthood-contraception-256732030

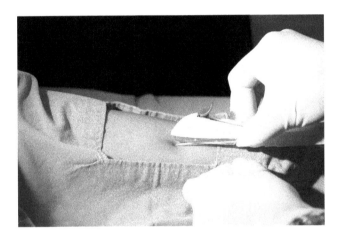

FIGURE 11.18B Insertion of contraceptive subdermal implant.

Source: www.shutterstock.com/image-photo/doctor-try-use-contraceptive-implant-on-668635678

acetate injections are among the instruments used for this purpose.[89] ESI is a scientifically safe and efficient form of contraception; however, lower continuation rates were observed after one year compared to the IUDs, often due to the disturbances in menstruation.[89] These devices require placement and withdrawal by an experienced professional.[90] Regular monitoring is always required to allow premature withdrawal, with immediate reversibility, in case of side effects or a wish to become pregnant.[89]

Conclusion and Future Recommendations

Technology has evolved exponentially over the last few decades, transforming our lives, often in a positive way; but it could also have drawbacks in some respects. The most common endocrine disorders such as diabetes and growth disorders are currently managed using simple and advanced medical devices. In order to achieve optimum therapeutic goals, knowing about current technology used

in the management of these conditions is essential. In addition, there are further ambitions for new technology such as sensor-augmented insulin and dual-hormone pumps to shape the future even better for our patients with diabetes. Furthermore, a future collaboration between health practitioners, health authorities, and pharmaceutical industries promises to improve care and protect the health of millions of people with diabetes and endocrine disorders around the globe.

REFERENCES

1. Paul S, Ali A, Katare R. Molecular complexities underlying the vascular complications of diabetes mellitus—a comprehensive review. J Diabetes Complications. 2020 Aug;34(8):107613. https://doi.org/10.1016/j.jdiacomp.2020.107613. Epub 2020 May 4. PMID: 32505477.

2. McCoy EK, Wright BM. A review of insulin pen devices. Postgrad Med. 2010 May;122(3):81–8. https://doi.org/10.3810/pgm.2010.05.2145. PMID: 20463417.

3. Shah RB, Patel M, Maahs DM, et al. Insulin delivery methods: past, present and future. Int J Pharm Investig. 2016;6(1):1–9. https://doi.org/10.4103/2230-973X.176456.

4. Giani E, Scaramuzza AE, Zuccotti GV. Impact of new technologies on diabetes care. World J Diabetes. 2015;6(8):999–1004. https://doi.org/10.4239/wjd.v6.i8.999.

5. Oyer D, Niemeyer M, Moses A. Empowering people with diabetes: improving perceptions and outcomes with technical advances in insulin pens. Postgrad Med. 2012;124(5):110–20.

6. Delvecchio M, Pastore C, Giordano P. Treatment options for MODY patients: a systematic review of literature. Diabetes Ther. 2020;11:1667–85. https://doi.org/10.1007/s13300-020-00864-4.

7. Da Costa S, Brackenridge B, Hicks D. A comparison of insulin pen use in the United States and the United Kingdom. Diabetes Educ. 2002 Jan–Feb;28(1):52–6, 59–60. https://doi.org/10.1177/014572170202800106. PMID: 11852744.

8. Bossi AC, Veronesi G, Poerio CS, et al. A prospective study for introducing insulin pens and safety needles in a hospital setting. The SANITHY study. Curr Diabetes Rev. 2016;12(4):460–7. https://doi.org/10.2174/1573399981166615 0806150210. PMID: 26245310; PMCID: PMC5112762.

9. Guerci B, Chanan N, Kaur S, et al. Lack of treatment persistence and treatment nonadherence as barriers to glycaemic control in patients with type 2 diabetes. Diabetes Ther. 2019;10:437–49. https://doi.org/10.1007/s13300-019-0590-x.

10. Miao R, Wei W, Lin J, et al. Does device make any difference? A real-world retrospective study of insulin treatment among elderly patients with Type 2 diabetes. J Diabetes Sci Technol. 2014;8(1):150–8. https://doi.org/10.1177/1932296 813516956.

11. Gnanalingham MG, Newland P, Smith CP. Accuracy and reproducibility of low dose insulin administration using pen-injectors and syringes. Arch Dis Child. 1998 Jul; 79(1):59–62.

12. Pfützner A, Bailey T, Campos C, et al. Accuracy and preference assessment of prefilled insulin pen versus vial and syringe with diabetes patients, caregivers, and healthcare professionals. Curr Med Res Opin. 2013 May; 29(5):475–81.

13. Ainscough LP, Ford JL, Morecroft CW, et al. Accuracy of intravenous and enteral preparations involving small volumes for paediatric use: a review. Eur J Hosp Pharm. 2018;25(2):66–71. https://doi.org/10.1136/ejhpharm-2016-001117.

14. American Diabetes Association. Insulin administration. Diabetes Care. 2004 Jan;27 Suppl 1:S106–9. https://doi.org/10.2337/diacare.27.2007.s106. PMID: 14693942.

15. ISO 11608-1:2012. Needle-based injection systems for medical use—requirements and test methods. Part 1: needle-based injection systems. Available from: www.iso.org.

16. Levemir® FlexTouch® instructions for use. Plainsboro, NJ: Novo Nordisk Inc.

17. Novolog® FlexTouch® instructions for use. Plainsboro, NJ: Novo Nordisk Inc.

18. Solbeck S, Nilsson CU, Engstrom M, et al. Dabigatran and its reversal with recombinant factor VIIa and prothrombin complex concentrate: a Sonoclot in vitro study. Scand J Clin Lab Invest. 2014;74(7):591–8.

19. Fiasp® FlexTouch® instructions for use. Plainsboro, NJ: Novo Nordisk Inc.

20. NovoLog® FlexPen® instructions for use. Plainsboro, NJ: Novo Nordisk Inc.

21. NovoLog® Mix 70/30 FlexPen® instructions for use. Plainsboro, NJ: Novo Nordisk Inc.

22. NNI. Novolin® 70/30 FlexPen® instructions for use. Plainsboro, NJ: Novo Nordisk Inc.

23. Novolin® R FlexPen® instructions for use. Plainsboro, NJ: Novo Nordisk Inc.

24. Novolin® N FlexPen® instructions for use. Plainsboro, NJ: Novo Nordisk Inc.

25. Lantus® prescribing information. Bridgewater, NJ: Sanofi US; July 2015.

26. Apidra® prescribing information. Bridgewater, NJ: Sanofi US; Feb 2015.

27. Toujeo® prescribing information. Bridgewater, NJ: Sanofi US; Mar 2019.

28. Humalog® prescribing information. Indianapolis, IN: Lilly USA, LLC; Nov 2015.

29. Humalog® Mix 75/25 prescribing information. Indianapolis, IN: Lilly USA, LLC; Feb 2015.

30. Humalog® Mix 50/50 prescribing information. Indianapolis, IN: Lilly USA, LLC; Feb 2015.

31. Humulin® 70/30 KwikPen® instructions for use. Indianapolis, IN: Lilly USA, LLC; Mar 2015.

32. Humulin® N KwikPen®. Indianapolis, IN: Lilly USA, LLC; Mar 2015.

33. Humalog® U200 KwikPen® instructions for use. Indianapolis, IN: Lilly USA, LLC; May 2015.

34. Basaglar® KwikPen® instructions for use. Indianapolis, IN: Eli Lilly and Company.

35. Humulin® R U500 KwikPen® instructions for use. Indianapolis, IN: Eli Lilly and Company.

36. Khan AM, Alswat KA. Benefits of using the i-Port system on insulin-treated patients. Diabetes Spectr. 2019 Feb;32(1):30–5. https://doi.org/10.2337/ds18-0015. PMID: 30853762; PMCID: PMC6380230.

37. Pickup JC. Is insulin pump therapy effective in Type 1 diabetes? Diabet Med. 2019 Mar;36(3):269–78. https://doi.org/10.1111/dme.13793. Epub 2018 Aug 29. PMID: 30098219.

38. American association of Diabetes Educators. Updated insulin pump comparisons and reviews. Diabetes Education Accreditation Program. Available from: https://integrateddiabetes.com/updated-insulin-pump-comparisons-and-reviews/.

39. Fowler MJ. Diabetes devices. Clin Diabetes. 2008 Jul;26(3):130–3. https://doi.org/10.2337/diaclin.26.3.130.

40. American Diabetes Association. Standards of medical care in diabetes—2008 [Position Statement]. Diabetes Care. 2008;31(Suppl. 1):S12–54.

41. Welschen LM, Bloemendal E, Nijpels G, et al. Self-monitoring of blood glucose in patients with type 2 diabetes who are not using insulin: a systematic review. Diabetes Care. 2005;28:1510–17.

42. Davis WA, Bruce DG, Davis TM. Does self-monitoring of blood glucose improve outcome in type 2 diabetes? The Fremantle Diabetes Study. Diabetologia. 2007;50:510–15.

43. Guerci B, Drouin P, Grange V, et al. Self-monitoring of blood glucose significantly improves metabolic control in patients with type 2 diabetes mellitus: the Auto-Surveillance Intervention Active (ASIA) study. Diabetes Metab. 2003;29:587–94.

44. Weitgasser R, Hofmann M, Gappmayer B, et al. New, small, fast-acting blood glucose meters—an analytical laboratory evaluation. Swiss Med Wkly. 2007;137:536–40.

45. Fink KS, Christensen DB, Ellsworth A. Effect of high altitude on blood glucose meter performance. Diabetes Technol Ther. 2002;4:627–35.

46. Thomas LE, Kane MP, Bakst G, et al. A glucose meter accuracy and precision comparison: the FreeStyle Flash versus the Accu-Chek Advantage, Accu-Chek Compact Plus, Ascensia Contour, and the BD Logic. Diabetes Technol Ther. 2008;10:102–10.

47. Heinemann L. Continuous Glucose Monitoring (CGM) or Blood Glucose Monitoring (BGM): interactions and implications. J Diabetes Sci Technol. 2018;12(4):873–9. https://doi.org/10.1177/1932296818768834.

48. Campos-Náñez E, Fortwaengler K, Breton MD. Clinical impact of blood glucose monitoring accuracy: an in-silico study. J Diabetes Sci Technol. 2017;11:1187–95.

49. Tanenbaum, M. Diabetes device use in adults with Type 1 diabetes: barriers to uptake and potential intervention targets. Diabetes Care. 2017 Feb;40(2):181–7.

50. Halford J. Determining clinical and psychological benefits and barriers with continuous glucose monitoring therapy. Diabetes Technol Ther. 2010:12(3). https://doi.org/10.1089/dia.2009.0121.

51. Wong J. Real-time continuous glucose monitoring among participants in the T1D exchange clinic registry. Diabetes Care. 2014. https://doi.org/10.2337/dc14-0303, Supplementary Data, Table 3.

52. McQueen R. Frequency of continuous glucose monitoring use and change in hemoglobin A1c for adults with Type 1 diabetes in a clinical practice setting. Endocr Pract. 2014. https://doi.org/10.4158/EP14027.OR.

53. De Block C. A review of current evidence with continuous glucose monitoring in patients with diabetes. J Diabetes Sci Technol. 2008;2(4):718–27.

54. DeSalvo D. Continuous glucose monitoring: current use and future directions. Curr Diab Rep. 2013 Oct;13(5):657–62.

55. Ives B. Practical aspects of real-time continuous glucose monitors: the experience of the Yale children's diabetes program. Diabetes Educ. 2010;36(1):53–62. https://doi.org/10.1177/0145721709352010.

56. Szypowska A. Beneficial effect of real-time continuous glucose monitoring system on glycemic control in Type 1 diabetic patients: systematic review and meta-analysis of randomized trials. Eur J Endocrinol. 2012;166:567–74.

57. Rosenfeld RG, Bakker B. Compliance and persistence in pediatric and adult patients receiving growth hormone therapy. Endocr Pract. 2008 Mar;14(2):143–54. https://doi.org/10.4158/EP.14.2.143. PMID: 18308651.

58. Mauras N, Attie KM, Reiter EO, et al. High dose recombinant human growth hormone (GH) treatment of GH-deficient patients in puberty increases near-final height: a randomized, multicenter trial. J Clin Endocrinol Metab. 2000;85:3653–60.

59. Dahlgren J. Easypod: a new electronic injection device for growth hormone. Expert Rev Med Devices. 2008 May;5(3):297–304. https://doi.org/10.1586/17434440.5.3.297. PMID: 18452378.

60. Kappor RR, Bruke SA, Sparrow SE et al. Monitoring of concordance in growth hormone therapy. Arch Dis Child. 2008 Feb;93(2):147–8.

61. Rosenfeld RG, Bakker B. Compliance and persistence in pediatric and adult patients receiving growth hormone therapy. Endocr Pract. 2008 Mar;14(2):143–54. https://doi.org/10.4158/EP.14.2.143. PMID: 18308651.

62. Bozzola M, Colle M, Halldin-Stenlid M, et al. Treatment adherence with the easypod™ growth hormone electronic auto-injector and patient acceptance: survey results from 824 children and their parents. BMC Endocr Disord. 2011 Feb 4;11:4. https://doi.org/10.1186/1472-6823-11-4. PMID: 21294891; PMCID: PMC3045978.

63. Norgren S. Adherence remains a challenge for patients receiving GH therapy. Pediatr Endocrinol Rev. 2009 Jun;6 Suppl 4:545–8.

64. Lee M, Lee H, Kim Y, et al. Mobile app-based health promotion programs: a systematic review of the literature. Int J Environ Res Public Health. 2018 Dec 13;15(12):2838. https://doi.org/10.3390/ijerph15122838. PMID: 30551555; PMCID: PMC6313530.

65. Kelly AS, Auerbach P, Barrientos-Perez M, et al. A randomized, controlled trial of liraglutide for adolescents with obesity. N Engl J Med. 2020 May 28;382(22):2117–28. https://doi.org/10.1056/NEJMoa1916038. Epub 2020 Mar 31. PMID: 32233338.

66. le Roux CW, Astrup A, Fujioka K, et al. 3 years of liraglutide versus placebo for type 2 diabetes risk reduction and weight management in individuals with prediabetes: a randomised, double-blind trial. Lancet. 2017 Apr 8;389(10077):1399–409. https://doi.org/10.1016/S0140-6736(17)30069-7. Epub 2017 Feb 23. Erratum in: Lancet. 2017 Apr 8;389(10077):1398. PMID: 28237263.

67. Davies M, Færch L, Jeppesen OK, et al. Semaglutide 2·4 mg once a week in adults with overweight or obesity, and type 2 diabetes (STEP 2): a randomised, double-blind, double-dummy, placebo-controlled, phase 3 trial. Lancet. 2021 Mar 13;397(10278):971–84. https://doi.org/10.1016/S0140-6736(21)00213-0. Epub 2021 Mar 2. PMID: 33667417.

68. Kasichayanula S, Grover A, Emery MG, et al. Clinical pharmacokinetics and pharmacodynamics of evolocumab, a PCSK9 inhibitor. Clin Pharmacokinet. 2018 Jul;57(7):769–79. https://doi.org/10.1007/s40262-017-0620-7. PMID: 29353350; PMCID: PMC5999140.

69. Toth PP, Worthy G, Gandra SR, et al. Systematic review and network meta-analysis on the efficacy of evolocumab and other therapies for the management of lipid levels in hyperlipidemia. J Am Heart Assoc. 2017 Oct 2;6(10):e005367. https://doi.org/10.1161/JAHA.116.005367. PMID: 28971955; PMCID: PMC5721820.

70. Makino H, Koezuka R, Tamanaha T, et al. Familial Hypercholesterolemia and Lipoprotein Apheresis. J Atheroscler Thromb. 2019 Aug 1;26(8):679–87. https://doi.org/10.5551/jat.RV17033. Epub 2019 Jun 22. PMID: 31231083; PMCID: PMC6711846.

71. Sampietro T, Tuoni M, Ferdeghini M, et al. Plasma cholesterol regulates soluble cell adhesion molecule expression in familial hypercholesterolemia. Circulation. 1997;96:1381–5.

72. Utsumi K, Kawabe M, Hirama A, et al. Effects of selective LDL apheresis on plasma concentrations of ICAM-1, VCAM-1 and P-selectin in diabetic patients with arteriosclerosis obliterans and receiving maintenance hemodialysis. Clin Chim Acta. 2007;377:198–200.

73. Hovland A, Hardersen R, Nielsen EW, et al. Hematologic and hemostatic changes induced by different columns during LDL apheresis. J Clin Apher. 2010;25:294–300.

74. Hara T, Kiyomoto H, Hitomi H, et al. Low-density lipoprotein apheresis for haemodialysis patients with peripheral arterial disease reduces reactive oxygen species production via suppression of NADPH oxidase gene expression in leucocytes. Nephrol Dial Transplant. 2009;24:3818–25.

75. Tamai O, Matsuoka H, Itabe H, et al. Single LDL apheresis improves endotheliumdependent vasodilatation in hypercholesterolemic humans. Circulation. 1997;95:76–82.

76. Tamura K, Tsurumi-Ikeya Y, Wakui H, et al. Therapeutic potential of low-density lipoprotein apheresis in the management of peripheral artery disease in patients with chronic kidney disease. Ther Apher Dial. 2013;17:185–92.

77. Makino H, Tamanaha T, Harada-Shiba M. LDL apheresis in Japan. Transfus Apher Sci. 2017;56:677–81.

78. Yuasa Y, Osaki T, Makino H, et al. Proteomic analysis of proteins eliminated by low-density lipoprotein apheresis. Ther Apher Dial. 2014;18:93–102.

79. Sathiyakumar V, Kapoor K, Jones SR, et al. Novel therapeutic targets for managing dyslipidemia. Trends Pharmacol Sci. 2018;39:733–47.

80. Tavori H, Giunzioni I, Linton MF, et al. Loss of plasma proprotein convertase subtilisin/kexin 9 (PCSK9) after lipoprotein apheresis. Circ Res. 2013;113:1290–5.

81. Hori M, Ishihara M, Yuasa Y, et al. Removal of plasma mature and furincleaved proprotein convertase subtilisin/kexin 9 by lowdensity lipoprotein-apheresis in familial hypercholesterolemia: development and application of a new assay for PCSK9. J Clin Endocrinol Metab. 2015;100:E41–E49.

82. Lambert G, Charlton F, Rye KA, et al. Molecular basis of PCSK9 function. Atherosclerosis. 2009;203:1–7.

83. Tang Z, Jiang L, Peng J, et al. PCSK9 siRNA suppresses the inflammatory response induced by oxLDL through inhibition of NF-kappaB activation in THP-1-derived macrophages. Int J Mol Med. 2012;30:931–8.

84. Waldmann E, Parhofer KG. Lipoprotein apheresis to treat elevated lipoprotein (a). J Lipid Res. 2016;57:1751–7.

85. Rogacev KS, Laufs U. Lipid-Management 2020—medikamentöse Therapie und Lipidapherese im Kontext [Lipid

management 2020—medical therapy and lipid apheresis in context]. Dtsch Med Wochenschr. 2020 Apr;145(7):464–9. German. https://doi.org/10.1055/a-0887-0595. Epub 2020 Apr 1. PMID: 32236927.

86. Wada T, Hara A, Muso E, et al. Effects of LDL apheresis on proteinuria in patients with diabetes mellitus, severe proteinuria, and dyslipidemia. Clin Exp Nephrol. 2021 Jan;25(1):1–8. https://doi.org/10.1007/s10157-020-01959-9. Epub 2020 Aug 28. PMID: 32857255.

87. Lindsay R, Krege JH, Marin F, et al. Teriparatide for osteoporosis: importance of the full course. Osteoporos Int. 2016 Aug;27(8):2395–410. https://doi.org/10.1007/s00198-016-3534-6. Epub 2016 Feb 22. PMID: 26902094; PMCID: PMC4947115.

88. Fan G, Zhao Q, Lu P, et al. Comparison between teriparatide and bisphosphonates for improving bone mineral density in postmenopausal osteoporosis patients: a meta-analysis. Medicine (Baltimore). 2020 Apr;99(15):e18964. https://doi.org/10.1097/MD.0000000000018964. PMID: 32282692; PMCID: PMC7220409.

89. Moray KV, Chaurasia H, Sachin O, et al. A systematic review on clinical effectiveness, side-effect profile and meta-analysis on continuation rate of etonogestrel contraceptive implant. Reprod Health. 2021 Jan 6;18(1):4. https://doi.org/10.1186/s12978-020-01054-y. PMID: 33407632; PMCID: PMC7788930.

90. Raccah-Tebeka B, Plu-Bureau G. Contraceptions de longue durée d'action réversibles [Long-acting reversible contraception]. Rev Prat. 2018 Apr;68(4):387–91. French. PMID: 30869384.

12 Medical Devices for Cardiology

Sowndramalingam Sankaralingam, Farhat Naz Hussain, and Ahmed Awaisu

CONTENTS

DOI: 10.1201/9781003002345-14

GENERAL INTRODUCTION AND CHAPTER OVERVIEW

Cardiovascular diseases (CVDs) are a group of disorders of the heart and blood vessels, comprising arteriosclerosis, coronary heart disease, cerebrovascular disease, rheumatic heart disease, aortic aneurysm, heart valve diseases, arrhythmias, heart failure, and others.[1,2] CVDs are a leading cause of morbidity and mortality worldwide with a projected substantial increase over the next decades.[1,2] According to the World Health Organization (WHO), about 17.5 million people die of CVDs annually. The use of medical devices plays an increasingly important role in the prevention, diagnosis, treatment, or rehabilitation procedures of CVDs. There is a wide range of cardiovascular diagnostic and therapeutic devices in contemporary clinical practice. Healthcare providers, including pharmacists, must be familiar with these devices, depending on their scope of practice, practice setting, and specialization. Access to a heart healthcare facility is a challenge in many developing countries due to financial constraints, poor facilities and infrastructure, and limited number of practicing cardiologists in hospitals.[3]

This chapter aims to provide an insight into the purpose, operation procedures, evidence of effectiveness, and important safety considerations for different cardiology devices commonly used in clinical practice. These include, but are not restricted to, sphygmomanometers and other blood pressure monitors, artificial heart valves, and some radiological investigation devices used in cardiology (e.g., electrocardiogram, echocardiogram, angiogram, X-rays, etc.).

BLOOD PRESSURE MONITORING DEVICES

BACKGROUND

Blood pressure (BP) is a vital sign and is one of the most commonly measured parameters in individuals visiting a healthcare facility.[4] BP is created by stretching of the arterial wall during the flow of blood with every cardiac cycle. In 2017, the Global Burden of Disease study found that high levels of systolic BP (SBP) were the leading modifiable risk factor for death globally.[5] Almost 10.4 million deaths were attributed to raised SBP annually. In addition, elevated SBP contributes to about 53–55% of the incidence of ischemic heart disease (IHD).[5] Moreover, among middle-aged individuals, reduction of SBP by only 2 mmHg could result in significant reductions in death due to stroke and IHD or other vascular causes by 7% and 10%, respectively.[6] Hypertension is a leading risk factor for cardiovascular diseases (CVD)s, including coronary artery disease (CAD), heart failure (HF), chronic kidney disease (CKD), stroke, heart attack, peripheral vascular disease. Therefore, it is essential to understand the devices used to measure BP and how to use them appropriately.

A BP device or monitor is also known as a sphygmomanometer. This chapter will discuss the various types of devices available to measure BP, the technology behind each one of them, and the techniques of BP measurement. BP devices can be classified as manual and digital or electronic devices. The manual devices include the mercury sphygmomanometer that is used as a reference standard and the aneroid sphygmomanometer. The auscultatory technique is used to measure BP using these devices. The digital or electronic devices are automated to measure BP. We will also discuss the types of BP cuffs and how they impact BP.

PURPOSE OF USE AND IMPORTANT FEATURES

BP is one of the vital signs and is therefore commonly measured on almost all individuals visiting a healthcare facility.[4,7] It is therefore essential for all healthcare providers including pharmacists to know the different devices, technologies, and techniques to measure BP. From a pharmacist point of view, accurate measurement of BP is essential to diagnose, and to guide treatment decisions, including when to start medications and when to adjust the dose. Inaccurate BP measurements can result in underdiagnosis and therefore complications or unnecessary treatment when not indicated.

Overview of Uses (Medical Conditions That They Help Treat/Diagnose)

The main use of a sphygmomanometer is to non-invasively measure BP.[8] It is used to diagnose high BP known as hypertension or to identify hypotension characterized by low BP, and to monitor response to therapy. In addition, it is also used to obtain an ankle-brachial index to determine peripheral arterial disease. Digital or electronic BP monitors are commonly used to perform home monitoring of blood pressure (HBPM), which is also known to be managed by pharmacists.

Description of Device Features

We will discuss three types of BP devices to monitor BP. The first one is the mercury sphygmomanometer; the second is the aneroid sphygmomanometer, and the third is a digital or electronic BP monitor. While the first two require manual techniques of BP measurement by the healthcare provider, the measurement of BP by the third digital or electronic monitor is automated.

The mercury manometer is the standard sphygmomanometer used to measure BP in clinics and hospitals[8–10] (Figure 12.1). It is also used as a gold standard reference device to calibrate other BP devices. It consists of a mercury column that rises within a glass chamber upon application of pressure using a bulb. The chamber is connected to a cuff that contains the bladder which gets filled with air upon inflation using the bulb that has a valve to control deflation of the cuff. The auscultatory technique is used to assess BP using this device which is discussed in the next section. The advantage of this device is that it does not require calibration and can be used readily as long as the meniscus is at 0 mmHg before each use. However, due to concerns of mercury contamination,[11] this device is being replaced by aneroid or digital automated BP devices in both clinics and hospitals.[12]

The aneroid sphygmomanometer has replaced the auscultatory mercury manometer in clinics and healthcare settings.[13] This is primarily due to environmental concerns of mercury in the manual mercury sphygmomanometers.

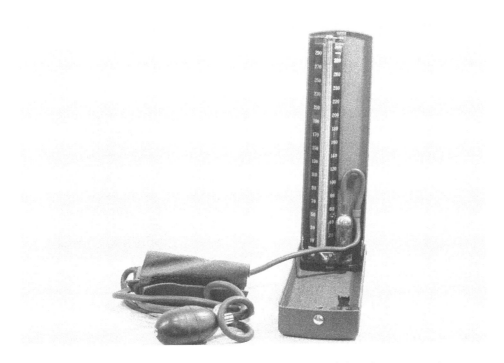

FIGURE 12.1   A mercury sphygmomanometer, a manual mercury BP device consisting of a mercury column, connected to the cuff that is inflated by a bulb-and-valve mechanism.

Source: https://image.shutterstock.com/image-photo/blood-pressure-cuff-called-sphygmomanometer-600w-692330830.jpg

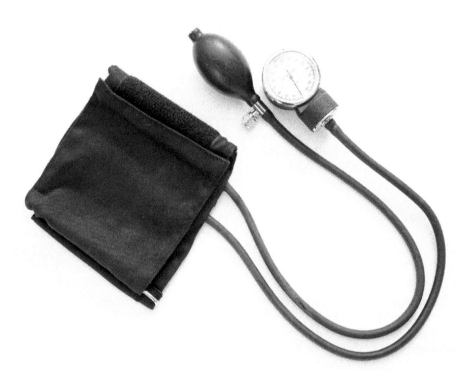

FIGURE 12.2 An aneroid sphygmomanometer, a manual BP device consisting of a calibrated dial connected to the cuff that is inflated by a bulb-and-valve mechanism.

Source: https://image.shutterstock.com/image-photo/hypertension-control-blood-pressure-measure-600w-1806966802.jpg

However, the digital or electronic BP monitor has also replaced the mercury manometers and are described in the next section. The aneroid manometer works on the same principle as the mercury manometer, except that instead of a mercury column it has an aneroid gauge that consists of a calibrated dial with a needle[8] (Figure 12.2). The needle moves like a watch connected to a compression cuff that is regulated by a bulb and a valve. When pressure is applied, movement of bellows rotates a gear-like part that turns the needle to indicate the pressure.

The digital or electronic BP monitor is a popular and widely available fully-automatic monitor that measures BP automatically without the need to manually inflate or deflate the cuff using a bulb and valve (Figure 12.3). The amplitude of oscillations in the lateral wall of the arm or limb as appropriate is estimated and BP readings are displayed according to a predetermined algorithm developed and set by the device manufacturer.[8,9] Simply, pressing a button or turning on a switch is sufficient to measure BP. The device is programmed by the manufacturer's algorithm to automatically determine inflation pressure, inflate, and deflate. The SBP, diastolic BP (DBP), and heart/pulse rate are displayed on the monitor screen.[12]

A modified and advanced form of digital BP monitor is used to serve as an automated office BP (AOBP) monitor.[8,14] This device is programmed to measure BP multiple times automatically during an encounter at predetermined intervals of 1–2 minutes. Once the BP cuff is applied and the device turned on, the observer will make sure the device functions normally during the first reading and will leave the patient or subject in a quiet room alone. The device measures BP 3–5 times and provides all individual readings as well as the average of all readings. This type of device is said to eliminate the "white-coat" effect, which is characterized by increased BP of an individual in a physician's office but lower BP at home. The average of the readings from this device correlates highly with awake ambulatory BP readings, which will be discussed next.

Another advanced type of digital monitor is the ambulatory BP monitor (ABPM) which is designed to measure BP over a 24-hour period during day and night at set intervals[8,15] (Figure 12.4). The 24-hour ABPM is the gold standard method for the diagnosis of hypertension and is also known to eliminate the "white-coat" effect. The device includes the monitor, the cuff, and the tubing. When the patient visits the healthcare provider, the device is programmed and is

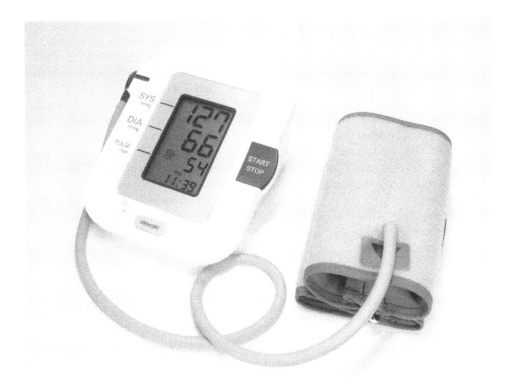

FIGURE 12.3   A d**igital blood pressure device,** an oscillometric automated BP device that is connected to a cuff and displays systolic and diastolic blood pressures and pulse rate.

Source: https://image.shutterstock.com/image-photo/modern-blood-pressure-monitor-cuff-600w-48115891.jpg

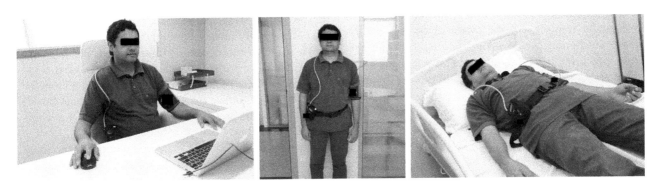

FIGURE 12.4   An ambulatory BP monitor (ABPM), a digital BP device that is programmed to measure BP at set intervals during the day and night for 24 hours.

applied on the patient as follows. The monitor is worn in the waist using the belt provided. A tube from the monitor runs behind the back around the side of the neck into the cuff on the arm on the opposite side. The cuff is designed differently with a sleeve-like pouch through which the arm is introduced and the cuff is wrapped around. Usually, BP is measured every 15 minutes during the day and every 30 minutes during the night and the output provides average values for day, night, and for the entire 24-hour duration.

A new type of digital or electronic BP monitor, known as the inflationary non-invasive blood pressure (iNIBP) device, is also available.[16] This device measures both SBP and DBP during inflation itself and has been shown to reduce pain and time taken to measure BP.

While in the foregoing section we have discussed the types of BP devices, it is also important to note that each of these devices should be used in conjunction with appropriately sized cuffs. In general, the width of the bladder should cover at least 40% of arm circumference and the length of the bladder should cover 80% of arm circumference.[8,17,18] Therefore, cuffs are available in various sizes from sizes for neonates to sizes for large adults. In addition, the type of cuff affects BP readings. Cuffs can be classified as one-piece and two-piece cuffs.[18] One-piece cuffs are the cuffs recently available that are provided along with digital devices in which the cuff itself inflates. On the other hand, the classical two-piece Baum® cuff contains a bladder within the cuff. The one-piece cuff is observed to provide lower BP readings compared to the standard two-piece cuffs.

In the next section, we will discuss the two techniques of non-invasive BP measurement; namely, manual auscultatory and the oscillometric methods.

Overview of Results Shown

Manual mercury or aneroid sphygmomanometers provide patient data on SBP and DBP only. However, the automated electronic devices that are oscillometric provide SBP and DBP as well as pulse rate. The disadvantage of using the automated oscillometric devices is that, in patients with atrial fibrillation, some of them do not provide BP readings at all (error message), while others are not accurate in measuring BP.[19,20] As indicated before, the 24-hour ABPM provides a 24-hour mean BP, as well as awake and nighttime BP readings that are used in the diagnosis of hypertension.

How to Operate/Use

While it is important to know how to operate the device, it is equally important to be aware of device quality, patient positioning, and other important precautions before measuring BP. BP should be measured using a calibrated and/or validated device.[8,19] Calibration of manual BP devices is important to ensure accuracy of measurement. BP devices are validated by organizations such as the American Heart Association (AHA), European Society of Hypertension (ESH), or British Hypertension Society (BHS). Validated devices are tested for accuracy and hence are most suitable for BP measurements. Unvalidated devices tend to be less accurate.[21] Mercury devices do not need calibration as long as the meniscus is at level 0 mmHg before beginning BP measurement. Aneroid devices may require calibration once every 6 months.[9,22] Digital or electronic devices need calibration and can be done only by the manufacturer. It is important to use validated digital monitors to ensure accuracy to provide the best evidence-based clinical care.

BP should be measured in a quiet room under comfortable temperature conditions.[8,12] The patient should not have smoked, had beverages containing caffeine, or exercised within the last 30 minutes. Upon arrival at a healthcare facility, the patient should relax for about 5 minutes before BP is taken. Patient should be seated comfortably with back supported, feet flat on the floor (no crossing of legs), and arm

supported at the level of the heart, and should not be talking during or in between measurements. An appropriately sized cuff should be used.[8,18,23] The width of the bladder should cover at least 40% of arm circumference and length of the bladder should cover at least 80% of arm circumference. The arterial index of the cuff should be in alignment with the location of the brachial artery. The lower border of the cuff should be at least 1 inch above the fold at the cubital fossa. At initial visit, BP should be measured from both arms and the arm with higher BP should be used for future measurements.

There are two techniques/methods to measure BP.[8,18] The auscultatory method is used to measure BP using the mercury or aneroid sphygmomanometers. The procedures for measuring BP are the same except that in the mercury manometer, the BP readings are observed in a mercury column, while in the case of aneroid manometer, the BP readings are measured on an aneroid dial with a pointer (or a needle). The oscillometric method is used in automated devices to measure BP without the need for auscultation for Korotkoff sounds.

Auscultatory Method of BP Measurement

It is important to ensure that the healthcare provider measuring BP has very good auditory and visual acuity, and manual dexterity to inflate and deflate the bulb.[12] This technique is ideally performed in a quiet room or room with little ambient noise, using a good-quality stethoscope. To perform the auscultatory method of BP measurement, first perform the palpatory method to determine maximal inflation pressure.[8,12] Once the cuff is applied to the arm, inflate the cuff, initially rapidly up to about 60 mmHg and then slowly in increments of about 10 mmHg while palpating the radial pulse. The pressure at which the radial pulse is obliterated is then determined. Now, deflate the cuff and wait for 1 minute. Then, inflate the cuff as described, about 20–30 mmHg above the pressure at which radial pulse was obliterated. Then, slowly deflate at about 2–4 mmHg per second, noting the pressure in mercury column. At the same time, listen to the low-pitched Korotkoff sounds using the bell of the stethoscope.[24] The onset of clear tapping sound (K1) known as Phase 1 sounds corresponds to the SBP. The last audible sound (K5) at which Korotkoff sounds disappear corresponds to the DBP. Occasionally, K5 will not be heard or will be heard at very low pressure levels. In such instances, the point at which the Korotkoff sound is muffled (K4) should be used as the DBP.[12] Using the manual method, the SBP and DBP are recorded to the nearest even number.

Oscillometric Method of BP Measurement

These devices are automated to measure SBP, DBP, and pulse rate.[8,12,25] The precautions listed previously and patient positioning should be taken into consideration. Upon application of the cuff, a button or switch is turned on. The cuff is automatically inflated, the maximal inflation pressure is determined, and is slowly deflated to provide SBP, DBP, and pulse rate. If it is necessary to repeat, then at least 1 minute of rest period must be provided before initiating measurement again. The cuff should be removed promptly.

Along with description of the AOBP and ABPM, the procedure of performing BP measurements is briefly described and therefore are not explained here.

EVIDENCE FOR EFFECTIVENESS

Brief Literature Review of Benefits/Advantages

One of the areas where assessment of BP has been shown to have advantages is in HBPM. A number of BP devices are available and sold in community pharmacies. Thus, pharmacists along with physicians may recommend and manage patients to monitor BP at home. Firstly, HBPM can aid in the diagnosis of hypertension especially among patients with "white-coat hypertension."[17] Second, HBPM has been shown to improve BP control and result in improved clinical outcomes.[26,27]

Economic Evaluations

Studies have shown that hypertension is the costliest of all CVDs. Individuals with hypertension have about $2,000 higher healthcare expenditure annually compared to non-hypertensive individuals.[28] A study assessed the roles of pharmacists on management of hypertension through medication therapy management (MTM). Compared with no MTM, the MTM clinic was cost-effective and achieved an incremental cost-effectiveness ratio of $38,798 per quality-adjusted life year (QALY) gained.[29]

IMPORTANT SAFETY ISSUES

When measuring BP non-invasively using a cuff, generally, there are no contraindications. During measurement of BP, when the cuff is fully inflated to obliterate arterial pulse, the venous drainage along with lymphatic drainage is also reduced. Therefore, one must avoid measuring BP in a limb that has lymphedema, or an arterial or venous cannula inserted, or with paresis or paralysis of limbs.

Adverse Effects Associated with Use

Measuring BP non-invasively following proper technique does not cause any adverse effects. However, measuring BP repeatedly or frequently in some individuals may cause discomfort or pain in upper limbs and some redness due to effect of cuff. Rarely, Rumpel-Leede (RL) phenomenon, known as acute dermis capillary rupture characterized by appearance of petechiae in the area of cuff application, can occur in patients with diabetes mellitus and hypertension, which usually resolves spontaneously within 10 days.[30] In some individuals with a latex allergy, use of cuff that is made of latex can cause rash or other allergic reactions.

STORAGE CONDITIONS AND MAINTENANCE

Manual BP monitors can be stored continuously at ambient temperature of 0–50°C and 15–90% relative humidity. These devices can be operated continuously in ambient temperature of 10–40°C and 15–90% relative humidity.[12] The digital or electronic BP monitors can be stored within a wide range of temperatures between –20°C to +60 °C and relative humidity of 10–95%, depending on the precautions and advice given in the user manual by each particular manufacturer.

IMPLICATIONS TO THE PHARMACY PROFESSION AND PRACTICE

Pharmacists, including community and hospital (clinical) pharmacists, are known to be involved in the MTM of hypertension. Their roles range from refilling prescriptions, assessing BP, and initiating antihypertensive therapy, to modification and monitoring of drug therapy. A recent systematic review of 35 studies has shown that pharmacist management of hypertension led to significant improvement in BP and medication adherence.[31]

CONCLUSION

BP devices are classified as mercury, aneroid, and digital or electronic devices. While the former two require the manual auscultatory method of BP measurement, the digital devices are automated to measure BP. BP devices are primarily used to measure BP, a vital sign. They are used to diagnose hypertension and monitor response to pharmacologic and nonpharmacologic therapy. The cuff application should be performed with caution in individuals allergic to the material of cuff and care must be taken to completely deflate the cuff between repeat measurements at intervals of at least 1 minute.

RADIOGRAPHIC FLUOROSCOPIC SYSTEM: X-RAY

BACKGROUND

The most important imaging service in the frontline of medical care is plain radiography. This section will provide a brief overview of application of radiography and its safety in cardiology. Radiography is considered one of the oldest imaging approaches used in diagnostic radiology and simply refers to the use of X-rays to generate images.[32] Terms such as plain film, conventional radiograph, and radiograph are commonly used to describe X-ray. Although projectional radiography may sometimes also refer to CT scan, fluoroscopy on the other hand is an application of projectional radiography that allows real-time observation of the internal structures of a patient.[32] X-ray has been discussed in more details in other chapters, particularly medical devices for respiratory and musculoskeletal conditions.

In particular, radiographic fluoroscopy is a type of medical imaging that shows a continuous X-ray image on a monitor, much like an X-ray movie.[33] An X-ray beam is passed through the body of the patient, during a fluoroscopy procedure. Consequently, the image is transmitted to a monitor such that the movement of the body part or contrast agent through the body can be visualized in detail. In this section, we will summarize the principle of operation of radiographic-fluoroscopic technology, evidence of effectiveness, important safety considerations, and application in cardiology.

PURPOSE OF USE AND IMPORTANT FEATURES

Overview of Uses

Radiographic-fluoroscopic system technology is effective and finds wide application in the diagnosis of several diseases including arthrography, bronchography, gastrointestinal studies, locating ingested foreign material, and diagnosis of congestive heart failure and ischemia. It is predominantly used in interventional radiology, gastrointestinal imaging, and musculoskeletal radiology. It is not within the scope of this chapter to describe the technology and physics of the radiographic-fluoroscopic system or the conventional X-ray tube in details. Nevertheless, we provide a brief description to help the reader and the user in conceptualizing the device.

Device Description and Important Features

Typically, this device (Figure 12.5) consists of a combination of a patient support unit (a table base and a movable table-top), an over- or under-table X-ray tube and holder, X-ray generators, a spot film device, radiation shields, an image intensifier, a film tray, an overhead X-ray tube and a ceiling support, and a control panel.[34]

The modern X-ray tube (Figure 12.6) is an evacuated chamber, containing cathode and anode electrodes, across which an electric potential is applied. The cathode contains a metal filament such as tungsten that is heated, releasing electrons through thermionic emission. The electric potential applied between the cathode and the anode draws the electrons toward the anode, thereby striking the anode disk, generating X-rays and a large amount of heat. The energy of the generated X-rays largely depends on the speed of the electrons as they migrate through the electrodes. On the other hand, the speed of the electrons depends on the strength of the electric potential between the electrodes (cathode and anode). The amounts of heating and electric potential are controlled on the X-ray control panel.

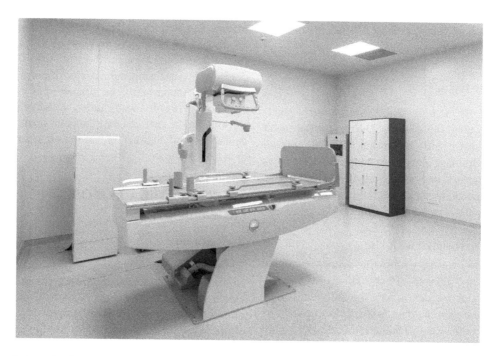

FIGURE 12.5   Schematic diagram of a diagnostic radiographic-fluoroscopic X-ray system.

X-RAY TUBE

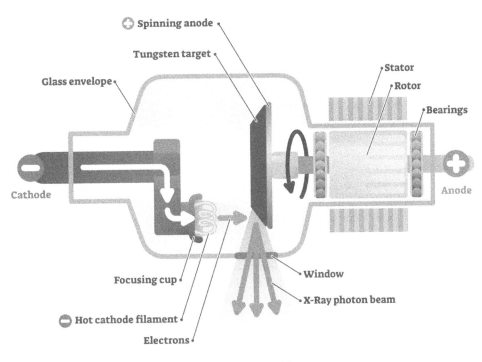

FIGURE 12.6   Schematic diagram of a conventional X-ray tube.

Royalty-free stock vector ID: 1610705320
X ray tube vector illustration. Radiology scan equipment structural scheme. Healthcare method for transparent body, luggage, or CT. Inside parts and process explanation with cathode and anode method.
Source: www.shutterstock.com/image-vector/x-ray-tube-vector-illustration-radiology-1610705320

PRINCIPLES OF OPERATION AND OPERATING PROCEDURES—HOW TO USE THE DEVICE

Most radiographic-fluoroscopic systems allow spot filming of the image to produce an X-ray film that is used for later detailed study by the radiologist and for film archiving. Typically, the system includes an under-table Bucky tray for use with an overhead X-ray tube. This is particularly applicable in routine radiography and follow-up X-ray scans after studies that use contrast media.[34] In general, the patient is positioned on the X-ray table and the scanner is used to produce fluoroscopic images. Depending on the procedure, a catheter may be inserted and a contrast media injected through an intravenous line in order to better visualize the organs or structures being examined.

The radiographs are produced by passing a beam generated by an X-ray tube through a patient using one of the techniques of capturing the attenuated beam. The image produced represents a "shadow" of the structures the X-ray beam passed through. It is worthwhile to note that the image contrast is produced by the ability of different materials to attenuate the X-ray beam. The X-rays may encounter resistance while passing through a particular organ and the degree of attenuation the of the X-ray beam varies from one organ to another.[32] For example, soft tissues such as the heart result in intermediate attenuation of the beam. This attribute is measured using "mass attenuation coefficient," expressed in cm^2/g. Different substances are used as contrast media to increase the contrast between different anatomical structures. Positive contrast agents such as barium sulfate and iodinated agents result in increased attenuation of X-rays and present as white on the X-ray film, while negative contrast agents such as CO_2 result in decreased attenuation of X-rays and appear as black or gray.

EVIDENCE OF EFFECTIVENESS

Radiography and other fluoroscopic procedures are not new in clinical practice and have long been proven to be effective in diagnosis of several diseases including CVDs.

Cost-effectiveness of other cardiac imaging procedures such as CT and MRI have been extensively studied.[35,36] However, evidence of cost-effectiveness and cost-benefit in radiography and X-ray is scanty. Plain radiograph/X-ray is a readily accessible imaging technique. It generally provides excellent imaging details of different areas of the body such as bones, joints, and the cardiopulmonary region. Considering that each radiographic test represents a cost, often a risk, and diagnostic hypothesis, it is obvious that every unnecessary or unjustifiable test adds to the burden of care. These negligible individual costs, risks, and wastes could translate to huge costs when multiplied by billions of examinations per year.[37] Therefore, it is necessary to quantify the costs and outcomes associated with these imaging studies.

Moores (2019) has proposed a comprehensive framework for cost-risk-benefit analysis for the protection of patients undergoing diagnostic radiology with special reference to the application of referral guidelines.[38] This investigation was an extension of previous work aimed to provide a theoretical framework that encompasses key factors that need to be considered in the optimization of patient protection from both diagnostic and radiation risk viewpoints. This may potentially guide economic evaluation approaches to diagnose CVDs using radiography and to inform cardiologists on how to use economic analyses for decision-making. Furthermore, Picano asserted that "increased awareness of economic, biologic, and environmental costs of cardiac imaging will hopefully lead to greater appropriateness, wisdom and prudence from both the prescriber and the practitioner."[37] In this way, the sustainability of cardiac imaging will eventually improve.

IMPORTANT SAFETY ISSUES

No significant short-term effects are associated with plain radiography/X-rays. For most plain radiographs, the radiation dose is no more than the ionizing radiation from the natural environment.

In general, the health benefits of an X-ray procedure are far more important than the small estimated risks. Despite this, the minimal risks of exposure to any type of diagnostic ionizing radiation from the X-rays needs to be weighed against the potential gain from the diagnostic information to be obtained. However, the doses are considerably higher for some CT scans and fluoroscopic procedures. Wallace and Cain have outlined the risks associated with radiation from diagnostic X-ray imaging and nuclear medicine procedures.[39] At the dose levels that are utilized in diagnostic radiography, there is little or no evidence of health effects.[40] Furthermore, scientific evidence has shown that there is a minimal increase in the possibility of cancer (stochastic or probabilistic effect) due to exposure to diagnostic radiation at lower doses. In addition, to a much lesser extent, there is a possibility of genetic alteration in future generations resulting in a new trait that can be inherited, for example physical or intellectual disability.[39,40] On the other hand, the potential risk of harmful effects from exposure to X-ray, CT, or nuclear medicine studies only becomes significant in most individuals after a substantial number of high-dose radiology procedures. Children and females are particularly more vulnerable to the effects of ionizing radiation. In addition, there are individuals with genetic predispositions to the long-term effects of ionizing radiation. The occurrence of deterministic effects, particularly tissue damage, is largely the result of long-term exposure or complex fluoroscopic diagnostic imaging procedures. Examples of tissue damage that occurs in higher doses than typically used in diagnostic imaging include skin erythema, necrosis, and hair loss.

The mechanism by which ionizing radiation can cause tissue or cell damage can simply be described as chemical reactions and alteration of the structure of macromolecules in human cells. Individuals that are particularly vulnerable to potential harm of ionizing radiation from radiography, CT, and nuclear medicine include the patient, technologist, and physician. Hence, it is always important to weigh the risk-to-benefit ratio of any imaging modality before recommending it for a patient. Moreover, clinicians are encouraged to always apply the principle of "as low as reasonably achievable" (ALARA) at all times in relationship to radiation dose. This implies using the lowest possible radiation exposure that is reasonably achievable to perform a study, while weighing the risk of the adverse effects of radiation against the benefit of a diagnosis that can influence therapy (see *Biological Effects of Radiation*).

This principle (ALARA) should begin by selecting an appropriate imaging study. Finally, minimization of the radiation dose is the ultimate responsibility of all healthcare professionals involved in the care of the patient, including, but not restricted to, the ordering clinician, the radiologist, the medical physicist, and the technologist who performs the procedure. An X-ray or any cardiac imaging study should only be requested if it directly influences patient care.

IMPLICATIONS TO THE PHARMACY PROFESSION AND PRACTICE

Pharmacists do not perform X-ray procedures, but may occasionally order these imaging studies in settings wherein they have direct patient care roles and where legislations and scope of their practice allow. The instances in which pharmacists may order such studies could include when monitoring the safety and efficacy of drug therapy; for example, when they anticipate that a drug may cause serious adverse effects (e.g., cardiomyopathy or pneumonitis caused by some anti-cancer agents). The pharmacist may also require X-rays to assess effectiveness (e.g., resolution of consolidation in patients with pneumonia or pulmonary tuberculosis). Therefore, it is important for the pharmacist to be familiar with the general knowledge of the operating procedures and mechanisms of the X-ray machines, as well as the associated risks and benefits of ordering the test. The ultimate responsibility of interpretation lies with the radiologist and other physicians.

CONCLUSION

Although there are more advanced cardiac imaging techniques such as ECG, CT, and MRI, plain radiography still has wide application in cardiology. In particular, radiographic fluoroscopy is a type of medical imaging that shows a continuous X-ray image on a monitor, much like an X-ray movie. Radiographic-fluoroscopic system technology is effective and finds wide application in the diagnosis of CVDs, including heart failure and ischemia. It is important for a pharmacist to understand the basic principles of operation of radiographic-fluoroscopic technology, evidence of its effectiveness, application in cardiology, and some important safety considerations. Pharmacists may utilize radiographs in monitoring the safety and efficacy of drug therapy. However, the onus of interpretation lies with the radiologist and other specialist physicians. The ability to order these radiographic procedures by a pharmacist will vary with the scope of pharmacy practice and legislations in a particular country and/or setting.

ELECTROCARDIOGRAM (ECG)

BACKGROUND

An electrocardiographic machine detects the electrical signals associated with cardiac activity and produces an electrocardiogram (ECG), which represents a graphic record of the electrical activities of the heart (voltage vs. time).[34] Multichannel electrocardiographs record signals from two or more leads simultaneously.[32,34] In addition, some electrocardiographs can perform automatic measurement and interpretation of the ECG as an optional feature. ECG is widely utilized in the diagnosis of several CVDs including arrhythmias and acute coronary syndromes (ACS). In this section, we will summarize the principle of operation of electrocardiography, evidence of its effectiveness in diagnosis, important safety considerations, and application in cardiology.

PURPOSE OF USE AND IMPORTANT FEATURES

Overview of Uses

ECG devices are used for the diagnosis and treatment of some CVDs including evaluation of chest pain to rule out cardiac conditions, arrhythmias, ACS, monitoring a patient's response to drug therapy, and observing trends in heart function.

Device Description and Important Features

An electrocardiograph consists of the ECG unit, the electrodes, and the cables. The instrumentation comprises the ECG machine with paper, the lead electrodes, and the adhesive electrode pads. The 12-lead ECG system comprises bipolar, unipolar, and precordial leads, with each of the 12 standard leads representing a different perspective of the heart's electrical activity.[32,34] This produces ECG waves

with varying polarity and amplitude: P waves, T waves, and QRS complex (Figure 12.7). An interpretive multichannel electrocardiograph acquires and analyzes the electrical signals, while a non-interpretive multichannel electrocardiograph only records the electric signals from the leads (electrodes) without their interpretation.

PRINCIPLES OF OPERATION AND OPERATING PROCEDURES—HOW TO USE THE DEVICE

Principles of Operation

Here we summarize the basic mechanism and principles of operation of an ECG. Typically, electrocardiograph measures and records a small amount of voltages (about 1 mV) that appears on the skin as a result of cardiac activities. The voltage differences between electrodes, which directly correspond to the heart's electrical activities, are measured. Each of the 12 standard leads represents a different perspective of the heart's electrical activity, thereby producing the ECG waveforms including the P waves and T waves (Figure 12.7).

Operating Procedures

It is worthwhile to note that most hospitals have fully automated ECG machines and a practitioner should become acquainted with the machine available in their facility. A general outline of operating procedures is presented here[41]:

- Establishing rapport and professional relationship: Establish rapport with the patient and explain the steps of the procedure in a language that is appropriate and clear to the patient.
- Environment and patient positioning: Instruct the patient to lie down in a comfortable recumbent position.
- Starting the ECG machine: Plug in the machine and turn it on.
- The electrodes and cables are attached as follows (Figure 12.8):
  - Cables: A conventional ECG machine has five lead cables/wires, with one for each limb and one for the chest leads. However, newer ECG machines may have six precordial electrodes, all of which are placed in the proper positions before the procedure. The cables may be color-coded in the following manner: right arm (white), left arm (black), right leg (green), left leg (red), and chest (brown).
  - Limb electrodes: Older ECG machines have flat, rectangular plates held in place by straps that encircle the limb, while newer machines have self-adhering electrode pads. Each electrode should be placed on the limb indicated, usually on the ventral surface.
  - Chest (precordial) electrodes: With newer machines, all leads can be placed before the

NORMAL ECG

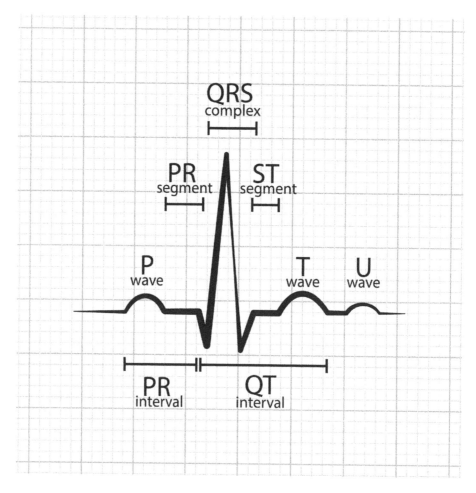

FIGURE 12.7A   A normal electrocardiogram showing different waves.

Source: www.shutterstock.com/image-vector/normal-ecg-electrocardiogram-p-wave-pr-403308226

Normal Sinus Rhythm

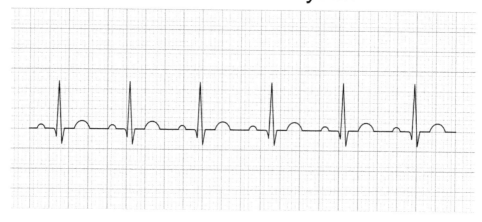

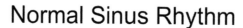

FIGURE 12.7B   A normal electrocardiogram showing different waves.

Source: www.shutterstock.com/image-vector/electrocardiogram-show-normal-heart-beat-line-1688917729

ECG is run with all pads applied simultaneously. However, older machines have a suction cup chest electrode that is designated by letter "C." The pericardial leads are placed as follows:

- V_1 = fourth intercostal space just to the right of the sternal border
- V_2 = fourth intercostal space intercostal space just to the left of the sternal border
- V_3 = midway between leads V_2 and V_4
- V_4 = mid-clavicular line in the fifth intercostal space
- V_5 = anterior axillary line at the same level as V_4
- V_6 = mid-axillary line at the same level as leads V_4 and V_5

- When everything is ready, the directions for a particular machine are followed to obtain the ECG tracing. It should include 12 leads: I, II, III, AVR, AVL, and V1—V6.
- For some machines, the operator can select the lead groupings, their sequence, and the recording duration for each group.
- The graphical presentation (i.e., the tracing) is labeled with the patient's information (e.g., name, date, and any other useful information). Typically, a routine 12-lead ECG procedure should take around 4–8 minutes.
- The basic ECG interpretation is beyond the scope of this chapter and can be found in other reference resources.

EVIDENCE OF EFFECTIVENESS

The utility and effectiveness of ECG in the diagnosis of several CVDs has long been documented. Similarly, there is overwhelming evidence of cost-effectiveness of ECG in different settings and populations, including, but not limited to, early (pre-hospital) diagnosis of ACS,[42] chronic stable angina,[35] diagnosis of arrhythmias,[43] screening programs for AFib,[44,45] stroke prevention,[46] prevention of sudden cardiac death,[47,48] and neonatal screening for long QT syndrome.[49]

A study conducted in urban Indian patients presenting first to a general practitioner with acute chest pain to determine the cost-effectiveness of a GP-performed ECG showed that this is a cost-effective strategy to reduce disability and mortality associated with ACS.[42] The ECG compared to no ECG costs an additional $12.65 per QALY gained and a cost-saving of $1,124/QALY. One study from Belgium evaluated whether an AFib screening program with a handheld ECG machine in a population-wide cohort has a high screening yield and is cost-effective.[45] The investigators used a Markov modeling analysis on 1,000 hypothetical individuals who matched the Belgian Heart Rhythm Week screening program. Overall, the study suggests that the use of a handheld ECG machine to identify subjects with newly diagnosed AFib was cost-effective in the general population, as well as in elderly population. Lowres and colleagues studied community screening for unknown AFib using an iPhone electrocardiogram (iECG) in community pharmacies in Australia, and determined the cost-effectiveness of this strategy.[46] The study found that screening with iECG in pharmacies with an automated algorithm is both feasible and cost-effective.

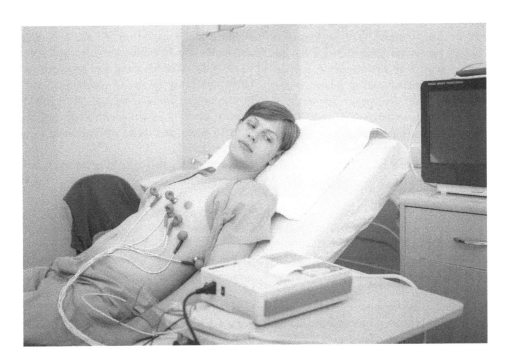

FIGURE 12.8 A 12-lead ECG system with the leads (electrodes) attached to the patient.

Source: www.shutterstock.com/image-photo/man-perform-electrocardiogram-381085723

The evidence of cost-effectiveness of ECG in diagnosis and prevention of different types of cardiac conditions is vast. However, what we provided in this section is only the tip of the iceberg.

IMPORTANT SAFETY ISSUES

In general, ECG is a non-invasive and safe procedure with no major health risks. The electrodes that connect the sensors to patient's chest do not send out electric shocks. Patients may develop mild rash or skin irritation where the electrodes are attached. This rash or irritation is usually transient and does not require any treatment.

IMPLICATIONS TO THE PHARMACY PROFESSION AND PRACTICE

It is not common for a pharmacist to conduct investigations using ECG machines; however, it is worthwhile to have the required competence and be familiar with the basic knowledge of operating procedures of the ECG machines as well as the interpretation of ECG.[50–52] Current practice and competency standards do not characterize the extent to which the pharmacists should know and be responsible for ECG.[51] However, there is increasing utility of point-of-care (POC) ECG devices in clinical as well as resource-constrained settings. Therefore, there is a potential for pharmacists to use these POC devices for assessment and subsequent referral to other healthcare practitioners and for monitoring drug therapy. Understanding these basic concepts by the pharmacist is important in different settings and environments. There are some common drug-induced ECG changes, some of which would require rapid identification and interpretation by a healthcare professional including the pharmacist. Examples include drug-induced QTc prolongation, ventricular arrhythmias, supraventricular tachycardia, etc. Pharmacists working in acute care environments, particularly those in emergency departments and intensive care units, are routinely faced with emergency scenarios in which they will need ECG tests to make decisions.[51,53] The role of the pharmacist in cardiac emergencies is also recognized as part of advanced cardiac life support programs.[50] This can promote safe drug preparation and administration, including changes in cardiac rhythm.[52]

CONCLUSION

Although the pharmacist has a limited role in diagnosing CVDs, there is a responsibility for pharmacists to understand essential diagnostic tests and cardiac imaging studies including ECG. This greatly influences pharmacotherapy decisions and therapeutic drug monitoring. Ultimately, pharmacists utilize ECG test procedures for monitoring the safety and efficacy of drug therapy related to some critical cardiac diseases such as ACS and arrhythmias. They also use it for assessment of drug-induced cardiac disorders. Continuing professional development programs and pharmacy curricula should establish minimum competency standards for understanding and interpreting ECG in an effort to produce pharmacists with the fundamental understanding of their role in monitoring drug therapy in cardiology settings.

ARTIFICIAL HEART VALVES

BACKGROUND

Valvular heart disease can result from cyclic stress and strain on native heart valves. Artificial heart valves, also known as prosthetic heart valves, can be used in patients with valvular heart disease to counteract stenosis or regurgitation, primarily in the aortic and mitral valves, and facilitate unidirectional blood flow.[54] The two main types of prosthetic heart valves available are mechanical and bioprosthetic (Figure 12.9), each having their own advantages and disadvantages.

Mechanical valves are composed of plastic and metal components. Three types of mechanical heart valves may be encountered in practice, each having improvements in flow patterns and reduced incidence of thrombogenicity[55]:

1. Ball-and-cage valves (these have been superseded by bileaflet valves and are no longer manufactured),
2. Monoleaflet valves (not implanted in current practice but still encountered in reoperations), and
3. Bileaflet mechanical valves (most common mechanical valve).

Bileaflet valves have more central blood flow mimicking the body's natural physiologic response. The advantages of using mechanical heart valves include structural stability and long-lasting effect, and bileaflet valves in particular are hemodynamically efficient; however, the increased risk of bleeding and requirement of anticoagulation can limit the use of mechanical valves, especially in women of childbearing age. Mechanical valves should be considered in patients with a life expectancy of greater than 15 years and those who are able to take vitamin K antagonists.

Bioprosthetic heart valves are made from animal species and include:

1. Porcine aortic valve tissue
2. Bovine pericardial tissue

Bioprosthetic heart valves have an advantage over their counterpart in that they do not require long-term anticoagulation post insertion, so there is a low risk of thromboembolism and valve failure. The greatest risk of a thromboembolic event is 3 months post insertion.[56,57] However, bioprosthetic valves deteriorate at a much quicker rate and must be replaced, with an increased risk of endocarditis; therefore these valves are preferred in patients with limited life expectancy.[58] In younger patients, the degradation of tissue

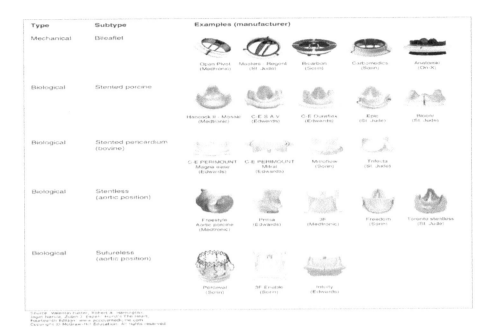

FIGURE 12.9 Types of surgical mechanical and bioprosthetic heart valves.

Source: Fuster V., Harrington R.A (Hurst's The Heart: Fourteenth Edition)[60]

valves is more evident presumably due to a higher cardiac output, because bioprosthetic valves cannot self-repair as can native valves.[59] Studies have shown that when inserted in patients younger than 40 years of age, the 10-year failure rate exceeds 42%. Due to a lower risk of thromboembolism, bioprosthetic heart valves should be considered in patients who are unwilling or unable to take vitamin K antagonists.

The choice of which specific valve should be used relies on a number of factors including personal preference, patient age, indication/contraindication for warfarin therapy, life expectance, and comorbidities.[57]

DEVICE DESCRIPTION/IMPORTANT FEATURES

Mechanical valves are composed of plastic and metal components such as stainless steel alloys, molybdenum alloys, and pyrolytic carbon which is used for the valve housings and leaflets.[61] Pyrolytic carbon was found to be a suitable component for mechanical valves by Bokros and Gott in 1966 and has now become the material of choice to design mechanical heart valves because of its extensive biocompatibility, thromboresistant and wear-resistant properties.[62,63] Mechanical valves have three main components: an occlude, an occlude restraint, and a sewing ring.[54] Ball-and-cage valves are not commonly seen in practice because they have been superseded by bileaflet valves. Production of the Starr Edwards ball-and-cage valves ceased in 2007 due to the high risk of thrombogenicity associated with more lateral rather than central blood flow.[64] Until that point, more than 500,000 of these valves were implanted between 1960 and 2007, with 300,000 implanted during the last 7 years of production.[65] In contrast, bileaflet heart

valves provide an increased central flow of blood closely mimicking the natural biological valve response.[54]

Ball-and-cage valves consist of a ball enclosed in a metal cage. Native heart valves produce central blood flow; however, with the ball –and-cage valve central flow is not acquired and may damage blood cells by colliding with the ball.[63,66]

Monoleaflet valves are composed of a single disc secured by metal struts. The opening angle of the disk results in two distinct orifices of different sizes.

Bileaflet valves designed by St. Jude Medical, Inc. consist of two semilunar discs attached to a valve ring by small hinges and the open valve consists of three orifices: a small, slit-like central orifice between the two open leaflets and two larger lateral semicircular orifices.[57] The disc can completely close the valve orifice in the closed position and tilts to an angle in the open position. The valve is packaged in a formaldehyde storage solution. The valve should be stored in the upright position at a temperature of 5°C to 25°C.

Bioprosthetic valves use several tissue types, mainly porcine valve and pericardium tissue. Both types of bioprosthetic heart valves are treated with glutaraldehyde solution. The use of glutaraldehyde in bioprostethic valves results in reduction of tissue degradation and increase in biological tissue stability.[63]

Porcine aortic valve tissue is composed of a glutaraldehyde-treated porcine aortic valve supported by a rigid ring with flexible posts. This is known as the Hancock porcine xenograft produced in 1970. A large quantity of porcine valves is required to produce prosthetic valves appropriate for insertion in humans in size and quality.

Bovine pericardial tissue is based on calf pericardial tissue and overcome the demands associated with porcine valve production. The Carpentier-Edwards pericardial valve, composed of bovine tissue and mounted on a flexible frame, was approved for commercial use in 1991. This valve provides better durability and greater hemodynamic performance compared to other pericardial valves. The Carpentier-Edwards valve should be stored at 10–25°C and kept in the original packaging.

EVIDENCE FOR EFFECTIVENESS

A retrospective cohort analysis of 2,727 patients who underwent bileaflet mechanical valve surgery between 1978 to 2012 was conducted. This study concluded with results showing a low late mortality and a low incidence of valve-related events associated with bileaflet mechanical valve replacement.[67]

A study conducted in 2013 with the aim to follow up elderly patients (65 to 80 years) who had undergone aortic valve replacement between 1991 and 1999 concluded that patients undergoing valve replacement for both reoperation (4%) and endocarditis (1.9%) were uncommon to 12 years. The risk of death (66.5%), stroke (14.1%), and bleeding (17.9%) was high. For patients who received a bioprosthetic heart valve (n = 14) compared to those with mechanical valves (n = 24), it was concluded that there was a higher risk of reoperation and endocarditis, but a lower risk of stroke and bleeding. These risks vary depending on the patient's age and comorbidities. Bioprosthetic patients aged 65 to 69 years had a 12-year absolute risk of reoperation of 10.5%. Long-term mortality rates were similar for those patients who received mechanical versus bioprosthetic valve replacement.[68]

More recently, a study conducted in 2020 observed a male patient who had a ball –and-cage valve inserted 40 years prior. Upon examination it was concluded that the valve is functioning normally, with no significant evidence of stenosis or regurgitation, highlighting the durability and longevity of the valve.[69]

IMPORTANT SAFETY ISSUES

Long-term effects associated with mechanical heart valves include thromboembolism, endocarditis, and hemorrhagic complications related to anticoagulation with vitamin K antagonists. Many factors are taken into consideration when determining the risk of thrombogenicity, including the type of valve, position of the valve, and other clinical characteristics.[64,70,71] Patients are at high risk of thrombogenicity with aortic mechanical heart valves, and therefore all require anticoagulation with vitamin K antagonists. Thrombogenicity and hemolytic anemia for bileaflet and tilting disk valves is markedly less prominent than ball-and-cage valves.[61]

Failure of the mechanical valves is rare; however, the bioprosthetic valves require monitoring and follow-up specifically around 7 years post implantation. An annual echocardiogram should be completed after this time. Bioprosthetic valves are prone to structural degeneration which in turn can lead to reoperation and associated risks.[72] The rate of infective endocarditis is similar for mechanical valves with anticoagulation and bioprosthetic valves, at an increase of 1%/year.[73,74] Patients who undergo dental procedures which may include gingival bleeding or penetration of the mucosa and may introduce the risk of systemic infection should be prescribed antibiotic prophylaxis to avoid infective endocarditis.

In pregnant women, cardiac valve surgery is a complex procedure preferable to be delayed until the fetus is viable or a cesarean section can be performed alongside the cardiac surgery. Pregnancy poses challenges in patients with prosthetic heart valves. Bioprosthetic valves degenerate rapidly especially during pregnancy, exposing the patient to the risk of reoperation. Mechanical valves are preferred but the need for anticoagulation can complicate a current or future pregnancy.[74,75] Warfarin, although the gold standard of treatment for anticoagulation, is a teratogen and contraindicated in pregnancy. A study completed in 2018 showed that there was an increased rate of pregnancy loss in patients with mechanical versus prosthetic valves (61% vs. 15%, respectively).[76] The lack of robust randomized control trial in pregnancy and anticoagulation leaves healthcare professionals with limited evidence-based options for therapy.

IMPLICATIONS TO THE PHARMACY PROFESSION AND PRACTICE

Pharmacists play a pivotal in the aftercare of patients with valvular heart disease who have undergone prosthetic heart valve surgery. Pharmacists are patient-facing healthcare professionals who can provide counseling on disease progression and self-monitoring, and advice on the appropriate use of medication such as anticoagulants. Pharmacists may also provide anticoagulation clinics and point-of-care testing for patients in the community. Patient education on adverse effects such as thromboembolism and raising awareness on the risks of complications such as infective endocarditis is of importance to allow patients to recognize early signs and symptoms. Knowledge surrounding the differences between mechanical and bioprosthetic heart valves is of importance so that pharmacists can counsel patients and monitor patients postoperatively. Pharmacists should ensure they are regularly updated on the effects associated with heart valve surgery and replacement and the pharmacotherapy associated with it.

CONCLUSION

There are a variety of mechanical and bioprosthetic heart valves available for use in clinical practice to treat valvular heart disease. The choice of which prosthetic valve is used depends on multiple factors including personal preference, patient age, indication/contraindication for warfarin therapy, life expectancy, and comorbidities.[57] Long-term effects must be taken into consideration including thromboembolism, endocarditis, and hemorrhagic complications related to anticoagulation with vitamin K antagonists. Pharmacists must ensure they are familiar with the pharmacotherapy associated with heart valve replacement to allow for optimal patient education and counseling.

PULSE OXIMETRY

BACKGROUND

Pulse oximetry is a painless, non-invasive diagnostic test used to determine hemoglobin oxygen saturation. The underlying principle of pulse oximetry is Beer's Law, which states that the concentration of an unknown substance dissolved in a solvent can be determined by its light absorption.[77] A pulse oximeter device is a small, clip-like device placed across the ear lobe, finger, toe, or any perfused tissue that can be transilluminated. Then, pulse oximetry works by using two light-emitting diodes, thus illuminating the skin and measuring the changes in light absorption of oxygenated (oxyhemoglobin) and deoxygenated (reduced hemoglobin) blood. It does so by using two different light wavelengths to detect the blood—660 nm (red) and 940 nm (infrared).

Oximetry relies on the observation that oxygenated and deoxygenated blood differ in their absorption of light; that is, the oxygenated blood absorbs more infrared light and deoxygenated blood absorbs more red light. The absorbance ratio of these wavelengths is calculated and aligned against direct measurements of arterial oxygen saturation

(SaO_2) to establish a measure of arterial saturation by pulse oximeter (SpO_2).[78] Critical to this measurement is pulsatile arterial flow by which the arterial signal can be identified and separated from the other factors that absorb the two wavelengths of light. The change in light absorption is the basis of oximetry determinations. The greater the ratio of red to infrared absorption, the lower is the arterial hemoglobin oxygen saturation.[79] The normal range of SpO_2 is considered between 97% and 99%, but those with lung conditions or smokers may exhibit lower readings. Readings below 90% may indicate the need for supplemental oxygen.[80] Two different probes are available in the clinical setting. Reusable clip probes can be rapidly used and are more cost-effective in a clinical outpatient setting because more patients can be tested and measured with the same probe. Single-patient adhesive probes reduce the risk of transmission of nosocomial infections and allow for secure placement of the probes during patient movements.[81]

PURPOSE OF USE AND IMPORTANT FEATURES

Pulse oximeters are used in a wide variety of healthcare settings and are often known as the "fifth vital sign."[82] This device is used in clinical practices such as general physical examination through to monitoring patients with lung and heart disorders who are at risk of low levels of blood oxygen (Figure 12.10). Pulse oximeters may be used before, during, and after surgery including anesthesia. Patients who have been diagnosed with sleep apnea can benefit from using pulse oximeters.

In light of the COVID-19 pandemic, there has been an increase in the use of home pulse oximeters in patients who have tested positive for COVID-19 but do not exhibit severe

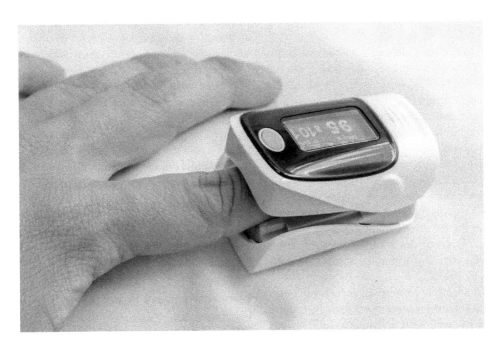

FIGURE 12.10 An example of a pulse oximeter.

Source: www.shutterstock.com/image-photo/pulse-oximeter-on-patients-hand-389892127

TABLE 12.1

Range of Values for Oxygen Saturation

SpO_2 %	Oxygenation status
95–100	Normal
91–94	Mild hypoxia
86–90	Moderate hypoxia
Less than 85	Severe hypoxia

symptoms and those who do not require hospitalization. This allows patients to continuously monitor their blood oxygen levels at home and present themselves to emergency care when they show evidence of hypoxia, in turn reducing the risk of complications such as unrecognized systemic organ dysfunction or cardiac arrest.[79]

Since 2013, the FDA announced that all medical-use pulse oximeters must report the root mean square of the differences between the measured and actual value (A_{RMS}).[83] This combines the bias (difference between the average of the measurements made by a monitor and the true value) and precision (how close repeated measures of the value are to each other) into a single measure reflecting the accuracy of the devices (how close the measured value is to the true value). The FDA requires that A_{RMS} values should be ≤ 3.0.[79]

The normal arterial oxygen saturation is considered to be between 97–99%; patients who smoke may have a lower reading between 93% and 95% (Table 12.1). Readings of less than 90% may indicate requirement of supplemental oxygen and further tests are required to confirm hypoxia. SpO_2 values of less than 70% are unreliable and further tests should be performed.

Evidence for Effectiveness

Pulse oximetry is widely available as a non-invasive test to determine blood oxygen saturation, compared to arterial blood gas measurement of oxygen saturation in which it is required to have blood drawn from the patient. In addition, arterial blood gas measurement requires specialist staff and equipment to analyze the samples and may result in procedure-related complications such as pain, bruising, and bleeding.[84] Using SpO_2 provides the clinical team serving the patient with continuous monitoring and the ability to highlight any sudden changes in oxygen saturation. Previous studies have suggested that pulse oximetry in patients who are in the intensive care unit may be suboptimal in its accuracy; however, deviations of the SpO_2 levels from the SaO_2 levels were still within the acceptable levels for FDA approval (≤ 3%).[84,85]

Literature independently examining the accuracy of finger oximeters in a clinical setting is scarce. One study by Lipnick et al. examined the accuracy of finger oximeters in 22 healthy individuals who compared six low-cost pulse oximeters (not approved by the FDA). From this study, only two pulse oximeters met the A_{RMS} value of < 3% at SaO_2 between 70% and

100%, thereby meeting the International Organization for Standardization's (ISO) criteria for accuracy.[86]

A recent study by Rauniyat et al. assessed arterial oxygen saturation by pulse oximetry and arterial blood gas of 101 patients in an intensive care unit. This study concluded that in patients who have measured an SpO_2 of > 90%, pulse oximetry can be used with high accuracy (83.2%) to determine SaO_2 instead of arterial blood gases. In patients with low oxygen saturation (SpO_2 < 90%), pulse oximetry is not a suitable alternative to measuring arterial oxygen saturation.[87]

Important Safety Issues

Pulse oximetry has been found to be a reliable measure of oxygen saturation at readings of 70–100% with a 95% confidence rate of ± 4%.[88] Pulse oximeters do not require calibration; therefore, it is important that users of the oximeter are aware of any device issues which may exhibit false readings. There are multiple conditions that can affect pulse oximetry readings. If a patient is wearing nail varnish (black, blue, or green), this can absorb light emitted by the oximeter and interfere with the detection of oxygenated blood.[79] The pulse oximeter may give an irregular reading if movement is detected, such as shivering, outputting an unstable waveform. Pulse oximeters rely on detection of pulsatile blood flow, to ensure that inaccurate readings from hemoglobin in the capillaries and venous blood are not detected. Poor peripheral perfusion, usually due to vasoconstriction from cold or hypovolemia, can result in failure of the oximeter to register a signal and provide a reliable reading due to reduced blood flow in the tissues and the difficulty in detecting a pulsatile signal of arterial blood flow.[79] Blood pressure readings less than 80 mmHg can cause inaccurate and unreliable oximeter readings.

Patients with abnormally high levels of carbon monoxide combined with hemoglobin (those who have been exposed to cigarette smoke or house fires) will result in inaccurate oximeter readings due to the presence of carboxyhemoglobin. More recent evidence suggests that skin pigmentation could give rise to inaccurate oximeter readings, with a study by Sjoding et al. suggesting that there is increasing failure to detect hypoxemia in black patients compared to white patients, with black patients having three times the frequency of hypoxemia detected by arterial blood gas but not detected by pulse oximetry, when compared to white patients.[89]

Storage Conditions and Maintenance

The pulse oximeter should be cleaned regularly with a damp cloth or alcohol swab.

Implications to the Pharmacy Profession and Practice

Considering the increasing prevalence of use of pulse oximeters at home in light of the COVID-19 pandemic, pharmacists play a pivotal role in ensuring patients are using the device correctly and counseling patients on how to ensure their readings are accurate and reliable. Use of over-the-counter oximeters has increased during the pandemic; however, the products sold in the pharmacy are not approved by the FDA and are not intended for medical care.[90] Limited data is available on the reliability and accuracy of pocket and smartphone oximeters. Because pharmacists have a patient care role, it is pivotal that pharmacists have extensive knowledge on how oximeters work, and the steps to be taken by the patient to ensure the most accurate results at home.

CONCLUSION

Pulse oximeters can be used in a wide variety of clinical settings for routine examination or for specific patient monitoring. Pulse oximeters determine the oxygen saturation level, with a normal range of 95–100% for healthy patients. The use of at-home pulse oximeters is rising; however, the accuracy of these devices should be carefully considered when interpreting results. A number of factors can give rise to erroneous readings (such as colored nail polish or if the patient is a smoker) and these should be taken into consideration when assessing a patient.

ANGIOGRAM

BACKGROUND

Invasive coronary angiography (ICA) was introduced by Mason Sones in 1958 and is a gold standard, invasive X-ray procedure used most commonly to diagnose and assess the severity of coronary artery disease (CAD), thus allowing physicians to make a decision on patient prognosis and treatment. Medical therapy and non-invasive tests are completed initially; followed by ICA which can diagnose CAD and assist physicians in assessing the most appropriate course of treatment such as revascularization by percutaneous coronary intervention or surgical intervention, if necessary.[91]

ICA is completed in a catheterization lab while the patient is under local anesthesia using a radiopaque contrast agent visible on X-rays (usually iodine dye) with X-ray pictures to determine if any blockage or narrowing of the coronary arteries is present (Figure 12.11).

PURPOSE OF USE AND IMPORTANT FEATURES

ICA is primarily used to identify and detect the prognosis of coronary artery disease. ICA may also be used to identify

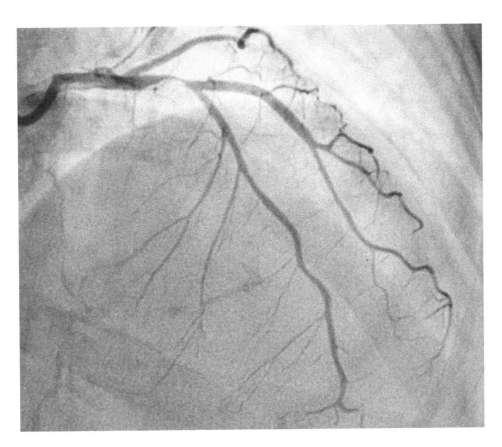

FIGURE 12.11 Radio contrast dye highlighting left coronary angiography.

Source: www.shutterstock.com/image-photo/coronary-angiography-left-stenosis-proximal-anterior-672940828

damage to blood vessels due to myocardial infarction and to assist diagnosis of angina. ICA may be used when the diagnosis of coronary disease is uncertain and cannot be excluded by non-invasive techniques. ICA should not be conducted in patients with angina who refuse invasive procedures, those who are not suitable candidates for percutaneous coronary intervention, and those who will not benefit from coronary revascularization.[92]

HOW TO OPERATE/USE

ICA is completed alongside cardiac catheterization in a catheterization lab, while the patient is under local anesthesia, by a fluoroscopy machine. Access to the artery is gained using the standard Seldinger technique. An incision is made into either the radial or femoral artery. Thereafter, a thin narrow tube known as a catheter (typically 1.7 mm) is inserted into an artery and guided to the area being examined. Using X-ray images as a guide, the tip of the catheter is guided to the heart and coronary arteries. A positive radiopaque contrast agent (usually iodine) is injected through the catheter and flows through the blood vessels; X-ray images are then taken to show detailed images of the heart (angiogram) and identify any blockage or narrowing of the arteries.[93] The radiopaque contrast agent is visible on the angiogram highlighting the blood vessels that the dye is flowing through to determine if any blockage of the coronary arteries is present.[91] X-ray is not the only method of screening; computed tomography (CT) angiography or magnetic resonance angiography (MRA) scan may also be used for angiography purposes. CT angiography is a safer, less invasive method of angiography; however, it is associated with a markedly high exposure to radiation. MRA angiography can be considered in patients who are susceptible to an allergic reaction with iodinated contrast agents; however, long image time, skilled operator dependency, and lower spatial image resolution limit its use.

Prior to the angiogram, patients are requested to refrain from eating and drinking 12 hours before the procedure. At the time of the procedure, patients are given an intravenous sedative to relax the body. Total procedure time is usually less than 1 hour and can be completed as an outpatient procedure. Patients may be admitted to a day clinic for further monitoring if required.

IMPORTANT SAFETY ISSUES

ICA, although invasive, is a relatively safe procedure (risk of major complication such as death, myocardial infarction, or major embolism is below 1%) which rarely causes serious side effects.[94] There has been a reduction in the number of complications associated with radial artery insertion and the main complication associated with femoral artery insertion (bleeding requiring blood transfusion) is 0.5–2%.[95,96] Complications which may occur include bleeding, allergic reactions to the radiopaque agent, infection, or blood vessel damage.[41] CT angiography does not require cardiac

catheterization and can be used to avoid invasive procedure complications. ICA can expose a patient to 350–750 times more radiation than a common X-ray of the chest; however, many different factors can affect the specific radiation dose such as operator technique and X-ray system set up.[97]

In pregnant women, iodine-based contrast agents have been found to cross the placenta and enter the fetus in measurable quantities; however, the effects on the fetus are inconclusive and not well understood.[98] After entering the fetal blood stream, iodinated agents will be excreted via the urine into the amniotic fluid and be subsequently swallowed by the fetus. It is then possible that a small amount will be absorbed from the gut of the fetus.[99] Therefore, the American College of Radiology manual on contrast media recommends that iodinated contrast agents be used only as needed in the imaging of pregnant patients.

IMPLICATIONS TO THE PHARMACY PROFESSION AND PRACTICE

Prior to and post ICA, patients are commonly placed on pharmacological cardiovascular medications (e.g., beta blockers, calcium antagonists, diuretics, aspirin, and ACE/ARBs) while waiting for a complete diagnosis of CAD. Pharmacists have a patient-facing role to ensure optimal disease management and medication education to increase adherence and promote safe medication use. Patients may also acquire knowledge and counseling from the pharmacist regarding their ICA procedure. Therefore, pharmacists should be well educated on the technique, benefits, and risks involved in ICA and cardiac catheterization.

CONCLUSION

An ICA is used to diagnose and assess the severity of coronary artery disease. The conventional angiography is by X-ray images in which the blood vessels are illuminated by an iodine dye injected through catheterization. Although invasive, complications from this procedure are rare and caution should be taken when conducting the procedure on any patient who is pregnant.

ECHOCARDIOGRAM

BACKGROUND

Echocardiography (ECHO) is the most widely used, non-invasive cardiac imaging technique. ECHO can be used to examine the heart for functional issues in the heart valves, blood clots in the heart chambers, and problems with the aorta, among many others. During the procedure, a probe called a transducer is placed on the patient's chest or esophagus (where there is no bone or lung tissue) at specific locations and angles, and high-frequency sound waves (ultrasound) are emitted which move through the skin to the heart. The transducers use piezoelectric crystals to generate and receive ultrasound waves.[100] The ultrasound waves are higher than 20 kHz and therefore unable to be heard by the human ear.[101] Once reaching the heart, the sound waves "echo" or bounce off the structure of the heart. The longer the time between the transmission of the sound wave and the arrival of the reflected waves, the deeper the structure is in the thorax. This can then be interpreted by a computer which can then create continuous, moving images of the heart chambers, valves, walls, and blood vessels (Figure 12.12).[102]

There are several types of ECHO, the most common being transthoracic (TTE) and transesophageal (TEE). ECHO may be used to detect damage from a myocardial infarction, heart failure, congenital heart disease, or cardiomyopathy. TTE—type of ECHO is conducted by applying the transducer to the chest to scan the heart.

PURPOSE OF USE AND IMPORTANT FEATURES

Transthoracic ECHO (TTE) is the primary non-invasive ECHO technique for evaluation of cardiac structure and function. Patients will be asked to remove any clothing. A lubricating gel is applied to the chest and the patient is requested to lie on the left side. The transducer will then be moved across the chest along the left or right sternal border, at the cardiac apex, suprasternal notch, or over the subxiphoid region. The recorded images will be displayed on the machine as either two- or three-dimensional tomographic images. The benefits of TTE are that it is a non-invasive technique, there is wide availability, and it bears a lack of exposure to harmful radiation.[103] There are four standard transducer locations used in a routine TTE examination: suprasternal, parasternal, apical, and subcostal.[104]

Transesophageal ECHO (TEE) is an invasive procedure in which a small transducer on the tip of an endoscope is passed through the esophagus providing a more detailed visualization of the heart. TEE is used when TTE is unsuitable such as in obese or COPD patients. Patients are provided with local anesthesia for the throat to avoid pain during the procedure. Due to the anatomical positioning of the transducer, TEE provides visualization of cardiac structures which cannot be seen through TTE due to the location.[105] Patients who experience dysphagia, esophageal disease, or severe pulmonary disease are unsuitable candidates for TEE.

There are a variety of modes for image display associated with ECHO: M-mode, Doppler, color Doppler, 2D ECHO, and 3D ECHO. M-mode is the first type of cardiac ultrasound and is the simplest, utilizing a single piezoelectric crystal. A single beam is directed towards the heart and signals are displayed on an oscillograph. This mode is useful for measuring or viewing the heart structure, but the real anatomy is not well visualized.[106] Doppler is used to assess the flow of blood through the heart chambers and valves

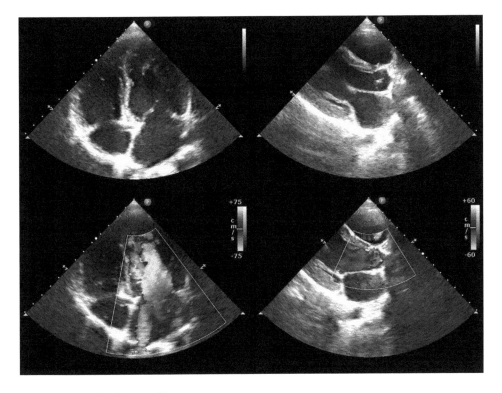

FIGURE 12.12 Echocardiography ultrasound images.

Source: www.shutterstock.com/image-photo/echocardiography-set-patterns-272661782

and can detect abnormal blood flow within the heart. An enhanced form of Doppler is color Doppler which illuminates the direction of blood flow in different colors. A 2D ECHO view is visualized by a "cone" shape on the computer and the real-time monitoring of the heart structures can be seen, providing information on the cardiac anatomy. A significant advance in the field of ECHO has resulted in the development of 3D ECHO which captures greater detail than 2D and allows for a more accurate assessment and interpretation of heart function, showing enhanced views of the heart chambers and valves.[105] 3D ECHO is useful for complex congenital heart disease due to its accuracy in displaying cardiac structure.[106,107]

Important Safety Issues

There are no known effects associated with TTE. There are minimal risks associated with TEE. Although the procedure is invasive, there is a low instance of major complications associated with it (0.18–0.5%) and only two deaths reported.[108,109]

Implications to the Pharmacy Profession and Practice

Pharmacists as healthcare professionals provide patients with a direct point of care, providing patient education and counseling. Therefore, pharmacists should ensure they are aware of the process by which ECHO is carried out to be able to provide patient education.

Conclusion

Echocardiogram is a widely used cardiac imaging technique to examine multiple functional issues with the heart. The most common types of ECHO used in clinical practice include TTE and TEE, with a variety of different imaging techniques available (most commonly 3D ECHO). Although there are no known safety issues with the use of ECHO, patients undergoing TEE should be questioned on allergic response to local anesthesia.

REFERENCES

1. World Health Organization. Cardiovascular diseases. Available from: www.who.int/health-topics/cardiovascular-diseases/#tab=tab_1.
2. Roth GA, Mensah GA, Johnson CO, et al. Global burden of cardiovascular diseases and risk factors, 1990–2019: update from the GBD 2019 study. J Am Coll Cardiol. 2020;76(25):2982–3021.
3. World Health Organization. WHO compendium of innovative health technologies for low-resource settings, 2016–2017. License: CC BY-NC-SA 3.0 IGO ed. Geneva: World Health Organization; 2018.
4. Magder S. The meaning of blood pressure. Crit Care. 2018;22(1):257.
5. Dai H, Much AA, Maor E, et al. Global, regional, and national burden of ischemic heart disease and its attributable risk factors, 1990–2017: results from the global Burden of Disease Study 2017. Eur Heart J Qual Care Clin Outcomes. 2020.
6. Lewington S, Clarke R, Qizilbash N, et al. Age-specific relevance of usual blood pressure to vascular mortality: a meta-analysis of individual data for one million adults in 61 prospective studies. Lancet. 2002;360(9349):1903–13.
7. Vousden N, Nathan HL, Shennan AH. Innovations in vital signs measurement for the detection of hypertension and shock in pregnancy. Reprod Health. 2018;15(Suppl 1):92.
8. Muntner P, Shimbo D, Carey RM, et al. Measurement of blood pressure in humans: a scientific statement From the American Heart Association. Hypertension. 2019;73(5):e35–e66.
9. Ogedegbe G, Pickering T. Principles and techniques of blood pressure measurement. Cardiol Clin. 2010;28(4):571–86.
10. SCENIHR (Scientific Committee on Emerging and Newly Identified Health Risks). Mercury sphygmomanometers in healthcare and feasibility of alternatives. 2009. Available from: https://ec.europa.eu/health/ph_risk/committees/04_scenihr/docs/scenihr_o_025.pdf.
11. UN Environment Programme. Overview of the Minamata convention on mercury activities. Switzerland. 3 Feb 2021.
12. World Health Organization. WHO technical specifications for automated non-invasive blood pressure measuring devices with cuff. Geneva: World Health Organization; 2020.
13. Pickering TG. What will replace the mercury sphygmomanometer? Blood Press Monit. 2003;8(1):23–5.
14. Myers MG, Godwin M. Automated office blood pressure. Can J Cardiol. 2012;28(3):341–6.
15. Shimbo D, Abdalla M, Falzon L, et al. Role of ambulatory and home blood pressure monitoring in clinical practice: a narrative review. Ann Intern Med. 2015;163(9):691–700.
16. Takahashi K, Asai T, Okuda Y. Efficacy of a new blood pressure monitor (inflationary non-invasive blood pressure, iNIBP): a randomised controlled study. Anaesthesia. 2020;75(1):37–44.
17. Rabi DM, McBrien KA, Sapir-Pichhadze R, et al. Hypertension Canada's 2020 comprehensive guidelines for the prevention, diagnosis, risk assessment, and treatment of hypertension in adults and children. Can J Cardiol. 2020;36(5):596–624.
18. Ringrose JS, McLean D, Ao P, et al. Effect of cuff design on auscultatory and oscillometric blood pressure measurements. Am J Hypertens. 2016;29(9):1063–9.
19. O'Brien E, Atkins N, Stergiou G, et al. European Society of Hypertension International Protocol revision 2010 for the validation of blood pressure measuring devices in adults. Blood Press Monit. 2010;15(1):23–38.
20. Stergiou GS, Karpettas N, Atkins N, et al. European Society of Hypertension International Protocol for the validation of blood pressure monitors: a critical review of its application and rationale for revision. Blood Press Monit. 2010;15(1):39–48.
21. Picone DS, Padwal R, Campbell NRC, et al. How to check whether a blood pressure monitor has been properly validated for accuracy. J Clin Hypertens (Greenwich). 2020;22(12):2167–74.

22. Turner MJ, Speechly C, Bignell N. Sphygmomanometer calibration—why, how and how often? Aust Fam Physician. 2007;36(10):834–8.

23. Pickering TG, Hall JE, Appel LJ, et al. Recommendations for blood pressure measurement in humans and experimental animals: part 1: blood pressure measurement in humans: a statement for professionals from the Subcommittee of Professional and Public Education of the American Heart Association Council on High Blood Pressure Research. Circulation. 2005;111(5):697–716.

24. Babbs CF. The origin of Korotkoff sounds and the accuracy of auscultatory blood pressure measurements. J Am Soc Hypertens. 2015;9(12):935–50e3.

25. Alpert BS, Quinn D, Gallick D. Oscillometric blood pressure: a review for clinicians. J Am Soc Hypertens. 2014;8(12):930–8.

26. Breaux-Shropshire TL, Judd E, Vucovich LA, et al. Does home blood pressure monitoring improve patient outcomes? A systematic review comparing home and ambulatory blood pressure monitoring on blood pressure control and patient outcomes. Integr Blood Press Control. 2015;8:43–9.

27. Green BB, Cook AJ, Ralston JD, et al. Effectiveness of home blood pressure monitoring, Web communication, and pharmacist care on hypertension control: a randomized controlled trial. JAMA. 2008;299(24):2857–67.

28. Kirkland EB, Heincelman M, Bishu KG, et al. Trends in healthcare expenditures among US adults with hypertension: national estimates, 2003–2014. J Am Heart Assoc. 2018;7(11).

29. Schultz BG, Tilton J, Jun J, et al. Cost-effectiveness analysis of a pharmacist-led medication therapy management program: hypertension management. Value Health. 2021;24(4):522–9.

30. Chester MW, Barwise JA, Holzman MD, Pandharipande P. Acute dermal capillary rupture associated with noninvasive blood pressure monitoring. J Clin Anesth. 2007;19(6):473–5.

31. Reeves L, Robinson K, McClelland T, et al. Pharmacist interventions in the management of blood pressure control and adherence to antihypertensive medications: a systematic review of randomized controlled trials. J Pharm Pract. 2021;34(3):480–92.

32. Zaer NF, Amini B, Elsayes KM. Overview of diagnostic modalities and contrast agents. In: Elsayes KM, Oldham SAA, editors. Introduction to diagnostic radiology. New York: McGraw-Hill Education; 2015.

33. Imaging Technology News. Radiographic fluoroscopy (RF). Available from: www.itnonline.com/channel/radiographic-fluoroscopy-rf.

34. World Health Organization. Core medical equipment. World Health Organization; 2011. Available from: www.who.int/medical_devices/en/index.html.

35. van Waardhuizen CN, Khanji MY, Genders TSS, et al. Comparative cost-effectiveness of non-invasive imaging tests in patients presenting with chronic stable chest pain with suspected coronary artery disease: a systematic review. Eur Heart J Qual Care Clin Outcomes. 2016;2(4):245–60.

36. Zeb I, Abbas N, Nasir K, et al. Coronary computed tomography as a cost-effective test strategy for coronary artery disease assessment—a systematic review. Atherosclerosis. 2014;234(2):426–35.

37. Picano E. Economic and biological costs of cardiac imaging. Cardiovasc Ultrasound. 2005;3:13–.

38. Moores BM. Cost-risk-benefit analysis in diagnostic radiology with special reference to the application of referral guidelines. Radiat Prot Dosim. 2019;186(4):479–87.

39. Wallace A, Cain T. InsideRadiology: radiation risk of medical imaging for adults and children. Available from: www.insideradiology.com.au/radiation-risk-hp/.

40. Australian Radiation Protection and Nuclear Safety Agency (ARPANSA). Radiation sources Australia 2021. Available from: www.arpansa.gov.au/understanding-radiation/what-is-radiation/ionising-radiation/health-effects.

41. Gomella LG, Haist SA. Chapter 13: bedside procedures. In: Clinician's pocket reference: the scut monkey, 11th edn. New York: The McGraw-Hill Companies; 2007.

42. Schulman-Marcus J, Prabhakaran D, Gaziano TA. Pre-hospital ECG for acute coronary syndrome in urban India: a cost-effectiveness analysis. BMC Cardiovasc Disord. 2010;10(1):13.

43. Krummen DE, Patel M, Nguyen H, et al. Accurate ECG diagnosis of atrial tachyarrhythmias using quantitative analysis: a prospective diagnostic and cost-effectiveness study. J Cardiovasc Electrophysiol. 2010;21(11):1251–9.

44. Aronsson M, Svennberg E, Rosenqvist M, et al. Cost-effectiveness of mass screening for untreated atrial fibrillation using intermittent ECG recording. EP Europace. 2015;17(7):1023–9.

45. Proietti M, Farcomeni A, Goethals P, et al. Cost-effectiveness and screening performance of ECG handheld machine in a population screening programme: the Belgian Heart Rhythm Week screening programme. Eur J Prevent Cardiol. 2019;26(9):964–72.

46. Lowres N, Neubeck L, Salkeld G, et al. Feasibility and cost-effectiveness of stroke prevention through community screening for atrial fibrillation using iPhone ECG in pharmacies. Thromb Haemost. 2014;111(06):1167–76.

47. Fuller CM. Cost effectiveness analysis of screening of high school athletes for risk of sudden cardiac death. Med Sci Sports Exerc. 2000;32(5):887–90.

48. Grazioli G, Sanz de la Garza M, Vidal B, et al. Prevention of sudden death in adolescent athletes: incremental diagnostic value and cost-effectiveness of diagnostic tests. Eur J Prevent Cardiol. 2020;24(13):1446–54.

49. Quaglini S, Rognoni C, Spazzolini C, et al. Cost-effectiveness of neonatal ECG screening for the long QT syndrome. Eur Heart J. 2006;27(15):1824–32.

50. Kronick SL, Kurz MC, Lin S, et al. Part 4: systems of care and continuous quality improvement: 2015 American Heart Association Guidelines update for cardiopulmonary resuscitation and emergency cardiovascular care. Circulation. 2015;132(18 Suppl 2):S397–413.

51. Noel ZR, Beavers CJ, Dunn SP, et al. Identifying core content for electrocardiogram instruction in doctor of pharmacy curricula. Am J Pharm Educ. 2018;82(10):7009–.

52. Zipes DP, Calkins H, Daubert JP, et al. 2015 ACC/AHA/HRS advanced training statement on clinical cardiac electrophysiology (a revision of the ACC/AHA 2006 update of the clinical competence statement on invasive electrophysiology studies, catheter ablation, and cardioversion). Heart Rhythm. 2016;13(1):e3–e37.

53. Bose DD. An elective course in cardiovascular electrophysiology for pharmacy learners. Am J Pharm Educ. 2016;80(8):130.

54. Mathew P, Kanmanthareddy A. Prosthetic heart valve. In: StatPearls. Treasure Island, FL: StatPearls Publishing. Copyright © 2021, StatPearls Publishing LLC.; 2021.

55. Chikwe J, Castillo JG. Prosthetic heart valves. In: Fuster V, Harrington RA, Narula J, et al., editors. Hurst's the heart, 14th edn. New York: McGraw-Hill Education; 2017.

56. Shapiro N, Hellenbart E. Thrombosis. In: Zeind C, Carvalho M, editors. Applied therapeutics: the clinical use of drugs, 11th edn. Philadelphia: Wolters Kluwer Health, Inc.; 2018.

57. Pibarot P, Dumesnil JG. Prosthetic heart valves: selection of the optimal prosthesis and long-term management. Circulation. 2009;119(7):1034–48.

58. Dixon B, Quader N. Pericardial and valvular heart disease. In: Crees Z, Fritz C, Heudebert A, Noé J, Rengarajan A, Wang X, editors. The Washington Manual® of medical therapeutics, 36th edn. Philadelphia: Wolters Kluwer Health; 2020.

59. David TE, Ivanov J, Armstrong S, et al. Late results of heart valve replacement with the Hancock II bioprosthesis. J Thoracic Cardiovasc Surg. 2001;121(2):268–77.

60. Fuster V, Harrington RA, Narula J, et al. Prosthetic heart valves. Hurst's the heart, 14th edn. New York: McGraw-Hill Education; 2017.

61. Lever MJ. 9—the cardiovascular system. In: Hench LL, Jones JR, editors. Biomaterials, artificial organs and tissue engineering. Cambridge: Woodhead Publishing; 2005. p. 90–6.

62. Bokros JC, Gott VL, La Grange LD, et al. Correlations between blood compatibility and heparin adsorptivity for an impermeable isotropic pyrolytic carbon. J Biomed Mater Res. 1969;3(3):497–528.

63. Dasi LP, Simon HA, Sucosky P, et al. Fluid mechanics of artificial heart valves. Clin Exp Pharmacol Physiol. 2009;36(2):225–37.

64. Bungard TJ, Sonnenberg B. Valvular heart disease: a primer for the clinical pharmacist. Pharmacotherapy. 2011;31(1):76–91.

65. Hirji SA, Kaneko T, Aranki S. The revolution and evolution of mechanical valves: the ball has left the cage. J Thorac Cardiovasc Surg. 2018;155(5):e149–e50.

66. Tashiro H, Popovic M, Dobrev I, et al. Artificial organs, tissues, and support systems. In: Popovic M, editor. Biomechatronics, 1st edn. London: Academic Press; 2019. p. 175–99.

67. Saito S, Tsukui H, Iwasa S, et al. Bileaflet mechanical valve replacement: an assessment of outcomes with 30 years of follow-up†. Interact CardioVascul Thorac Surg. 2016;23(4):599–607.

68. Brennan JM, Edwards FH, Zhao Y, et al. Long-term safety and effectiveness of mechanical versus biologic aortic valve prostheses in older patients: results from the Society of Thoracic Surgeons Adult Cardiac Surgery National Database. Circulation. 2013;127(16):1647–55.

69. Powell S, Choxi R, Gunda S, Jovin IS. A 43-year-old functional Starr—Edwards ball and cage mechanical aortic valve. Gen Thorac Cardiovasc Surg. 2021;69(1):97–9.

70. Cannegieter SC, Rosendaal FR, Wintzen AR, et al. Optimal oral anticoagulant therapy in patients with mechanical heart valves. New Engl J Med. 1995;333(1):11–17.

71. Bonow RO, Carabello BA, Chatterjee K, et al. 2008 Focused update incorporated into the ACC/AHA 2006 guidelines for the management of patients with valvular heart disease: a report of the American College of Cardiology/American Heart Association Task Force on Practice Guidelines (Writing Committee to Revise the 1998 Guidelines for the Management of Patients With Valvular Heart Disease): endorsed by the Society of Cardiovascular Anesthesiologists, Society for Cardiovascular Angiography and Interventions, and Society of Thoracic Surgeons. Circulation. 2008;118(15):e523–661.

72. Jaffer IH, Whitlock RP. A mechanical heart valve is the best choice. Heart Asia. 2016;8(1):62–4.

73. Wilson W, Taubert KA, Gewitz M, et al. Prevention of infective endocarditis: guidelines from the American Heart Association: a guideline from the American Heart Association Rheumatic Fever, Endocarditis, and Kawasaki Disease Committee, Council on Cardiovascular Disease in the Young, and the Council on Clinical Cardiology, Council on Cardiovascular Surgery and Anesthesia, and the Quality of Care and Outcomes Research Interdisciplinary Working Group. Circulation. 2007;116(15):1736–54.

74. Nishimura RA, Carabello BA, Faxon DP, et al. ACC/AHA 2008 guideline update on valvular heart disease: focused update on infective endocarditis: a report of the American College of Cardiology/American Heart Association Task Force on Practice Guidelines: endorsed by the Society of Cardiovascular Anesthesiologists, Society for Cardiovascular Angiography and Interventions, and Society of Thoracic Surgeons. Circulation. 2008;118(8):887–96.

75. Dore A, Somerville J. Pregnancy in patients with pulmonary autograft valve replacement. Eur Heart J. 1997;18(10):1659–62.

76. Batra J, Itagaki S, Egorova NN, et al. Outcomes and long-term effects of pregnancy in women with biologic and mechanical valve prostheses. Am J Cardiol. 2018;122(10):1738–44.

77. Wemple M, Benditt JO. Oxygen therapy and toxicity. In: Grippi MA, Elias JA, Fishman JA, et al., editors. Fishman's pulmonary diseases and disorders, 5th edn. New York: McGraw-Hill Education; 2015.

78. Jubran A. Pulse oximetry. Crit Care (London, England). 2015;19(1):272.

79. Luks AM, Swenson ER. Pulse oximetry for monitoring patients with COVID-19 at home. potential pitfalls and practical guidance. Ann Am Thorac Soc. 2020;17(9):1040–6.

80. DeMeulenaere S. Pulse oximetry: uses and limitations. J Nurse Pract. 2007;3(5):312–17.

81. Chan ED, Chan MM, Chan MM. Pulse oximetry: understanding its basic principles facilitates appreciation of its limitations. Respir Med. 2013;107(6):789–99.

82. Neff TA. Routine oximetry. A fifth vital sign? Chest. 1988;94(2):227.

83. Pulse Oximeters—Premarket notification submissions [510(k)s]: guidance for Industry and Food and Drug Administration Staff. In: Health CfDaR, editor. 2013. p. 19.

84. Philip KEJ, Bennett B, Fuller S, et al. Working accuracy of pulse oximetry in COVID-19 patients stepping down from intensive care: a clinical evaluation. BMJ Open Respir Res. 2020;7(1).

85. Van de Louw A, Cracco C, Cerf C, et al. Accuracy of pulse oximetry in the intensive care unit. Intensive Care Med. 2001;27(10):1606–13.

86. Lipnick MS, Feiner JR, Au P, et al. The accuracy of 6 inexpensive pulse oximeters not cleared by the food and drug administration: the possible global public health implications. Anesth Analg. 2016;123(2):338–45.

87. Rauniyar NK, Pujari S, Shrestha P. Study of oxygen saturation by pulse oximetry and arterial blood gas in ICU

patients: a descriptive cross-sectional study. JNMA J Nepal Med Assoc. 2020;58(230):789–93.

88. Chan MM, Chan MM, Chan ED. What is the effect of fingernail polish on pulse oximetry? Chest. 2003;123(6):2163–4.

89. Sjoding MW, Dickson RP, Iwashyna TJ, et al. Racial bias in pulse oximetry measurement. N Engl J Med. 2020;383(25):2477–8.

90. Pulse Oximeter Accuracy and Limitations: FDA Safety Communication: FDA. 2021. Available from: www.fda. gov/medical-devices/safety-communications/pulse-oximeter-accuracy-and-limitations-fda-safety-communication.

91. Kočka V. The coronary angiography—an old-timer in great shape. Cor et Vasa. 2015;57(6):e419–e24.

92. Corrigendum to: 2019 ESC Guidelines for the diagnosis and management of chronic coronary syndromes. Eur Heart J. 2019;41(44):4242–.

93. Zaer N, Amini B, Elsayes K. Overview of diagnostic modalities and contrast agents. In: Elsayes K, Oldham S, editors. Introduction to diagnostic radiology. New York: McGraw Hill; 2014. p. 1–51.

94. Carrozza J. Complications of diagnostic cardiac catheterization. In: Cutlip D, editor. UpToDate. 2021. Available from: https://www.uptodate.com/contents/complications-of-diagnostic-cardiac-catheterization.

95. Mason PJ, Shah B, Tamis-Holland JE, et al. An update on radial artery access and best practices for transradial coronary angiography and intervention in acute coronary syndrome: a scientific statement from the American Heart Association. Circ Cardiovasc Interv. 2018;11(9):e000035.

96. Arora N, Matheny ME, Sepke C, et al. A propensity analysis of the risk of vascular complications after cardiac catheterization procedures with the use of vascular closure devices. Am Heart J. 2007;153(4):606–11.

97. Crowhurst JA, Whitby M, Thiele D, et al. Radiation dose in coronary angiography and intervention: initial results from the establishment of a multi-centre diagnostic reference level in Queensland public hospitals. J Med Radiat Sci. 2014;61(3):135–41.

98. Webb JA, Thomsen HS, Morcos SK. The use of iodinated and gadolinium contrast media during pregnancy and lactation. Eur Radiol. 2005;15(6):1234–40.

99. on AC, Contrast Da, Media. ACR Manual on Contrast Media. 2021.

100. Patel A. Echocardiography essentials: physics and instrumentation. UpToDate. 2021. Available from: https://www.uptodate.com/contents/echocardiography-essentials-physics-and-instrumentation.

101. Mohamed AA, Arifi AA, Omran A. The basics of echocardiography. J Saudi Heart Assoc. 2010;22(2):71–6.

102. Rotzenberg K, Aulie R, Breslow R, et al. Diagnostic procedures boh's pharmacy practice manual: a guide to the clinical experience, 4th edn. Philadelphia: Wolters Kluwer Health; 2015.

103. Patel A. Transthoracic echocardiography: normal cardiac anatomy and tomographic views. UpToDate. 2021. Available from: https://www.uptodate.com/contents/transthoracic-echocardiography-normal-cardiac-anatomy-and-tomographic-views.

104. Malik SB, Chen N, III RAP, et al. Transthoracic echocardiography: pitfalls and limitations as delineated at cardiac CT and MR imaging. 2017;37(2):383–406.

105. Mayer P. At the heart of the matter: an overview of adult echocardiography for the non-cardiac sonographer. J Diagnost Med Sonogr. 2015;31(4):221–32.

106. Maleki M, Esmaeilzadeh M. The evolutionary development of echocardiography. Iran J Med Sci. 2012;37(4):222–32.

107. Mor-Avi V, Lang RM. Three-dimensional echocardiography. In: Yeon SB, editor. UpToDate. 2021. Available from: https://www.uptodate.com/contents/three-dimensional-echocardiography.

108. Frazin L, Talano JV, Stephanides L, et al. Esophageal echocardiography. Circulation. 1976;54(1):102–8.

109. Seward JB, Khandheria BK, Oh JK, et al. Critical appraisal of transesophageal echocardiography: limitations, pitfalls, and complications. J Am Soc Echocardiogr: Off Publ Am Soc Echocardiogr. 1992;5(3):288–305.

13 Medical Devices for Surgery

Kadir Alam and Subish Palaian

CONTENTS

DOI: 10.1201/9781003002345-15

GENERAL BACKGROUND

Surgery is the branch of medicine employing operations for treating a disease or injury. A surgery normally involves one or more steps such as cutting, abrading, suturing, and sometimes changing the body tissues and organs physically. A medical professional who performs surgery is recognized as a surgeon. There are also surgeons in podiatry, dentistry, and veterinary medicine. Surgical procedures commonly involve bleeding due to incisions made in the body surface that result in damage to the blood vessels. A few commonly performed surgical procedures are appendectomy, cesarean section, cholecystectomy, debridement of wound, burn, or infection. A surgical procedure can be performed in any part of the body and can be categorized as cardiac surgery (heart), gastric surgery (gastrointestinal tract), etc. These days there are surgical procedures involving laparoscopic surgeries and robotic surgeries that cause minimal harm to the body surface and hence are often preferred by patients over the conventional open surgeries.

From a pharmacist's perspective, it is important to be knowledgeable of devices and consumables used in the surgical procedures for three reasons: 1) a pharmacist is involved in selecting vendors, assessing quality in coordination with surgeons, comparing costs, storage, and distribution of these devices and consumables within hospital, 2) a pharmacist often sells these devices and consumables directly to patients while they use these items in their homes, 3) a pharmacist in primary care may use few of these products (e.g., wound dressing materials) directly on their patients. In addition, as it is accepted, a pharmacist is expected by both medical professionals and patients to sell medicines and accessories with "information" and this largely determines whether the patients choose to visit the pharmacies to buy these items instead of a supermarket. In this chapter of the book, authors discuss the surgical items under four categories: sutures, wound care and dressing materials, suction and drainage tubes, and miscellaneous items. The items discussed under this chapter are often considered "general surgical items" because they are used very often. More specialized items used in more specific surgical disciplines, such as cardiac surgery, gastric surgery etc., are discussed elsewhere in this book and hence beyond the scope of this chapter.

DEVICE 1: SURGICAL SUTURES

A. BACKGROUND

Surgical sutures are sterilized threads used to sew skin and other body tissues together after a surgical incision or a tear occurring due to an injury.[1] Sutures are applied using a surgical needle to secure with a surgical knot (Figure 13.1). Sutures minimize the risk of bleeding and infection and facilitate the healing process. In the past, various materials were used for this purpose, which include intestinal tissues and tendons of a large animal, thread derived from fibers of vegetable, camel and horse hair, human hair, metallic wire, and synthetic thread.[1,2] Sutures are sterile in nature and any contamination increases the risk of infection and hence delayed wound healing and other related complications. Often, metallic sutures called as skin staplers and other methods that use glue are employed and are beyond the scope of this chapter.[3,4]

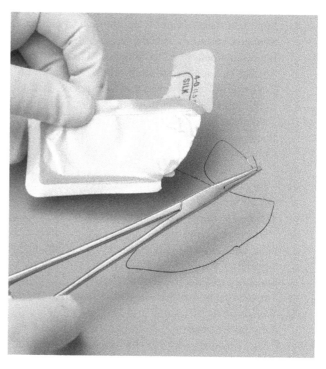

FIGURE 13.1   A sterile suture needle and suture.

Source: www.shutterstock.com/image-photo/surgical-technologist-loading-silk-suture-on-177265151

TABLE 13.1
Brief Description and Indications of Commonly Used Sutures

Type of suture		Feature and application
Absorbable sutures (are absorbed into body)	Catgut e.g., Chromic Gut (Ethicon), Trugut (Suture India)	Natural monofilament. Used for repairing internal soft tissue wounds or lacerations. Not suitable for cardiovascular or neurological procedures.
	Polydioxanone e.g., PDS (Ethicon), MonoPlus (B*Braun)	Synthetic monofilament used for soft tissue wound repair (such as abdominal closures) as well as pediatric cardiac procedures.
	Poliglecaprone e.g., Monocryl (Ethicon), Monoglyde (Suture India)	Synthetic monofilament used for soft tissue repair. Most commonly used to close skin in an invisible manner.
	Polyglactin e.g., Vicryl (Ethicon), Maxon (Covidien)	Synthetic braided suture used for repairing hand or facial lacerations. Not used for cardiovascular or neurological procedures.
Nonabsorbable sutures	Nylon e.g., Ethilon Nylon (Ethicon), Dafilon (B*Braun)	Indicated in general soft tissue approximation and/or ligation. Used in cardiovascular, neurological, and eye procedures.
	Polypropylene e.g., Prolene (Ethicon), Trulene (Suture India)	Used in skin closure during cardiovascular, ophthalmic, and neurological procedures.
	Silk e.g., Silk (Ethicon), Sofsilk (Covidien)	Used in general soft tissue approximation and/or ligation, cardiovascular, ophthalmic, and neurological procedures.

B. DEVICE DESCRIPTION/IMPORTANT FEATURES

Sutures are broadly classified as absorbable and nonabsorbable based on their ability to be absorbed into the human body. Brief descriptions on the common types of surgical sutures are provided in Table 13.1.[1,2,3,4] More details are provided by manufacturers in the form of a manual.[5]

A more detailed classification of suture materials is available in literature and can be read from here.[6,7]

i. Suture Nomenclature[8,9]

Since sutures are of different natures and sizes and often with very slight differences, it is important to know their nomenclature. The size of sutures refers to the diameter of the suture strand (the smaller the suture, the larger the number). A few of the salient features of suture nomenclature are as follows:

1. As per the USP scale, 11–0 (smallest) to #7 (largest). Zeros are written as 2–0 for 00 and 3–0 for 000, etc., for convenience and clarity.
2. From sizes 0 to 11–0, each extra zero corresponds to a unit decrease in diameter (e.g., 0, 00, 000, etc. until the smallest size of eleven zeroes is reached). More zeros mean smaller (and hence weaker) the suture diameter.
3. The smallest sutures such as 10–0 are tiny in nature and are mostly applied during microvascular surgery.
4. The biggest size is 00 that is commonly applied in abdominal wall closure.
5. The most commonly used sutures are sized between 3–0 and 6–0.

In summary, small sutures such as 5–0 and 6–0 are applied in facial surgery and the bigger ones such as 3–0 and 4–0 are applied in body parts.

ii. Categorization of Suture Needle Attached to the Sutures

Normally, sutures are available along with a needle attached to the length of thread. The needle facilitates placing the suture correctly in the tissue and carrying through with minimal trauma. While understanding the suture, it is also important to know the nature and categorization of the suture needle. The ideal qualities of a suture needle are available in literature.[8,10,11] The most commonly used suture needles are made of stainless steel.

Needle bodies can be categorized into round, cutting, reverse cutting, and/or tapered.[8,10,11] They are used for stitching soft tissues like liver and kidney, tough tissues like sternum, tough tissues like tendon, and subcutaneous tissues respectively [Figure 13.2].

C. PURPOSE AND HOW TO USE

The pharmacist should know how to describe the use of the suture so that they can understand and help surgeons select the appropriate ones, and use the sutures correctly while performing first aid themselves. The common steps involved in a simple surgical suturing are as follows:[12]

Step I: A needle holder is used to grasp the needle at the distal portion of the body, one half to three quarters of the distance from the tip of the needle.

Step II: The needle holder is tightened by squeezing it until the first ratchet catches.

TYPES OF SURGICAL NEEDLES

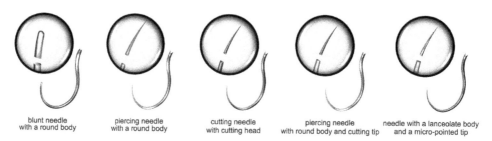

blunt needle   piercing needle   cutting needle   piercing needle   needle with a lanceolate body
with a round body   with a round body   with cutting head   with round body and cutting tip   and a micro-pointed tip

FIGURE 13.2   Depictions of different types of surgical suture needles.

Source: www.shutterstock.com/image-vector/vector-illustration-types-surgical-needles-1046743390

Step III: The needle is held vertically and longitudinally perpendicular to the needle holder.

Step IV: The needle is placed vertically and longitudinally perpendicular to needle holder.

Step V: The needle holder is held through loops between thumb and fourth finger, and index finger rests on fulcrum of instrument.

More details on the use of sutures can be viewed from the YouTube link provided [13] and text books.[4]

D.   IMPORTANT SAFETY ISSUES (CAUTIONS AND COMMON ADVERSE EFFECTS)

In general, sutures do not carry any major side effects. However, at times they may cause some allergic reaction. Unexpected tissue reactions like inflammation, granuloma, extrusion, fistula, and abscess have been reported with absorbable surgical suture.[14] Similarly, inconvenience, pain, and specific morbidity were reported with nonabsorbable suture (retention suture).[15] A delayed skin reaction to synthetic suture poliglecaprone 25 has been reported.[16] A rare severe inflammatory reaction to nylon sutures has also been documented.[17] Conclusively, sutures are safe but sometimes they may produce an allergic reaction like itching in some patients. Mostly it is self-limited but in case of serious reaction, the patient should be advised to report to the surgeon at the earliest opportunity.

E.   STORAGE CONDITIONS AND MAINTENANCE

Sterilized surgical suture should be protected from light and stored in a cool and dry place. It should be packed in an air-tight container with moisture content less than 0.1%. If not stored properly, sutures may lose their strength. The shelf life of sutures is usually long (4–5 years or more). After expiry, they breakdown and become unusable.[18]

F.   IMPORTANT FEATURES (CAPABILITIES AND LIMITATIONS) AND SPECIAL ADVANTAGES

The choice of suture material depends on type of tissue, wound, and place to be stitched, and is always decided by the surgeon. Comparing different sutures is very difficult because there is no consensus among the different users. Many surgeons prefer nonabsorbable suture material because it is easy to tie and less likely to break prematurely, and it generates minimal inflammatory response. Others prefer absorbable sutures because they do not have to be removed, saving time and reducing patient anxiety and discomfort.[19]

G.   SPECIAL TIPS FOR PATIENT COUNSELING

Since sutures are not used by patients at their own will, there are only a few counseling points. However, after suturing the wound, care and protection should be done by the patient as suggested by the surgeon. Following are a few tips for counseling a patient who has recently undergone wound closure by suture:

1. Keep wound area dry for the first 24 hours and protect from water.
2. Apply antibiotic ointment for 48 hours, after which it can be left uncovered.
3. Patient may shower if permitted by the surgeon but only after the wound has healed.
4. A wet dressing promotes bacterial growth and hence should be avoided while sutures are still on the body.
5. Any signs of infection such as fever, increased redness, swelling, tenderness, pus at the suture site, etc. should be immediately reported to the surgeon.
6. Return to hospital for suture removal as advised by the surgeon.

H.   EVIDENCE OF EFFECTIVENESS AND SAFETY

Surgical sutures are usually safe and effective, but some of the common issues related to surgical sutures are listed in Table 13.2. The standards/quality of sutures are normally established based on the certifications obtained by specific suture brands.

TABLE 13.2

Evidence of effectiveness and safety of sutures

Authors	Objective	Major findings
Burute SB, Karan A, Puri M, Sansare S[20]	Efficacy of different types of sutures in wound closure	• No significant difference between absorbable (Polyglactin 910) suture and nonabsorbable (Nylon) suture in terms of wound complication was observed. • Common side effects seen with these sutures were a rise in temperature, itching at suturing site, mild rigor, and yellowish discharge.
Kailas CT, Naik CG[21]	Comparison of efficacy of two suture materials, the delayed-absorbable polydioxanone (PDS) versus nonabsorbable suture polypropylene (PPL) in abdominal wound closure	• PDS was found superior to nonabsorbable PPL while used in cases of midline laparotomy incision closure and preventing wound complications.
Gokarneshan N[22]	Review of new-generation surgical sutures	• Medicated suture and smart sutures are more effective in achieving target drug delivery at surgical site and are able to reduce surgical site infection, inflammation, and pain.

I. ECONOMIC EVALUATION

Cost comparison of sutures is crucial since they contribute to a major portion of the surgical procedure cost. Hence, a careful consideration of suture cost should be made within the same brand and among different brands. Table 13.3 lists few studies comparing the cost of sutures.

J. IMPLICATION TO THE PHARMACY PROFESSION AND PHARMACY PRACTICE

Sutures are essential products available in any pharmacy and often a pharmacist manages suture inventory in the operation theatre. A pharmacy practitioner should be aware of the following information about sutures:

1. Nomenclature: Pharmacists are expected to handle sutures in various settings and are hence expected to know the suture nomenclature and description of each type.

2. Counseling patients: Pharmacists should know special counseling points on sutures in terms of their storage and uses.

3. Direct use by pharmacists: While pharmacists use sutures in primary care, they should be knowledgeable on the natures of the suture materials and should be able to choose the most suitable one for a given condition.

4. Cost comparison of sutures: Economic analyses of sutures can be performed by pharmacists and can thus help in cost containment through effective procurement procedures.

5. Storage and inventory management: Sutures generally have a five-year shelf life and pharmacists can play an important role in proper inventory management.

6. Substitution of sutures: Since sutures are often replaceable with a different brand of the same size and type and even with different sizes, pharmacists can play an important role in substitution of sutures. However, such substitutions can be done only after being approved by the operating surgeon.

TABLE 13.3

Studies Comparing the Costs of Different Sutures

Authors	Objective	Major findings
Elmallah RK et al.[23]	Cost comparison using barbed versus conventional interrupted sutures	Barbed sutures reduce surgery time and thus total cost in comparison to interrupted sutures. The postoperative complications remain the same for both types.
Gokani SA et al.[24]	Economic evaluation of small bite sutures versus large bite sutures in the closure of midline laparotomies	Reduction in SSI rates and herniation leading to cost savings was reported with small bite sutures.

K. CHALLENGES TO PHARMACISTS AND USERS

The major challenges are lack of product knowledge on handling of suture materials and understanding their nomenclature. In addition, at times different surgeons in different hospitals prefer different brands of sutures leading to overstocking of sutures, which can be another challenge to the pharmacy managers.

L. RECOMMENDATIONS: THE WAY FORWARD

Since sutures are commonly handled by pharmacists, pharmacists are expected to be knowledgeable on their chemical nature, nomenclature, storage, indications, and other aspects of sutures. These aspects will further enhance cost effective and proper utilization by surgeons and other health professionals. It is also recommended that pharmacy curricula address adequate emphasis on technical aspects of handling sutures; experiential learning programs cover these aspects. In addition, more research is needed on exploring the scope of pharmacists in handling of suture materials.

M.   Conclusions

It is learned that there are enough technical aspects on suture materials making it essential for pharmacists to be involved actively in handling sutures, such as procurement, storage, distribution, and educating other health professionals and patients. Pharmacists can also help cost-containment of sutures in multiple ways. More research on efficacy and economic effects of sutures is needed and can be coordinated by pharmacists.

N.   Lessons Learned

- Sutures are important surgical items needed for all surgical procedures involving manipulation in the human body.
- Pharmacists should have a thorough understanding of the nomenclature and procurement standards of sutures.
- There is considerable scope for substitution of sutures in different procedures and thus pharmacists can contribute a great deal towards minimizing economic losses due to expiry.

DEVICE 2: WOUND CARE AND DRESSING MATERIAL

A.   Background

Wounds are injuries in body tissue caused by a cut, blow, or other impact leading to disruption in the protective function of the skin.[25,26] Wounds can lead to complications, such as infections, and often lead to permanent damage to the affected area. Wounds are of different types and this chapter of the book deals only with open wounds requiring dressing. Wound care is the critical step in the treatment of wounds and requires adequate pharmacological care and dressing to be followed. Many times, patients with wounds receive care from a pharmacist, be it a new fresh wound or an old one, like in the case of diabetic foot. Proper wound care consists of dressing materials, antimicrobials, and other supportive treatments targeting hygiene and inhibition of microbial population at the site of wound.

Currently, large numbers of dressing materials are used for wound care and range from conventional dressing materials to newer materials. Generally, dressings are of different types. Primary dressing is the layer which is in direct contact with the wound, secondary dressing is the layer covering primary dressing for further care, and island dressing involves an absorbent core and a transparent layer with an adhesive on it.[27j]

B.   Device Description and Important Features

Traditionally, wound dressing materials are classified based on the type of material and at times based on their mechanism of wound protection as passive, interactive, and bioactive products. An ideal dressing material should be sterile and hypoallergenic, and should offer protection to the wounds from bacteria and foreign particles.[28] This chapter of the book describes only the most common types of dressing materials available on the market (Table 13.4). A more detailed description of the dressing materials is available in literature. [27,28,29,30,31,32]

C.   Purpose of Use

Wound dressings are designed to facilitate the healing process by providing a favorable wound environment. The purpose/indications of various types of dressing materials are given here in Table 13.5.

TABLE 13.4
Various Dressing Materials[27,28,29,30,31,32]

Name of the dressing material	Description
Gauze dressing	Traditionally used materials are made of cotton or polyester fibers available in different shapes (common size: 4"x4") and sizes.

FIGURE 13.3   A roll of cotton gauze for wound dressing.
Source: www.shutterstock.com/image-photo/white-medical-cotton-gauze-bandage-on-52306123
Common brands: Bactisafe gauze dressing, Bactigras gauze dressing

Name of the dressing material	Description
Composite dressing	This dressing consists of a combination of different types of dressing like gauze and foam, alginate, and carboxymethyl cellulose sodium (CMC), and silver ion dressing. It is available in multiple sizes such as 2"x3", 3(1/5)"x4", 3(1/5)"x6", 4"x4", 4"x8", 4"x10", 4"x12", 4"x14", 6"x6". Common brands: COVRSITE* Plus composite dressing, Cardinal Health™ composite dressings, etc.
Foam dressing	These are made from sheet of polymer materials consisting of three layers: anti-adhesion layer that remains in contact with wound, infiltration layer, and waterproof layer. They are highly absorbent leading to less risk of maceration, and the foams provide a moist environment to the wound. This dressing is available in multiple sizes of 2"x2", 4"x4" and 6"x6". Common brand: Allevyn adhesive foam dressing
Alginate dressing	This consists of extracts of naturally occurring polysaccharide derived from seaweed. It absorbs fluid from wounds and forms a gel-like substance. They are available in different sizes of 2"x2", 4"x4". Common brands: Algisite M calcium alginate dressing, Cutimed alginate calcium wound dressing
Hydrogel dressing	This dressing is made up of CMC, pectin, or propylene glycol. It is a hydrophilic gel pad, having high water content and thus showing weak exudate absorptive capacity. It provides a moist environment for wounds that are dry in nature. Available in tube as well as in the dressing sheet of 2"x2" and 4"x4". Common brands: Cutimed Hydro B, DynaGel
Hydrocolloid dressing	This consists of CMC along with gelatin, pectin, elastomers, and plasticizer. It forms a hydrated gel over wound surface and is available commonly as 2"x2" and 4"x4". Common brands: DynaDerm hydrocolloid dressing, Hydraseal hydrocolloid dressing
Antibacterial wound dressing	This contains antibacterial substances which work against a wide range of bacteria and fungi. It kills or inhibits bacteria, fungus, protozoa, viruses, and prions. It is available in different sizes of 1"x3", 2"x2", 4"x5", 6"x6", 8"x12", and many more sizes.

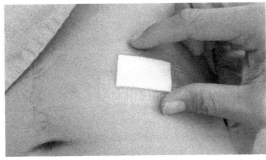

FIGURE 13.4 An antibacterial wound dressing.
Source: www.shutterstock.com/image-photo/surgical-wound-715785931
Common brands: Areza antibacterial dressing, Covidien Kendall AMD antimicrobial dressing

Iodine dressing	This three-dimensional polysaccharide lattice of iodine dressing contains 0.9% iodine and is available in sizes of 2"x2" and 4"x4".

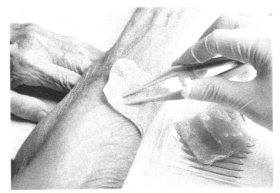

FIGURE 13.5 An iodine lattice dressing.
Source: www.shutterstock.com/image-photo/wound-dressing-doctor-cleaning-wash-infected-1770239339
Common brands: Inadine Dressing, Iodoflex Dressing

TABLE 13.5

Purpose of Use of Dressing Materials[27,28,29,30,31,32]

Name of the dressing material	Purpose of use
Gauze dressing	Used for providing first aid to any injury and is preferred in cleaning local wounds.
Composite dressing	Most commonly used in wounds of infectious origin, surgical wounds, chronic wounds, and grade II and II burns.
Foam dressing	Used in wounds of partial or full-thickness injury origin.
Alginate dressing	Indicated in venous ulcers, sinus wounds, and severely exudating wounds.
Hydrogel dressing	Preferred in wounds leaking fluid, wounds that are painful or necrotizing, pressure ulcers, second-degree burns, and wounds that are infected.
Hydrocolloid dressing	Applied in burns, wounds that emit liquid, necrotizing wounds, and pressure and venous ulcers.
Iodine dressing	Provides a moist wound-healing environment by gradually releasing iodine into the wound; usually used in infected wounds with moderate amounts of exudate and sloughy wounds.
Antibacterial wound dressing	Applied on infectious wounds, especially serious wounds that need to be taken care for recovery and in case of germ infection.

D. IMPORTANT SAFETY ISSUES (CAUTIONS AND COMMON ADVERSE EFFECTS)

Usually, wound care dressings are safe but they have a potential risk to health. Common adverse drug reactions (ADRs) include adverse tissue reaction (e.g., toxicity, allergic reaction), delayed wound healing, retention of dressing material in wound especially with solid wound dressing, incompatibility with other therapy, risk of infection, microbial growth within product due to infective antimicrobial activity and lack of preservative effectiveness, and/or product degradation during shelf storage.[33]

However, ADRs observed with the use of antimicrobial dressing are allergic reaction (including anaphylaxis), rashes, erythema, infection, blistering, tissue damage, skin irritation, burning sensation, and cellulitis. In addition to all, there is growing concern of antimicrobial resistance.[33]

E. STORAGE CONDITIONS AND MAINTENANCE[34]

Like any other surgical materials, wound dressings should be stored in temperatures not exceeding 25°C and in a ventilated, dry place. Improper storage can lead to development of ADRs, especially upon long storage, and can make them brittle, perished, stained, and malodorous. Any damaged or wet packaging should be discarded. Readers are further advised to refer to the product leaflets for more specific information on storage of specific products.

F. IMPORTANT FEATURES (CAPABILITIES AND LIMITATIONS) AND SPECIAL ADVANTAGES

The choice of dressing materials depends upon the nature of the wound and is mainly based on the wound characteristics; these are discussed in literature.[29,30,31,35,36] While selecting the appropriate wound dressing materials, it is important to consider the important features and special

advantages and limitations of various surgical dressings given in Table 13.6.

G. SPECIAL TIPS FOR PATIENT COUNSELING

The procedures followed in wound dressing are beyond the scope of this chapter. Counseling the patients on proper use of dressing materials is important. In general, the patients should be provided counseling on:

1. Aspects related to wound care and wound hygiene depending upon the nature of the wounds.
2. Storage of dressing materials.
3. Choice of wound dressing materials based on the nature of the wound.

H. EVIDENCE OF EFFECTIVENESS AND SAFETY

A common problem with wound care is lack of evidence on the efficacy of different types of wound procedures and wound dressing products. It is recommended to develop a suitable design for establishing evidences and to establish an international working group focusing on these issues.[7] There are a few studies that compare the safety and efficacy of wound dressing materials.[38,39]

I. IMPLICATION TO THE PHARMACY PROFESSION AND PHARMACY PRACTICE

Wound care can be considered an extended community pharmacy service by the pharmacists, and hence pharmacists should be knowledgeable on various types of wound care products that are available. Wound care can be a niche area for community pharmacists.[40] A detailed role of the pharmacist in wound care is discussed by Susie Jin.[41] In addition, a pharmacist should know the choice of dressing materials for a given type of wound. Pharmacists can

TABLE 13.6
Advantages and Limitations of Various Surgical Dressings

Name of the device	Advantages	Limitations
Gauze dressing	Cheap, easy to use, and used with simple solutions such as normal saline, topical antimicrobial, gel, etc., and along with other dressing materials.	Disrupts wound healing if it becomes dry; often requires secondary dressing and must be removed carefully. In addition, it may cause maceration of skin and is not suitable for highly exudating wounds. It also requires frequent dressing, which is time consuming.
Foam dressing	Available in many different shapes and sizes, highly absorbent, and very protective.	May prevent occurrence of autolysis.
Alginate dressing	Generates moist environment to nerve endings and reduces pain. Suitable for wounds that bleed.	Used only in wounds with exuding nature. Sometimes the dressing adheres to wound surface leading to stinging and discomfort.
Hydrogel dressing	Some of the dressing allows wound visualizing. It keeps nerve ending moist and hence reduces pain.	Can cause maceration of the nearby skin and the presence of preservatives poses hypersensitivity risk for predisposed individuals.
Hydrocolloid dressing	Being waterproof it allows patients to shower, absorbs exudate, provides moist wound environment, and thus promotes formation of new tissue.	Favors growth of anaerobic bacteria and at times possesses malodor often mistaken for pus.
Antibacterial wound dressing	Absorbs exudate and bacteria, can reduce hypergranulation.	Patients may experience transient stinging or burning upon application.
Iodine dressing	Easy to use, has broad spectrum antiseptic effects, and is used prophylactically against bacteria, protozoa, and fungi.	Contraindicated in thyroid disorder (due to interference with thyroid level), pregnancy, and lactating women.

also conduct safety and efficacy studies for commonly used wound dressing materials.

J. CHALLENGES TO PHARMACISTS AND USERS

The major challenge is choosing the most appropriate ones for different type of wounds. Another challenge is applying the dressing materials in proper form.

K. RECOMMENDATIONS: THE WAY FORWARD

Pharmacy curricula should train pharmacists on wound care, an achievable patient care activity with minimal resources, and can be helpful for patients to a larger extent. There is also a need for research to compare the safety and effectiveness of various dressing materials, and pharmacists can collaborate such research efforts.

L. CONCLUSIONS

Considering that wound care can be a niche area for community pharmacists and wound care can be often easy and deliverable with minimal resources at pharmacies, this service can be promising for pharmacists.

M. LESSONS LEARNED

- There are different types of wound dressing materials which often requires careful selection.

- Wound care can be a niche area for community pharmacists.
- More research is needed on comparative safety and efficacy of available wound dressing materials.

DEVICE 3: SURGICAL DRAIN AND DRAINAGE CATHETERS

A. BACKGROUND

Most wounds produce some exudate and discharges usually described as serosanguineous, and it contains both blood and blood serum (a clear yellow liquid) that needs to be drained. The nature of the wound drain is described by type, color, amount, and odor. Most common type of drainage is described as serous if it is clear and thin, which may be present in a healthy, healing wound; or serosanguineous if it contains blood, which may also be present in a healthy, healing wound; or sanguineous, which primarily contains blood; or purulent, which describes thick, white, pus-like exudate indicating infection and should be cultured.[42,43] It is undoubtedly clear that any wound exudate should be drained in order to facilitate the healing process. This part of the chapter mentions various drainage materials used by surgeons after performing surgery, or at times any drainage process, such as pleural tapping.

B. DEVICE DESCRIPTION AND IMPORTANT FEATURES

Surgical drains are small plastic tubes placed in the site of the wound during the surgery and remain until removed, which normally takes a few days. The drainage tubes are connected to a small plastic bag that collects any fluid or air that has drained away from the site of wound. The necessity of placing a drain is decided by the surgeon after several factors are assessed.[44] Commonly used drains include closed wound suction, chest drains, and abdominal drains. The important features of surgical drain items are given in Table 13.7.

C. PURPOSE AND HOW TO USE

The purpose and use of common surgical drain items are described in Table 13.8.

D. IMPORTANT FEATURES (CAPABILITIES AND LIMITATIONS) AND SPECIAL ADVANTAGES OF DRAINAGE CATHETERS

The ideal drain fits the following criteria:[55]

- It should be neither too rigid nor too soft.
- It should be smooth to facilitate easy removal after use.
- It should be made up of non-decomposing and non-disintegrating materials to avoid leaving foreign bodies in the patient after removal.
- It should be wide enough and patent to prevent blockage by effluents.
- It should not have electrolytic properties.
- It should be non-carcinogenic and non-thrombogenic while being used in vascular surgeries.

TABLE 13.7

Important Features of Surgical Drain Items

Device	Descriptions
Closed wound suction	This drain consists of a rubber tube connected to a soft, round squeeze bulb at one end, another end is kept on the site where fluid is expected to build up, and the last end outside the body through a small incision (cut). The medium-level vacuum created by the squeeze bulb results in drainage of serosanguineous fluid from the wound.[45,46]

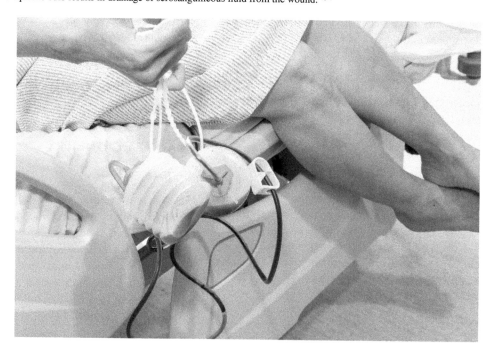

FIGURE 13.6 A closed wound suction device.
Source: www.shutterstock.com/image-photo/patient-holding-surgical-blood-drainage-collection-1867258393
Size of chamber: 600 and 800 mL
Sizes for tubes: 6, 8, 10, 12, 14, 16, and 18 FG
Examples of commercially available device are available here.[47]

Chest drainage catheter/chest tubes	These are hollow flexible tubes placed between ribs and into the space between the inner lining and the outer lining of chest to drain fluid, blood, or air from thoracic cavity region. The tube may be connected to a machine to help with the drainage.[48] Examples of commercially available tubes are present here.[49]

Device	Descriptions
Abdominal catheter/ suprapubic catheter	This is a soft and smooth catheter with large atraumatic eyes with a radiopaque line throughout for X-ray visualization. It is specially designed for postoperative abdominal drainage with very smooth kink resistance tubing that ensures uniform flow rate.

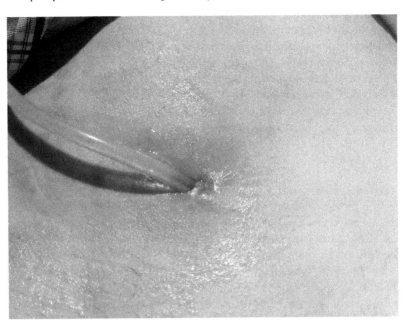

FIGURE 13.7 An abdominal catheter.
Source: www.shutterstock.com/image-photo/suprapubic-catheter-inserted-urinary-retention-patient-1548776237
The bag capacity is about 2 L and length of tube is about 50 cm.
Available sizes are 16 FG, 20 FG, 24 FG, 28 FG, and 32 FG.
Examples of commercially available suprapubic catheters are available here.[50]

TABLE 13.8
Purpose of Use of Surgical Drains

Device	Purpose of use
Closed wound suction	Used to drain surgical wounds with serosanguineous fluid. Helps preventing infections, hematomas, and other factors interfering with the healing of wound. The main indications are to prevent accumulation of fluid and air.[51]
Chest drainage catheter	Applied to drain fluid and air from the pleural space[52] in pneumothorax, hemothorax, chylothorax, pleural effusions, and postoperatively, e.g., after cardiac surgery or thoracotomy.[53]
Abdominal catheter	Use to drain fluid from abdomen accumulated due to inflammation, infection, and traumatic injury.[54]

E. SPECIAL TIPS FOR PATIENT COUNSELING

The patients on chest drainage system should be told not to lie on the tube and to keep the collection part upright and below the chest. The drainage should be kept clean and dry. Patients on a chest tube should be instructed to perform coughing and breathing exercises. More information can be obtained here.[56]

F. EVIDENCE OF EFFECTIVENESS AND SAFETY

Authors	Objectives	Major findings
Tanaka K et al.	To study appropriate management of abdominal drains and their effectiveness	Abdominal drains were found effective in postoperative monitoring as well as in morbidity treatment.[57]
Alcalá-Cerra G	Meta-analysis to analyze safety and efficacy of subdural drains	Insertion of a subdural drain reduces the risk recurrence and need of surgical interventions.[58]
Wakai S et al.	To study efficacy of closed-system drainage in treating chronic subdural hematoma	Findings concluded that it reduces the recurrence rate of chronic subdural hematoma.[59]
Cafarotti S et al.	To study safety and effectiveness of chest drains in pneumothorax, malignant effusions, and pleural empyema	Well-tolerated and acceptable morbidity in treating pneumothorax. It is not indicated for the treatment of empyema.[60]

G. IMPLICATION TO THE PHARMACY PROFESSION AND PHARMACY PRACTICE

Often patients with wounds might require these devices attached while receiving home care. Hence, the pharmacist should be knowledgeable about the use of the devices and should be able to instruct patients regarding the same. Similarly, a pharmacist working in hospitals must be knowledgeable on the purpose of these devices, their description, and instructions for use. Pharmacists involved in procurement should also be aware of the quality considerations while choosing a cost-effective, high-quality product.

H. CONCLUSIONS

Often surgical wounds exudate, and specialized devices are needed to remove these exudates. Similarly, fluid accumulation in body cavities needs removal using specialized drainage devices. These devices are of different types and specifications. A well-chosen drainage item, as normally performed by surgeons, can substantially influence the wound-healing process. Upon fixing the suction and drainage system, patients must ensure that it is being maintained in a proper manner, and any abnormalities in the system should be identified and repaired. The availability of cost-effective, good-quality suction and drainage systems within the hospital lies in the hands of pharmacists involved in procurement.

I. LESSONS LEARNED

- Wound drainage devices facilitate wound healing and should be of good quality.
- Pharmacists have a crucial role in ensuring cost-effective, good-quality suction and drainage devices.

DEVICE 4: MISCELLANEOUS SURGICAL DEVICES

A. BACKGROUND

In this part of the chapter, authors categorize some other surgical devices that are not grouped under previous sections. These items are related to transfusion, infusion, central venous catheterization, and others. These devices maybe important from a pharmacist's perspective since some of them are very commonly used in hospitals and a thorough product knowledge among pharmacists is considered crucial.

B. DEVICE DESCRIPTION AND IMPORTANT FEATURES

The features of selected devices are described here.

i. Intravenous Infusion Set (IV Set/ Blood Transfusion Set)[61,62,63,64]

This device enables delivery of liquid dosage forms directly into the patient's vein through an IV cannula. Broadly, they are used for two purposes: either to infuse blood, or non-blood products such as saline, which may be often mixed with other drugs. Based on the purpose of use, IV sets may be micro (small quantity, accurate dosing, and usually delivers 1 mL in 60 drops) and macro (large volume at rapid rate and usually delivers as few as 10 drips to infuse one mL). (Figure 13.8)

Different types of IV sets available in the markets are:

1. Filtered IV sets: These have a filter as small as 0.22 micron–5.0 microns enabling filtering of microorganisms and large particles.

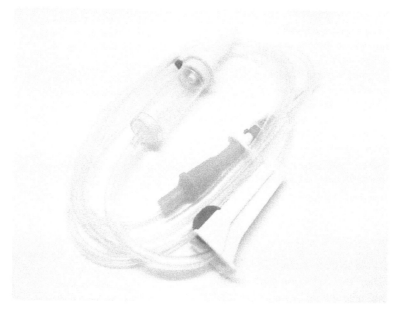

FIGURE 13.8 An intravenous infusion set (also known as an "IV line").

2. Vented IV sets: These have a small vent that can be opened and closed allowing air to enter and displace the fluid from the IV container.

3. Non-vented IV sets: These allow a vacuum to be created inside the plastic IV bag enabling it to collapse as it is emptied.

4. Gravity tubing: These devices rely upon gravity and flow rate regulators to infuse the fluid. They can be set in drops per minute, which can be equated to mL/hour infusion rate.

5. IV set with extension line: These are used to extend IV lines without risk of contamination.

A list of commercially available IV sets can be read here.[65]

ii. Three-Way Stopcock[66,67]

This device regulates the flow of fluid through a tube. A stopcock is a form of valve used to control the flow of a liquid or gas. The valve is designed to completely stop the flow when closed fully. The three-way stopcock with extension tube is also available for improved use (Figure 13.9).

iii. IV Cannula[68,69]

IV cannulas are placed inside a vein to get venous access in patients. Once placed, IV cannulas allow blood withdrawal for tests, administration of fluids, medications, parenteral nutrition, chemotherapy, and blood products. IV cannulas

are available in different gauges ranging from 14 G to 26 G with lengths varying between 25–44 mm. Each gauge by a manufacturer has color coding, e.g., 14 G (orange), 16 G (gray), 18 G (green), 20 G (pink), 22 G (blue), 24 G (yellow), and 26 G (purple). The IV cannulas are also available as Safety IV cannulas, which offer safety to the nurse using them. A detail on Safety IV cannulas is available here.[70] (Figure 13.10)

iv. Central Venous Catheter[71,72,73]

Also known as a central line, this is a thin, flexible tube inserted into a large vein in the neck, chest, groin, or arm. It is mostly placed below the right collarbone and guided (threaded) into a large vein above the right side of the heart called the superior vena cava. These catheters are very important in patients receiving Intensive Care Unit (ICU) care.

v. Ambu Bag/Self-Inflating Bag[74,75,76]

This device is used for providing artificial respiration for a deteriorating patient facing breathing difficulties. It provides oxygen via an endotracheal tube or face mask in emergencies. This device is a compressible, self-inflating bag made up of silicone connected with a one-way valve that only allows entry of air. Air from bag is pushed into throat by pressing the bag to ultimately reach the lungs, thus providing artificial ventilation (Figure 13.11).

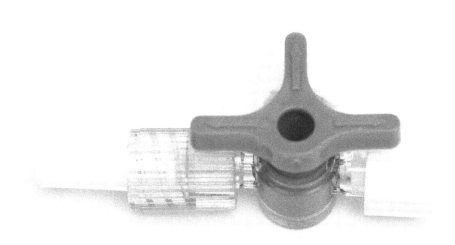

FIGURE 13.9 A three-way stopcock apparatus.

Source: www.shutterstock.com/image-photo/3-way-stop-cock-isolated-on-766121614

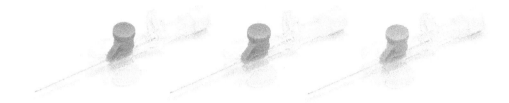

FIGURE 13.10   A set of IV cannulas.

Source: www.shutterstock.com/image-photo/iv-catheter-intravenous-needle-stabbing-blood-1203964825

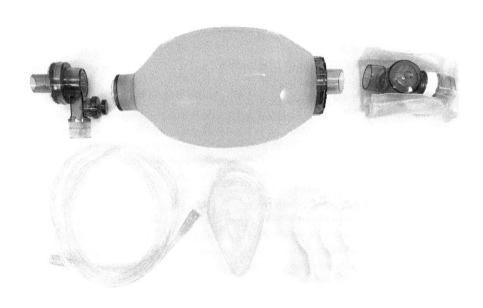

FIGURE 13.11   The components of a self-inflating bag (known widely by the original proprietary name Ambu bag).

Source: www.shutterstock.com/image-photo/medical-breathing-devices-called-ambu-placed-1696596571

D.   IMPLICATION TO THE PHARMACY PROFESSION AND PHARMACY PRACTICE

These devices actually contribute to the majority of the surgical devices sold in a hospital pharmacy. These devices are further available from different manufacturers with different specifications. Often a slight change in the specifications makes a huge difference in the price. A careful consideration of cost versus specifications and quality should be considered by the pharmacists while procuring these devices. Since they are commonly moving items, a bulk purchase can be cost-effective.

E.   CONCLUSIONS

The aforementioned miscellaneous devices account for a vast majority of surgical items used in a hospital and hence the pharmacist should be knowledgeable regarding these devices. There is a large scope of saving costs by having adequate knowledge of these products. In addition, an Ambu bag is used while transferring patients from one ward to another, while transferring the patients for X-rays, CT scan, MRI, etc., and at times while transferring patients from one hospital to another hospital. It is recommended that every health professional in a hospital learns to use this device. At times, patients are trained to use this device by pharmacists and hence pharmacists should be knowledgeable about these devices and their correct use and function.

F.   LESSONS LEARNED

- These devices form a major portion of surgical items sold in a hospital pharmacy.
- A bulk purchase can be more profitable and cost-effective.

ACKNOWLEDGMENT

Authors would like to acknowledge Dr. Gani Alam, Senior Resident, Department of Surgery, Western Regional Hospital, Pokhara Academic Health and Sciences, Pokhara, Nepal, for reviewing the scientific contents and suggesting modifications.

REFERENCES

1. Cooper J, Gunn C. Surgical ligatures and sutures. In: Carter SJ, editor. Tutorial pharmacy. New Delhi, India: CBS Publishers and Distributors; 1986. p. 429–32.

2. Rawlins EA. Suture and ligatures. In: Bentleys textbook of pharmaceutics, 8th edn. London, England: Bailliére Tindall; 1995. p. 626–37.

3. Azmat CE, Council M. Wound closure techniques [updated 2020 Jun 28]. In: StatPearls [Internet]. Treasure Island, FL: StatPearls Publishing; 2020 Jan. Available from: www.ncbi.nlm.nih.gov/books/NBK470598/

4. Williams N, Connell RO, McCaskie A, editors. Baily and Love's short practices of surgery, 27th edn. Boca Raton: CRC Press; 2017.

5. Dunn DL, Phillips J, editors; Ethicon INC. Wound Closure Manual. Available from: www.uphs.upenn.edu/surgery/Education/facilities/measey/Wound_Closure_Manual.pdf (accessed 11 Nov 2020).

6. Suture Materials. Available from: https://coreem.net/core/suture-materials/ (accessed 11 Nov 2020).

7. Malmö BZ. Choice of suture materials for wound closure. Eur Surg RCS. 1983;15:57–8. Available from: www.karger.com/Article/PDF/128333 (accessed 11 Nov 2020).

8. TeachMe Surgery. Suture materials. Available from: https://teachmesurgery.com/skills/theatre-basics/suture-materials/ (accessed 28 Oct 2020).

9. University of Saskatchewan. Lab 4. Part 4—suture size. Available from: https://wcvm.usask.ca/vsac205/Lab4/suture-size.php (accessed 28 Oct 2020).

10. Thrive AP. Suturing 101: needles size and material. Available from: https://thriveap.com/blog/suturing-101-needles-sizes-and-materials#:~:text=Most%20commonly%2C%20you%20will%20use,concern%20such%20as%20the%20extremities (accessed 28 Oct 2020).

11. Ratner D. Edited by Dirk M Elston. What are the types of needle points and when are they used in suturing? Emedicine. Available from: www.medscape.com/answers/1824895-32116/what-are-the-types-of-needle-points-and-when-are-they-used-in-suturing (accessed 28 Oct 2020).

12. Ratner D. Edited by Dirk M Elston. What are the steps in suture placement? Available from: www.medscape.com/answers/1824895-32123/what-are-the-steps-in-suture-placement (accessed 28 Oct 2020).

13. Basic suturing: how to suture. Available from: www.youtube.com/watch?v=DJMf0vN8fkw.

14. Holzheimer RG. Adverse events of sutures: possible interactions of biomaterials? Eur J Med Res. 2006;10:521–6.

15. Rink AD, Goldschmidt D, Dietrich J, et al. Negative side-effects of retention sutures for abdominal wound closure. A prospective randomised study. Eur J Surg. 2000;166:932–7.

16. Bali R, Kankam HKN, Agrawal A. A rare reaction to synthetic mono-filament sutures: a report of two cases. J Perioper Pract. 2018;28(1&2):27–30.

17. Yip C, Bowen K, Chew BK. A report of rare adverse tissue reaction to Ethilon® Nylon Suture. J Surg Case Rep. 2018;3:1–2.

18. Howard. Shelf life of sutures. Preparedness advice. 2011 June 6. Available from: https://preparednessadvice.com/medical/shelf-life-of-sutures/#:~:text=Absorbable%20sutures%20are%20marked%20with,years%20from%20date%20of%20manufacturer (accessed 29 Oct 2020).

19. Parell GJ, Becker GD. Comparison of absorbable with non-absorbable sutures in closure of facial skin wounds. Arch Facial Plast Sur. 2003;5(6):488–90. https://doi.org/10.1001/archfaci.5.6.488.

20. Burute SB, Karan A, Puri M, et al. Efficacy of different types of sutures materials used in the wound closure of pfannenstiel skin incision by subcuticular technique in cesarean section. Int J Clin Obstetr Gynaecol. 2019;3(1):150–3. https://doi.org/10.33545/gynae.2019.v3.i1c.26.

21. Kailas CT, Naik CG. A randomised control trial comparison the efficacy between delayed-absorbable polydioxanone and non-absorbable suture material in abdominal wound closure. Int Surg J. 2017;4:153–6.

22. Gokarneshan N. Review article new generation surgical sutures. Glob J Oto. 2018;16(2):555932. https://doi.org/10.19080/GJO.2018.16.555932.

23. Elmallah RK, Khlopas A, Faour M, et al. Economic evaluation of different suture closure methods: barbed versus traditional interrupted sutures. Ann Transl Med. 2017;5(Suppl 3):S26. https://doi.org/10.21037/atm.2017.08.21.

24. Gokani SA, Elmqvist KO, El-Koubani O, et al. A cost-utility analysis of small bite sutures versus large bite sutures in the closure of midline laparotomies in the United Kingdom National Health Service. Clinicoecon Outcomes Res. 2018;10:105–17. Published 2018 Feb 19. https://doi.org/10.2147/CEOR.S150176.

25. Wounds and Injuries. Available from: https://medlineplus.gov/woundsandinjuries.html (accessed 6 Nov 2020).

26. Mercandetti M. Edited by Molinar JA. Wound healing and repair. Emedicine. Available from: https://emedicine.medscape.com/article/1298129-overview (accessed 6 Nov 2020).

27. Sharma S, Dua A, Malik A. Third generation materials for wound dressings. Int J Pharm Sci Res. 2014;5(6):2113–24. https://doi.org/10.13040/IJPSR.0975-8232.5(6).2113-24.

28. Foutsizoglou S. A practical guide to the most commonly used dressings in wound care. The PMFA J. 2018;6(1). Available from: www.thepmfajournal.com/features/post/a-practical-guide-to-the-most-commonly-used-dressings-in-wound-care (accessed 11 Nov 2020).

29. Lei J, Sun L, Li P, et al. The wound dressings and their applications in wound healing and management. Health Sci J. 2019;13(4):662.

30. Edwards H, Gibb M, Finlayson K, et al. Wound dressing guide. In: Champions for skin integrity. Brisbane: Queensland University of Technology; 2013. ISBN 978-1-921897-79-5.

31. Mulder, M., Small, N., Botma, Y. et al. Basic principles of wound care. Cape Town: Pearson Education; 2002.

32. Sood A, Granick MS, Tomaselli NL. Wound dressings and comparative effectiveness data. Adv Wound Care. 2014;3(8):511–29. https://doi.org/10.1089/wound.2012.0401.

33. FDA Executive Summary. Classification of Wound Dressings Combined with Drugs. Prepared for the Meeting of the General and Plastic Surgery Devices Advisory Panel. 2016 Sept 20–21. Available from: www.fda.gov/media/100005/download (accessed 6 Nov 2020).

34. British Pharmacopoeia Commission. British pharmaco-poeia 1993, Vols I & II. London: Her Majesty's Stationery Office, 1993. p. 1249–50.

35. Hampton S. Selecting wound dressings for optimum heal-ing. Nurs Times. 2015;111(49/50):20–3.

36. Dabiri G, Damstetter E, Phillips T. Choosing a wound dressing based on common wound characteristics. Adv Wound Care (New Rochelle). 2016;5(1):32–41. https://doi.org/10.1089/wound.2014.0586.

37. Gottrup F. Evidence is a challenge in wound management. Int J Low Extrem Wounds. 2006;5(2):74–5.

38. Zhang L, Yin H, Lei X, et al. A systematic review and meta-analysis of clinical effectiveness and safety of hydrogel dressings in the management of skin wounds. Front Bioeng Biotechnol. 2019 Nov 21;7;342. https://doi.org/10.3389/fbioe.2019.00342. PMID: 31824935; PMCID: PMC6881259.

39. Chamorro AM, Vidal Thomas MC, Mieras AS, et al. Multicenter randomized controlled trial comparing the effectiveness and safety of hydrocellular and hydro-colloid dressings for treatment of category II pressure ulcers in patients at primary and long-term care institu-tions. Int J Nurs Stud. 2019 Jun;94:179–85. https://doi.org/10.1016/j.ijnurstu.2019.03.021. Epub 2019 Apr 4. PMID: 31048187.

40. Radzi S. Wound care can be a successful niche for a com-munity pharmacy. Available from: https://today.mims.com/wound-care-successful-niche-community-pharmacy.

41. Jin S. A day in the life: a pharmacist's role in wound care. Wound Care Canada. 2015;13(2). Available from: www.woundscan ada.ca/docman/public/wound-care-canada-magazine/2015-vol-13-no-2/540-wcc-fall-2015-v13n2-day-in-the-life/file.

42. Panasci K. Burns and wounds. In: Acute care handbook for physical therapists, Vol. 7. St. Louis, MO: Elsevier Saunders; 2013. p. 283.

43. Wound Source Editors. Identifying the different types of wound drainage. Available from: www.woundsource.com/blog/identifying-different-types-wound-drainage (accessed 8 Nov 2020).

44. Starr R. Surgical drains. Available from: https://patient.info/treatment-medication/surgical-drains (accessed 8 Nov 2020).

45. Fatal air embolism from misuse of closed-wound suction units. Hazard [Health Devices. May–Jun 1990;19(5–6):200–2]. Available from: www.mdsr.ecri.org/summary/detail.aspx?doc_id=8241#:~:text=The%20closed%2Dwound%20suction%20unit,up%20to%20the%20indicator%20ring (accessed 8 Nov 2020).

46. Chinn SD, Burns A. Closed wound suction drainage. J Foot Surg. 1985 Jan–Feb;24(1):76–81. PMID: 3973352.

47. Polymed Medical Devices. Closed wound suction unit. Available from: www.polymedicure.com/closed-wound-suction-units/ (accessed 9 Nov 2020).

48. Physiopedia contributors. Chest Drains. Physiopedia. Available from: www.physiopedia.com/index.php?title=Chest_Drains&oldid=223501 (accessed 9 Nov 2020).

49. Utah Medical Products INC. Chest drainage catheters. Available from: www.utahmed.com/thora-cath.html (accessed 9 Nov 2020).

50. Bladder and Bowel Community. Supra pubic catheter. Available from: www.bladderandbowel.org/surgical-treatment/suprapubic-catheter/ (accessed 10 Nov 2020).

51. Imm N. Surgical drains—indications, management and removal. Available from: https://patient.info/doctor/surgi-cal-drains-indications-management-and-removal (accessed 9 Nov 2020).

52. Mattox KL, Allen MK. Systematic approach to pneumotho-rax, haemothorax, pneumomediastinum and subcutaneous emphysema. Injury. 1986 Sep. 17(5):309–12.

53. Clinical Guidelines (Nursing). Chest drain management. Available from: www.rch.org.au/rchcpg/hospital_clinical_guideline_index/Chest_drain_management/ (accessed 9 Nov 2020).

54. Abdominal drainage (paracentesis). Available from: www.stanfordchildrens.org/en/topic/default?id=abdominal-drainage-paracentesis-22-abdominaldrainage (accessed 9 Nov 2020).

55. Makama JG, Ameh EA. Surgical drains: what a resident needs to know. Niger J Med. 2008;17:244–50.

56. Maliakal M. Chest tubes. Patient education series. Nursing. 2011;33. https://doi.org/10.1097/01.NURSE.0000398453.60078.49.

57. Tanaka K, Kumamoto T, Nojiri K, et al. The effectiveness and appropriate management of abdominal drains in patients undergoing elective liver resection: a retrospective analysis and prospective case series. Surg Today. 2013;43:372–80. https://doi.org/10.1007/s00595-012-0254-1.

58. Alcala-Cerra G, Young AM, Moscote-Salazar LR, et al. Efficacy and safety of subdural drains after burr-hole evac-uation of chronic subdural hematomas: systematic review and meta-analysis of randomized controlled trials. World Neurosurg. 2014;82:1148–57.

59. Wakai S, Hashimoto K, Watanabe N, et al. Efficacy of closed-system drainage in treating chronic subdural hematoma: a pro-spective comparative study. Neurosurgery. 1990;26(5):771–3. https://doi.org/10.1227/00006123-199005000-00006.

60. Cafarotti S, Dall'Armi V, Cusumano G, et al. Small-bore wire-guided chest drains: safety, tolerability, and effective-ness in pneumothorax, malignant effusions, and pleural empyema. J Thorac Cardiovasc Surg. 2011;141:683–7.

61. Scales K. Intravenous therapy: a guide to good practice. Br J Nurs. 2008 Oct 23–Nov 12;17(19):S4–S12. https://doi.org/10.12968/bjon.2008.17.Sup8.31469. PMID: 18974684.

62. The simple IV giving set. Available from: www.dsmedi-cal.co.uk/the-simple-iv-giving-set-i34#:~:text=In%20modern%20day%20medical%20practice,gravity%2C%20often%20called%20gravity%20infusion.

63. What is IV therapy?—Ware, Brenda Lesson 7, Chapter 30; Study.com. Available from: https://study.com/academy/les-son/what-is-iv-therapy-definition-history-types-complica-tions.html (accessed 11 Nov 2020).

64. The different types of IV sets and their uses. Available from: www.wolfmed.com/blog/the-different-types-of-iv-sets-and-their-uses/ (accessed 11 Nov 2020).

65. BD. IV administration set. Available from: www.bd.com/en-us/offerings/capabilities/infusion-therapy/iv-adminis-tration-sets (accessed 11 Nov 2020).

66. Instruction of use for 3-way stop cock. Available from: http://euromed.com.eg/sites/default/files/files/Instruction%20For%20Use%20Of%20%20STPO%20COCK.pdf (accessed 11 Nov 2020).

67. Three way stopcock. Available from: www.medidex.com/datacards/45-iv/665-three-way-stopcock453.html#:~:text=It%20provides%203%2Dway%20flow,the%20attachment%20of%20extension%20lines (accessed 11 Nov 2020).

68. Shlamovitz GZ. Edited by Rowe VL. Intravenous cannulation. Emedicine. Availalble on https://emedicine.medscape.com/article/1998177-overview#a1 (accessed 11 Nov 2020).

69. Size of cannula. Available from: www.maxhealthcare.in/sites/default/files/Sizes-of-IV-Cannulas-and-Flow-Rate-Calculations.pdf (accessed 11 Nov 2020).

70. B Braun. Safety IV catheter. Available from: www.bbraun.com/en/products-and-therapies/product-catalog/infusion/peripheral-venouscatheters/safety-iv-catheter.html (accessed 11 Nov 2020).

71. Roe EJ. Edited by Rowe VL. What is central venous catheterization? Emedicine. Availalble on www.medscape.com/answers/80336-117529/what-is-central-venous-catheterization (accessed 11 Nov 2020).

72. Kolikof J, Peterson K, Baker AM. Central venous catheter [updated 2020 May 24]. In: StatPearls [Internet]. Treasure Island, FL: StatPearls Publishing; 2020 Jan. Available from: www.ncbi.nlm.nih.gov/books/NBK557798/

73. Smith RN, Nolan JP. Central venous catheters. BMJ. 2013;347:f6570. https://doi.org/10.1136/bmj.f6570

74. AMBU bag—the principle of work. Available from: https://westmedgroup.ru/en/ambu-bag-the-principle-of-work (accessed 11 Nov 2020).

75. Ambu bag/self inflating bag. Available from: www.pediatriconcall.com/medical-equipment/critical-care/8/ambu-bag-self-inflating-bag/22 (accessed 11 Nov 2020).

76. Sheela NNJ. Ambu bag artificial maneuver breathing unit. Narayana Nurs J. 2013;1(3):62–4.

14 Medical Devices for Infectious Diseases

Elhassan Hussein Eltom and Mohamed Awad Mousnad

CONTENTS

DOI: 10.1201/9781003002345-16

INTRODUCTION

Historically, infectious diseases have been the primary source of mortalities in the ancient world and have been responsible for massive mortalities via endemic and epidemic incidences. In the modern era, infectious diseases remain a significant cause of death in low-income countries in Africa, Asia, and Latin America, in the form of endemic illnesses like yellow fever, hepatitis, and cholera, as well as globally in notorious pandemic outbreaks, such as those for Ebola virus disease (EVD) and various strains of the coronavirus (including SARS, MERS, and COVID-19).

Pharmacists are involved in infectious diseases as active members of the multidisciplinary medical team. Specialized clinical pharmacists are involved in selecting, monitoring, and controlling antimicrobial drugs and associated medical devices. During epidemics and pandemic waves, all healthcare workers (HCWs), including pharmacists, are empowered to fight against infectious diseases to control their spread and reduce catastrophic outcomes. Pharmacists need to understand and be familiar with a broad array of medical devices used to combat infectious diseases in the field to protect themselves, their patients, and the community. Pharmacists can also play a significant role in counseling and teaching the community in this regard.

Decision-making should evaluate the impact of healthcare technology through applying Health Technology Assessment (HTA). HTA deals with clinical effectiveness and economic effectiveness and includes four dimensions: medical, social, ethical, and economic. This chapter of the book consists of two main parts. The first part deals with personal protective equipment (PPE) because of its importance in controlling infectious diseases in healthcare delivery institutions and society. This part dealt with seven of the most important PPE devices (goggles, face shields, gloves, masks, gowns, coveralls, and aprons). A detailed discussion is provided for each one, including a description of the device, its purpose and main features, the various available versions, the most important safety standards, storage and maintenance methods, special counseling tips for users, the available evidence on the effectiveness of the device, and an economic evaluation of the device's performance. The first part concludes with implications for the pharmacy profession and practice, challenges for the pharmacist and user recommendations, and a general conclusion.

The second part of this chapter deals with four important rapid diagnostic tests (RDTs)—for HIV/AIDS, malaria, syphilis, and tuberculosis. First, a detailed discussion of each item is presented, ending with implications and challenges for the pharmacists and other users and a general conclusion.

1. PERSONAL PROTECTIVE EQUIPMENT

BACKGROUND

In highly contagious diseases epidemics and pandemics, frontline HCWs (including pharmacists) are at high risk of infection due to their direct contact with patients. In such circumstances, PPE is highly recommended to control the transmission of infection. PPE selection, best practices for donning and doffing, and methods for determining that HCWs are using PPE appropriately remain challenging for policymakers and stakeholders.[1] High-quality simulation studies are needed to determine the best PPE combination to provide the best possible protection because inadequate training in PPE and a lack of resources have been partially associated with the high number of HCW mortalities in Africa.[2] Documentation and follow-up of PPE use by HCWs should be routine discipline to control infection.[3] Since December 2019, HCWs globally face the COVID-19 pandemic, which has continued even as a vaccine has become available and protecting HCW during this pandemic is crucial.[4]

The OSHA Technical Manual (Section VIII, Chapter 1, Part C) defines four levels of protection against both skin and respiratory exposures. Level A offers maximum protection for the skin and respiratory system. Level B is used when there is a high need for respiratory protection. Level C is "non-encapsulated clothing" used for known airborne substances. Finally, Level D is work clothing used for "nuisance contamination (i.e., non-protective)," and it should not be worn when there is a respiratory or skin hazard.[5]

1.1. GOGGLES

a. Device Description

Medical goggles may be reusable or disposable. They should have a flexible frame that easily fits all face contours without too much pressure, cover the eyes and surrounding areas while accommodating prescription glasses, and form a good seal with the skin of the face. Medical goggles must be fog- and scratch-resistant. They have an adjustable band that can be firmly secured so they do not come loose during clinical activity and have indirect venting to reduce fogging. Medical goggles should comply with the EU standard directive 86/686/EEC, EN 166/2002, ANSI/ISEA Z87.1–2010, or equivalent standards.[6]

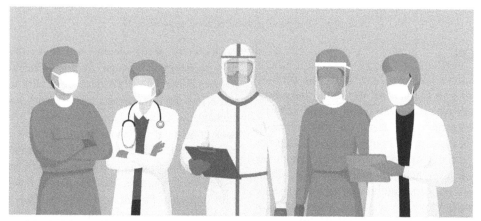

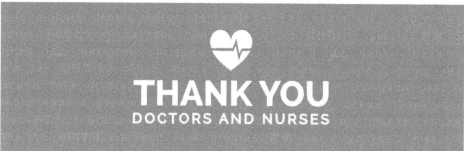

FIGURE 14.1   Figure illustrating different types of personal protective equipment (PPE).

Source: https://www.shutterstock.com/image-illustration/doctor-health-care-provider-wearing-personal-1970507342

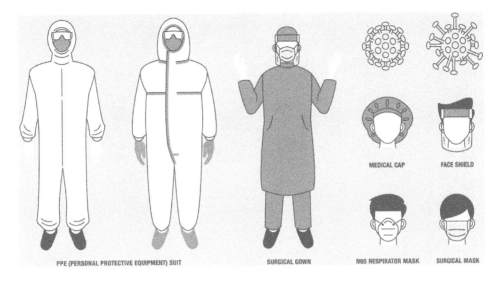

FIGURE 14.2   A complete set of PPE.

Source: [www.shutterstock.com/image-vector/nice-vector-set-equipments-protect-coronavirus-1730561998]

b.   Versions/Generations

Two versions of eye protection are available: hermetically and non-hermetically sealed goggles.[7]

c.   Purpose of Use

The need for safe eyewear is growing. It is estimated that, by 2025, the US eyewear market will grow to around $669 million.[8] The purpose of goggles as PPE during an epidemic or pandemic is to protect the eyes and prevent mutual contamination of HCWs' eyes and hands.[9] To put goggles on appropriately, "Apply goggles and (ask a buddy to check that there is no skin exposed), to take off goggles, close eyes and remove the goggles, pulling them forward, so they are free from the face, gently pulling them off. Discard goggles in the chlorine bucket, wash hands."[10]

d.   Important Safety Issues

The individual PPE pieces and ensembles required for infection control should achieve a low probability of penetration.[11] One piece of PPE can negatively affect the performance of other pieces where they join, and an N95 respirator or face shield can be negatively affected by adding goggles inappropriately.[11] Fogging is another safety issue for goggles, and it has been reported that they are more likely to become fogged than face shields are.[12]

e.   Storage Conditions and Maintenance

Most goggles and safety glasses can technically last up to 3 years, but there is an intractable area between usability and safety-compromising, especially during emergencies. In high-dust environments, safety eyewear can gradually become scratched over time, creating a haze that affects visibility.[13] It is important to check for damage

regularly—before each shift at a minimum. Any pitted, scratched, broken, bent, or ill-fitting goggles should be replaced immediately.

f.   Important Features

Novel features that improve the usability of medical goggles include the development of durable goggles, easily manufactured and marketed and cost-effective; providing interchangeable mesh screens in the eye shield; making frames that easily fit different faces; providing a fogless screen to cope with ambient moisture; and solving the problem of the smudged eye shield.[14]

g.   Special Tips for Patient Counseling

Many factors have a direct effect on the decision to use PPE among HCWs. These factors include "accident experience, attitude towards using PPE, habituation, risk perception, safety consciousness, safety knowledge, outcome expectations, perceived ease of use, perceived usefulness, social influence, safety management system, time pressure and workplace conditions."[15]

h.   Available Evidence for Effectiveness and Safety

The assortment of public healthcare guidelines is mainly due to the lack of a united standard for protecting the eyes and face from biological hazards.[16] Combining face shields with other PPE such as goggles and face masks was reported to decrease the inhalation contact threat.[12] Gala et al.[17] reported that the transmission risk was 43% in the control group versus 6% in the intervention group using medical goggles (χ^2: $P = 0.04$). The evidence for medical goggle effectiveness was also found in two studies out of four that used methods to avert respiratory syncytial virus (RSV) transmission to staff.[18]

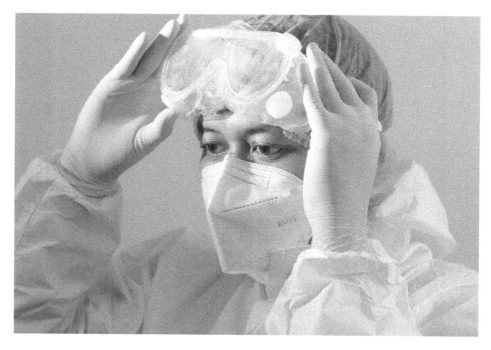

FIGURE 14.3 A medical protective goggle.

Source: [www.shutterstock.com/image-photo/concept-health-protection-medical-worker-wearing-1876816000]

i. Economic Evaluation

There is insufficient evidence of the economic evaluation of medical goggles and their impact on preventing infection transmission.

1.2. FACE SHIELDS

a. Device Description

Face shields can be disposable, recyclable, and consumable. The face shield is composed of a visor, frame, and suspension system. Visors are the lenses of the face shield and are produced from different materials such as polyethene terephthalate and polyvinyl glycol chloride. Face shield frames are generally manufactured from plastic and can be either modifiable or non-modifiable. Continuous improvements in suspension systems have appeared on the market with a range of complete to partial circumferential attachments. The physical features and quality specifications for face shields are specified through the ANSI/ISEA Z.87.1–2015 standard in the US,[19] with similar standards existing globally. Face shields are categorized as Class I medical devices, "the least-regulated FDA category."[20]

b. Versions/Generations

Face shields are available in different forms, but all have the same feature of providing a transparent covering for the user's face.[21] In emergencies, face shield production lines can be rearranged rapidly because no special material is needed.[22] Although the face shield is a simple device

subjected to regulation, because of the PPE shortage due to the COVID-19 pandemic, the "FDA as of April 2020 has provided guidance that it does not intend to object to individuals' distribution and use of improvised PPE when no alternatives, such as FDA-cleared masks or respirators, are available."[20]

c. Purpose of Use

Face shields are used mainly to protect the eyes, nose, and mouth from hazardous contamination[19]; they are categorized as adjunctive PPE because a face shield should be used in conjunction with other items of PPE.[12]

d. Important Safety Issues

Light reflection, fogging, optical defectiveness, improperly fitting with respirators, and poor peripheral fit compared to face masks are factors negatively affecting the safety and efficacy of face shields.[23,24]

e. Storage Conditions and Maintenance

In general, face shields will last for years if stored in perfect storage conditions. Spare face shield visors are available and can be replaced when needed.

f. Important Features

It is easy to clean to face shields with soap and water and available disinfectants, which offers an advantage over medical masks with limited durability. Self-contamination is negligible when comparing a face shield to a medical mask. It is not important to remove the face shield when talking to others, since it allows for perfect communication because the visor is transparent.[22]

g. Special Tips for Patient Counseling

i. Ensure that your face has been covered entirely by the face shield.

ii. Avoid touching the inside and outside surfaces of the face shield.

iii. To prevent the face shield from falling, adjustable straps should be used to make it fit. Use the adjustable straps to fit it comfortably to the forehead.

h. The Available Evidence for Effectiveness and Safety

A face shield effectively reduces the respirator or mask surface by 97%, and it can reduce the potential for HCWs to inhale contaminant droplets by 96%.[23] However, to date, there is no evidence comparing face shield and goggle use in preventing virus transmission to HCWs. The CDC, therefore, recommends a mutual use of each device according to user preferences.[6]

i. Economic Evaluation

There is a high potential for infection transmission in transferring patients from the operating theater to the recovery area. One study found that using a disposable face shield while transferring patients offers good protection for anesthesia staff while maintaining overall cost-effectiveness, usability, and infection control.[25]

1.3. FLUID-RESISTANT SURGICAL OR MEDICAL FACE MASK

a. Device Description

A surgical mask is a device that protects the mucous membranes of the mouth and nose from potential contamination

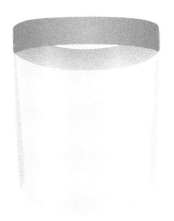

FIGURE 14.4 Medical face shield, a transparent plastic helmet.

Source: [www.shutterstock.com/image-vector/medical-face-mask-shield-transparent-plastic-1701090961]

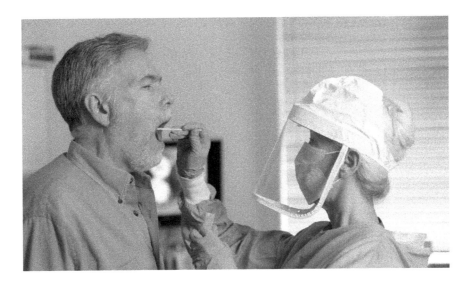

FIGURE 14.5 Importance of protective garb for healthcare worker performing swab test.

Source: [www.shutterstock.com/image-photo/mature-caucasian-man-clinical-setting-being-1675328332]

from the surrounding environment. They are often called face masks, and one important feature of the face mask is that it is loose and does not form a seal around the mouth and nose. An N95 respirator is a type of face mask that is close-fitting and provides airborne filtration; it should form a good seal around the mouth and nose.

b. Versions/Generations

There are two types of face masks. Type I masks are used by patients and aim to control the contamination source. Type II or Type IIR (R stands for "resistant") masks are used by HCWs at different levels of the healthcare setting and operation theaters. Bacterial filtration efficiency remains the primary determinant of mask efficacy, so Type IIR is the only mask that can protect against splashes.[26] Another important type of face mask is the filtering facepiece respirator (FFR), which is registered as an inhalational protective device. FFRs have different labels according to their filtration characteristics, and these labels vary by region or country. In the European Union, FFR2 are able to decrease aerosol concentration by 94%, while FFR3 reduce aerosol concentration by 99%. Worldwide, FFR corresponds to European FFR2 are as follows: "N95 (United States), KN95 (China), P2 (Australia/New Zealand), DS (Japan), and Korea 1st class (Korea)".[27]

c. Purpose of Use

Face masks and FFRs are used to protect the face against liquid contamination and airborne particles.[28] The combination of intrusions across the infection levels is crucial for optimal control of airborne transmission.[29]

d. Important Safety Issues

Patients suffering any medical condition that affects breathing should consult their healthcare provider before using any N95 respirator because it may affect the wearer's breathing.[30] The N95 model containing exhalation valves can make breathing easier, but it should not be used for aseptic techniques.[31] The respirator should be replaced when it is impaired or if it causes breathing difficulties.[32] To discard the safety mask, put the mask in a plastic container, place the container in the trash, and then wash hands.[33] There is no suitable N95 design for children and bearded persons.[34]

e. Storage Conditions and Maintenance

In response to the COVID-19 pandemic emergency, the CDC recommends using N95 masks even if they have exceeded their shelf life because the US authorities believe that even expired respirators offer more protection than a plain surgical mask. It is not, however, recommended to use expired respirators for surgical settings.

f. Important Features

Face masks play a pivotal role in preventing and containing infectious disease transmission. The use of face masks became a norm among the general public after COVID-19 based on the varying recommendations by healthcare authorities. However, effective educational intervention for the general public and HCWs is needed regarding different face masks according to different settings.[35] Importantly, particulate respirators must be kept for HCWs, and they should be apprised of the potential harms associated with those respirators. Particulate respirators are also expensive and can provide a false sense of security, particularly since more tests are needed to improve how they fit the face, including (potentially) people with beards.[36]

g. Special Tips for Patient Counseling

The COVID-19 pandemic highlighted the need for cloth face masks. Thus, practical guidelines regarding fabrics and designs for cloth face masks should be provided to the public.[37] The protection efficiency of different fabrics varies broadly; for example, cotton blend T-shirt material is more effective than pure cotton, while scarves and silk perform poorly.[38] The most desirable cloth mask consists of two to three layers of hydrophobic fabric.[37] To prevent auto-contamination, daily washing of cloth masks is recommended. It is also essential to keep in mind the false sense of security provided by the mask, which may increase the risk of infection.[39]

h. The Available Evidence for Effectiveness and Safety

Studies have reported that a combination of hand hygiene and masks are more effective in transmission control than hand hygiene alone,[40] although there have been no RCTs to measure the effect of masks alone.[37] Rigorous RCTs are therefore required to provide evidence concerning such interventions.[41] However, there is dubious evidence that there is no difference between medical masks and respirators in prevention against infection transmission for HCWs during procedures that do not involve aerosol generation.[42]

i. Economic Evaluation

Masks and respirators have been stated to be cost-effective and cost-saving when matched to no intervention or other infection control measures.[43] Among the various types of masks, N95 masks cost US$490 in preventing clinical respiratory illness, which is less expensive than medical masks, which cost US$1,230.[44]

1.4. Gloves

a. Device Description

Medical gloves are a disposable device used to prevent mutual contamination between HCWs and patients.[45] For the European Union, "the selected glove must conform to EN 374 European standard, and they must also be CE marked for specific use with biological agents."[46]

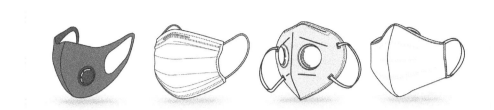

FIGURE 14.6   Different type of medical face masks.

Source: [www.shutterstock.com/image-vector/medical-face-mask-safety-breathing-fashion-1682221543]

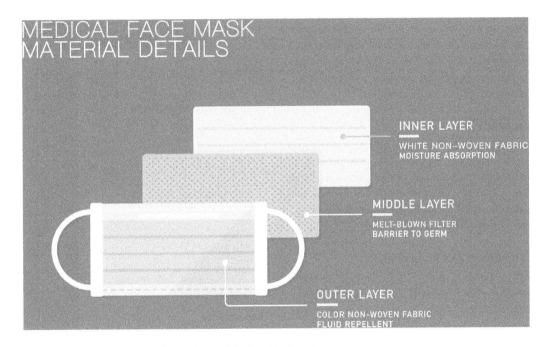

FIGURE 14.7   Figure illustrating the design and material of medical mask.

Source: [www.shutterstock.com/image-vector/vector-medical-surgical-maskfunctions-illustrating-three-1664219023]

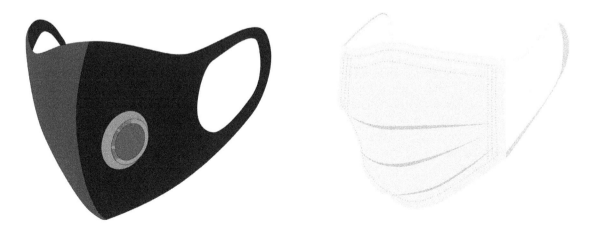

FIGURE 14.8   N95 mask versus medical respiratory mask.

Source: [www.shutterstock.com/image-vector/safety-breathing-masks-industrial-n95-mask-1555079888]

b. Versions/Generations

Medical gloves are made of different polymers, "including latex, nitrile rubber, polyvinyl chloride, polyurethane, and neoprene."[47] Latex and vinyl gloves are touch-sensitive and offer modest protection. Vinyl gloves are the least durable, while nitrile gloves offer the maximum protection and durability.[47] However, in a specific condition, when the procedures need high sensitivity, powder-free latex gloves are preferred.[46]

c. Purpose of Use

In healthcare settings, HCWs use gloves to protect themselves from contamination with patient body fluids, prevent the release of microorganisms from the hand into the sterile work area during aseptic techniques, protect from chemicals, and protect against radiation. These different uses demand various qualities from the gloves.[48] The potential for HCW self-contamination when removing gloves in routine contact precautions is of great concern, so methods for donning and removing gloves are standardized.[49]

d. Important Safety Issues

Some adverse skin reactions have been reported in the use of different kinds of gloves, including but not limited to irritant contact dermatitis, allergic contact dermatitis, and contact urticaria.[47] "Other adverse effects of gloves are discomfort, reduced visibility, high temperature, humidity, gloves perforation, and self-contamination."[50]

e. Storage Conditions and Maintenance

Gloves should be stored in a dry, cool place, in a ranging temperature between 10°C and 22°C. Gloves should not be stored close to any source of physical or chemical contamination.

f. Important Features

Although powdered gloves have the advantage of keeping the user's hand(s) dry for ease of wear and removal, the powder can cause respiratory irritation.

g. Special Tips for Patient Counseling

The CDC recommends wearing gloves in public when providing care or cleaning for a patient[51,52] and touching or handling patients' medicines.[53] Gloves are not disinfectable or reusable and must be disposed of in a suitable trash receptacle after use.[54]

h. The Available Evidence for Effectiveness and Safety

Natural rubber latex (NRL) gloves remain the first choice because they protect effectively against bloodborne viruses and other contaminated fluids while also providing user dexterity.[55] Due to their susceptibility to damage and permeability, polyethylene gloves are not appropriate for medical use.[56] Because nitrile gloves have had the lowest failure

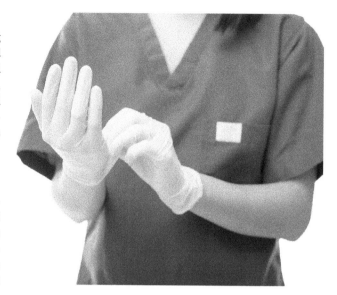

FIGURE 14.9   Putting on/donning surgical gloves.

Source: [www.shutterstock.com/image-photo/closeup-nurse-scrubs-putting-surgical-gloves-566726986]

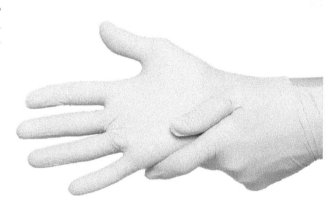

FIGURE 14.10   Protective blue gloves.

Source: [www.shutterstock.com/image-photo/doctor-putting-on-protective-blue-gloves-1380369467]

rate, they remain an adequate substitute for NRL gloves.[28] One study found a synergistic effect of combining different infection control measures. It stated that using gloves alone can offer a transmission risk reduction by 55%, mask plus hand hygiene combine for a 68% reduction, while combining all mentioned measures contributed a 91% reduction.[57]

i. Economic Evaluation

Due to NRL's allergy and asthma concerns, policymakers have recommended non-latex gloves—"safe latex"—be used, although the cost exceeds that of NRL gloves.[58] One study found that using disposable gloves was cost-effective compared to reprocessing and recycling gloves even in "resource-limited settings."[59]

1.5. DISPOSABLE GOWNS

a. Device Description

In healthcare facilities, gowns are recognized as second to gloves in general PPE use.[60] According to the Guideline for Isolation Precautions from the CDC, isolation gowns are an element of PPE that protects the arms and exposed body areas of HCWs from patient excretions.[61] Gowns are categorized into different types according to their resistance to body fluids, permeability, and the material of they are made.[62]

b. Versions/Generations

Isolation gowns on the market are manufactured mainly from different fabrics and other fiber types[62] and are classified as "disposable/single-use" or "reusable/multi-use." According to one source, "Around 80% of hospitals in the US use single-use gowns and drapes."[63]

c. Purpose of Use

"When applying Standard Precautions (minimum infection prevention practices that apply to all patient care, regardless of suspected or confirmed infection status of the patient), isolation gowns (and gloves) are worn only if contact with blood or body fluid is anticipated."[64]

d. Important Safety Issues

Some factors positively affect the effectiveness and usability of gowns, including design, size, interfaces, fit, and fabric characteristics; other factors that affect the selection of gowns are the level of potential contact with contagious substances, the anticipated volume of body fluids, and the duration of patient/HCW interaction.[62]

e. Storage Conditions and Maintenance

It is recommended to store medical gowns below 37°C, and they should not be used after their expiry date unless there is exemption stockpiling due to emergencies.[65]

f. Important Features

Efficacy in offering adequate protection against liquids and microorganisms remains the most important feature of an isolation gown. Thus, the vital safety and performance properties may include "stain resistance, strength, pilling, softness graze resistance, drapeability, breathability, flammability, susceptibility for linting and electrostatic charge."[66]

g. Special Tips for Patient Counseling

In high demands and scarcity conditions, a surgical gown that exceeds its shelf life can be used as an isolation gown that will still provide an excellent physical barrier.[65] For patients in the same area and with the same diagnosis, the HCW can look after them using the same gown.[67] However, if there is a coexisting infection among patients in the same area, wearing the same gown between treating patients is not recommended.[68]

h. The Available Evidence for Effectiveness and Safety

There is no evidence supporting the reduction of filovirus transmission to HCWs using coveralls; however, from the literature evaluation, there is concrete evidence that coveralls and gowns are equal in providing adequate body protection and can be used interchangeably according to the preferences of the HCWs.[6]

i. Economic Evaluation

A study conducted to estimate the cost-benefit of wearing a medical gown by HCWs and visitors to ICU patients to avoid nosocomial infection found that the gown policy has an annual net benefit of $419,346, with a $1,897 cost per case avoided of VRE; therefore, it is a cost-saving policy for avoiding nosocomial infection, which is an economic and clinical burden.

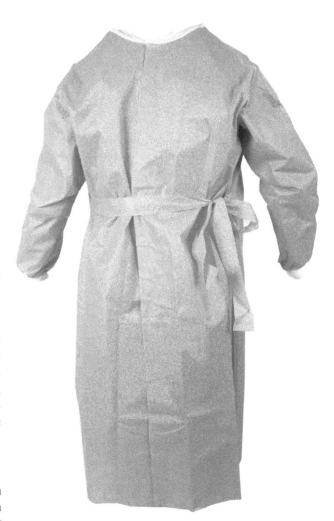

FIGURE 14.11 Disposable surgical gown.

Source: [www.shutterstock.com/image-photo/disposable-surgical-gown-surgery-1626497422]

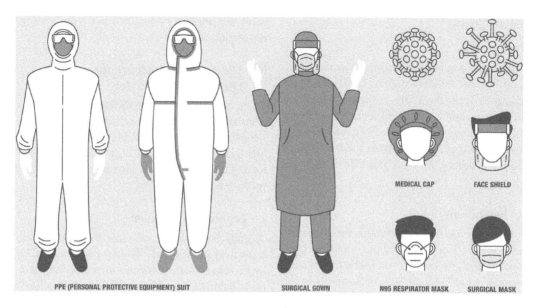

FIGURE 14.12   PPE including surgical gown.

Source: [www.shutterstock.com/image-vector/nice-vector-set-equipments-protect-coronavirus-1730561998]

1.6.   DISPOSABLE COVERALLS

a.   Device Description

Medical coveralls are an essential item of PPE in all settings of suspected contamination to workers or when there is a chance of transfer of contaminants to patients. Medical coveralls are mainly fabricated from cotton or a polyester/cotton mix according to directive 89/686/EEC.[70]

b.   Versions/Generations

According to the level of protection, protective suits can be categorized into different groups ranging from 1 to 6, wherein type 1 provides the highest level of protection[71]:

> Type 1: Gas-proof suits: Fully sealed suits; Type 2: Limited gas-tightness: Suits prevent dust, liquids, and vapors from penetrating at overpressure; Type 3 and 3B: Liquid-proof protection: Suits are approved to withstand compressed fluids; Type 4 and 4B: Splash-proof protection: Suits are approved for the saturation of a liquid that can condense on the suit and Type 4B protects against biologically contaminated particles; Type 5 and 5B: Protect against harmful substances and type 5B protects against biologically contaminated particles; Type 6 and 6B: Limited splash-proof protection: Protect when there is a risk of splashing on the suit; type 6B protects against biologically contaminated particles.

c.   Purpose of Use

> "Coveralls are used to protect against biological, radioactive, and environmental hazards."[72]

d.   Important Safety Issues

There are risk factors associated with coverall use, such as heat stress, heart rate, core temperature, oral temperature, and dehydration.[73,74]

e.   Storage Conditions and Maintenance

Coveralls should be stored in a cool, dry place according to the manufacturer's recommendations and supplied in individual, sealed polyethylene bags.

f.   Important Features

The selection of appropriate coveralls depends upon the following safety features: heavy-duty fabrics, elasticity, flame resistance, insulation, waterproof, and visibility.

g.   Special Tips for Patient Counseling

i.   Coveralls without joined covers are preferred.

ii.   Coveralls with or without assimilated snaps are suitable.

iii.   Coveralls and gowns should be available in well-fitting sizes to ensure forearms are covered.

iv.   Coveralls with thumb hooks are preferred to ensure sleeves are secure over the inner gloves.

v.   When removing coveralls and gowns, care should be taken that taped gloves do not tear the gloves, coveralls, or gown.

vi.   Taping can increase the risk of cross-contamination, so some facilities have recognized ways to improve tape use in attaching sleeves over inner gloves.

h. The Available Evidence for Effectiveness and Safety

Using an air-purifying respirator with coveralls "provides better protection than an N95 mask and gown (risk ratio [RR] 0.27, 95% confidence interval [CI] 0.17 to 0.43) but the earlier was more difficult to don (noncompliance: RR 7.5, 95% CI 1.81 to 31.1). In one RCT (59 participants), less contamination had been documented among those using long gowns in comparison to those using coveralls (low-certainty evidence)."[75]

i. Economic Evaluation

A study of the provided low-certainty evidence found that better protection is achieved when more parts of the body are covered. However, the difficulty of donning/removal and comfort remain.[75]

1.7. WATERPROOF APRONS

a. Device Description

A device that ties around the waist to protect the user's clothes is called an apron.

b. Versions/Generations

The apron is categorized into two main types: reusable, subjected to washing after use; and disposable, made of nonwoven material and discarded after use.[76]

c. Purpose of Use

A single-use plastic apron is recommended whenever direct contact with a patient is suspected or there is a contamination hazard from patient body fluids.[28]

d. Important Safety Issues

An apron's lead-containing shields are a potential source of lead toxicity and should be handled with care.[77]

e. Storage Conditions and Maintenance

Manufacturers recommend storing aprons and gowns in a clean, wall-mounted storage unit.

f. Important Features

Important features of medical aprons that make their use comfortable are: easy to put on, made from recyclable material, free size (fits all), waterproof, and lightweight.

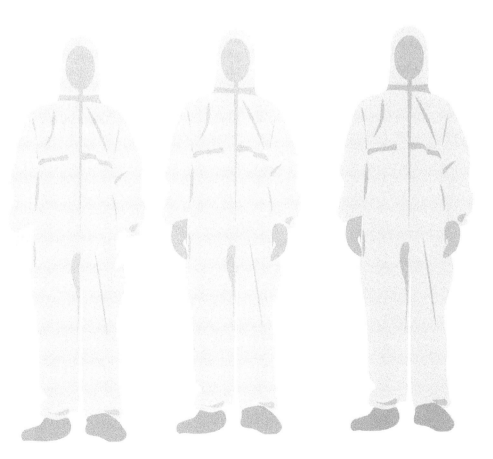

FIGURE 14.13 Person wearing protective suits and coveralls.

Source: [www.shutterstock.com/image-vector/coverall-protective-suit-medical-personnel-coveralls-1711498327]

g. Special Tips for Patient Counseling

i. Aprons/gowns should be changed between caring for different patients and different procedures for the same patient.

ii. Removal of the apron/gown requires special care so as not to touch the outer surface.

iii. Discard the used apron/gown immediately after use.

iv. Hand hygiene is essential after apron/gown removal.

h. The Available Evidence for Effectiveness and Safety

According to US CDC Guidelines, aprons are an alternative to gowns in shortage circumstances.[78] However, a recent review reported that there is no study comparing the effectiveness of aprons with gowns. For aerosol-generating procedures, the CDC recommends using aprons on top of a gown as a synergistic measure.[79]

i. Economic Evaluation

Although Morgan et al. stated that the labor cost increases with the desirable use of disposable plastic aprons and gloves, another study found that overall economic efficiency improved when changing the apron and gloves for each patient.[80]

1.8. Implications for the Pharmacy Profession and Practice Regarding PPE

Before and after the COVID-19 pandemic, pharmacists had and have a vital role in infection control in different healthcare facilities; as a member of the infection control team, the pharmacist is responsible for promoting the rational use of antibiotics, the selection and procurement of PPE, the education of HCWs and the community about the rational use of PPE, and the management of PPE stockpiles.

1.9. Challenges to Pharmacists and Users Regarding PPE

The most important challenges that face the pharmacist as a frontline HCW are the inquiries of the community and colleagues about the effective use of different PPE devices and PPE shortages during emergencies.

1.10. Recommendations: Ways Forward

- Availability of PPE should be optimized through the appropriate use of PPE, supply chain coordination, and needs minimization.
- Provide assistance and support for vulnerable countries when there is a disruption in the PPE supply chain.
- "Irrespective of the measure implemented, health care workers must have the required IPC education and training about the correct use of PPE and other IPC precautions, including demonstration of competency in appropriate procedures for putting on and removing PPE."[16]

1.11. Conclusions

The selection of PPE depends upon the hazard of exposure and the route of transmission. The degree of protection offered by PPE varies depending on the setting and procedures.[81] Evidence-based studies about the efficacy and safety of PPE in different settings would therefore be highly appreciated, for the ideal selection, procurement, and distribution of PPE.

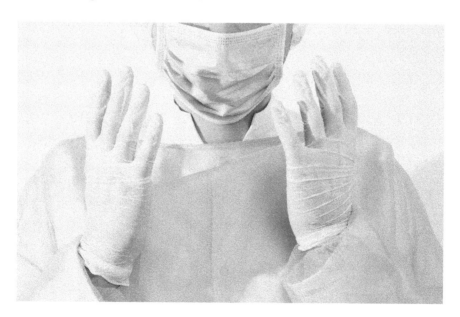

FIGURE 14.14   Green surgical apron.

Source: [www.shutterstock.com/image-photo/man-dressed-green-surgical-apron-mask-1471952111]

2. RDTS AND POINT OF CARE TESTS

2.1. HIV RDT

a. Background

Human immunodeficiency virus infection and acquired immune deficiency syndrome (HIV/AIDS) is a syndrome caused by the human immunodeficiency virus (HIV).[82] HIV/AIDS has caused a globally catastrophic pandemic, which has created a rigorous distortion in the demographics of the affected communities.[83] As of 2018, about 77.3 million HIV victims and about 35.4 million individuals died from illnesses allied to AIDS.[84] In 2006, there were 1.9 million predicted deaths due to HIV/AIDS, which declined afterwards.[83] In 2017, there was a 51% drop in AIDS-related deaths compared to 2006.[84] Between 1992 and 2013, 60% of mortalities in some north and south African regions were attributed to HIV.[85] There was also an increase in male mortality rates in some Eastern Mediterranean regions due to HIV/AIDS, with an increase of 6.7% annually since 1990.[83] In 2014, "the Joint United Nations Programme on HIV/AIDS (UNAIDS) and partners set the 90–90–90 target for the year 2020: diagnose 90% of all people living with HIV (PLHIV); treat 90% of people who know their status, and suppress the virus in 90% of people on treatment. In 2015, countries began reporting to UNAIDS on progress against 90–90–90 using standard definitions and methods."[86]

The most common route for HIV diagnosis is through blood tests,[87] using the enzyme-linked immunosorbent assay (ELISA) RDT. If the ELISA test is positive, the diagnosis is confirmed through a Western blot test.[88] To ensure accurate diagnosis and epidemic control, the "U.S. President's Emergency Plan for AIDS Relief (PEPFAR) recommends that all countries use World Health Organization (WHO) pre-qualified RDTs within the recommended strategies and algorithms for HIV testing."[89]

b. Device Description

HIV RDTs are immunoassay tests that can be performed easily, accurately, and with no need for laboratory equipment.[90] They resolve many problems in HIV diagnosis, particularly in remote areas that are not well equipped. However, RDTs may be fraught, which stands as a challenge for purchasing and interpreting the result.[90]

c. Versions/Generations

Table 14.1 shows the different types of WHO prequalified HIV RDT.

d. Purpose of Use

For communities with a high risk of HIV, self-testing provides a novel strategy for infection control.[91]

TABLE 14.1
WHO Prequalified HIV RDT by Year

Year prequalified	Type of assay	Product name	Manufacturer
2020	HIV RDT	STANDARD Q HIV 1/2 Ab 3-Line Test	SD Biosensor, Inc.
2019	HIV RDT	SURE CHECK HIV Self-Test	Chembio Diagnostic Systems, Inc.
2019	HIV RDT	*First Response HIV 1–2.O Card test (Version 2.0)	Premier Medical Corporation Private Limited
2019	HIV RDT	*Mylan HIV Self Test	Atomo Diagnostics, Ltd.
2019	HIV RDT	*ONE STEP Anti-HIV (1&2) Test	InTec PRODUCTS, INC.
2018	HIV RDT	*INSTI® HIV Self-Test	bioLytical Laboratories, Inc.
2018	HIV RDT	One Step HIV1/2 Whole Blood/Serum/Plasma Test	Guangzhou Wondfo Biotech Co., Ltd.
2017	HIV RDT	Genie™ Fast HIV 1/2	Bio-Rad
2017	HIV RDT	*OraQuick HIV Self-Test	OraSure Technologies, Inc.
2016	HIV RDT	Diagnostic kit for HIV (1+2) antibody (colloidal gold) V2	Shanghai Kehua Bio-engineering Co., Ltd.
2016	HCV RDT	*SD BIOLINE HCV	Standard Diagnostics, Inc.
2016	HIV RDT	Alere™ HIV Combo	Alere Medical Co., Ltd.
2016	HIV RDT	DPP® HIV 1/2 Assay	Chembio Diagnostic Systems, Inc.
2016	HIV RDT	*OraQuick HIV 1/2 Rapid Antibody Test	OraSure Technologies, Inc.
2016	HIV RDT	Rapid Test for Antibody to Human Immunodeficiency Virus (HIV) (Colloidal Gold Device)	Beijing Wantai Biological Pharmacy Enterprise Co.
2014	HIV RDT	*SURE CHECK® HIV 1/2 Assay	Chembio Diagnostic Systems, Inc.
2014	HIV RDT	*ABON™ HIV 1/2/O Tri-Line Human Immunodeficiency Virus	ABON Biopharm (Hangzhou) Co. Ltd.
2013	HIV RDT	VIKIA HIV 1/2	bioMérieux SA
2013	HIV RDT	*INSTI HIV-1/HIV-2 Antibody Test	bioLytical Laboratories, Inc.
2013	HIV RDT	SD BIOLINE HIV-1/2 3.0	Standard Diagnostics, Inc.
2012	HIV RDT	*Uni-Gold™ HIV	Trinity Biotech Manufacturing, Ltd.
2012	HIV RDT	HIV 1/2 STAT-PAK®	Chembio Diagnostic Systems, Inc.
2011	HIV RDT	Alere™ Determine HIV-1/2	Alere Medical Co., Ltd.
2011	HIV RDT	HIV 1/2 STAT-PAK® Dipstick	Chembio Diagnostic Systems, Inc.

e. Interpretation of Readings

The most important feature of the HIV RDT is that the user can visually interpret it. When the control and test lines appear simultaneously, that main result is positive; otherwise, this signifies a negative result when only the control line appears. An incorrect interpretation has been associated significantly with educational level.[91]

f. Important Safety Issues

The WHO has adopted algorithms for HIV RDT result interpretation; unfortunately, the performance failed to reflect the expectations and thresholds targeted, with high rates of false results.[92] This is mainly due to population and geographical variation among the individuals performing the test, which needs to be locally designed, but with standardized algorithms to comply with scores adopted by the WHO.[93]

g. Storage Conditions and Maintenance

For quality assurance measures, the recommended temperature for device storage must be confirmed, which ranges from 2°C to 30 °C, or 2°C to 8 °C for different prequalified tests.

h. Important Features

Although there have been developments in HIV RDTs, a gap remains in qualitative point-of-care (POC) applications. First, acute infected HIV patients remain seronegative, with a high viral load; this makes them unintentionally infectious. Second, infants born to an infected mother may test serologically positive while they may not be infected. Third, appropriate tests for those vaccinated with experimental HIV antigens in clinical trials should be developed: "In each of these cases, new rapid molecular POC HIV screening tests will fill an important diagnostic gap."[94] Due to confidentiality, convenience, and lower stigma, self-testing was preferred to facility-based testing.[95]

i. Special Tips for Users Counseling

POC users should:

  i. Follow safety guidelines.
 ii. Sustain organized care points.
iii. Follow guidelines for disposing of used materials.
 iv. Follow guidelines for handling accidental contact with infectious, hazardous materials.
  v. Collect blood from a client's finger-prick accurately and confidently.

j. The Available Evidence for Effectiveness and Safety

Generally, the RDT algorithm was highly accurate, but sensitivity was lower than anticipated, so post-HIV test counseling is essential to decrease the probability of false negative results.[93]

k. Economic Evaluation

"Home-based Voluntary Counseling and Testing VCT" provides the lowest cost for patient testing, along with cost-effectiveness in determining "HIV seropositive" patients in rural areas; the promotion of this strategy may facilitate timely determination of patients eligible for treatment[96] and could provide a cost-effective, affordable alternate for people living in rural areas. It should be treated as part of "community outreach programs"[97] because such programs were found to be cost-effective in populations with high HIV prevalence.[98]

2.2. Malaria RDT

a. Background

Malaria is a significant cause of morbidity and mortality globally, and environmental changes are likely to increase its importance in the coming years. Malaria diagnosis is not easy and requires highly reputable skills, especially in non-endemic countries.[99] The clinical presentation of malaria ranges from mild illness with minor symptoms to a very severe, fatal course of illness.[100] HCWs should be well trained to face the challenges of malaria's erratic epidemiology.[99] Reports from 2017 indicate that malaria was endemic in more than 91 countries, with about 219 million diagnosed cases and 435,000 deaths reported.[101] For appropriate diagnosis of malaria, thick and thin films are considered the gold standard tests.[102] In this technique, by allowing one drop of blood to be dry on a film, the lysed erythrocytes free the parasite, stained with Giemsa. Trained personnel can estimate the parasite density.[103] Currently, the RDT is recommended to guide diagnosis and treatment.[104]

b. Device Description

Malaria RDTs are "lateral flow immuno-chromatographic antigen-detection tests." Dye-labeled antibodies bind to a parasite antigen and are detected as a visible band on a nitrocellulose strip which forms a test line in the resulting outlet along with a control line in response to antibody-dye conjugation.

c. Versions/Generations

"Parascreen—Rapid test for Malaria Pan/Pf" and "FalciVax—Rapid test for Malaria Pv/Pf" are 2020 WHO prequalified malaria RDTs.

d. Purpose of Use

A test with a sensitivity of 82–97% and an accuracy of 98–100% is used to diagnose Plasmodium falciparum and other forms of plasmodial infections,[105] and the existence or nonexistence of a visible band in the test and control area are used to determine positive and negative results.[106]

e. Interpretation of Readings

Comparing RDT with microscopy, the interpretation of results remains a challenge; sometimes, the RDT is positive when no parasite is seen under a microscope and vice versa, so the interpretation of results should be made carefully to guarantee good treatment outcomes.[107] The practitioner should not ignore causes of fever other than malaria in positive RDT results to control fatal outcomes for the patient.[108]

f. Important Safety Issues

Introducing the malaria RDT to guide treatment and optimize therapy may end up with irrational use of antibiotics to control fever in negative RDT results. There has been an overprescription of antibiotics in 69% of patients with negative RDT results.[109]

g. Storage Conditions and Maintenance

For quality measures, all tests should be stored in the temperature limits specified by the manufacturer, such as 2°–30°C or 2°–8°C.

h. Important Features

The performance of RDTs is safe and effective by expert HCWs. Tests are generally precise across situations, but lower specificities were noticed through drug shops. Test use by HCWs remains in inquiry due to issues related to blood safety, interpretation of results, and obedience to treatment guidelines.[110]

i. Special Tips for Patient Counseling

WHO has Global Malaria Programme, FIND, and their collaborators have set a precise guideline for malaria RDT supply management, with deep concern about handling test kits such as buffer packaging, packaging of alcohol swabs, and the utility of the blood transfer device (BTD).[111]

j. The available Evidence for Effectiveness and Safety

Malaria RDT "is cost-effective, simple to perform, easy to interpret, and easy to transport and is recommended for situations exceeding microscopic capability such as an outbreak"[112] in which the use of malaria RDTs by HCWs as a cost-effective intervention in the moderate-to-high transmission area, but it is not a low-cost intervention in low transmission areas.[113] Based on available evidence, malaria "RDT had the potential to be more cost-effective than either microscopy or presumptive diagnosis."[114]

k. Economic Evaluation

One review reported fifteen studies that evaluated the malaria RDT in comparison to other diagnostic methods from an economic point of view; most studies were of high to moderate quality, ten of which stated the cost-efficacy of RDT compared to other methods[114]: "A study in Myanmar evaluated the effectiveness of financial incentives *vs* information, education and counseling (IEC) in driving the proper use of subsidized malaria RDTs among informal private providers. This cost-effectiveness analysis compares intervention options. In conclusion, private provider subsidies with IEC or a combination of IEC and financial incentives may be a good investment for malaria control."[115]

2.3. SYPHILIS RDT

a. Background

Treponema pallidum (TP) is responsible for the systemic disease commonly called syphilis. The disease has been divided into ordinal stages based on clinical outcomes, guiding the management and follow up. Those stages are primary syphilis characterized by ulcers at the site of infection; secondary syphilis, which manifests in skin rash, mucocutaneous lesions, and lymphadenopathy; and tertiary syphilis, which is characterized by cardiac symptoms, gummatous lesions, tabes dorsalis, and general paresis. Instances of the disease lacking clinical manifestations are referred to as latent infections and can be detected by serologic testing. The central nervous system can be affected by TP, resulting in neurosyphilis, which can appear at any of the three stages of syphilis. "Cranial nerve dysfunction, meningitis, stroke, acute altered mental status, and auditory or ophthalmic abnormalities" are the early neurologic clinical symptoms, and they usually present within the first few months or years of infection, while tabes dorsalis and general paresis are late neurologic symptoms that occur 10–30 years after infection.[116] Currently, the WHO estimates that, worldwide, about 17.7 million individuals in the age group 15–49 years had syphilis in 2012, with a predicted 5.6 million new cases annually. There is variation in prevalence and incidence by region or country, with the highest prevalence in Africa.[117] Early syphilis is mainly diagnosed using darkfield examinations and tests to detect TP directly from lesion exudate; unfortunately, there is no available commercial test to detect TP, although validated PCR tests can detect bacterial DNA. There are two types of tests for presumptive diagnosis of syphilis: a nontreponemal test (i.e., Venereal Disease Research Laboratory [VDRL] or Rapid Plasma Reagin [RPR]) and a treponemal test—that is, "fluorescent treponemal antibody absorbed [FTA-ABS] tests, the *T. pallidum* passive particle agglutination [TP-PA] assay, various enzyme immunoassays [EIAs], chemiluminescence immunoassays, immunoblots, or rapid treponemal assays." Because of the false and false positive results associated with only one serological test, a person with a reactive nontreponemal test should always receive a treponemal test to confirm the diagnosis of syphilis.[118] A rapid syphilis diagnostic test is used; it is easy to perform, and the result may be easily interpreted within 30 minutes.

b. Device Description

The syphilis RDT is used to identify TP antibodies in whole blood, serum, or plasma; the principle of the test depends upon the interaction between the patient sample and the syphilis antigen stationary to the test line, and it is formulated to detect both TP antibodies (IgG and IgM). A coloured line will appear in the test line region if the sample contains TP antibodies, which indicates a positive result. If there are no TP antibodies in the sample, the visible line will appear only in the control line region, indicating a negative result.

c.   Versions/Generations

2020 WHO prequalified syphilis RDTs are the "First Response® HIV1+2/Syphilis Combo Card Test, STANDARD Q HIV/Syphilis Combo Test, and SD BIOLINE HIV/Syphilis Duo."

d.   Purpose of Use

There are more than 20 syphilis RDTs marketed; there are some differences in the processing instructions, but most tests have 3–4 steps as follows: "1. Remove the test from the wrapper and place on a flat surface; 2. Add a specified amount of patient sample (whole blood, plasma or serum) to the sample well S; 3. Add a specified amount of diluent buffer to sample well S; 4. Read the results after a specified time (usually 15–20 mins) as shown in Figure 14.2: (C=control line; T=test line)."[119]

e.   Interpretation of Readings

A visible band in both the test and control regions indicates a positive result, while a visible band appearing only in the control region indicates a negative result.

f.   Important Safety Issues

Users should be very conscious that the visible band can be challenging to observe, making the interpretation of the results very difficult, and may cause some false positive/negative results.[120]

g.   Storage Conditions and Maintenance

Manufacturers recommend storing the syphilis RDTs between 4°–30°C. Because the shelf life is less than 18 months, it is recommended not to supply the rural areas to reduce the chances of overwhelming the supply chain and avoid waste due to expiration.[119]

h.   Important Features

The syphilis RDT detects TP antibodies but not TP or its related antigen; therefore, the syphilis diagnosis remains challenging. Nontreponemal antibodies are a part of most algorithms designed to diagnose syphilis, which raises the research question of whether this new rapid treponemal test could be expanded to improve syphilis treatment affordability.[121]

i.   Special Tips for Patient Counseling

To perform the test appropriately and safely, the user should adhere to the following tips:

  i.   Open the alcohol swab pad.
  ii.   Clean the finger.

  iii.   Knob off the lancet.
  iv.   Press the lancet to the cleaned finger.
  v.   Collect 1–2 blood drops using the micropipette.
  vi.   Place one drop in the sample well.
  vii.   Add 2–4 drops of the provided diluent.
  viii.   Read the result after 10 minutes.

j.   The Available Evidence for Effectiveness and Safety

Available evidence reported equitable performance of syphilis RDTs with "median sensitivity of 86%, specificity of 99% and positive predictive values >80% when prevalence was >0.3%"[122] compare the performance of two rapid syphilis diagnostic tests: Hexagon and the SD Bioline against *Treponema pallidum* hemagglutination assay (TPHA) reference test." Both tests show good performance with negative and positive concordance.[123] The use of a syphilis RDT along with the "venereal disease research laboratory (VDRL) test" improved the number of patients diagnosed effectively.[124]

k.   Economic Evaluation

There is concrete evidence that the prevention of congenital syphilis through prenatal screening programs is cost-effective. However, the implementation is low due to the lack of screening tools in primary healthcare settings.[125] Increasing the availability of screening tools along with a dual HIV and syphilis test could result in a cost-savings outcome when matched to other screening policies.[126]

2.4.   Tuberculosis RDT

a.   Background

The causative agent of tuberculosis (TB) is *Mycobacterium tuberculosis*, most commonly spread by cough aerosols.[127] TB was estimated to kill more than 1.5 million persons worldwide in 2016, despite available effective treatment.[128] A partnership between Stop TB and Millennium Development Goals (MDGs) has stated a universal goal of reducing the epidemiological affliction of TB between 2015 and 2050. Achieving this goal will reflect the global efforts in controlling TB and guide future planning and investments.[129] An RDT relay on the mycobacterial lipoarabinomannan (LAM) antigen in urine has been developed to facilitate urgent diagnosis of TB.[130] However, this test is not appropriate for the entire population because of its suboptimal sensitivity,[131] although new evidence justifies its applicability in a wide range of the population.[132] In addition, "a new urine-based test—the Fujifilm SILVAMP TB LAM, Tokyo, Japan (FujiLAM)—has been developed, and preliminary evaluation shows promising results."[132]

b.   Device Description

Most TB diagnostic tests depend on sputum samples, but it can be challenging to obtain samples from children, immunocompromised patients, and patients with disseminated

TB. This could negatively affect the initiation of the treatment, so "the WHO calls for the development of a rapid, biomarker-based, non-sputum test capable of detecting all forms of TB at the point of care to enable immediate treatment initiation."[133]

c. Versions/Generations

The Alere Determine™ TB LAM Ag is an RDT recommended by the WHO to detect TB comorbidity in the HIV positive population.[134] A novel rapid lateral flow assay test from Fujifilm named "SILVAMP TB LAM (SILVAMP-LAM)" can detect the presence of TB LAM in urine with superior sensitivity to that of the previous test.[135]

d. Purpose of Use

The main goal of the TB RDT is to attain a quick, simple, specific test with high sensitivity and affordability for optimal diagnosis and treatment outcomes.[133]

e. Interpretation of Readings

The TB RDT is run by adding 60 μL of unprocessed urine to the test strip, then incubated for 25 minutes. The eye then checks the strip for the appearance of bands. The result depends on the visible band intensity of a scale card provided by the manufacturer. The current manufacturer recommendations use a four-band scale; all bands graded 1 or higher reflect a positive result.[132]

f. Important Safety Issues: None
g. Storage Conditions and Maintenance

To the end of their shelf life, all TB RDTs should be stored at 2°–30°C and should be handled and stored as recommended by the manufacturer. Test kits are stable until their expiry date. Spoiled devices should not be used unless otherwise directed.[136]

h. Important Features

A study conducted in Kenya, South Africa, and Uganda that used the LF-LAM showed a significant dissimilarity in populations in whom the diagnosis of TB is difficult. The test characteristics, sample, time shift, usability, cost, set-up, and maintenance necessities were reviewed by study participants, who agreed that the LF-LAM is a usable RDT, requires minor logistics, and, the most important feature, it depends on urine—the safest available sample—rather than sputum.[132]

i. Special Tips for Patient Counseling

For inpatient and outpatient settings and HIV-positive patients in different age categories, there is a strong recommendation by the WHO to use LF-LAM to support active TB diagnosis.

j. Available Evidence for Effectiveness and Safety

Testing the FujiLAM POCT AlereLAM in a multicenter cohort study in Peru and South Africa found that the FujiLAM POCT was 98.9% specific to identify 53.2% of positive tuberculosis cases, which represents a five-fold increase in sensitivity among HIV negative encounters.[137]

k. Economic Evaluation

The costs, cost-effectiveness, and affordability of urine-based LF-LAM to diagnose active TB in HIV-positive individuals have been reviewed. All six studies found steady trends, reporting that LF-LAM is cost-effective in adult Africans living with HIV.[132]

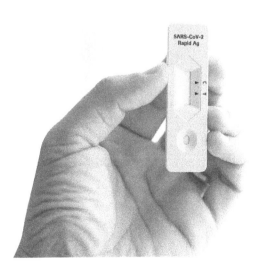

FIGURE 14.15 Hand holding a rapid COVID-19 diagnostic self-test.

Source: [www.shutterstock.com/image-photo/geneva-switzerland-2-may-2021-hand-1966332004]

2.5. Implications for the Pharmacy Profession and Practice

The need for pharmacists to assist in screening for infectious disease is vast and crucial. However, many barriers negatively affect the role of pharmacists in POC testing, such as "lack of test familiarity, physical assessment skills, specimen collection techniques, reimbursement, patient awareness, data sharing and follow-up, and patient acceptance."[138]

There is a need for decision-making to establish priorities in selecting and managing medical devices by adopting Health Technology Assessments (HTAs). HTAs deal with clinical effectiveness and economic effectiveness and include four dimensions: medical, social, ethical, and economic. HTA helps in medical device regulations to ensure the appropriate use of medical devices for the patients.[139-140]

2.6. Challenges to the Pharmacist and Users

Community awareness about pharmacist capability in conducting POC testing is of great concern,[141] while other challenges include legislative and administrative barriers.

2.7. Recommendations: Ways Forward

- Training and education programs are highly appreciated in undergraduate curricula and continuous education programs to overcome pharmacist barriers to POC testing.
- Build a collaborative relationship between the community pharmacist and other HCWs to facilitate POC testing in community pharmacies.
- Tailor education programs to community need about the capabilities of the pharmacist in conducting POC screening.
- Prioritize the availability of RDTs for infectious diseases according to prevalence.
- Assure quality standards when performing RDTs in community pharmacies.
- Promote adopting Health Technology Assessments tools for medical devices.

2.8. Conclusions

RDTs are essential for better treatment outcomes, formulating public health policies, and preventing outbreaks of communicable diseases. It is time to fulfill the need for technological advancements in RDTs through research and development centers to improve the efficacy, sensitivity, reliability, usability, and affordability of these tests.

REFERENCES

1. Verbeek JH, Ijaz S, Mischke C, et al. Personal protective equipment for preventing highly infectious diseases due to exposure to contaminated body fluids in healthcare staff. Cochrane Database Syst Rev. 2016/04/20. 2016;4:Cd011621.
2. Poller B, Tunbridge A, Hall S, et al. A unified personal protective equipment ensemble for clinical response to possible high consequence infectious diseases: a consensus document on behalf of the HCID programme. J Infect. 2018/09/04. 2018;77(6):496–502.
3. Verbeek JH, Rajamaki B, Ijaz S, et al. Personal protective equipment for preventing highly infectious diseases due to exposure to contaminated body fluids in healthcare staff. Cochrane Database Syst Rev. 2019/07/02. 2019;7:Cd011621.
4. Lockhart SL, Duggan LV, Wax RS, et al. Personal protective equipment (PPE) for both anesthesiologists and other airway managers: principles and practice during the COVID-19 pandemic. Can J Anaesth. 2020/04/25. 2020;
5. van Wely E. Current global standards for chemical protective clothing: how to choose the right protection for the right job? Ind Health [Internet]. 2017/10/17. 2017 Dec 7;55(6):485–99. Available from: https://pubmed.ncbi.nlm.nih.gov/29046493.
6. World Health Organization. Personal protective equipment for use in a filovirus disease outbreak: rapid advice guideline. Institutional Respiratory for Information Sharing, iris. Geneva, Switzerland: World Health Organization; 2016.
7. Douglas D, Douglas R. Addressing the corona virus pandemic: will a novel filtered eye mask help? Int J Infect Dis [Internet]. 2020/04/22. 2020 Jun;95:340–4. Available from: https://pubmed.ncbi.nlm.nih.gov/32334119.
8. Simkin JP, Darnay A. Manufacturing & distribution USA: industry analyses, statistics and leading companies [Internet]. Farmington Hills, MI: Gale, Cengage Learning; 2015. (Manufacturing & Distribution USA; 8th edn). Available from: http://sdl.edu.sa/middleware/Default.aspx?USESDL=true&PublisherID=AllPublishers&BookURL=https://sdl.idm.oclc.org/login?url=http://search.ebscohost.com/login.aspx?direct=true&db=edsebk&AN=1077930&site=eds-live.
9. Morgan JS. Personal protective equipment. In: Hewlett A, K. Murthy AR, editors. Bioemergency Plan: A Guid Healthc Facil [Internet]. 2018 Jul 7;169–82. Available from: www.ncbi.nlm.nih.gov/pmc/articles/PMC7121970/.
10. Christensen L, Rasmussen CS, Benfield T, et al. A randomized trial of instructor-led training versus video lesson in training health care providers in proper donning and doffing of personal protective equipment. Disaster Med Public Health Prep [Internet]. 2020 Mar 30;1–15. Available from: https://pubmed.ncbi.nlm.nih.gov/32223776
11. Jones RM, Bleasdale SC, Maita D, et al. A systematic risk-based strategy to select personal protective equipment for infectious diseases. Am J Infect Control [Internet]. 2019/07/27. 2020 Jan;48(1):46–51. Available from: https://pubmed.ncbi.nlm.nih.gov/31358421.
12. Roberge RJ. Face shields for infection control: a review. J Occup Environ Hyg. 2016;13(4):235–42.
13. Roth L, Sobey A, Young R. JEM-EUSO baseline optical design lens and frame stress and dynamics analysis. 2012. Available from: https://ntrs.nasa.gov/api/citations/20120014854/downloads/20120014854.pdf.
14. Lopez JA. Goggles. Google Patents; 1999.
15. Wong TKM, Man SS, Chan AHS. Critical factors for the use or non-use of personal protective equipment amongst construction workers. Saf Sci [Internet]. 2020;126:104663. Available from: www.sciencedirect.com/science/article/pii/S0925753520300606.

16. World Health Organization. Rational use of personal protective equipment for coronavirus disease (COVID-19) and considerations during severe shortages: interim guidance, 6 April 2020. World Health Organization; 2020.

17. Gala CL, Hall CB, Schnabel KC, et al. The use of eye-nose goggles to control nosocomial respiratory syncytial virus infection. JAMA. 1986;256(19):2706–8.

18. French CE, McKenzie BC, Coope C, et al. Risk of nosocomial respiratory syncytial virus infection and effectiveness of control measures to prevent transmission events: a systematic review. Influenza Other Respi Viruses [Internet]. 2016/03/24. 2016 Jul;10(4):268–90. Available from: https://pubmed.ncbi.nlm.nih.gov/26901358.

19. Mostaghimi A, Antonini M-J, Plana D, et al. Regulatory and safety considerations in deploying a locally fabricated, reusable face shield in a hospital responding to the COVID-19 pandemic. Med (NY) [Internet]. 2020 Jun 19; Available from: www.ncbi.nlm.nih.gov/pmc/articles/PMC7304404/.

20. Mostaghimi A, Antonini M-J, Plana D, et al. Rapid prototyping and clinical testing of a reusable face shield for health care workers responding to the COVID-19 pandemic. medRxiv Prepr Serv Heal Sci [Internet]. 2020 Apr 15;2020.04.11.20061960. Available from: https://pubmed.ncbi.nlm.nih.gov/32511612

21. Cuttino M. Management of ventilation during resuscitation. In: Cardiopulmonary resuscitation. Humana Press; 2005. p. 95–110.

22. Perencevich EN, Diekema DJ, Edmond MB. Moving personal protective equipment into the community: face shields and containment of COVID-19. JAMA [Internet]. 2020 Jun 9;323(22):2252–3. https://doi.org/10.1001/jama.2020.7477.

23. Lindsley WG, Noti JD, Blachere FM, et al. Efficacy of face shields against cough aerosol droplets from a cough simulator. J Occup Environ Hyg. 2014;11(8):509–18.

24. Farrier SL, Farrier JN, Gilmour ASM. Eye safety in operative dentistry—a study in general dental practice. Br Dent J. 2006;200(4):218–23.

25. Ko-Keeney EH, Saran MS, McLaughlin K, et al. Improving protection from bioaerosol exposure during postoperative patient interaction in the COVID-19 era, a quality improvement study. Am J Otolaryngol. 2020;41(6):102634.

26. Administration OS and H. Assigned protection factors for the revised respiratory protection standard. Maroon Ebooks; 2015.

27. Atkinson J, Chartier Y, Pessoa-Silva CL, et al., editors. Natural ventilation for infection control in health-care settings. Geneva: World Health Organization; 2009. PMID: 23762969.

28. Loveday HP, Wilson JA, Pratt RJ, et al. epic3: national evidence-based guidelines for preventing healthcare-associated infections in NHS hospitals in England. J Hosp Infect [Internet]. 2014 Jan;86 Suppl 1:S1–70. Available from: https://pubmed.ncbi.nlm.nih.gov/24330862.

29. Lammers MJW, Lea J, Westerberg BD. Guidance for otolaryngology health care workers performing aerosol generating medical procedures during the COVID-19 pandemic. J Otolaryngol Head Neck Surg [Internet]. 2020 Jun 3;49(1):36. Available from: https://pubmed.ncbi.nlm.nih.gov/32493489.

30. Fisher EM, Shaffer RE. Considerations for recommending extended use and limited reuse of filtering facepiece respirators in health care settings. J Occup Environ Hyg [Internet]. 2014;11(8):D115–28. Available from: https://pubmed.ncbi.nlm.nih.gov/24628658.

31. Galloro G, Pisani A, Zagari RM, et al. Safety in digestive endoscopy procedures in the COVID era recommendations in progres of the Italian Society of Digestive Endoscopy. Dig Liver Dis [Internet]. 2020 May 13;10.1016/j.dld.2020.05.002. Available from: https://pubmed.ncbi.nlm.nih.gov/32405285

32. Chochoms M. Respirators: air purifying, self-study, course 40723. Los Alamos, NM: Los Alamos National Lab (LANL); 2017.

33. Broadwater K, Grimes GR, Wiegand DM. Evaluation of laser coding particulate composition, health effects, and safety climate at a brewery. 2019. Available from: https://stacks.cdc.gov/view/cdc/78671.

34. Carver BR. Analysis of user preference with n95 and powered air-purifying respirators in a healthcare work environment. Morgantown, West Virginia: West Virginia University; 2019.

35. Azap A, Erdinç FŞ. Medical mask or N95 respirator: when and how to use? Turkish J Med Sci. 2020;50(SI-1):633–7.

36. Conly J, Seto WH, Pittet D, et al. Use of medical face masks versus particulate respirators as a component of personal protective equipment for health care workers in the context of the COVID-19 pandemic. Antimicrob Resist Infect Control [Internet]. 2020 Aug 6;9(1):126. Available from: https://pubmed.ncbi.nlm.nih.gov/32762735.

37. Raina MacIntyre C, Jay Hasanain S. Community universal face mask use during the COVID 19 pandemic—from households to travellers and public spaces. J Travel Med [Internet]. 2020 May 18 [cited 2020 Jun 17];27(3). Available from: https://academic.oup.com/jtm/article/doi/10.1093/jtm/taaa056/5822103.

38. Lustig S, Biswakarma JJH, Rana D, et al. Effectiveness of common fabrics to block aqueous aerosols of virus-like nanoparticles. ACS Nano. 2020;4(6):7651–8.

39. Raina MacIntyre C, Jay Hasanain S. Community universal face mask use during the COVID 19 pandemic—from households to travellers and public spaces. J Travel Med [Internet]. 2020 Apr 18;27(3). https://doi.org/10.1093/jtm/taaa056.

40. Aiello AE, Perez V, Coulborn RM, et al. Facemasks, hand hygiene, and influenza among young adults: a randomized intervention trial. PLoS One [Internet]. 2012/01/25. 2012;7(1):e29744–e29744. Available from: https://pubmed.ncbi.nlm.nih.gov/22295066.

41. Chu DK, Akl EA, Duda S, et al. Physical distancing, face masks, and eye protection to prevent person-to-person transmission of SARS-CoV-2 and COVID-19: a systematic review and meta-analysis. Lancet (London, England) [Internet]. 2020/06/01. 2020 Jun 27;395(10242):1973–87. Available from: https://pubmed.ncbi.nlm.nih.gov/32497510.

42. Bartoszko JJ, Farooqi MAM, Alhazzani W, et al. Medical masks vs N95 respirators for preventing COVID-19 in healthcare workers: a systematic review and meta-analysis of randomized trials. Influenza Other Respi Viruses [Internet]. 2020/04/21. 2020 Jul;14(4):365–73. Available from: https://pubmed.ncbi.nlm.nih.gov/32246890.

43. Mukerji S, MacIntyre CR, Newall AT. Review of economic evaluations of mask and respirator use for protection against respiratory infection transmission. BMC Infect Dis [Internet]. 2015 Oct 13;15:413. Available from: https://pubmed.ncbi.nlm.nih.gov/26462473.

44. Mukerji S, MacIntyre CR, Seale H, et al. Cost-effectiveness analysis of N95 respirators and medical masks to protect healthcare workers in China from respiratory infections. BMC Infect Dis [Internet]. 2017 Jul 3;17(1):464. Available from: https://pubmed.ncbi.nlm.nih.gov/28673259.

45. Trapp R. Medical examination or objective medical evidence: what is the correct procedure to determine if an employee infected with the HIV virus presents a direct threat under the Americans with Disabilities Act-EEOC v. Prevo's Family Market, Inc. Creight L Rev. 1998;32:1585.

46. Pastorino B, de Lamballerie X, Charrel R. Biosafety and biosecurity in European Containment Level 3 Laboratories: focus on french recent progress and essential requirements. Front Public Health [Internet]. 2017 May 31;5:121. Available from: https://pubmed.ncbi.nlm.nih.gov/28620600.

47. Tabary M, Araghi F, Nasiri S, et al. Dealing with skin reactions to gloves during the COVID-19 pandemic. Infect Control Hosp Epidemiol [Internet]. 2020 May 8;1–2. Available from: https://pubmed.ncbi.nlm.nih.gov/32381129.

48. Kramer A, Assadian O. Indications and the requirements for single-use medical gloves. GMS Hyg Infect Control [Internet]. 2016 Jan 12;11:Doc01–Doc01. Available from: https://pubmed.ncbi.nlm.nih.gov/26816673.

49. Baloh J, Reisinger HS, Dukes K, et al. Healthcare workers' strategies for doffing personal protective equipment. Clin Infect Dis [Internet]. 2019 Sep 13;69(Suppl 3):S192–8. Available from: https://pubmed.ncbi.nlm.nih.gov/31517970.

50. World Health Organization. Preferred product characteristics for personal protective equipment for the health worker on the frontline responding to viral hemorrhagic fevers in tropical climates. World Health Organization; 2018.

51. Woolley K, Smith R, Arumugam S. Personal Protective Equipment (PPE) guidelines, adaptations and lessons during the COVID-19 pandemic. Lignes directrices sur l'équipement Prot Individ pendant la pandémie COVID-19 leçons Adapt [Internet]. 2020 Jan 1; Available from: http://10.0.3.248/j.jemep.2020.100546.

52. Srivastav A, Santibanez TA, Lu PJ, et al. Preventive behaviors adults report using to avoid catching or spreading influenza, United States, 2015–16 influenza season. PLoS One. 2018 Mar 30;13(3):e0195085.

53. GAETZ PBYS. Keep children—and adults—healthy: prevent and curb common infections. Available from: http://www.childcarequarterly.com/pdf/summer20_infections.pdf.

54. Prevention C for DC and. Considerations for events and gatherings. 2020. Available from: https://www.cdc.gov/coronavirus/2019-ncov/community/large-events/considerations-for-events-gatherings.html.

55. DRAFT C. Australian guidelines for the prevention and control of infection in healthcare. 2010. Available from: https://www.nhmrc.gov.au/about-us/publications/australian-guidelines-prevention-and-control-infection-healthcare-2010.

56. Ward D. Community infection control: what is the evidence? Br J Community Nurs [Internet]. 2002 Jun;7(6):304. Available from: http://sdl.edu.sa/middleware/Default.aspx?USESDL=true&PublisherID=AllPublishers&BookURL=https://sdl.idm.oclc.org/login?url=http://search.ebscohost.com/login.aspx?direct=true&db=edb&AN=106958749&site=eds-live.

57. Deepthi R, Masthi NRR, Nirmala CJ, et al. Personal Protective Equipments (PPE)—prerequisites, rationale and challenges during COVID 19 pandemic. Indian J Community Heal [Internet]. 2020 Jan 2;32(2):196. Available from: http://sdl.edu.sa/middleware/Default.aspx?USESDL=true&PublisherID=AllPublishers&BookURL=https://sdl.idm.oclc.org/login?url=http://search.ebscohost.com/login.aspx?direct=true&db=edb&AN=143065531&site=eds-live.

58. Phillips VL, Goodrich MA, Sullivan TJ. Health care worker disability due to latex allergy and asthma: a cost analysis. Am J Public Health [Internet]. 1999 Jul;89(7):1024–8. Available from: https://pubmed.ncbi.nlm.nih.gov/10394310.

59. Arora P, Kumari S, Sodhi J, et al. Gloves reprocessing: does it really save money? Indian J Surg. 2015;77(3):1291–4.

60. Gruendemann BJ. Taking cover: single-use vs. reusable gowns and drapes. Infect Control Today. 2002;6(1):32–4.

61. Siegel JD, Rhinehart E, Jackson M, et al. 2007 Guideline for isolation precautions: preventing transmission of infectious agents in health care settings. Am J Infect Control [Internet]. 2007 Dec;35(10 Suppl 2):S65–164. Available from: https://pubmed.ncbi.nlm.nih.gov/18068815.

62. Kilinc FS. A review of isolation gowns in healthcare: fabric and gown properties. J Eng Fiber Fabr [Internet]. 2015 Sep;10(3):180–90. Available from: https://pubmed.ncbi.nlm.nih.gov/26989351.

63. Gupta BS. The effect of structural factors on the absorbent characteristics of nonwovens. Tappi J. 1988;71(8):147–52.

64. Anagnostopoulos-King F, Rodriguez DS. Infection control standards of care: a global perspective. In: Infection control in the dental office. Cham: Springer; 2020. p. 63–75.

65. Bauchner H, Fontanarosa PB, Livingston EH. Conserving supply of personal protective equipment—a call for ideas. JAMA. 2020;323(19):1911.

66. Kilinc Balci FS. Isolation gowns in health care settings: laboratory studies, regulations and standards, and potential barriers of gown selection and use. Am J Infect Control [Internet]. 2015/09/26. 2016 Jan 1;44(1):104–11. Available from: https://pubmed.ncbi.nlm.nih.gov/26391468.

67. McNeary L, Maltser S, Verduzco-Gutierrez M. Navigating Coronavirus Disease 2019 (Covid-19) in physiatry: a CAN report for inpatient rehabilitation facilities. PM&R. 2020;12(5):512–15.

68. Simpson C. Reusable PPE. Re: optimizing the supply of Personal Protective Equipment (PPE) during the COVID-19 pandemic as you know, the response to the COVID-19 pandemic is causing shortages of personal protective equipment (PPE) around the world. Here in Ontario, we continue to. Health (Irvine Calif). 2020.

69. Puzniak LA, Gillespie KN, Leet T, et al. A cost-benefit analysis of gown use in controlling vancomycin-resistant Enterococcus transmission: is it worth the price, Infect Control Hosp Epidemiol. 2004 May;25(5):418–24.

70. Lebesc N, Bouneb F, Piketty H, et al. Performance of textile and non-woven materials against penetration and permeation of liquid pesticides. J fuer Verbraucherschutz und Leb [Internet]. 2015 Dec;10(4):307. Available from: http://sdl.edu.sa/middleware/Default.aspx?USESDL=true&PublisherID=AllPublishers&BookURL=https://sdl.idm.oclc.org/login?url=http://search.ebscohost.com/login.aspx?direct=true&db=edb&AN=111241135&site=eds-live.

71. Wang Y, Zhang J, Zhao X, et al. Selection of emergency medical protective equipment for harsh environment: a study of effectiveness evaluation method on the basis of connection numbers. Ekoloji. 2018;27(106):1227–34.

72. Bhuiyan MAR, Wang L, Shaid A, et al. Advances and applications of chemical protective clothing system. J Ind Text [Internet]. 2019 Jul;49(1):97. Available from: http://sdl.edu.sa/middleware/Default.aspx?USESDL=true&PublisherID=AllPublishers&BookURL=https://sdl.idm.oclc.org/login?url=http://search.ebscohost.com/login.aspx?direct=true&db=edb&AN=136890140&site=eds-live.

73. Fletcher OM, Guerrina R, Ashley CD, et al. Heat stress evaluation of two-layer chemical demilitarization ensembles with a full face negative pressure respirator. Ind Health [Internet]. 2014/04/05. 2014;52(4):304–12. Available from: https://pubmed.ncbi.nlm.nih.gov/24705801.

74. Coca A, Quinn T, Kim J-H, et al. Physiological evaluation of personal protective ensembles recommended for use in West Africa. Disaster Med Public Heal Prep. 2017;11(5):580–6.

75. Verbeek JH, Rajamaki B, Ijaz S, et al. Personal protective equipment for preventing highly infectious diseases due to exposure to contaminated body fluids in healthcare staff. Cochrane Database Syst Rev. 2020;(4).

76. Pissinati P de SC, Haddad M do CL, Rossaneis MÂ, et al. Costs of reusable and disposable aprons in a public teaching hospital. Rev da Esc Enferm da USP. 2014;48(5):915–21.

77. Burns KM, Shoag JM, Kahlon SS, et al. Lead aprons are a lead exposure hazard. J Am Coll Radiol. 2017;14(5):641–7.

78. Hegde S. Which type of personal protective equipment (PPE) and which method of donning or doffing PPE carries the least risk of infection for healthcare workers? Evid Based Dent [Internet]. 2020 Jun;21(2):74–6. Available from: http://sdl.edu.sa/middleware/Default.aspx?USESDL=true&PublisherID=AllPublishers&BookURL=https://sdl.idm.oclc.org/login?url=http://search.ebscohost.com/login.aspx?direct=true&db=cmedm&AN=32591668&site=eds-live.

79. Coles B, Burton C, Khunti K, et al. What is the effectiveness of protective gowns and aprons against COVID-19 in primary care settings? Available from: https://www.researchgate.net/profile/Trisha-Greenhalgh/publication/340934176_What_is_the_effectiveness_of_protective_gowns_and_aprons_against_COVID-19_in_primary_care_settings/links/5ea5b9a2a6fdccd79457227c/What-is-the-effectiveness-of-protective-gowns-and-aprons-against-COVID-19-in-primary-care-settings.pdf.

80. Seko T, Tachi T, Kawashima N, et al. Economic evaluation of infection control activities. J Hosp Infect [Internet]. 2017;96(4):371–6. Available from: www.sciencedirect.com/science/article/pii/S0195670117302827.

81. Park SH. Personal protective equipment for healthcare workers during the COVID-19 pandemic. Infect Chemother [Internet]. 2020 Jun;52(2):165–82. Available from: https://pubmed.ncbi.nlm.nih.gov/32618146.

82. Sepkowitz KA. AIDS—the first 20 years. N Engl J Med. 2001;344(23):1764–72.

83. Gao D, Zou Z, Dong B, et al. Secular trends in HIV/AIDS mortality in China from 1990 to 2016: gender disparities. PLoS One [Internet]. 2019 Jul 18;14(7):e0219689–e0219689. Available from: https://pubmed.ncbi.nlm.nih.gov/31318900.

84. HIV Glasgow 2018, 28–31 October 2018, Glasgow, UK. J Int AIDS Soc [Internet]. 2018 Oct;21(Suppl 8):e25187—e25187. Available from: https://pubmed.ncbi.nlm.nih.gov/30362663.

85. Mee P, Kahn K, Kabudula CW, et al. The development of a localized HIV epidemic and the associated excess mortality burden in a rural area of South Africa. Glob Heal Epidemiol Genom. 2016;1.

86. Marsh K, Eaton JW, Mahy M, et al. Global, regional and country-level 90–90–90 estimates for 2018: assessing progress towards the 2020 target. AIDS [Internet]. 2019 Dec 15;33 Suppl 3(Suppl 3):S213–26. Available from: https://pubmed.ncbi.nlm.nih.gov/31490781.

87. Miller JM, Binnicker MJ, Campbell S, et al. A guide to utilization of the microbiology laboratory for diagnosis of infectious diseases: 2018 update by the Infectious Diseases Society of America and the American Society for Microbiology. Clin Infect Dis [Internet]. 2018 Aug 31;67(6):e1–94. Available from: https://pubmed.ncbi.nlm.nih.gov/29955859.

88. Alexander TS. Human immunodeficiency virus diagnostic testing: 30 years of evolution. Clin Vaccine Immunol [Internet]. 2016 Apr 4;23(4):249–53. Available from: https://pubmed.ncbi.nlm.nih.gov/26936099.

89. Kravitz Del Solar AS, Parekh B, Douglas MO, et al. A commitment to HIV diagnostic accuracy—a comment on "Towards more accurate HIV testing in sub-Saharan Africa: a multi-site evaluation of HIV RDTs and risk factors for false positives "and" HIV misdiagnosis in sub-Saharan Africa: a performance of diagno. J Int AIDS Soc [Internet]. 2018 Aug;21(8):e25177–e25177. Available from: https://pubmed.ncbi.nlm.nih.gov/30168275.

90. Chiu Y-HC, Ong J, Walker S, et al. Photographed rapid HIV test results pilot novel quality assessment and training schemes. PLoS One [Internet]. 2011 Mar 31;6(3):e18294–e18294. Available from: https://pubmed.ncbi.nlm.nih.gov/21483842.

91. Tonen-Wolyec S, Batina-Agasa S, Longo JDD, et al. Insufficient education is a key factor of incorrect interpretation of HIV self-test results by female sex workers in Democratic Republic of the Congo: a multicenter cross-sectional study. Medicine (Baltimore) [Internet]. 2019 Feb;98(6):e14218–e14218. Available from: https://pubmed.ncbi.nlm.nih.gov/30732137.

92. Kosack CS, Shanks L, Beelaert G, et al. HIV misdiagnosis in sub-Saharan Africa: performance of diagnostic algorithms at six testing sites. J Int AIDS Soc. 2017;20(1):21419.

93. Kosack CS, Page A-L, Beelaert G, et al. Towards more accurate HIV testing in sub-Saharan Africa: a multi-site evaluation of HIV RDTs and risk factors for false positives. J Int AIDS Soc [Internet]. 2017 Mar 24;19(1):21345. Available from: https://pubmed.ncbi.nlm.nih.gov/28364560.

94. Haleyur Giri Setty MK, Hewlett IK. Point of care technologies for HIV. AIDS Res Treat [Internet]. 2014/01/21. 2014;2014:497046. Available from: https://pubmed.ncbi.nlm.nih.gov/24579041.

95. Qin Y, Han L, Babbitt A, et al. Experiences using and organizing HIV self-testing. AIDS [Internet]. 2018 Jan 28;32(3):371–81. Available from: https://pubmed.ncbi.nlm.nih.gov/29194120.

96. Mulogo EM, Batwala V, Nuwaha F, et al. Cost effectiveness of facility and home based HIV voluntary counseling and testing strategies in rural Uganda. Afr Health Sci. 2013;13(2):423–9.

97. Tabana H, Nkonki L, Hongoro C, et al. A cost-effectiveness analysis of a home-based HIV counselling and testing intervention versus the standard (facility based) HIV testing strategy in rural South Africa. PLoS ONE [Internet].

2015 Aug 14;10(8):e0135048–e0135048. Available from: https://pubmed.ncbi.nlm.nih.gov/26275059.

98. Maheswaran H, Clarke A, MacPherson P, et al. Cost-effectiveness of community-based human immunodeficiency virus self-testing in Blantyre, Malawi. Clin Infect Dis [Internet]. 2018 Apr 3;66(8):1211–21. Available from: https://pubmed.ncbi.nlm.nih.gov/29136117.

99. Hidalgo J, Arriaga P, Concejo BA (Hidalgo J, Woc-Colburn L, editors). Malaria. Highly Infect Dis Crit Care A Compr Clin Guid [Internet]. 2020 Jan 3;213–34. Available from: www.ncbi.nlm.nih.gov/pmc/articles/PMC7120402/.

100. Mirzaian E, Durham MJ, Hess K, et al. Mosquito-Borne illnesses in travelers: a review of risk and prevention. Pharmacother J Hum Pharmacol Drug Ther. 2010;30(10):1031–43.

101. Parselia E, Kontoes C, Tsouni A, et al. Satellite earth observation data in epidemiological modeling of malaria, dengue and West Nile Virus: a scoping review. Remote Sens. 2019;11(16):1862.

102. Birnbaumer DM, Rutkowski A. Malaria: a comprehensive review for the emergency physician. Adv Emerg Nurs J. 2003;25(1):2–12.

103. Hommel M. Diagnostic methods in malaria. Essent Malariol. 2002;4:35–58.

104. McMorrow ML, Aidoo M, Kachur SP. Malaria rapid diagnostic tests in elimination settings—can they find the last parasite? Clin Microbiol Infect [Internet]. 2011/09/13. 2011 Nov;17(11):1624–31. Available from: https://pubmed.ncbi.nlm.nih.gov/21910780.

105. Gatton ML, Rees-Channer RR, Glenn J, et al. Pan-Plasmodium band sensitivity for Plasmodium falciparum detection in combination malaria rapid diagnostic tests and implications for clinical management. Malar J [Internet]. 2015 Mar 18;14:115. Available from: https://pubmed.ncbi.nlm.nih.gov/25889624.

106. Nkrumah B, Acquah SE, Ibrahim L, et al. Comparative evaluation of two rapid field tests for malaria diagnosis: Partec Rapid Malaria Test® and Binax Now® Malaria Rapid Diagnostic Test. BMC Infect Dis [Internet]. 2011 May 23;11:143. Available from: https://pubmed.ncbi.nlm.nih.gov/21605401.

107. Orish VN, De-Gaulle VF, Sanyaolu AO. Interpreting rapid diagnostic test (RDT) for Plasmodium falciparum. BMC Res Notes [Internet]. 2018 Dec 4;11(1):850. Available from: https://pubmed.ncbi.nlm.nih.gov/30509313.

108. Bisoffi Z, Gobbi F, Buonfrate D, et al. Diagnosis of Malaria Infection with or without Disease. Mediterr J Hematol Infect Dis [Internet]. 2012/05/09. 2012;4(1):e2012036—e2012036. Available from: https://pubmed.ncbi.nlm.nih.gov/22708051.

109. Hopkins H, Bruxvoort KJ, Cairns ME, et al. Impact of introduction of rapid diagnostic tests for malaria on antibiotic prescribing: analysis of observational and randomized studies in public and private healthcare settings. BMJ [Internet]. 2017 Mar 29;356:j1054–j1054. Available from: https://pubmed.ncbi.nlm.nih.gov/28356302.

110. Boyce MR. Use and limitations of malaria rapid diagnostic testing in sub-Saharan Africa. Duke University; 2017. Available from: https://dukespace.lib.duke.edu/dspace/bitstream/handle/10161/15227/Boyce_duke_0066N_13842.pdf?sequence=1.

111. Harvey SA, Incardona S, Martin N, et al. Quality issues with malaria rapid diagnostic test accessories and buffer packaging: findings from a 5-country private sector project in Africa. Malar J [Internet]. 2017 Apr 20;16(1):160. Available from: https://pubmed.ncbi.nlm.nih.gov/28427428.

112. Hansen KS, Grieve E, Mikhail A, et al. Cost-effectiveness of malaria diagnosis using rapid diagnostic tests compared to microscopy or clinical symptoms alone in Afghanistan. Malar J [Internet]. 2015 May 28;14:217. Available from: https://pubmed.ncbi.nlm.nih.gov/26016871.

113. Hansen KS, Ndyomugyenyi R, Magnussen P, et al. Cost-effectiveness analysis of malaria rapid diagnostic tests for appropriate treatment of malaria at the community level in Uganda. Health Policy Plan [Internet]. 2017 Jun 1;32(5):676–89. Available from: https://pubmed.ncbi.nlm.nih.gov/28453718.

114. Ling X-X, Jin J-J, Zhu G-D, et al. Cost-effectiveness analysis of malaria rapid diagnostic tests: a systematic review. Infect Dis Poverty [Internet]. 2019 Dec 30;8(1):104. Available from: https://pubmed.ncbi.nlm.nih.gov/31888731.

115. Chen IT, Aung T, Thant HNN, et al. Cost-effectiveness analysis of malaria rapid diagnostic test incentive schemes for informal private healthcare providers in Myanmar. Malar J [Internet]. 2015 Feb 5;14:55. Available from: https://pubmed.ncbi.nlm.nih.gov/25653121.

116. Workowski KA, Bolan GA. Prevention C for DC and sexually transmitted diseases treatment guidelines, 2015. Morb Mortal Wkly report Recomm reports [Internet]. 2015 Jun 5;64(RR-03):1–137. Available from: https://pubmed.ncbi.nlm.nih.gov/26042815.

117. Newman L, Rowley J, Vander Hoorn S, et al. Global estimates of the prevalence and incidence of four curable sexually transmitted infections in 2012 based on systematic review and global reporting. PLoS One [Internet]. 2015 Dec 8;10(12):e0143304–e0143304. Available from: https://pubmed.ncbi.nlm.nih.gov/26646541.

118. APHL. Laboratory diagnostic testing for Treponema pallidum. In Expert Consultation Meeting Summary Report, January 13–15, 2009, Atlanta, GA. 2009.

119. Initiative STDD, UNICEF. The use of rapid syphilis tests. World Health Organization. 2006.

120. Van Den Heuvel A, Smet H, Prat I, et al. Laboratory evaluation of four HIV/syphilis rapid diagnostic tests. BMC Infect Dis. 2019;19(1):1.

121. Peterman TA, Fakile YF. What is the use of rapid syphilis tests in the United States? Sex Transm Dis [Internet]. 2016 Mar;43(3):201–3. Available from: https://pubmed.ncbi.nlm.nih.gov/26859809.

122. O'Donnell CJ, Lindpaintner K, Larson MG, et al. Evidence for association and genetic linkage of the angiotensin-converting enzyme locus with hypertension and blood pressure in men but not women in the Framingham Heart Study. Circulation. 1998;97(18):1766–72.

123. Dlamini NR, Phili R, Connolly C. Evaluation of rapid syphilis tests in KwaZulu-Natal. J Clin Lab Anal [Internet]. 2014/01/02. 2014 Jan;28(1):77–81. Available from: https://pubmed.ncbi.nlm.nih.gov/24395488.

124. Gallo Vaulet L, Morando N, Casco R, et al. Evaluation of the utility of a rapid test for syphilis at a sexually transmitted disease clinic in Buenos Aires, Argentina. Sci Rep [Internet]. 2018 May 15;8(1):7542. Available from: https://pubmed.ncbi.nlm.nih.gov/29765114.

125. Peeling RW, Holmes KK, Mabey D, et al. Rapid tests for sexually transmitted infections (STIs): the way forward.

Sex Transm Infect [Internet]. 2006/12/06. 2006 Dec;82 Suppl 5(Suppl 5):v1–6. Available from: https://pubmed. ncbi.nlm.nih.gov/17151023.

126. Bristow CC, Larson E, Anderson LJ, et al. Cost-effectiveness of HIV and syphilis antenatal screening: a modelling study. Sex Transm Infect [Internet]. 2016/02/26. 2016 Aug;92(5):340–6. Available from: https://pubmed. ncbi.nlm.nih.gov/26920867.

127. Cohen KA, Manson AL, Desjardins CA, et al. Deciphering drug resistance in *Mycobacterium tuberculosis* using whole-genome sequencing: progress, promise, and challenges. Genome Med [Internet]. 2019 Jul 25;11(1):45. Available from: https://pubmed.ncbi.nlm.nih.gov/31345251.

128. Petersen E, Blumberg L, Wilson ME, et al. Ending the Global Tuberculosis Epidemic by 2030—the Moscow declaration and achieving a major translational change in delivery of TB healthcare. Int J Infect Dis. 2017;65:156–8.

129. Glaziou P, Sismanidis C, Floyd K, et al. Global epidemiology of tuberculosis. Cold Spring Harb Perspect Med [Internet]. 2014 Oct 30;5(2):a017798—a017798. Available from: https://pubmed.ncbi.nlm.nih.gov/25359550.

130. Sarkar P, Biswas D, Sindhwani G, et al. Application of lipoarabinomannan antigen in tuberculosis diagnostics: current evidence. Postgrad Med J. 2014;90(1061):155–63.

131. Shah M, Variava E, Holmes CB, et al. Diagnostic accuracy of a urine lipoarabinomannan test for tuberculosis in hospitalized patients in a High HIV prevalence setting. J Acquir Immune Defic Syndr. 2009;52(2):145.

132. World Health Organization. Lateral flow urine lipoarabinomannan assay (LF-LAM) for the diagnosis of active tuberculosis in people living with HIV: policy update 2019. World Health Organization. 2019.

133. Bulterys MA, Wagner B, Redard-Jacot M, et al. Point-of-care urine LAM tests for tuberculosis diagnosis: a status update. J Clin Med [Internet]. 2019 Dec 31;9(1):111. Available from: https://pubmed.ncbi.nlm.nih.gov/31906163.

134. Bjerrum S, Schiller I, Dendukuri N, et al. Lateral flow urine lipoarabinomannan assay for detecting active tuberculosis in people living with HIV. Cochrane database Syst Rev [Internet]. 2019 Oct 21;10(10):CD011420–CD011420. Available from: https://pubmed.ncbi.nlm.nih.gov/31633805.

135. Broger T, Nicol MP, Székely R, et al. Diagnostic accuracy of a novel tuberculosis point-of-care urine lipoarabinomannan assay for people living with HIV: a meta-analysis of individual in- and outpatient data. PLoS Med [Internet]. 2020 May 1;17(5):e1003113—e1003113. Available from: https://pubmed.ncbi.nlm.nih.gov/32357197.

136. World Health Organization. The use of lateral flow urine lipoarabinomannan assay (LF-LAM) for the diagnosis and screening of active tuberculosis in people living with HIV: policy guidance. World Health Organization; 2015.

137. Broger T, Nicol MP, Sigal GB, et al. Diagnostic accuracy of 3 urine lipoarabinomannan tuberculosis assays in HIV-negative outpatients. J Clin Invest. 2020;130(11).

138. McCants H. Role of pharmacist-provided point-of-care testing. J Am Pharm Assoc. 2015;55(6):576.

139. HTA Glossary. International Network of Agencies for Health Technology Assessment and Health Technology Assessment international. Available from: www.htaglossary.net/ (accessed Apr 2021).

140. Garrido V, et al. Health technology assessment and health policy-making in Europe: current status, challenges, and potential. No. 14. WHO Regional Office Europe; 2008.

141. Bastianelli KMS, Nelson L, Palombi L. Perceptions of pharmacists' role in the health care team through student-pharmacist led point-of-care screenings and its future application in health care. Curr Pharm Teach Learn. 2017;9(2): 195–200.

15 Medical Devices for Oncology

Sunil Shrestha, Asmita Priyadarshini Khatiwada, Binaya Sapkota, Sajin Rajbhandari, and Bhuvan KC

CONTENTS

BACKGROUND

There are various types of medical devices available to treat cancer and manage adverse drug reactions due to chemotherapy. Medical oncologists, nurses, pharmacists, and other concerned health professionals should select the appropriate device for each cancer patient's condition and counsel them on their proper application. Here, we discuss in depth devices applicable from the pharmacy's and pharmacist's points of view.

CHAPTER OBJECTIVES

At the end of the chapter, the readers will be able to understand the details of the following devices:

1. Patient-controlled analgesia
2. Domicile oxygen therapy for cancer patients (oxygen cylinder)
3. Intravenous pumps (digital and manual)
4. Automatic compounding system for oncology patients
5. Biological safety cabinet (BSC)
6. IV admixture unit for chemotherapy
7. Peripheral venous catheter
8. Central venous catheter
9. Peripherally inserted central catheter line
10. Port line
11. Devices used for pressure ulcers
12. Implantable pain medication pump
13. Hair wigs
14. Ryle's tube (nasogastric tubes)
15. Postmastectomy devices (inner wears, artificial breast)
16. Pill pulverizer
17. Bone marrow aspiration syringe
18. Intravenous cannula
19. Personal protective equipment (PPE; relevant to the BSC)
20. Automated compounding devices (ACDs) for total parenteral nutrition (TPN)
21. Other devices used in medical oncology
    a. Face mask (surgical)
    b. Thermometer
    c. Bed
    d. Incontinence products
    e. Adult diapers
    f. Wheelchair

DEVICE 1: PATIENT-CONTROLLED ANALGESIA

A) BACKGROUND

Patient-controlled analgesia (PCA) is an excellent alternative to traditional methods of medication administration to patients. It can be used to manage acute, chronic, labor, and postoperative pain.[1] The method is beneficial in patients who are unable to take medication orally. Additionally, with the patient having the control to administer the medicine at the desired time, the nursing staff's workload is reduced. Patients with pain associated with phantom limb syndrome, metastatic cancer, trauma, burns, complex regional pain syndrome, labor, and post-surgery pain are eligible for PCA.[2] The management of chronic pain in patients with cancer requires analgesics, and an effective way to manage the pain is patient-controlled analgesia (PCA).[3,4] PCA is a pain management approach that allows patients to decide the time of pain medication.[2,5] The patients are given the liberty to administer the preset doses of pain medications at their desired time. However, medication and dose per day are determined by the prescribers.[6] The use of PCA in cancer management and other chronic pain primarily focuses on the noninvasive and anticipatory application of appropriate analgesics.[3]

PCA can be delivered in various ways, including pumps. The use of infusion pumps for the delivery of analgesics by the patients themselves is quite common. PCA pumps are the computerized system delivering the medicine at the press of a button at specified intervals. The pump is connected to the intravenous (IV) line of the patients and contains a syringe containing the prescribed drug that delivers the programmed and locked dose of drugs directly to the veins through IV lines with each press of the button.[2] The pump delivers the medicine either in the form of a continuous infusion or a single shot bolus. Even when receiving the medicine continuously in a constant flow, sometimes a patient may desire an extra dose because of the severe pain. The dose is administered by pressing the pump button by the patients themselves or the individual authorized to give the medicine to the patient.[7] The medicines delivered may be opioids, such as morphine and fentanyl. PCA can be administered through various approaches, including intravenous lines, central lines, epidural catheters, peripheral nerve catheters, or transdermal delivery systems.

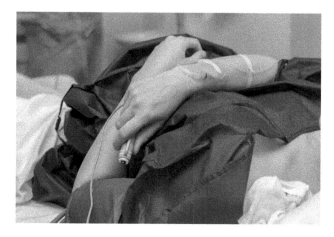

FIGURE 15.1   Patient-controlled analgesia pump.

Source: www.shutterstock.com/image-photo/woman-delivery-room-dropper-presses-remote-1300531705

B)   DEVICE DESCRIPTION

PCA pumps consist of a locking system, medication chamber, programming settings, display, and patient button; most PCA systems have these components in common. However, the pumps available on the market may vary in their appearances and sizes.[2]

A variety of pain medications can be administered using PCA, depending on the PCA routes chosen. Some of these medications include opioids and local anesthetics. Medications such as ketamine, naloxone, clonidine, and ketorolac may be used for IV PCA to enhance pain control and reduce unwanted effects.[2]

C)   TYPES OF PCA DEVICES

Both types of devices have a drug reservoir and patient-controlled button.

1. Electronic PCA device

   This type of pump is commonly used for inpatients in hospitals or bedridden patients. A constant background infusion can be delivered by an electronic PCA device with flexibility in terms of the timing of the medicine delivery. These devices have a higher volume capacity than disposable PCA devices, and the amount of the medicines delivered can vary, as necessary. A pump with the prescribed medicine and regimen is fitted to the patient's bed side, and a handheld button connected to the pump is made available to the patients. These devices are usually tamper-proof, and the medication is not easily accessible (e.g., bedside infusion pump).[8]

2. Disposable PCA device

   These devices deliver a fixed, usually small, quantity of medications with each press of the patient

demand button. Compared to tamper-proof electronic devices, the medicine in the disposable PCA device reservoir is easily accessible. Disposable PCA devices are portable, simple, and easily disposable. One type is a wrist-worn device. This device is designed so that it can be tied around the wrist like a watch. It can provide both bolus doses and continuous infusion, and the desired pain medication regimens can be easily programmed. The pump cartridge volume capacity for the analgesics may vary from 10–20 ml; the total capacity is not usually more than that for the wrist-worn pump. However, devices containing a cartridge with greater capacity can be worn on a belt, a harness, or pocket. Medications can be added to the pump just before administration, or prefilled pumps may also be available for use with compatible and stable medicines.[9]

D)   PURPOSES OF USE, HOW TO USE/OPERATE PROPERLY, AND OPERATIONAL REQUIREMENTS (SUPPORTED WITH PICTURES AND DRAWINGS)

PCA is commonly used in hospitals as a pain management approach for postsurgical pain, caesarian pain, or chronic pain patients. When appropriate candidates are chosen, PCA is safe in children, adults, and adolescents.[10-12] PCA has an additional benefit of determining the suitable time for medication administration when the patient needs it the most. Patients can determine the extent of their pain and need for pain relief. The workload of nursing staffs is reduced with the provision of PCA in hospitalized patients.[13,14]

A treatment regimen is prescribed for individual patients by oncologists. The prescribers evaluate appropriate patients for PCA. The medication is loaded into the pump according to the prescription. The dose and frequency of medicine administration are set as per the prescription. PCA is facilitated with a locking system and various alarms to prevent medicine overdose and other possible accidents. The healthcare staff (the nurse in most cases) educate the patient on the PCA and how to initiate medicine administration by pressing the hand-held button, after which the medicine is self-administered by the patients. However, arrangements are usually made beforehand by the healthcare staff. The daily dose of the medicine is predetermined and loaded into the pump. The pump is programmed to deliver the initial loading dose, lockout interval, infusion rate, PCA dose, and so on. The patients can administer the medications whenever they desire, but they cannot choose the dose and amount of medicine per day. Sometimes, PCA may be adjusted to provide a low dose of continuous pain medication to establish a base level of pain control.[2,15,16]

Patients may be administered IV fluid between the doses of pain medication to keep the patient hydrated.

E) IMPORTANT SAFETY ISSUES

PCA is usually a safe and effective approach for pain management. In addition to the technical issues related to PCA administration, the specific pain medications administered (opioids usually) may add to unwanted effects of PCA. The associated issues with PCA are mentioned here:

- The PCA infusion lines should be kept near the bedside and be appropriately labeled to avoid any confusion. If feasible, information on PCA pump programming should be made available at the patient's bed to help any staff who do not regularly initiate PCA.
- Physicians should independently evaluate the changes in programming and settings of the PCA, medicines and doses to avoid errors.
- As soon as the patient's updated report is available, the PCA settings should be verified and changed if required.
- Respiratory depression (breathing difficulties): In hospitalized patients, the nursing staff needs to check on the patients frequently for breathing problems.[15]
- Elderly patients, patients with existing respiratory diseases (such as asthma or other lung problems), obese patients, patients with sleep apnea, patients who have not been previously exposed to opioids, and patients prescribed with a higher dose of pain medication should be monitored carefully for respiratory problems.[15,17]
- Patients should also be monitored for any allergic reactions, hypotension, constipation, sedation, nausea, or vomiting while on opioids.
- The risk of under-treatment or over-treatment is lower with PCA, because the patient himself/herself is responsible for medicine administration at the time of need. However, if family or friends are to administer medicine, the chance of over-sedation and breathing difficulties increases. The family, friends, and staff involved in patient care should be alert for signs of over sedation.[15]
- Contraindications: sleep apnea; chronic kidney disease; bleeding disorders, or concurrent use of antithrombotic agents; hypersensitivity to any pain medication; systemic or local infection, burns, or trauma at the preferred area of PCA placement; neural impairment in the preferred site for indwelling nerve catheter; raised ICP (in case of epidural catheter placement).[2,18-21]
- Simultaneous administration of other analgesics should be avoided.

F) STORAGE CONDITIONS AND MAINTENANCE

Protect the equipment from moisture and humidity.

G) IMPORTANT FEATURES (CAPABILITIES AND LIMITATIONS) AND SPECIAL ADVANTAGES (SUCH AS THE SMALL SIZE, BEING USER FRIENDLY, AND PORTABILITY)

PCA is a preferred method of analgesic administration over traditional intermittent injections.[22] Pre-evaluation of patients to ensure their cognitive and physical ability to activate the dosing button needs to be done to determine whether they understand the need to press a dosing button for pain relief. Therefore, people with cognitive impairment and children below five years of age are not appropriate candidates for PCA.[22,23]

H) BENEFITS

- The patients do not need to be dependent on others for medicine administration. PCA ensures the safe administration of medications by patients themselves when they require pain relief.[2,16]
- Since portable pumps are also available for PCA, they do not restrict the patients' movement.
- An electronic PCA device allows the delivery of a precise amount of medicine, as well as the ability to adjust basal and bolus infusion rate and set a lock-out time, making the device safe. Additionally, it allows recording of the pattern of analgesic usage by the patients.
- The device is user friendly. The patients and authorized patient party can efficiently operate the device with an initial orientation on its use by healthcare professionals.
- Disposable pumps used in PCA have benefits such as ease of use, light weight, small size, no requirement for an external power supply, elimination of programming errors, and disposability.[24]
- PCA through various routes, such as epidural and intravenous routes, can help identify drug interactions among pain medications, such as IV morphine and clonidine, morphine and diclofenac, and oxycodone and diclofenac.[25]
- Workload for nurses or other attending staff is reduced.[2]

I) LIMITATIONS

- Disposable pumps used in PCA have a fixed reservoir volume and may have inaccurate flow rates and limited ability to change the flow rate and bolus-dose volume. Additionally, information on the prior analgesia on demand of the patient may not be available. Finally, PCA disposable pumps may not be combined with continuous background infusions, and they have a high long-term cost. In absence of an appropriate alarm system, any errors in the disposable PCA device may go unnoticed by the patients and/or healthcare professionals.[24]

- PCA by proxy is an alternative to PCA by the patient. The proxy can be a family member or friend authorized to administer medications to the patient in addition to the patient. However, the chance of overdose and oversedation increases.[15,26]
- Patients should be critically evaluated under the criteria for PCA eligibility. Elderly patients with disease conditions that alter mental status and memory are not eligible for PCA.
- Uninterrupted facility electricity is necessary for electronic PCA devices. These devices may also have errors in the alarming, display screen, and battery maintenance.
- Overflow of medication can occur for various reasons, including unintentional electrical short circuits and device malfunctions.[4]

J) COMPLICATIONS

Complications from PCA are usually related to the procedure and the medications used. Some of the complications associated with PCA are mentioned here[2,4]:

1. PCA by proxy: If the button is pressed by people other than the patient (family, friends, healthcare providers) when they think the patient is in pain, it is considered PCA by proxy. This might lead to overdose and thus increase the risk of respiratory problems in the patient, accordingly.
2. Failure to use anti-reflux valves: In the absence of the anti-reflux valve, the chance of reflux of the medication into the fluid infusion line increases. This might prevent the patient from obtaining the required dose at that moment. Additionally, if the IV line is then flushed, the medications collected in the infusion line (because of the reflux) may get delivered to the patient all at once, leading to overdose and undesired effects.
3. Error in syringe placement: Incorrect placement of syringe in the PCA pump might lead to an error in administering the medicine. The medication loaded in the syringe may flow into infusion line because of gravity, administering an excess dose of the medicine to the patient—precautions such as keeping the machine below a level of the patient's IV catheter and clamping the tubing from the PCA syringe should be taken while adding the pumps' syringes, to avoid any mishaps.
4. Machine tampering: Only authorized health personnel should be allowed to program and access the medication in PCA pumps to prevent tampering so that any deviations can be identified and dealt with.
5. Run-away pumps: Sometimes, pain medications might be delivered to patients at irregular intervals and times because of mechanical disruptions. This can result in excess dose delivery and fatal

consequences. Although a rare complication, patients on PCA should be monitored periodically for any adverse outcomes.
6. Indwelling nerve and epidural catheters may be associated with complications such as infection, medication leakage, nerve damage, hypersensitivity, and catheter dislodgment.[18,19]
7. Nausea, vomiting, constipation, urinary retention, pruritis, and respiratory depression may be seen in patients with PCA, depending on the medicines used.[2,18,21]

K) SPECIAL TIPS FOR PATIENT COUNSELING IF A DEVICE IS USED FOR SELF-CARE (FOR EXAMPLE, IF THE PATIENT CHANGED A DEVICE AND THE READINGS ARE DIFFERENT, ETC.)

Since PCA patients self-administer medication, patient counseling on the rational use of medication is crucial. Counseling on the appropriate use of PCA can be done by nurses, pharmacists, or the physician themselves. Points for patient counseling are listed here:

- Skin irritation or infection may occur at the site of catheter placement; patients should be asked to inform healthcare professionals immediately if infection is suspected.
- Treatment with PCA may be long term. In case of long-term use of PCA, the catheter may have to be changed on a regular interval. Therefore, the patients should be advised to keep the information on treatment safe for future use.[2]
- Patients should be counseled on the complications associated with PCA.
- Patients or their proxies should be properly instructed about the PCA operating procedures by healthcare staff.
- Periodic evaluation of infusion lines and pumps should be performed.

L) AVAILABLE EVIDENCE ON THE EFFECTIVENESS AND SAFETY OF PCA

PCA is a safe, effective, and well-accepted approach for pain management by patients.[2,9] The efficacy of PCA may rely on various factors, such as severity of the pain, PCA settings, potency of the analgesics administered in single and combination forms, type of PCA device used, medical history of patients, and psychological factors.[25] Patients are satisfied with pain relief using PCA with programmable pumps and self-administration buttons, and they prefer PCA over the traditional method of delivering medicines by nurses when required.[27]

Additionally, patients admire the easy use of portable, electrochemically driven wrist-worn infusion pump for PCA. The miniature pump in the wrist-worn device is as effective as the routine PCA device. It is more convenient than larger systems with complex features.[9] Although medications are self-administered by the patient, and there is a high chance of excess administration of opioids, serious complications have not been reported with PCA.[2] However, careful monitoring of the patients' condition, awareness of the staff, and selecting the right patients for PCA are necessary to prevent any undesired complications.[25,27]

m) Economic Evaluation (Including Pharmacoeconomics of the Device Compared to Less Expensive Methods of Drug Therapy)

Usually, the cost variations in different pain management approaches are due to differences in the cost of medicines, consumables, equipment, and labor. The economic evaluation of PCA has been debatable. There is no doubt that an extra cost is incurred for the equipment and infusion lines, maintenance, medications, and personal staff for monitoring. Nevertheless, the benefits of PCA regarding a shorter hospitalization duration, prevention from complications, easy application, and patient satisfaction cannot be overlooked.[4] Even though the cost of pain management using PCA is higher than that with traditional intermittent administration of pain medication, patient satisfaction in terms of pain relief and ease of use cannot be ignored for the sake of cost.[28,29]

n) Implications for the Pharmacy Profession and Pharmacy Practice

Along with other healthcare professionals, pharmacists have a crucial role in PCA. Minimizing errors in programming and early detection of problems can be achieved via a pharmacist's active involvement.[30] The preparation of medicines for administration as per the prescriber's instructions is one of the critical responsibilities of pharmacists.[2] Pharmacists also have a role in the appropriate dispensing of medications via PCA. Pharmacists are responsible for the accurate concentration, correct labeling, identification of any drug interactions, identification of any allergies to the medication prescribed, reviewing PCA orders before administration, and obtaining the patient medication history. In case of unavailability of the prescribed concentration of the medication commercially, it should be prepared in-house and well labeled by a pharmacist. Special precautions about the medications, including dosage adjustments, complications, and adverse reactions, should be well communicated with the healthcare team and the patients, wherever appropriate, by the pharmacists.[17] Pharmacists should be competent to suggest alternative drugs in case the prescribed drugs are unavailable.

Pharmacists can also be involved in educating healthcare professionals and patients about the device and medications.

o) Challenges to the Pharmacists and Users

PCA operation requires a collaborative approach by the healthcare team, including pharmacists, nurses, and physicians.[2] Many hospitals lack pharmacists on their clinical team, leading to inadequate pain control and poor patient outcomes. The healthcare staff should be aware of PCA operating procedures, medications, doses, adverse outcomes and complications, criteria for assessing patients before and after PCA, and expected outcomes. Pharmacists and nurses should double-check the dosing regimens, loaded medication, dose, programmed lockout period, and infusion rate. While continuous monitoring is not required, periodic PCA monitoring needs to be done to ensure safe drug delivery and adjust the dose of medications per the patient's needs.[2]

Errors in the operation/settings of PCA, such as misprogramming of the infusion pump, and device-related errors, such as switches, display screens, motors, batteries, and software, may result in harmful consequences. However, it is shown that even with a higher percentage of errors in operation, PCA has fortunately resulted in a significantly lesser percentage of patient harm.[31]

Educating the patients on medications and PCA, programming and setting up the device, periodic monitoring, controlling overflow of medications, adjusting doses, and changing medications in the infusion pump may be challenging for healthcare team members.

Inability to use the device effectively (even after receiving education), control overflow, notice any unwanted effects, and notice any problems with the infusion pump, especially in cases of ambulatory PCA, are potential challenges on the patient side.

p) Recommendations: Way Forward

- Mandatory audible safety alarm systems and mechanical safety devices should be incorporated into the PCA system (electronic and disposable) to detect any deviation from its operation.
- Stringent eligibility criteria should be followed when identifying patients eligible for PCA.
- Devices used for PCA should be appropriately evaluated for their safety and effectiveness beforehand.
- Pharmacists should be engaged directly in programming the pump with the right medication, dose, infusion rate, duration, and patient counseling regarding the medications and the device itself.
- Interdisciplinary involvement in PCA for better pain management is highly recommended.

q) Conclusions

PCA is an effective, safe, and preferable means of pain management. All PCA devices have a drug reservoir and a patient control system. However, the various PCA devices available have pros and cons. Considering the need of an individual patient, a suitable type of device can be selected. The collaboration of healthcare professionals during PCA use will lead to better pain control and patient outcomes. Pharmacists on the healthcare team have a pivotal role in PCA and can contribute to patient counseling and medication and PCA device evaluation.

R) LESSONS LEARNED

- The choice of appropriate PCA for an individual patient is crucial for better pain relief.
- Pre-assessment should be performed to evaluate the patients' cognitive and physical functioning to check the eligibility for PCA.
- Post assessment should be done for patients who used PCA for the first time to learn about any required adjustments and changes in the device settings or the dose of the medications.
- PCA is an individualized treatment for patients with several types of pain, including chronic cancer pain.

DEVICE 2: DOMICILE OXYGEN THERAPY FOR CANCER PATIENTS [OXYGEN CYLINDER]

A) BACKGROUND

Shortness of breath or respiratory depression can be a common issue in patients with advanced cancer because of multiple factors. While it occurs as a mainstay symptom in lung cancer or cancer involving the thorax and respiratory tract, respiratory depression or breathlessness can be observed as a metastatic cancer effect, as a side effect of cancer treatment (chemotherapy-induced fibrosis), or as a result of comorbid conditions such as infections, anemia, pulmonary embolism, heart disease, asthma/COPD, or anxiety.[32] Breathlessness in terminally ill patients or patients with advanced cancer and palliative care is caused by the severe weakness of respiratory muscles.[33] The management of respiratory depression/shortness of breath often involves using oxygen therapy in the hospital and identifying and managing the underlying causes.[34,35] Oxygen therapy in palliative care is shown to be prescribed for refractory dyspnea.[34] The use of oxygen therapy is a preferable management approach in patients who have failed available pharmacological and non-pharmacological approaches. Depending on the severity of the patient's condition, and after evaluating possible existence of any reversible causes of breathlessness, home oxygen therapy or domicile oxygen therapy may also be prescribed on discharge.

Oxygen therapy refers to administering oxygen at a concentration higher than that of room air for therapeutic purposes. Oxygen therapy is an effective way to treat hypoxemia associated with COPD and other respiratory and non-respiratory conditions, including cancer.[34,36] The decision to prescribe domicile oxygen therapy should be based on the appropriate indication for oxygen therapy, selection of the

right device system/right source for oxygen, and titration of the oxygen flow. Cost, technical issues, patient satisfaction and requirements, and adaptability should be considered when deciding the oxygen source.[34,36,37] The concentration of oxygen use depends on the oxygen saturation of the patients.[38] Oxygen therapy can be prescribed for short-term or long-term use in patients.

Domicile oxygen therapy for cancer patients is oriented towards the prevention and treatment of possible hypoxia.[39] Furthermore, portable devices used as a source of oxygen promote a better quality of life in cancer patients. There are various available devices for home oxygen therapy. Some of them include oxygen concentrators, compressed gas cylinders, and liquid oxygen systems.[40]

B) DEVICE DESCRIPTION

An oxygen cylinder, also called an oxygen tank, is a metal cylinder and contains 99.5% pure oxygen gas in compressed form under high pressure.[41] It is equipped with a pressure valve near the cylinder's opening, which estimates the oxygen pressure in the cylinder. The oxygen cylinder size varies widely from ambulatory cylinders to large stationary cylinders with a capacity range of approximately 164 liters to 2,000 liters.[40,42] The variations in sizes mirror the volume of gas that the cylinder holds and the duration of time before which the cylinder

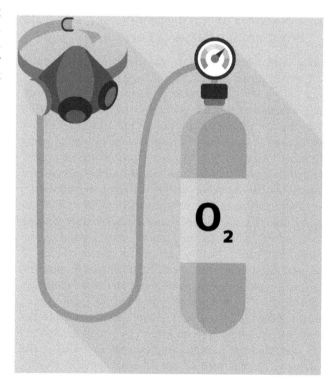

FIGURE 15.2 Various sizes of oxygen cylinders used in domicile oxygen therapy.[45]

Source: www.shutterstock.com/image-vector/flat-medical-oxygen-cylinder-vector-icon-1316392604

runs out of oxygen. The flow of oxygen from the cylinder to the patient is controlled by a regulator fitted to the top of the cylinder. It acts as a tap, and when opened, it delivers oxygen to the patients via an oxygen administration device such as a nasal cannula, face mask, or transtracheal catheter.[40] These regulators convert the cylinder's pressure unit to liters/min, which is the pressure generally used in prescriptions.[41] The regulator can also use oxygen-conserving devices; in the absence of these devices the patient will receive a continuous oxygen flow. In the presence of an oxygen-conserving device within the regulator, oxygen is delivered to the patient when he/she inhales, and the flow is cut off when he/she exhales.[43] There are two types of regulators that differ based on how the oxygen is delivered to the patient: continuous and pulse-dose flow.[41] The oxygen tank is sometimes connected to an oxygen concentrator. The oxygen concentrator takes room air, purifies it for delivery as pure oxygen, stores it in the tank, and decreases the need for constant replacement of empty oxygen cylinders.[44] To make the oxygen cylinders easy to identify, the cylinders are usually colored white.[40]

c)   TYPES

1. Portable oxygen cylinders

   The cylinders filled with oxygen that can be carried along with the patients are portable or ambulatory oxygen cylinders, which allow patients to perform their daily activities. These portable cylinders can also be carried using trolleys, backpacks, or wheeled carts, depending on the cylinder's size and weight.[40] The portable cylinders are small to medium in size, and when set to deliver 2 liters oxygen/min, the cylinder may last for approximately 4–6 hours.

2. Static oxygen cylinders

   Static oxygen cylinders are stationary cylinders kept at home. These cylinders are larger in size and volume than portable cylinders. Small-sized portable cylinders can be filled with oxygen from these large tanks. These can be kept as an oxygen backup.[44]

d)   PURPOSES OF USE, HOW TO USE/OPERATE PROPERLY, AND OPERATIONAL REQUIREMENTS

Domicile oxygen therapy is generally most suitable for patients who spend most of the time in home and have less mobility.[40] Home oxygen therapy aims to prevent and treat hypoxemia and avoid any harmful consequences of hypoxemia while the patients is in the home. These are prescribed for patients with respiratory and non-respiratory diseases that affect breathing. The prescription of oxygen varies depending on the individual requirements of oxygen delivery. The oxygen cylinders serve as back-ups and are also used to provide palliative oxygen in the home.[46]

e)   IMPORTANT SAFETY ISSUES (INCLUDING HAZARDS AND COMMON ADVERSE EFFECTS)

1. Fire: Oxygen is a combustible gas, and when stored in a cylinder under high pressure, it tends to increase the risk of catching fire. If the regulator is opened rapidly, it may cause particle impact ignition, leading to fire hazards.[47]

2. There are chances of confusing gas cylinders containing carbon dioxide and oxygen if they are not color-coded distinctly. In cases of mix-ups, the patient may end up being administered the wrong gas.[47]

3. Since the oxygen cylinder is opaque, it may sometimes be mistaken for being empty when it is full. This may occur when the pressure gauge is not working correctly or when the cylinder and regulator valves are dysfunctional. In such cases, the full cylinder might be kept in places where empty cylinders are stored and treated with less care than the full cylinder, resulting in unwanted hazards.[47]

4. Any flammable liquids or cleaners, smoking, or alcohol use should be avoided around the oxygen cylinder to prevent a fire hazard.[44]

5. Side effects of oxygen therapy may include claustrophobia, dry nose/eyes/mouth, drowsiness, fire risk, hypercapnic respiratory failure, loss of independence, pressure sores on the ears or nose, psychological dependence, and reduced mobility.[48]

f)   STORAGE CONDITIONS AND MAINTENANCE

- The cylinders should be stored away from stoves, heaters, open flames, and electronic devices.
- Regular monitoring for any pressure leaks should be done using a gauge.[40]

g)   IMPORTANT FEATURES AND SPECIAL ADVANTAGES

Benefits

- Large domicile oxygen cylinders can act as a back-up system when the electricity goes off or in the case of concentrator failure.[46]
- The large cylinders act as a reservoir and are used to fill the small portable cylinders whenever necessary.
- Domiciliary oxygen delivery can be performed using both static and portable compressed gas cylinders.
- Without any complex system involved in their use, oxygen cylinders are user-friendly.
- Compared to liquid oxygen, if compressed gas cylinders are attached to oxygen concentrators and used, the cost will be lower.

Disadvantages

- When filled with oxygen, even portable cylinders are heavy and might sometimes be challenging to carry. Additionally, extra equipment such as trolleys, wheeled carts, or back packs might be needed.
- Because the gas is under high pressure, it may be associated with fire hazards.
- The oxygen in portable cylinders does not last much longer than liquid oxygen, thus limiting the ability of patients to visit the outdoors.
- If the cylinder is attached to oxygen concentrators, it requires continuous electricity or internal batteries to work, which may reduce patient mobility.
- Depending on the cylinder's size, the amount of oxygen supply is limited compared to oxygen concentrators.
- The refilling and transport of the cylinder may be costly.

H) Special Tips for Patient Counseling if a Device Is Used for Self-Care (For Example, if the Patient Changed a Device and the Readings Are Different, etc.)

- Patients and patient caregivers should be educated by healthcare professionals about the properties of the gas, proper use and handling of the cylinders, cleaning of the administering devices (canula, masks, tubing), preventive measures to take in case of emergency, monitoring any pressure leaks in the cylinder, and filling of the portable oxygen cylinders from the static cylinders.[40,49]
- Patients should be appropriately counseled about possible fire hazards.
- Patients and their caregivers should be told to avoid smoking, using flammable liquids or cleansers, oil, or using petroleum-based creams and ointments in the vicinity of the cylinder.
- Fire alarms and smoke detectors can be installed as a measure of precaution.
- The cylinders should be kept away from any electronic devices, such as heaters or dryers.[50]
- Patients should be counseled not to alter the flow rate of the cylinder without consulting their physicians.

I) Available Evidence on the Effectiveness and Safety

Oxygen therapy is effective in the management of dyspnea at rest in patients with advanced cancer.[51] Regarding safety concerns, the use of domicile oxygen therapy is associated with fire hazards.[46] However, the use of oxygen therapy to relieve dyspnea in patients with hypoxemia is safe if proper precautions are considered.[52–54] Dyspnea can occur because of various physical and psychosocial reasons, such as anxiety in cancer patients. Therefore, not all cases of dyspnea require oxygen therapy. It is preferable to use oxygen therapy in patients with cancer-specific respiratory tract issues and other comorbid conditions directly affecting respiration, such as COPD.[52,53]

J) Economic Evaluation

The complications that may arise from decreased oxygenation will be prevented with home oxygen therapy, which ultimately reduces the cost of treatment in the broader picture.[55] The combined use of portable and stationary oxygen therapy has been shown to promote quality of life.[46] Compared to other devices for home oxygen therapy, including oxygen concentrators and liquid oxygen, compressed oxygen cylinders seem to be less expensive. The oxygen concentrators have associated costs for continuous power supply, installation, servicing, and maintenance. Liquid oxygen also has associated costs, including electricity, acquisition cost, and metering gas to the patients. However, when the long-term use and cost, and ease of use are considered, liquid oxygen and oxygen concentrators are preferable to the compressed cylinder.[46,55]

K) Implication to the Pharmacy Profession and Pharmacy Practice

Pharmacists can be involved in counseling patients on the proper use and maintenance of domicile compressed oxygen cylinders and oxygen properties. Since community pharmacists are easily approachable and the first contact of healthcare professionals, oxygen cylinders for home oxygen therapy can be cost-effectively provided by pharmacies.[56] They can extend their services with home deliveries, adjustments for regulators, and maintaining the flow rate of oxygen required by the patient, which may promote better patient outcomes. However, an appropriate medication history should be taken before oxygen prescription, and in case of any complications, the pharmacists should refer the patient to the physicians. In addition to services regarding oxygen therapy, pharmacists can provide other medication-related information and advice on alternative oxygen delivery devices[56] such that the patients will receive different services regarding their health at a single place. Pharmacists can also monitor the overall progress or adverse outcomes associated with oxygen therapy.

L) Challenges to the Pharmacists and Users

If community pharmacies start to provide oxygen cylinders, it will be cumbersome for pharmacists, because extra precautions should be taken to store cylinders. Educating patients on the use of oxygen cylinders is a crucial task because, in addition to the information about medication, patients need to know about the technical matters related to the cylinder, pressure valve, regulators, and tubing, which are parts of the cylinder that should be closely monitored for proper functioning to avoid any mishaps.

The use of oxygen is also associated with many health hazards. The underuse of oxygen can worsen hypoxemia and might also lead to ischemic cell death. On the other hand, overuse of oxygen therapy can cause organ and tissue damage.[57] Therefore, use of oxygen in the exact required amount is essential. Regular assessment of oxygen saturation and consultation with physicians in case of fluctuations may be challenging for users. Additionally, the mobility of patients may wane when compressed oxygen cylinders are used.

M) RECOMMENDATIONS: WAYS FORWARD

- Modification of the cylinders by adding an oxygen concentrator to synergistically improve the benefit of home oxygen therapy.
- Direct involvement of pharmacists in home oxygen delivery for better patient outcomes.

N) CONCLUSION

Domicile oxygen therapy is an essential approach in managing the associated breathlessness in advanced cancer patients. In addition to compressed oxygen cylinders, home oxygen therapy is delivered using oxygen concentrators and liquid oxygen, both of which can be available as either a portable or stationary device. These devices are comparatively more beneficial, preferable, and cost-effective than oxygen cylinders in long-term oxygen therapy. However, considerably larger static compressed oxygen cylinders serve as a back-up device in a power cut. Although oxygen therapy is associated with some hazards, it is safe and effective in managing cancer patients' breathlessness.

O) LESSONS LEARNED

- Because of oxygen's combustible nature, compressed oxygen cylinders containing oxygen under high pressure should be handled very carefully.
- Patients should be counseled to seek immediate medical attention if any adverse outcomes of overuse or underuse of oxygen therapy are detected.
- Routine assessment of oxygen saturation in patients should be performed for those on oxygen therapy.

DEVICE 3: IV PUMPS (DIGITAL AND MANUAL)

A) BACKGROUND

Various treatment strategies and plans are optimized for individual cancer patients. The use of chemotherapeutic agents and their doses vary among individuals. These chemotherapeutic agents can be administered through various routes, such as topical, oral, intravenous, intramuscular, intra-arterial, or site-specific routes, depending on the type

of cancer.[58,59] One of the common methods for intravenous administration is using an intravenous pump (IV pump). IV pumps are used in the medical field to deliver various types of fluids, medications, blood products, nutrients, hormones, and so on and are used in hospitals, clinics, nursing homes, and patient homes. Chemotherapy can be delivered as an IV, push, IV infusion, or continuous IV infusion for an extended period.[60] IV pumps deliver a controlled amount of medication to the bloodstream at a regulated rate.[61] The amount of medication delivery and the rate of infusion can be set in the infusion pump. Chemotherapy is delivered through a central or peripheral line. Thin tubing, called a catheter, is connected to the infusion pump. Towards the end of the catheter, a needle is attached, which is inserted to the vein, artery, body cavity, or body part, leaving the catheter in place for drug delivery; the catheter is removed after therapy.[62]

The chemotherapy session can be minutes, hours, or a few days long (in case of continuous infusion). Therefore, the use of IV pumps for infusion of chemotherapy is widely applicable due to its user-friendly nature. Moreover, the application of smart IV pumps, with absolute safety software, for chemotherapy infusion is shown to prevent IV medication administration errors.[63]

B) DEVICE DESCRIPTION (DESCRIPTION OF THE GENERAL STRUCTURE AND MAIN PARTS SUPPORTED WITH PICTURES AND DRAWINGS)

The IV pump is a widely applicable device in oncology settings. It is used to deliver the specified amount of chemotherapy to the patient in a controlled fashion, either continuously or intermittently. The IV pump is linked to IV bag, and it delivers medication through the catheter. The pump contains a user interface or displays to program the rate, flow, and duration of medication delivery. Additionally, alarm system, control circuit, motor, and infusion mechanism are incorporated within the pump.[64]

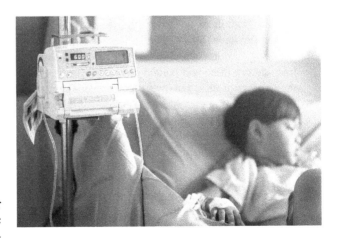

FIGURE 15.3 Intravenous pump.

c) Types

IV pumps can be of various types, such as large- and small-volume infusion pumps, elastomeric pumps, syringe pumps, ambulatory pumps, and electronic pumps. Furthermore, IV pumps can be classified based on portability and functioning.

Based on Portability

1. Ambulatory IV pumps

    These are portable or wearable pumps that ease the delivery of chemotherapy to patients. The patients can use it in the home after appropriately being instructed on its use. The majority of these pumps are usually small and can be carried in a bag or with a belt holster. These pumps are either continuous pressure pumps that do not require batteries for their function or battery-operated pumps.[65]

2. Continuous ambulatory delivery device (CADD)

    With CADD, continuous delivery of the medication to the patient is ensured without the patient's need to be hospitalized or in nursing homes for chemotherapy infusion. The device can be used for the administration of 5-fluorouracil, which requires continuous infusion over an extended period.[66,67] Patients need to carry the IV bag and pump in a bag pack for mobility. In addition to continuous infusion, intermittent boluses can also be scheduled with CADD.[64,67]

3. Elastomeric pumps

    Elastomeric pumps are generally used for continuous infusion in the ambulatory setting and are lightweight and small. The pump has a balloon that contains chemotherapy and a flow restrictor that controls the rate of chemotherapy infusion. The medication moves from the balloon with the help of pressure generated by an elastomeric reservoir. The elastomeric pump has a fill port, infusion line, clamp, filter, and patient connector. Some of the benefits of these pumps include reduced errors related to pump programming, easy patient education and operation, lightweight design, and lack of noise generation. However, the safety risk is an issue with these pumps, because they lack alarm alerts.[68–71]

4. Stationary pumps

    These are mainly used in hospitalized or bedridden patients. The pump is placed at bedside of the patient. However, an IV pump can also be attached to the drip stand with wheels, ensuring that the patient can walk along with it.[61]

5. Electronic IV pumps

    The use of electronic IV pumps depends on the availability of a continuous power supply for their function. The operation of these electronic pumps is generally based on peristaltic movement, which pushes the medication forward through the appendages.[70] These pumps often have an alarm and alert systems for functioning errors such as blockages, battery issues, and fluctuations in the flow rates. Medications can be programmed to be delivered as a continuous or intermittent infusion with the electronic IV pump.[70]

6. Syringe pumps

    Usually, the maximum volume of a syringe pump is 50 ml. Therefore, it is used for medications that require a small hourly volume (e.g., less than 5 ml/hr).[72]

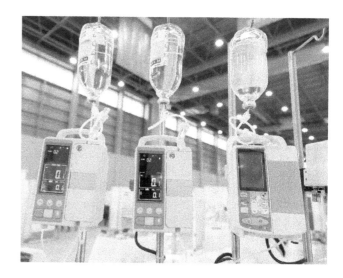

FIGURE 15.4   Electronic IV pumps.

Source: www.shutterstock.com/image-photo/modern-digital-infusion-pump-medical-purposes-770896198

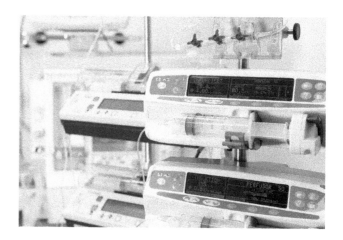

FIGURE 15.5   Syringe electronic pumps.

Source: www.shutterstock.com/image-photo/medical-perfusion-pump-188164115

D) Purposes of Use, How to Use/Operate Properly, and Operational Requirements (Supported with Pictures and Drawings)

IV pumps are used to deliver the prescribed chemotherapy to the patient in a controlled and regulated manner over some time.[73] IV pumps are attached to venous catheters, which are of various types, namely, peripherally inserted central catheters (PICCs), implanted ports, and tunneled chest catheters.[71] Electronic IV pumps can be tricky to use and require trained users to operate. With the use of a software interface in the IV pump, the user can set the duration, amount, and rate of medication delivery to the patient.[74] The IV pumps' operation differs according to their types, and the medications can be delivered in the form of continuous or intermittent infusion.

E) Important Safety Issues (Including Hazards and Common Adverse Effects)

The battery status and programming of the flow rate and duration of chemotherapy in the electronic IV pump will be ensured by healthcare providers. If they fail to do so, the administration and effect of the medication will not be as desired. The IV lines should be flushed before and after administration to avoid any contamination.[74]

Also, there is a risk of catheter-related complications such as pneumothorax (subclavian catheter) and cellulitis (Broviac catheter in a patient with leukopenia).[75] Needles and catheters can cause scarring of skin and damage to veins used for continuous chemotherapeutic infusion.

F) Storage Conditions and Maintenance

IV pumps should be stored in a safe place and protected from humidity.[76]

Elastomeric pumps should be kept away from direct sunlight, and extremely hot and cold temperatures should be avoided.

G) Important Features (Capabilities and Limitations) and Special Advantages (Such as Having a Small Size, Being User Friendly, and Being Portable)

Accidental overdose and toxicity due to a higher flow rate and dose of medication than prescribed and selection of appropriate IV pumps and material should be considered when using IV pumps. IV pumps offer various advantages, as mentioned here:

Capabilities and advantages:

1. Desired amounts of fluids/medications can be delivered at a controlled rate using IV pumps.[74]
2. Elastomeric pumps are small and lightweight, do not require a power supply to work, decrease the chance of programming mistakes, and are preferred by patients for ambulatory purposes.[70]
3. Flexibility to change the flow rate or duration of the medication therapy.[76]
4. There is flexibility to use a wide range of chemotherapy and volume of fluids/medications from small bolus doses to large continuous dosing with pumps.[67]
5. Safe use of the device is ensured by equipping IV pumps with an alarm system. This system provides alerts for various situations, such as air entrapment or any blockage in the tubing, battery issues, alteration in set infusion rate, etc.[74]
6. Smart IV pumps have a system to alert the user and healthcare providers about the risk of adverse drug reactions.[74]
7. Ambulatory IV pumps have been shown to improve patient tolerance of chemotherapy, and they are technically more feasible.[77]

Limitations:

- The elastomeric pump does not have any alert system; the pump function is affected by external factors such as temperature and backpressure.[70]
- Liable to user error, software problems, mechanical or electrical failures, user interface issues, alarm defects, fire sparks, charring or shock while plugging or unplugging from the electrical outlets, battery failures, and broken components.[74]
- Electronic pumps are noisy compared to elastomeric pumps, are sensitive to radiation, and require well-trained people for effective operation.[70]
- Limitation of portable pumps: variation in flow rate, venous complications, drug cartridge failure.[78]

H) Special Tips for Patient Counseling if a Device Is Used for Self-Care

1. Patients should be appropriately counseled for safe use of ambulatory IV pumps and provided with an instruction manual written in simple language.
2. Patients should be educated about the things to consider while wearing the pump. For example, positioning of the pump higher or lower on the parts of body can affect the flow rate (in case of the elastomeric pump).[71]
3. Patients should be counseled about the complications and possible problems that may arise during the use of IV pumps and should be informed to contact the healthcare provider in case of any issues, such as leakage from the pump, duration of the infusion less or more than suggested, or the occurrence of pain, swelling, or accumulation of fluids around the site of infusion.[71]
4. Patients should be educated about the drug they are receiving via a pump, the dose and volume

of the medication, duration of infusion, routine checking of the tubing for any blockage, and the remaining volume of medication in the pump.[70]

5. For elastomeric pumps, direct sun exposure and extreme temperatures (hot and cold) should be avoided.

6. The battery function and availability of a spare battery should be ensured while using electronic IV pumps.

7. In case of any alerts, the instruction displayed on the screen should be carefully read, and necessary actions should be taken.

8. Regular activities such as taking a shower, sleep, and other daily activities can be performed, but the pump should be protected from being wet.

9. IV pumps and tubing should be protected from pets and should be kept out of reach of children.[67]

I) AVAILABLE EVIDENCE ON THE EFFECTIVENESS AND SAFETY

Portable infusion pumps are considered safe and were well accepted by the patients. The use of these devices can reduce the duration of hospitalization and hospital admissions for only chemotherapy infusion purposes.[79] Smart IV pumps with alarm systems and safety software reduce errors in intravenous medication administration, thereby promoting the safe use of high-risk medications.[63,80,81]

J) ECONOMIC EVALUATION

The use of elastomeric pumps is less expensive than using electronic IV pumps.[82]

K) IMPLICATION TO THE PHARMACY PROFESSION AND PHARMACY PRACTICE

Pharmacists can be involved in choosing the appropriate IV pump for the individual patient based on the type of therapy, presence of any physical disability in the user that might affect the operation of the pump, disease state, cost, and so on. Pharmacists can initiate the use of a standard label for chemotherapy infusion, including all vital information (such as the name of drug, dose, volume, concentration, flow rate, estimated duration, etc.) about the infusion for easy medication information access for the patient and for cross-checking of the prescribed medication by the medical team. The shift of IV pumps from hospital settings to outpatient and home settings has remarkably increased.[83] With this, the role of pharmacists becomes critical in ensuring the safe use of ambulatory IV pumps. The pharmacists can educate the patients about the medication they are receiving, the operation of the pump, its maintenance, and the provision of a validated instruction manual for the IV pump.[70] Pharmacists can be engaged in identifying, reporting, and monitoring adverse drug reactions and complications with medication use through IV pumps. Additionally,

the calibration of various IV pumps can be performed by pharmacists. The pharmacists should ensure that the right drug is being infused into the patient according to the prescribed flow rate. Pharmacists should be involved in double-checking the safety cabinets, mixing process, flow rate, duration of infusion, and status of the IV pump used to ensure safe delivery of chemotherapy.[74,84]

L) CHALLENGES TO THE PHARMACISTS AND USERS

Challenges to the Pharmacists

Since elastomeric pumps vary according to the flow restrictor diameter and the pressure generated by the elastomeric membrane, so does the flow rate of the infusion. The choice of an appropriate elastomeric pump for ambulatory use to ensure that the prescribed flow rate of infusion is being delivered to the patient may be challenging for pharmacists. Errors in pump selection can result in the delivery of more or less of the medication than prescribed, leading to treatment hazards.[69,84] The different pump models should be stored sequentially based on the volume and flow rate they can offer for easy identification.

Challenges to Users

The IV pump's programming for its flow rate and duration is challenging for those who have difficulty understanding the necessary operational procedures of the pump. The troubleshooting of IV pump malfunctions is another challenge for users.

M) RECOMMENDATIONS: WAYS FORWARD

- The pharmacists and other healthcare staff who operate the IV pumps should be educated and trained for appropriate selection and operation of the IV pumps.
- IV pumps that are not affected by radiation in patients taking simultaneous radiation therapy should be explored. Additionally, other possible alternatives for easing therapy in such patients can be studied.

N) CONCLUSIONS

IV pumps are a widely applicable device for administration of chemotherapeutic agents. In combination with other accessories, these pumps are used to deliver the chemotherapeutic infusion at a prescribed flow rate and duration. Different types of IV pumps are available to be used in a hospital setting and in home settings, thereby offering the flexibility of safe use by the patients.

O) LESSONS LEARNED

- Many IV pumps, which differ in their functions and offer benefits, are available on the market. Therefore, the appropriate IV pump choice for the individual patient is critical to ensure accurate drug delivery.

- The safe use of IV pumps should be ensured by a collaborative approach between the healthcare team and patients. On occurrence of any complications with IV pumps, such as pain, swelling, redness at the IV site, and hypersensitivity, patients should immediately contact healthcare professionals.
- The users of IV pumps (healthcare personnel) should know the available and updated guidelines and safety procedures for pump operation. They should educate the patients accordingly.

DEVICE 4: AUTOMATIC COMPOUNDING DEVICES FOR ONCOLOGY PATIENTS

A) BACKGROUND

Chemotherapy stands as an essential treatment approach for cancer in addition to radiation and surgery. The treatment of cancer with chemotherapy depends on the stages and types of cancer.[59,85] Sooner or later, chemotherapy is prescribed to patients with cancer, tailored to individual patient requirements. For each individual's requirements, chemotherapy is compounded in the cancer care center or hospitals. Chemotherapy compounding is routine work in an oncology setting. Compounding involves combining medications to create individualized therapy for patients.[59,86] Usually, compounding is done manually by trained staff in a sterile environment, preferably under a laminar flow hood. However, manual compounding of chemotherapy is accompanied by a greater risk of errors.[87] Humans tend to make mistakes during compounding, even when working meticulously. The reasons may be broad, including stress, fatigue, workload, insufficient experience, mistakes in calculation of dose and dispensing, and so on. Errors in the compounding process have a direct or indirect negative impact on patient outcomes.[88] Errors such as incorporating the wrong type or volume of diluent for the drugs to be reconstituted, misplacing of vials, misreading of the prescription, errors in dosing and labeling of the compounded drugs, and product contamination may occur with manual compounding.[87] Additionally, issues such as exposure hazards to the operator, a high chance of drug waste, increased cost, longer average wait time for patients, and stress due to continuous repetitive procedures for the operators are associated with manual compounding.[89–91] Furthermore, the compounded medications are not legally approved by authorized national or international bodies. Therefore, the quality of medication may be questioned.

To overcome the shortcomings of manual compounding, provide patients with a medication of quality, and ensure the safety of involved healthcare professionals, automatic compounding is introduced. Automatic compounding devices mix, reconstitute, dilute, or transfer chemotherapeutic agents to form a new mixture in a sterile environment. These automatic systems can read the prescription, compound the desired dose and quantity of medications with more accuracy, and pack medications in suitable final containers. Furthermore, labels are also made and attached to the final container by the system. Ultimately, human-induced errors seem to decline by using automatic compounding devices.[92] Developments in the compounding of chemotherapy are impressive and have enhanced the quality of compounded drugs, reducing the work burden of compounding pharmacists or nurses.[93,94]

B) DEVICE DESCRIPTION (DESCRIPTION OF THE GENERAL STRUCTURE AND MAIN PARTS SUPPORTED WITH PICTURES AND DRAWINGS)

The automatic compounding devices are used in various departments of the hospital, including oncology. The system has advanced features to ease the compounding process. The automation of compounding process involves the use of either robots or special compounding devices. The robotic system consists of an automated robotic hand/s for compounding the medications. One example of a robotic compounding system is KIRO Oncology. It consists of an air treatment area, user interface, compounding area, and waste area. The air treatment area has HEPA filters incorporated within and the negative pressure in the recirculation chamber for environmental protection. The compounding area consists of two robotic arms, a carousel to hold vials in use, a syringe holder, a syringe capping station, a preparation bay, a holding area for partially used vials, the gravimetric device for in-process weighing, a peristaltic pump for diluent filling and reconstitution, cameras for syringe and vial identification, a barcode reader for product identification, and a touchpad for entering validation parameters. The user interface includes a user touchscreen, barcode reader, label printers, and gravimetric device to double-check the weights. Last, the waste area consists of disposal units and filters for cleaning the air before recirculation.[95]

Automated compounding equipment, such as the Pharmoduct, is used to prepare the final patient-specific mixture of chemotherapeutic agents. The equipment consists of an automatic ozone cleaning system, negative pressure laminar airflow, a touch screen monitor, a thermal transfer printer for personalized labels, a barcode identification system for the diluent kit, a radiofrequency identification system for consumable kits, an upper rotating assembly for drug vials, a label identification system for vials, a gravimetric scale for the multidose bag, peristaltic pumps for liquid transfer, a lower rotating assembly for final containers, and a segregated waste area with bag heat sealing.[94]

C) PURPOSES OF USE, HOW TO USE/OPERATE PROPERLY, AND OPERATIONAL REQUIREMENTS (SUPPORTED WITH PICTURES AND DRAWINGS)

An automatic compounding device is used to minimize or omit the factors affecting the compounded product's compounding process and quality. The ultimate purpose of automatic compounding is to avoid human-related errors in any step of the compounding process. Some automatic systems can read electronic prescriptions and automatically gather those with the same active ingredients. However, the robotic compounding system lacks integration with the e-prescription platform.[94] The equipment is then loaded with the required vials of medications, diluents, and other consumable kits. The equipment identifies these through automatically reading labels or barcodes. Also, the different variants of the final containers are also identified through barcode reading by the equipment. The vials loaded in the system are emptied into a mixing arrangement, and empty vials are directed to the waste-collecting compartment. The powders are reconstituted by the system itself beforehand. The final product is prepared by adding diluents to the drug mixture. Throughout the process, the gravimetric scale is used to check the dosage in real time. The final containers are filled with the required quantity of the product. A suitable label for the container, which includes the drug and patient details, is generated by the system and attached to the container immediately by the operator.[94]

D) IMPORTANT SAFETY ISSUES (INCLUDING HAZARDS AND COMMON ADVERSE EFFECTS)

Chemotherapies are cytotoxic agents, and exposure to these agents results in a significant health hazard to the pharmacists and nurses involved in their compounding and administration.[96] Since the automatic compounding device does not require the operator to be directly exposed to the chemotherapeutic drug during mixing and waste disposal, the risk of health hazards is reduced. However, it is always better to wear personal protective equipment while working with high-risk medications.

E) STORAGE CONDITIONS AND MAINTENANCE

The device should be kept near plugs and a power supply for easy access to electricity.

The operators (pharmacists or nurses) should monitor the device and check all parts for compliance with the advised standard operation to avoid any potential system errors. The device may need to be calibrated once in a while.[97]

F) IMPORTANT FEATURES (CAPABILITIES AND LIMITATIONS) AND SPECIAL ADVANTAGES

With an automatic compounding device, patient-specific chemotherapy is mixed and packed in an IV bag or syringe aseptically within the device. The system offers various advantages and also has certain limitations. The benefits and limitations of automatic compounding are mentioned here.

Advantages:

- There is little to no chance of particle contamination with automatic systems. The medications are reconstituted, mixed, or diluted in a sterile and clean environment.
- The automatic compounding device ensures better dose accuracy and quality. The dose in the final container complies with the prescription.[94,95]
- The waiting time for patients is also not as long as that with manual compounding.[98]
- There is less exposure hazard than with manual compounding since the system itself packs the final product, disposes of the waste materials, and cleans the system.[95]
- The system incorporates the flexibility of using various types of final containers, such as syringes, IV bags, elastomeric pumps, bottles, and cassettes.[93]
- The cost per dose of chemotherapy is lower with an automatic compounding device since the partially used vials are not wasted; instead, they are held in the cabinet for further use. The operator need not sit and watch the overall process and can perform other work during the compounding process. Therefore, it is a more economical approach.[95]

Limitations:

- An automatic system requires a continuous power supply to function.
- Automated equipment requires trained and knowledgeable human resources to be available to troubleshoot minor operating problems quickly.
- Automated systems also require periodic updates of installed system software.
- The automatic system device is more expensive and requires more maintenance. Additionally, it carries the risk of failure.
- Switching the products or adding new vials may be complicated, and there is a risk of new errors.[99]

Limitations of the robotic system[94]:

1. Low control of drug waste and related costs
2. Inability to be integrated with the e-prescribing system
3. Impossibility to use bags as drug sources
4. Incompatibility with several types of final containers
5. Difficult to clean the conjunctions of the robotic arms

A study has shown that the robot compounding system was associated with mechanical issues (e.g., robot arm-clamping failures), robot downtime, and the need to recalibrate the device periodically.[100]

G) AVAILABLE EVIDENCE ON EFFECTIVENESS AND SAFETY

The automatic compounding device is shown to have better accuracy than the manual process. Different studies have shown this to be true for robotic systems (a type of automatic compounding equipment). The studies found that the robotic system can compound medications with improved accuracy (±10%) and precision compared to the manual process.[98,101] However, a three-year study revealed limited efficiency of the robotic system for compounding chemotherapy.[102] Considering the safety aspects, the combination of chemotherapy is safe when performed with the robotic system.[98] The self-cleaning function of the automatic compounding device reduces operator exposure hazards.[103]

H) ECONOMIC EVALUATION (INCLUDING PHARMACOECONOMICS OF THE DEVICE COMPARED TO LESS EXPENSIVE METHODS)

Even though installing an automatic compounding device is associated with more significant investment costs, and the maintenance or operation cost also seems high, the return on investment is appreciable.[104] The use of an automatic system saves operator time, and it can be utilized to perform other essential activities. The automation of the chemotherapy compounding process is cost-effective because the cost per dose and preparation time are less with the automatic system. Additionally, the remaining amount of the drugs in the vial is not wasted; instead, it is preferably used to prepare other batches without being contaminated. This reduces the waste of expensive drugs.[95] Compared with the manual process of compounding, an automatic compounding device has less exposure risk and ensures maintenance of the final product quality, thereby providing a positive financial impact.[105]

I) IMPLICATION TO THE PHARMACY PROFESSION AND PHARMACY PRACTICE

The automatic compounding device introduced to pharmacy practice in oncology settings has many benefits and positive perspectives.[106] The system has improved the compounding process that was previously done manually by pharmacists and nurses. Even if the compounding is done by a very experienced or sharp pharmacist or pharmacy technician, there is still a chance of error. With introduction of the automatic system, human-induced errors are minimized, and the pharmacists' work burden is reduced. Pharmacists can better focus on medication utilization and drug therapy management since the automatic system is less time-consuming.[107] In addition to the traditional roles of pharmacists, such as compounding, packaging, and distributing medicines, the automatic system allows pharmacists to perform their clinical roles. All these factors directly affect the quality of health services being provided to the patients. Furthermore, the automatic

compounding device ensures that the correct drug is being used in a sterile and clean environment in every compounding step. Thus, medication and patient safety should be considered.[90]

J) CHALLENGES TO THE PHARMACISTS AND USERS

Special training on the operation of the device is required. This demands time for understanding the system and its operation. Additionally, the operator should be aware of the technical information about software updates and troubleshooting. Relying totally on the automatic system might not be wise because if there is device failure or breakdown, then the whole workflow is disrupted. Therefore, the operator should always be prepared with a back-up plan while using the automatic system in case of any crisis.

K) RECOMMENDATIONS: WAYS FORWARD

- Data from institutions using the automatic compounding device for chemotherapy should be published to obtain more evidence on the practical use of this system.
- The automation of the compounding process is still evolving, and new technologies overcoming the disadvantages of the existing technologies can be introduced and backed up with evidence of actual use.

L) CONCLUSIONS

Compounding chemotherapy using an automatic compounding device is a new achievement in oncology. Despite the high investment and maintenance cost of the system, it undoubtedly provides better product quality and ensures patient safety. The automatic compounding device can be put into best use by routinely training, educating, and monitoring the respective operators regarding the device's operation software updates. However, for institutions that cannot afford the installation of an automatic system, the traditional manual compounding process remains a good alternative.

M) LESSONS LEARNED

The automatic compounding device is a novel technology with advanced features for compounding chemotherapy.

- Automatic compounding devices minimize the main drawback of manual compounding, i.e., human-induced errors in various compounding steps.
- The automatic system's other benefits include less exposure hazard with improved safety, efficiency, cost-effectiveness, dose accuracy, and quality maintenance throughout the process.

DEVICE 5: BIOLOGICAL SAFETY CABINET

To overcome issues related to biohazards, various biosafety levels were established by the Centers for Disease Control and Prevention (CDC) and the National Institutes of Health (NIH).

- Biosafety level 1: The technician operates with necessary safety instruments and facilities pertinent to working with specific and identified lethal strains of microbes that do not cause any infection in healthy humans.
- Biosafety level 2: The technician operates with necessary safety instruments and facilities pertinent to working with a broad spectrum of native microbes having an average probability of causing infections of different severity in humans.
- Biosafety level 3: The technician operates with necessary safety instruments and facilities pertinent to working with primordial microbes having a high probability of causing deadly infections through respiratory transmission.
- Biosafety level 4: The technician operates with necessary safety instruments and facilities pertinent to working with lethal agents that could threaten life through aerosol transmission.

Biological safety cabinets represent an instrument within an enclosed space in the laboratory or pharmacy equipped with HEPA filter(s) that protect personnel, products, and the environment from biohazardous matters.[108]

- Class I Biological safety cabinet:

    Inside the Class I cabinet, the flowing air consists of a mist produced during microbiological manip-

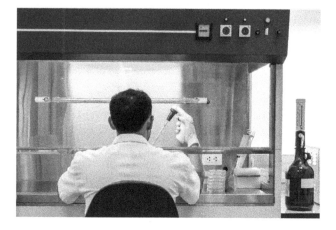

FIGURE 15.6   Biological safety cabinet.

Source: www.shutterstock.com/image-photo/working-biological-safety-cabinets-laminar-air-533631763

ulation, which is then allowed to pass through filters (prefilters and HEPA filters) to confine all the germs and particles and ultimately pass clean air out of the cabinet. However, this system does not prevent the specimen inside the cabinet from being contaminated with matter present in the surroundings. Class I cabinets are only acceptable for working with microorganisms designated for biosafety levels 1, 2, and 3.

- Class II Biological safety cabinet:

    Inside the Class II cabinet, the flowing air consists of a mist produced during microbiological manipulation that prevents particles from getting away through the front opening. However, in Class II cabinets, impure air cannot enter the work zone; hence, the specimen present inside the cabinet is not contaminated with matter present in the surroundings. Class II cabinets are only acceptable for working with microorganisms designated for biosafety levels 1, 2, and 3.

  - Class II Type A (A1/A2) Biological safety cabinets: The most conventional type of biological safety cabinet, in which 30% of the inlet air is dissipated to the outer space and 70% is rereleased in the interior working area. Type A1 cabinets are maintained at positive pressure, and type A2 cabinets are maintained at negative pressure.
  - Class II Type B Biological safety cabinets: These cabinets function via an outer blower that dissipates its inlet air to the surroundings through the duct system and provides extra safety to the operator.
  - Class II Type B1 Biological safety cabinets: These cabinets allow 70% of inlet air to be dissipated to the outer space and 30% to be rereleased in the interior working area.
  - Class II Type B2 Biological safety cabinets: The inlet air is dissipated into the surroundings only after passing across the HEPA filters without rerelease; this is the most appropriate cabinet type to work with toxic chemicals.

- Class III Biological safety cabinet:

  - This cabinet gives the highest degree of safety among all biological safety cabinets. It is constructed out of metals and is maintained at negative pressure. It is most appropriate for working with very lethal agents.[108]
  - The biological safety cabinet protects technicians from the exposure hazards of cytotoxic drugs and lower the risk of particle contamination during chemotherapy compounding.[109]

DEVICE 6: IV ADMIXTURE UNIT FOR CHEMOTHERAPY

Chemotherapy usually contains a combination of two or more medications.[110] IV admixtures are aseptic solutions prepared by combining one or more medications within different IV solutions delivered to patients via the venous route using intravenous administration sets. It is a very complex process that mandates correct administration since any error could be fatal.[111]

Pharmacists and nurses are exposed continuously to biohazards while compounding and delivering chemotherapy to the patients.[112] The IV admixture unit should ensure that the product's contamination is minimal and that the quality is maintained. To reduce medication errors, the use of telepharmacy and barcode technology has been evolving for a few years. In telepharmacy, the composition process is viewed through digital images from which a pharmacist ensures that an accurate proportion of medicine has been conveyed from the primary source to the secondary container. Barcode technology is an electronic operation technique that validates the right medicine at the start of the preparation process.[113]

DEVICE 7: PERIPHERAL VENOUS CATHETER

A peripheral venous catheter is a thin device that withdraws blood or administers medications or IV fluids.[114] It is used for hydration, delivering nutrition supplements, medication therapy, and transfusion of blood products and has been gaining popularity in chemotherapy administration.[115]

Pharmacists are responsible for confirmation that the medication is correct, properly labeled, and accurately dispensed. Additionally, delivering accurate information to members of the healthcare system regarding improved utilization of chemotherapy drugs and safety guidelines on the application of chemotherapeutics remains a major

responsibility of the pharmacist.[116] Some of the key points to consider include the following:

- The catheter must be handled only with clean hands.
- The catheter tip should not be held when the lid is closed.
- The region should be regularly cleaned, and dressing directions must be appropriately followed.
- Catheter fixation must be rigidly tightened except during therapy.
- Any cracks or fractures in the catheter should be avoided.
- The catheter must be flushed regularly, as instructed.[117]

DEVICE 8: CENTRAL VENOUS CATHETER

Sometimes, patients manifest various complications that demand administration of medications through the IV route for longer duration, such as total parenteral nutrition, and short-term access to kidney dialysis, which imposes repeated invasion in the body that could be tedious and irritating. A central venous catheter is available; this device is a thin, flexible tube placed inside the skin and into a large vein that can be positioned in the same place for days or months. These are mostly preferred in patients requiring antibiotics or chronic pain medicines during chemotherapy. However, placing a foreign object in the body for therapeutic purposes always requires a special care to prevent any infection or blockage.[118,119]

To prevent blockage, the catheter must be repeatedly flushed with aseptic solutions. Additionally, special emphasis must be given to the clamping of catheter with its tip shielded.[120]

The central venous catheter is different from the peripherally inserted catheters since the central catheters are placed in larger central veins in the upper chest, neck, or groin region. Compared to peripherally inserted catheters, central catheters can remain in the body for a longer duration, enabling chemotherapy delivery. The risk of damage to the blood vessel is less than that with peripheral catheters

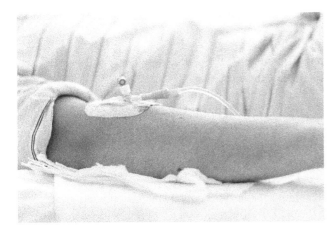

FIGURE 15.7　Peripheral venous catheter.

Source: www.shutterstock.com/image-photo/peripheral-venous-catheter-vein-human-hand-569303755

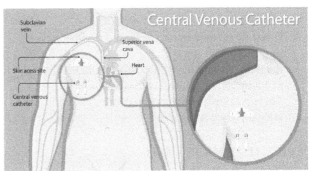

FIGURE 15.8　Central venous catheter.

Source: www.shutterstock.com/image-vector/central-venous-catheter-cvc-picc-line-1093816661

because larger veins can withstand the catheters for a longer period than smaller veins. In addition, the central line gives freedom of easy mobility to patients receiving chemotherapy.[121] However, there is comparatively less risk of catheter-related infection with peripherally inserted catheters.[122]

Since the catheter line is short in peripheral catheters and comparatively longer in central venous catheters, the former facilitates faster delivery of drugs and liquids in contrast to central venous catheters.[64]

DEVICE 9: PERIPHERALLY INSERTED CENTRAL CATHETER LINE

Central venous catheters can be divided into three major classes. One of them is a peripherally inserted central catheter (PICC line). The PICC line is placed in a vein located near the elbow.[120,123,124] The line passes through a larger vein in the heart (superior vena cava) to deliver a chemotherapeutic agent to the targeted site. It prevents frequent vein invasion for medicinal purposes and has been less irritating than the IV route. However, the possibility for infection rises when foreign matter is placed inside the body.[125] Moreover, a thrombus may form within the end of the tube.[126] Additionally, medication therapy failure due to catheter dysfunction arises when the line is dislocated from its original placement.[125]

Special care must be taken by the patients who have PICCs inserted within their arms:

- Lifting heavy objects should be avoided.
- Blood pressure measurement on the PICC arm should be avoided.
- The area should be covered with a protective cloth (available in a medical store) while bathing, because the insertion site should not get wet.[125]
- Additionally, the line should be flushed regularly with anti-clot agents such as heparin or saline water.[127]

DEVICE 10: PORT LINE

A port line is a type of central catheter consisting of an accumulation space with a rubber top.[120] It is placed under the skin on the right side of the body. It has certain advantages over PICC lines.[128]

- Ports can be used inside the body for a long period (if possible).
- Ports do not require regular flushing as PICCs do, and they can be cleaned once a month.
- The area in which the port has been placed is not affected, even when wet.[128]

DEVICE 11: DEVICES USED IN PRESSURE ULCERS

Pressure ulcer may be defined as an abrasion of the skin and/or its fundamental tissue over a bony prominence due to pressure or pressure and shear.[129] Pressure ulcers can occur when medical instruments such as nasogastric tubes and ventilation masks composed of rubber, plastic, or silicone create friction and cause pressure on soft tissues.[130] Device-related pressure ulcers have been most frequently seen in the head and neck region.[131] According to a study by Hendrichova et al., pressure ulcers were present in 22.9% of cancer patients in Italy,[132] and according to Brink et al., 10.5% of seriously ill patients had pressure ulcers.[133]

Some devices have been designed to prevent device-related pressure ulcers:

- Offloading footwear: This material assists in pressure redistribution and hence reduces injury.
- Protectors: Mostly worn on the elbows and heels, the material lowers abrasion risk due to medical devices.
- Positioners: By modifying the body area's location through suspension or elevation, the pressure is reduced.[134]

DEVICE 12: IMPLANTABLE PAIN MEDICATION PUMP

An implantable pain medication pump is used to manage severe pain in cancer patients. It is surgically implanted inside the body and carries and supplies pain medications through the attached catheter. One of the implantable medication pumps currently being used is an intrathecal pump. The battery-operated pump is surgically placed under the skin in the abdominal region and is connected to a thin catheter that reaches out to the spinal entry, thus delivering the pain medication into the spinal fluid. This technique can be incorporated for drugs with a complicated dosing regimen.[135] It has proven to be advantageous over large doses of pain medications that also come with a higher risk of side effects.[136] However, a periodic refill of implanted pain medication pumps (approximately every 1–3 months) is needed.[137]

The device consists of two parts, namely, a pump and a catheter.

- The pump is a round device that usually carries the medication.
- The catheter, which is connected to the pump, delivers medication to the target site.
- Implanted intrathecal drug pumps could be a better choice for patients who experience severe pain in advanced cancer or patients who are receiving palliative care.[138]

Implantable medication pumps provide quick and effective pain relief and are safe when used appropriately. Therefore, they have reasonable patient satisfaction. Additionally, since the drug is delivered to the spinal fluid itself and does not get distributed in the body through blood, typical side effects of pain medications, such as constipation and nausea, can be avoided.[136] However, implanted intrathecal pumps are associated with a risk of infection during or after surgery, headache, and spinal fluid leakage. Resolution of any device-related problems requires surgery, which can be risky in patients, and the patients should be cautious about different alarm or alert sounds from the device.[136,139]

DEVICE 13: HAIR WIGS

Patients undergoing cancer treatments may lose confidence due to alopecia, which occurs as a side effect of anticancer drugs. In such cases, hair wigs are widely used as a management option.[140] These hair wigs are not used as accessories but are a fundamental requirement, similar to using prosthetic devices in patients requiring them.[141] The product is used to enhance quality of life in patients with severe alopecia areata (AA) by boosting their self-confidence and helping them gain normal treatment in society.[142] According to a study by Park et al., along with boosted self-confidence, an optimistic effect on psychosocial features has been seen in patients with severe AA when hair wigs are used for more than an accessory or cosmetic purpose, which has been supported by parameters such as the Psychosocial Impact of Assistive Device Scale (PIADS) and Hair Specific Skindex-29.[143]

The types of hair wigs available are described here:

*   Real hair wigs: These appear to be like the patient's hair, but they are expensive compared to synthetic hair wigs.
*   Synthetic hair wigs: These are comparatively less expensive and made out of acrylic fibers.[144]

DEVICE 14: RYLE'S TUBE (NASOGASTRIC TUBES)

Ryle's tube is a narrow tube inserted through the nasal region into the stomach to provide necessary nutrients and supplements to patients who cannot take foods and drinks orally. The tube is made out of materials such as polyurethane and silicone, which have minimum interaction with gastric acid; these tubes can be used for up to six weeks.[145]

Two types of Ryle's tubes are commonly used in the medical field.

*   Wide bore tubes used in gastric drainage
*   Fine bore tubes used in artificial feeding[146]

Some salient features of Ryle's tube include the following:

*   The tubes are smooth-surfaced, which lessens the risk of tissue irritation.
*   The presence of a thermosensitive material on the tube surface soothes with increased body temperature.
*   Ryle's tubes align with the shape of gastro tubes.[147]

However, in patients highly prone to aspiration, such as individuals with gastroesophageal reflux and upper gastrointestinal stricture, the use of Ryle's tube is contraindicated.[148]

DEVICE 15: POSTMASTECTOMY DEVICES (PROSTHESES, ARTIFICIAL BREASTS)

Postmastectomy devices are prosthetic devices worn after mastectomy to compensate for the tissues removed during breast cancer surgery.[149] These devices are also known as external breast prostheses; they help the patient look more natural and enhance body posture. According to a study

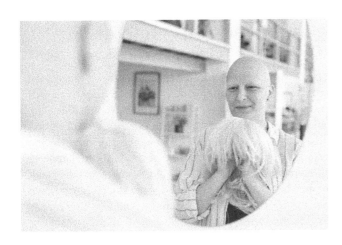

FIGURE 15.9 Hair wigs.

Source: www.shutterstock.com/image-photo/reflection-portrait-bald-adult-woman-looking-1783780490

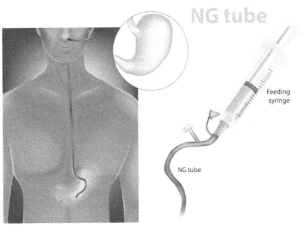

FIGURE 15.10 Ryle's tube.

Source: www.shutterstock.com/image-vector/nasogastric-intubation-tube-ng-1374322184

conducted by Borghesan et al. in Brazil, 56.6% of the women were contented with prosthetic substitutes.[150]

Breast prostheses are available as adhesive types and conventional types.

- The adhesive prostheses are connected to the breast tissues through adherents.
- The conventional prostheses are worn inside the bra.[151]
- Prostheses are made from several materials to enhance the patient's natural tissues, such as silicone and non-silicone materials fabricated with foams.[152]

Additionally, breast prosthetics are available as:

- Full prosthetics that restore intact breast tissues.
- Partial prosthesis that fulfills only the removed tissues.
- Shell prosthetics that assist remodeled breasts.
- Prosthetics for nipple and areola.[153]

DEVICE 16: PILL PULVERIZER

To ease drug intake, maceration of two or more tablets, without amending much of the effectiveness of each tablet, is sometimes preferred. For the pulverization of drug tablets, a pill pulverizer can be used. The crushed product is then taken along with food, water, juice, milk, or other substances, or through tubes. A variety of pill pulverizers are available on the market. However, a certain fraction of drug loss has been observed in the process.[154] According to a study by Palese et al., drug loss due to crushing of tablets using mortar and pestle was found to be 0.7%, and using a pill pulverizer, was found to be 0.6%.[155]

According to some studies, following some rules might help in reducing drug loss:

- Putting some water into the crusher and ingesting medication directly through the vessel, followed by a second rinse, could be very useful.
- When mixing crushed tablets with food items is preferred, highly viscous items such as honey, yoghurt, and jam should be favored, because they reduce the likelihood of aspiration.
- The device should be cleaned after crushing the tablets.[154]

DEVICE 17: BONE MARROW ASPIRATION SYRINGE

Bone marrow aspiration refers to the process of sampling soft tissues located inside the bones when any blood test performed previously shows exceptional levels of blood components, and hence, assists in the diagnosis of hematological and nonhematological malignancies or any other abnormalities.[156,157] Tissue specimens are typically taken

from the posterior or anterior iliac region. A syringe different from that used in the bone marrow biopsy is recommended for bone marrow aspiration. A 20 ml syringe is generally used to remove 0.3 ml of aspirate.[158] The syringe is composed of a stylet in the interior and a cannula at the exterior part. The stylet prevents possible blockage by the cannula and body tissues.[159] However, a large-volume syringe (50 ml) is associated with a risk of blood dilution of the bone marrow aspirate. According to a study performed by Hernigou et al., when aspirates were withdrawn from 50 ml and 10 ml syringes, the concentration of mesenchymal stem cells from the bone marrow was 300% greater in the latter group.[160] Additionally, using tiny-volume syringes (1 ml–4 ml) might mandate repeat biopsies, which can be disadvantageous.[160]

DEVICE 18: IV CANNULA

Chemotherapy is usually given via the intravenous route, and the use of an IV cannula is common.[161] Patients are administered drugs with cannulas of different gauge sizes, such as larger[20,22] and smaller[24,26] cannulas. A smaller gauge is recommended when a patient experiences any complications, such as phlebitis and extravasation, with an IV cannula.[162] The IV cannula allows easy and effective drug administration to the patient without the intense pain of an injection every time the drug needs to be administered. Patients might feel pain while the cannula is fixed in their hands (venipuncture) only. Drug administration through an IV cannula is an integrated approach when patients need to be administered intravenously over a long period.[163] An authorized person with preinjection, injection, and postinjection skills is compulsory when inserting and using a cannula for drug administration.[164] In addition to drug administration, an IV cannula can be used for fluid therapy, electrolyte solution administration, and emergency venous access.[163]

DEVICE 19: PERSONAL PROTECTIVE EQUIPMENT (PPE) (RELEVANT TO THE BIOLOGICAL SAFETY CABINET [BSC])

The use of personal protective equipment is necessary while working with high-risk cytotoxic medications. All health workers, including pharmacists, have mandated the application of chemotherapy-tested gloves, one-use throwaway gowns, face cover masks, and eye shields.[165] In the oncology department, sensitivity lies in both the handling of chemotherapeutic drugs by health workers and the weak immune health of cancer patients. Many studies have shown that carelessness in personal care by health workers leads to problems in the reproductive system, sporadic cancers, respiratory infections, and many more.[166] Antineoplastic guidelines have been developed, which mandate Class II biological safety cabinets, a face mask, two pairs of gloves, a head cap, and a gown as a single set of PPE. In the case of

Class II safety cabinet scarcity, Class III cabinets can also be used as a substitute.[166] The guidelines for working with chemotherapeutic drugs mostly obligate working within the boundaries created by the Oncology Nursing Society (ONS), American Society of Health-System Pharmacists (ASHP), Occupational Safety and Health Administration (OSHA), and National Institute for Occupational Safety and Health (NIOSH).[167]

DEVICE 20: AUTOMATED COMPOUNDING DEVICES (ACD) FOR TOTAL PARENTERAL NUTRITION (TPN)

Pharmacists are responsible for the extemporaneous preparation of many products in pharmacies. Traditionally, these works were performed manually by preparing liquid mixtures of large volumes that consumed labor and time. Nevertheless, with time, automated devices have emerged. The required solution can be conveyed from the primary container to the final container using a volumetric or gravimetric fluid pump system. Moreover, software for receiving, delivering, and storing all the necessary information also adds to the technology's crucial role. In a volumetric system, a specific volume of solution is transferred from one container to the other using a rotary pump, while in a gravimetric system, a specific volume of solution to be transferred is determined by specific gravity.[168] An automated compounding system saves the operator's time and effort and provides a good-quality final product compounded in a clean environment within the system.

MINOR DEVICES USED IN MEDICAL ONCOLOGY

In addition to the aforementioned medical devices, other medical devices are commonly used in medical oncology.

FACE MASK (SURGICAL)

Cancer patients are more prone to infections because of their weakened immune systems. Surgical masks, also known as isolation or procedure masks, help restrict microbe spread when a person coughs, sneezes, or talks. However, medical experts suggest that these masks are only for one-time use.[169,170]

THERMOMETER

Many cancer patients have deficient neutrophils levels, which account for fever and may signal serious health hazards. Oral thermometers are commonly used to measure a patient's temperature.[171] Nevertheless, for patients in whom oral thermometers are prohibitive, noninvasive methods are preferred, such as:

- A tympanic artery thermometer determines temperature by measuring the amount of infrared heat produced in the tympanic artery located in the ear that connects to the hypothalamus, a temperature regulator of the body.
- A temporal artery thermometer determines the temperature from the temporal artery located in the forehead and behind the ear by slow scanning and direct skin contact.[172]

HOSPITAL BED

A hospital bed is a useful piece of furniture in inpatient care.[173] It should be available to every admitted patient in a pure form with proper safety rules followed. Recommended beds include the following:

- Conventional types that are confined within one room
- Electric beds that can be moved from one place to other
- Healing facilitation beds that help the patient recover from bedsores that occur when they stay in one position for a longer period
- Bed with rails to ensure that the patient does not fall while resting[174]

INCONTINENCE PRODUCTS

These products are mostly made for patients who deal with urinary incontinence. Some of the products include the following:

- Pantyliners for women who experience insignificant incontinence.
- Guards for men who require protection against incontinence.
- Incontinence underwear for patients who are not developed enough to detect the urinary urge.
- Cleansing creams and wipes for cleaning the intimate areas and removing such problems to stay healthy[175]

ADULT DIAPERS

Adults wear these products; they differ from baby diapers in size and function. These diapers are used when a patient is unaware of the urinary urge, cannot move out of bed, or has diarrhea. Adult diapers are also sometimes worn by pregnant women.[176] They are available in both pull-up and tabbed versions and different sizes.[176] These diapers provide protection ranging from 8–12 hours.

WHEELCHAIRS

Some people struggle with walking. For these patients, wheelchairs, consisting of a seating facility and wheels, are available to ease moving from one place to another, either with the help of a caretaker or by one's self, to enhance the quality of life. Wheelchairs allow postural support as well as independence. These wheelchairs are available in many sizes and for people of all age groups,[177] and prescriptions are made based on an individual level.[178]

Wheelchairs come in different types:

- Manual wheelchair: This wheelchair is moved manually by the patient or pushed by the caretaker.
- Electric wheelchair: This wheelchair is set in motion with the help of a battery or motor. It can quickly move upstairs and does not show any problem with traveling in graveled areas.
- Sports wheelchair: This is an appropriate device for people with walking disabilities and a particular enthusiasm for sports. They are used for games such as tennis, wheelchair basketball, etc.[179]

REFERENCES

1. Mann C, Ouro-Bang'na F, Eledjam JJ. Patient-controlled analgesia. Curr Drug Targets. 2005;6(7):815–19.
2. Pastino A, Lakra A. Patient controlled analgesia. [Updated 2021 Jul 24]. In: StatPearls [Internet]. Treasure Island, FL: StatPearls Publishing; 2021 Jan. Available from: https://www.ncbi.nlm.nih.gov/books/NBK551610/.
3. Ferrell BR, Nash CC, Warfield C. The role of patient-controlled analgesia in the management of cancer pain. J Pain Sympt Manag. 1992;7(3):149–54.
4. Macintyre PE. Safety and efficacy of patient-controlled analgesia. Br J Anaesth. 2001;87(1):36–46.
5. Patak LS, Tait AR, Mirafzali L, et al. Patient perspectives of patient-controlled analgesia (PCA) and methods for improving pain control and patient satisfaction. Reg Anesth Pain Med. 2013;38(4):326–33.
6. Málek J, Ševčík P, Bejšovec D, et al. Postoperative pain management. 3rd updated edition. Mladá Fronta. 2017. Available from: https://management.ind.in/forum/attachments/f2/39049d1586398178-postoperative-pain-postoperative-pain.pdf.
7. Patient-Controlled Analgesia (PCA) [cited 2020 Dec 18]. Available from: www.webmd.com/pain-management/guide/pca.
8. UWHealth. Patient Controlled Analgesia (PCA) by Proxy [cited 2020 Dec 18]. Available from: www.uwhealth.org/healthfacts/pain/7697.pdf.
9. O'Keefe D, O'herlihy C, Gross Y, et al. Patient-controlled analgesia using a miniature electrochemically driven infusion pump. Br J Anaesth. 1994 Dec;73(6):843–6.
10. Macintyre PE. Safety and efficacy of patient-controlled analgesia. BJA: Br J Anaesth. 2001;87(1):36–46.
11. Tesoro S, Mezzetti D, Marchesini L, et al. Clonidine treatment for agitation in children after sevoflurane anesthesia. Anesth Analg. 2005;101(6).
12. Allegretta G. Safety issues in pediatric patient-controlled analgesia by proxy. Safety. 2005;7(2–3).
13. Wells N, Pasero C, McCaffery M. Improving the quality of care through pain assessment and management. In: Hughes RG, editor. Patient safety and quality: an evidence-based handbook for nurses. Rockville, MD: Agency for Healthcare Research and Quality (US); 2008 Apr. Chapter 17. Available from: https://www.ncbi.nlm.nih.gov/books/NBK2658/.
14. Wirz S, Conrad S, Shtrichman R, et al. Clinical evaluation of a novel technology for oral patient-controlled analgesia, the PCoA® Acute device, for hospitalized patients with postoperative pain, in pilot feasibility study. Pain Res Manag. 2017; 7962135.
15. Patient-Controlled Analgesia Pumps [cited 2020 Dec 9]. Available from: www.hopkinsmedicine.org/health/treatment-tests-and-therapies/patientcontrolled-analgesia-pumps.
16. Fernandes MTP, Hernandes FB, de Almeida TN, et al. Patient-controlled analgesia (PCA) in acute pain: pharmacological and clinical aspects, pain relief—from analgesics to alternative therapies. Cecilia Maldonado: IntechOpen. https://doi.org/10.5772/67299. Available from: https://www.intechopen.com/chapters/54018
17. Grissinger M. Safety and patient-controlled analgesia: part 2: how to prevent errors. P T. 2008;33(1):8–9.
18. Maddali P, Moisi M, Page J, et al. Anatomical complications of epidural anesthesia: a comprehensive review. Clin Anat. 2017;30(3):342–6.
19. Ilfeld BM. Continuous peripheral nerve blocks: an update of the published evidence and comparison with novel, alternative analgesic modalities. Anesth Analg. 2017;124(1):308–35.
20. Jamison RN, Mao J. Opioid analgesics. Mayo Clin Proc. 2015;90(7):957–68.
21. Dickerson DM, Apfelbaum JL. Local anesthetic systemic toxicity. Aesthet Surg J. 2014;34(7):1111–19.
22. Cooney MF, Czarnecki M, Dunwoody C, et al. American Society for Pain Management Nursing position statement with clinical practice guidelines: authorized agent controlled analgesia. Pain Manag Nurs. 2013;14(3):176–81.
23. Licht E, Siegler EL, Reid MC. Can the cognitively impaired safely use patient controlled analgesia? J Opioid Manag. 2009;5(5):307.
24. Skryabina EA, Dunn TS. Disposable infusion pumps. Am J Health-System Pharm. 2006;63(13):1260–8.
25. Lehmann KA. Recent developments in patient-controlled analgesia. J Pain Sympt Manag. 2005;29(5):72–89.
26. Ocay DD, Otis A, Teles AR, et al. Safety of patient-controlled analgesia after surgery in children and adolescents: concerns and potential solutions. Front Pediatr. 2018;6:336.
27. McNicol ED, Ferguson MC, Hudcova J. Patient controlled opioid analgesia versus non-patient controlled opioid analgesia for postoperative pain. Cochrane Database Syst Rev. 2015(6).
28. Choiniere M, Rittenhouse Brian E, Perreault S, et al. Efficacy and costs of patient-controlled analgesia versus regularly administered intramuscular opioid therapy Anesthesiology. 1998;89(6):1377–88.
29. Colwell CW, Jr., Morris BA. Patient-controlled analgesia compared with intramuscular injection of analgesics for the management of pain after an orthopaedic procedure. JBJS. 1995;77(5).

30. Grass JA. Patient-controlled analgesia. Anesth Analg. 2005;101(5S):S44–S61.

31. Son H-J, Kim S-H, Ryu J-O, et al. Device-related error in patient-controlled analgesia: analysis of 82,698 patients in a tertiary hospital. Anesth Analg. 2019;129(3).

32. Booth S, Wade R. Oxygen or air for palliation of breathlessness in advanced cancer. J R Soc Med. 2003;96(5):215–18.

33. Dudgeon DJ, Lertzman M, Askew GR. Physiological changes and clinical correlations of dyspnea in cancer outpatients. J Pain Sympt Manag. 2001;21(5):373–9.

34. Criner GJ. Ambulatory home oxygen: what is the evidence for benefit, and who does it help? Respir Care. 2013;58(1):48–64.

35. Marciniuk DD, Goodridge D, Hernandez P, et al. Managing dyspnea in patients with advanced chronic obstructive pulmonary disease: a Canadian Thoracic Society clinical practice guideline. Can Respir J. 2011;18(2):69–78.

36. Ortega Ruiz F, Díaz Lobato S, Galdiz Iturri JB, et al. Continuous home oxygen therapy. Arch Bronconeumol. 2014;50(5):185–200.

37. Díaz Lobato S, Mayoralas Alises S. Mobility profiles of patients with home oxygen therapy. Arch Bronconeumol. 2012;48(2):55–60.

38. Bateman N, Leach R. Acute oxygen therapy. BMJ. 1998;317(7161):798–801.

39. Moen I, Stuhr LE. Hyperbaric oxygen therapy and cancer—a review. Target Oncol. 2012;7(4):233–42.

40. Hardavella G, Karampinis I, Frille A, et al. Oxygen devices and delivery systems. Breathe. 2019;15(3):e108–e16.

41. Overview of oxygen tanks or cylinders [cited 2020 Dec 11]. Available from: www.oxygenconcentratorstore.com/breathe-easy/equipment-info/oxygen-tanks.

42. Srivastava U. Anaesthesia gas supply: gas cylinders. Indian J Anaesth. 2013;57(5):500.

43. Palwai A, Skowronski M, Coreno A, et al. Critical comparisons of the clinical performance of oxygen-conserving devices. Am J Respir Crit Care Med. 2010;181(10):1061–71.

44. Oxygen tanks and how to choose one [cited 2020 Dec 11]. Available from: www.webmd.com/lung/oxygen-tanks-how-to-choose.

45. McCoy RW. Options for home oxygen therapy equipment: storage and metering of oxygen in the home. Respir Care. 2013;58(1):65.

46. Hardinge M, Annandale J, Bourne S, et al. British Thoracic Society guidelines for home oxygen use in adults: accredited by NICE. Thorax. 2015;70(Suppl 1):i1.

47. VA National Center for Patient Safety [cited 2020 Dec 11]. Available from: www.patientsafety.va.gov/professionals/hazards/oxygen.asp.

48. Scott A, Robinson C, Thompson A, et al. Guidelines for the use of oxygen in palliative care. Cheshire and Merseyside Palliative and End of Life Care Strategic Clinical Network. Available from: www nwcscnsenate nhs uk/files/9814/5684/6563/Oxygen_in_Palliative_Care_FINAL pdf (accessed Jan 2019).

49. Compressed medical oxygen. Essential safety information [cited 2020 Dec 11]. Available from: www.bochealthcare.co.uk/en/images/507770-Healthcare%2520Oxygen%2520MGDS%2520Rev4%2520%2528Nov%25202016%2529%2520_tcm409-54070.pdf.

50. Home oxygen therapy [cited 2020 Dec 11]. Available from: www.nhs.uk/conditions/home-oxygen-treatment/.

51. Booth S, Kelly MJ, Cox NP, et al. Does oxygen help dyspnea in patients with cancer? Am J Respir Crit Care Med. 1996;153(5):1515–18.

52. Kamal AH, Maguire JM, Wheeler JL, et al. Dyspnea review for the palliative care professional: treatment goals and therapeutic options. J Palliat Med. 2012;15(1):106–14.

53. Kloke M, Cherny N. Treatment of dyspnoea in advanced cancer patients: ESMO Clinical Practice Guidelines. Ann Oncol. 2015;26(suppl_5):v169–v73.

54. O'driscoll B, Howard L, Davison A. BTS guideline for emergency oxygen use in adult patients. Thorax. 2008;63(Suppl 6):vi1–vi68.

55. McCoy RW. Options for home oxygen therapy equipment: storage and metering of oxygen in the home. Respir Care. 2013;58(1):65–85.

56. The Pharmaceutical Journal. Value of pharmacists' oxygen role [cited 2020 Dec 11]. Available from: www.pharmaceutical-journal.com/value-of-pharmacists-oxygen-role/20001580.article?firstPass=false.

57. Budinger GS, Mutlu GM. Balancing the risks and benefits of oxygen therapy in critically Ill adults. Chest. 2013;143(4):1151–62.

58. Jin J-F, Zhu L-L, Chen M, et al. The optimal choice of medication administration route regarding intravenous, intramuscular, and subcutaneous injection. Patient Prefer Adherence. 2015;9:923–42.

59. Understanding chemotherapy: American Society of Clinical Oncology (ASCO) [cited 2020 Dec 12]. Available from: www.cancer.net/navigating-cancer-care/how-cancer-treated/chemotherapy/understanding-chemotherapy.

60. American Cancer Society. Getting IV or injectable chemotherapy [cited 2020 Dec 12]. Available from: www.cancer.org/treatment/treatments-and-side-effects/treatment-types/chemotherapy/getting-chemotherapy.html.

61. Cancer Research UK. Chemotherapy pumps [cited 2020 Dec 12]. Available from: www.cancerresearchuk.org/about-cancer/cancer-in-general/treatment/chemotherapy/how-you-have/into-your-vein/pumps#:~:text=Chemotherapy%20pumps%20are%20also%20called,very%20slowly%20into%20your%20bloodstream.

62. American Cancer Society. Getting IV or injectable chemotherapy [cited 2020 Dec12]. Available from: www.cancer.org/treatment/treatments-and-side-effects/treatment-types/chemotherapy/getting-chemotherapy.html.

63. Garrido M, Faus V, Lopez-Martin C, et al. GRP-175 Smart infusion pumps in chemotherapy administration. Eur J Hosp Pharm: Sci Pract. 2013;20(Suppl 1):A63–A.

64. Cassano-Piché A, Fan M, Sabovitch S, et al. Multiple intravenous infusions phase 1b: practice and training scan. Ontario Health Technol Assessm Ser. 2012;12(16):1.

65. Rapsilber LM, Camp-Sorrell D. Ambulatory infusion pumps: application to oncology. Semin Oncol Nurs. 1995;11(3):213–20.

66. Chavis-Parker P. Safe chemotherapy in the home environment. Home Healthcare Now. 2015;33(5):246–51.

67. Thomas SAS. Chemotherapy pumps: preparation and counseling. J Carcinogen Mutagen Res. 2019;1(1):2–6.

68. Hobbs JG, Ryan MK, Ritchie B, et al. Protocol for a randomised crossover trial to evaluate patient and nurse satisfaction with electronic and elastomeric portable infusion pumps for the continuous administration of antibiotic therapy in the home: the Comparing Home Infusion Devices (CHID) study. BMJ Open. 2017;7(7):e016763–e.

69. Thiveaud D, Demazieres V, Lafont J. Comparison of the performance of four elastomeric devices. Eur J Hosp Pharm Pract. 2005;11:54–6.

70. Which ambulatory infusion pump is best for 5-FU? [cited 2020 Dec 17]. Available from: https://voice.ons.org/news-and-views/which-ambulatory-infusion-pump-is-best-for-5-fu.

71. Continuous Infusion with Your Elastomeric Pump [cited 2020 Dec 17]. Available from: https://www.mskcc.org/pdf/cancer-care/patient-education/continuous-infusion-elastomeric-pump.

72. MedView Systems. Infusion pumps [cited 2020 Dec 18]. Available from: www.medviewsystems.com/instructions-for-iv-pumps/.

73. Cancer Research UK. Chemotherapy pumps [cited 2020 Dec 17]. Available from: www.cancerresearchuk.org/about-cancer/cancer-in-general/treatment/chemotherapy/how-you-have/into-your-vein/pumps#:~:text=Chemotherapy%20pumps%20are%20also%20called,very%20slowly%20into%20your%20bloodstream.

74. USFDA. Infusion pumps [cited 2020 Dec 17]. Available from: www.fda.gov/medical-devices/general-hospital-devices-and-supplies/infusion-pumps.

75. Plasse T, Ohnuma T, Bruckner H, et al. Portable infusion pumps in ambulatory cancer chemotherapy. Cancer. 1982;50(1):27–31.

76. CS/09—GT1 Metrology in Health. Metrology in health—Good practices guide—Part II. Infusion pumps edition Portuguese Institute for Quality. 2018 Portuguese Institute for Quality. Ministry of Economy Sectoral Comission on Health (CS/09). ISBN 978-972-763-172-8 [cited 2020 Dec 17]. Available from: https://www.ordemfarmaceuticos.pt/fotos/qualidade/good_practices_metrology_in_health_guide_infusion_pumps_12797950485cb5de48431c1.pdf.

77. Lokich JJ, Perri J, Bothe A, et al. Cancer chemotherapy via ambulatory infusion pump. Am J Clin Oncol. 1983;6(3):355–63.

78. Dorr RT, Trinca CE, Griffith K, et al. Limitations of a portable infusion pump in ambulatory patients receiving continuous infusions of anticancer drugs. Cancer Treat Rep. 1979;63(2):211–13.

79. Díaz I, Hoyos MT, Arredondo A, et al. Acceptance of portable infusion pumps for chemotherapy in patients with metastatic colorectal cancer. Atencion Farmaceutica. 2014;16:95–101.

80. Hertzel C, Sousa V. The use of smart pumps for preventing medication errors. J Infus Nurs: Off Publ Infusion Nurses Soc. 2009;32:257–67.

81. Giuliano KK. IV smart pumps: the impact of a simplified user interface on clinical use. Biomed Instrum Technol. 2015;Suppl:13–21.

82. Salman D, Biliune J, Kayyali R, et al. Evaluation of the performance of elastomeric pumps in practice: are we under-delivering on chemotherapy treatments? Curr Med Res Opin. 2017;33(12):2153–9.

83. Rapsilber LM, Camp-Sorrell D. Ambulatory infusion pumps: application to oncology. Sem Oncol Nurs. 1995;11(3):213–20.

84. Hall KK, Shoemaker-Hunt S, Hoffman L, et al. Making healthcare safer III: a critical analysis of existing and emerging patient safety practices [Internet]. Rockville, MD: Agency for Healthcare Research and Quality (US); 2020 Mar. Available from: https://www.ncbi.nlm.nih.gov/books/NBK555526/.

85. Arruebo M, Vilaboa N, Sáez-Gutierrez B, et al. Assessment of the evolution of cancer treatment therapies. Cancers. 2011;3(3):3279–330.

86. Ma CS. Role of pharmacists in optimizing the use of anti-cancer drugs in the clinical setting. Integr Pharm Res Pract. 2014;3:11–24.

87. Gilbert RE, Kozak MC, Dobish RB, et al. Intravenous chemotherapy compounding errors in a follow-up pan-Canadian observational study. J Oncol Pract. 2018;14(5):e295–e303.

88. McDowell S, Ferner H, Ferner R. The pathophysiology of medication errors: how and where they arise. Br J Clin Pharmacol. 2009;67:605–13.

89. Gorman T, Dropkin J, Kamen J, et al. Controlling health hazards to hospital workers: a reference guide. New Solut: J Environ Occup Health Pol. 2014;23(1_suppl):1–169.

90. Hospital News. Automated pharmacy compounding essential to patient safety. Available from: https://hospitalnews.com/automated-pharmacy-compounding-essential-to-patient-safety/.

91. Connor TH, DeBord DG, Pretty JR, et al. Evaluation of antineoplastic drug exposure of health care workers at three university-based US cancer centers. J Occup Environ Med. 2010;52(10).

92. Minghetti P, Pantano D, Gennari CGM, et al. Regulatory framework of pharmaceutical compounding and actual developments of legislation in Europe. Health Pol. 2014;117(3):328–33.

93. From manual to automated systems [cited 2020 Dec 19]. Available from: www.todaysmedicaldevelopments.com/article/tmd0915-automatic-solution-compounding-processes/.

94. Pharmoduct: automatic pharmacy compounding system [cited 2020 Dec 21]. Available from: www.comecer.com/pharmoduct-automatic-compounding-system/.

95. Automated compounding for intravenous chemotherapy [cited 2020 Dec 18]. Available from: www.grifols.com/documents/10192/1227732/kiro-oncology-grifols-brochure/fcb0997a-1c48-4f5f-97dd-605c98808f22.

96. Simegn W, Dagnew B, Dagne H. Knowledge and associated factors towards cytotoxic drug handling among University of Gondar Comprehensive Specialized Hospital health professionals, institutional-based cross-sectional study. Envir Health Prev Med. 2020;25(1):11.

97. Pharmacists ASoH-S. ASHP guidelines on the safe use of automated dispensing devices. Am J Health-Syst Pharm. 2010;67(6):483–90.

98. Iwamoto T, Morikawa T, Hioki M, et al. Performance evaluation of the compounding robot, APOTECAchemo, for injectable anticancer drugs in a Japanese hospital. J Pharm Health Care Sci. 2017;3:12.

99. Soumoy L, Hecq J-D. Automated compounding of intravenous therapy in European countries: a review in 2019. Pharm Technol Hosp Pharm. 2019;4(2):51–7.

100. Nurgat Z, Faris D, Mominah M, et al. A three-year study of a first-generation chemotherapy-compounding robot. Am J Health-Syst Pharm: AJHP: Off J Am Soc Health-Syst Pharm. 2015;72:1036.

101. Geersing TH, Klous MG, Franssen EJF, et al. Robotic compounding versus manual compounding of chemotherapy: comparing dosing accuracy and precision. Eur J Pharm Sci. 2020;155:105536.

102. Nurgat Z, Faris D, Mominah M, et al. A three-year study of a first-generation chemotherapy-compounding robot. Am J Health-Syst Pharm. 2015;72(12):1036–45.

103. Telleria N, García N, Grisaleña J, et al. Evaluation of the efficacy of a self-cleaning automated compounding system for the decontamination of cytotoxic drugs. J Oncol Pharm Pract. 2020:1078155220951866.

104. M Boyd A, W Chaffee B. Critical evaluation of pharmacy automation and robotic systems: a call to action. Hosp Pharm. 2019;54(1):4–11.

105. Masini C, Nanni O, Antaridi S, et al. Automated preparation of chemotherapy: quality improvement and economic sustainability. Am J Health Syst Pharm. 2014;71(7):579–85.

106. Yaniv AW, Knoer SJ. Implementation of an iv-compounding robot in a hospital-based cancer center pharmacy. Am J Health-Syst Pharm. 2013;70(22):2030–7.

107. Schneider PJ. The impact of technology on safe medicines use and pharmacy practice in the US. Front Pharmacol. 2018;9:1361.

108. ESCO. A guide to biosafety & biological safety cabinets [cited 2020 Dec 21]. Available from: www.escoglobal.com/resources/pdf/biosafety-booklet.pdf.

109. The Class II Biosafety Cabinet in a pharmaceutical laboratory [cited 2020 Dec 21]. Available from: https://www.labconco.com/articles/the-class-ii-biosafety-cabinet-in-a-pharmaceutic.

110. Lokich JJ. Admixtures of chemotherapy agents by continuous infusion. In: Concomitant continuous infusion chemotherapy and radiation. Springer; 1991. p. 49–55.

111. Farhan YM. Medical assistants' knowledge about preparation and administration of intravenous admixtures in the teaching hospitals of Alanbar governorate. Int J Pharm Phytopharmacol Res. 2018;8(5):31–4.

112. Patel S. Safe handling of chemotherapy for pharmacists. 2014 [cited 2020 Dec 21]. Available from: www.uspharmacist.com/article/safe-handling-of-chemotherapy-for-pharmacists.

113. Innovations in chemotherapy preparation safety use of telepharmacy and barcode technology in the IV admixture area [cited 2020 Dec 16]. Available from: www.gerpac.eu/innovations-in-chemotherapy-preparation-safetyuse-of-telepharmacy-and-barcode-technology-in-the-iv-admixture-area.

114. Beecham GB, Tackling G. Peripheral line placement. In: StatPearls [Internet]. Treasure Island, FL: StatPearls Publishing; 2019.

115. Kapucu S, Özkaraman AÖ, Uysal N, et al. Knowledge level on administration of chemotherapy through peripheral and central venous catheter among oncology nurses. Asia-Pacific J Oncol Nurs. 2017;4(1):61–8.

116. Cassagnol MM, McBride A. Management of chemotherapy extravasations. 2009 [cited 2020 Dec 2]. Available from: www.uspharmacist.com/article/management-of-chemotherapy-extravasations.

117. Catheters and Ports in Cancer Treatment. 2019 [cited 2020 Dec 2]. Available from: https://www.cancer.net/navigating-cancer-care/how-cancer-treated/chemotherapy/catheters-and-ports-cancer-treatment.

118. Hartl WH, Jauch KW, Parhofer K, et al. Complications and monitoring—guidelines on parenteral nutrition, chapter 11. Ger Med Sci. 2009;7:Doc17–Doc.

119. Taylor RW, Palagiri AV. Central venous catheterization. Crit Care Med. 2007;35(5):1390–6.

120. Central Venous Catheters and IV Ports 2016 [cited 2020 Dec 2]. Available from: www.uspharmacist.com/article/central-venous-catheters-and-iv-ports.

121. American Thoracic Society. Patient education | Information Series. Central Venous Catheter [cited 2020 Dec 2]. Available from: www.thoracic.org/patients/patient-resources/resources/central-venous-catheter.pdf.

122. Fang S, Yang J, Song L, et al. Comparison of three types of central venous catheters in patients with malignant tumor receiving chemotherapy. Patient Prefer Adherence. 2017;11:1197.

123. Jonczyk M, Gebauer B, Schnapauff D, et al. Peripherally inserted central catheters: dependency of radiation exposure from puncture site and level of training. Acta Radiol. 2018;59(6):688–93.

124. Gonzalez R, Cassaro S. Percutaneous central catheter. In: StatPearls [Internet]. Treasure Island, FL: StatPearls Publishing; 2021 Jan. Updated 2020 Sep 7. Available from: https://www.ncbi.nlm.nih.gov/books/NBK459338/.

125. What's the difference between a CVC and a PICC? [cited 2020 Dec 2]. Available from: www.azuravascularcare.com/infodialysisaccess/difference-between-cvc-and-picc/.

126. Peripherally inserted central catheter (PICC) line [cited 2020 Dec 2]. Available from: www.mayoclinic.org/tests-procedures/picc-line/about/pac-20468748.

127. PICC lines (peripherally inserted central catheter) [cited 2020 Dec 2]. Available from: www.cancerresearchuk.org/about-cancer/cancer-in-general/treatment/chemotherapy/how-you-have/into-your-vein/picc-lines.

128. Central venous catheters: PICC lines versus ports. Available from: www.healthline.com/health/breast-cancer-navigator/central-venous-catheters-picc-lines-versus-ports#comparison.

129. Bhattacharya S, Mishra RK. Pressure ulcers: current understanding and newer modalities of treatment. Indian J Plast Surg. 2015;48(1):4–16.

130. Bhattacharya S, Mishra R. Pressure ulcers: current understanding and newer modalities of treatment. Indian J Plast Surg: Off Publ Assoc Plastic Surgeons of India. 2015;48(1):4.

131. Black J, Kalowes P. Medical device-related pressure ulcers. Chronic Wound Care Manag Res. 2016;3:91–9.

132. Hendrichova I, Castelli M, Mastroianni C, et al. Pressure ulcers in cancer palliative care patients. Palliat Med. 2010;24(7):669–73.

133. Brink P, Smith TF, Linkewich B. Factors associated with pressure ulcers in palliative home care. J Palliat Med. 2006;9(6):1369–75.

134. Tools of the trade: pressure injury/ulcer prevention and medical devices [cited 2020 Dec 6]. Available from: www.woundsource.com/blog/tools-trade-pressure-injuryulcer-prevention-and-medical-devices#:~:text=Pressure%20

Injury%20Prevention%20Devices&text=Protectors%20 %E2%80%93%20Protectors%20are%20devices%20 that,position%20of%20the%20body%20area.

135. Knight KH, Brand FM, McHaourab AS, et al. Implantable intrathecal pumps for chronic pain: highlights and updates. Croatian Medical J. 2007;48(1):22–34.

136. Medtronic. Benefits and risks—drug pumps chronic pain [cited 2020 Dec 6]. Available from: www.medtronic.com/ uk-en/patients/treatments-therapies/drug-pump-chronic-pain/drug-pumps-benefits-risks.html.

137. Memorial Sloan Kettering Cancer Center. About your intrathecal pump [cited 2020 Dec 6]. Available from: www.mskcc.org/cancer-care/patient-education/intrathecal-pump-treatment-pain.

138. Bhatia G, Lau ME, Koury KM, et al. Intrathecal Drug Delivery (ITDD) systems for cancer pain. F1000Res. 2013;2:96.

139. Pain pump (intrathecal drug pump) [cited 2020 Dec 7]. Available from: https://mayfieldclinic.com/pe-pump. htm.

140. Inui S, Inoue T, Itami S. Psychosocial impact of wigs or hair-pieces on perceived quality of life level in female patients with alopecia areata. J Dermatol. 2013;40(3):225–6.

141. Park J, Kim D-W, Park S-K, et al. Role of hair prostheses (wigs) in patients with severe alopecia areata. Ann Dermatol. 2018;30(4):505–7.

142. Messenger AG, McKillop J, Farrant P, et al. British Association of Dermatologists' guidelines for the management of alopecia areata 2012. Br J Dermatol. 2012;166(5):916–26.

143. Park J, Kim D-W, Park S-K, et al. Role of hair prostheses (wigs) in patients with severe alopecia areata. Ann Dermatol. 2018;30(4):505–7.

144. Head covers for hair loss from chemotherapy. Available from: www.verywellhealth.com/head-covers-for-hair-loss-from-chemotherapy-2249232.

145. Henderson R. Nasogastric (Ryles) tubes. Available from: https://patient.info/doctor/nasogastric-ryles-tubes.

146. Higgins D. Nasogastric tube insertion. 2005. Available from: www.nursingtimes.net/clinical-archive/gastroenterology/ nasogastric-tube-insertion-13-09-2005/.

147. Ryles tube. Available from: www.angiplast.com/product/ gastroenterology/ryles-tube.

148. Nasogastric (ryles) tubes [cited 2020 Dec 11]. Available from: https://patient.info/doctor/nasogastric-ryles-tubes.

149. Gardner KE. Hiding the scars: a history of post-mastectomy breast prostheses, 1945–2000. Enterp Soc. 2000;565–90.

150. Borghesan DH, Gravena AA, Lopes TC, et al. Variables that affect the satisfaction of Brazilian women with external breast prostheses after mastectomy. Asian Pac J Cancer Prev. 2014;15(22):9631–4.

151. Jetha ZA, Gul RB, Lalani S. Women experiences of using external breast prosthesis after mastectomy. Asia-Pacific J Oncol Nurs. 2017;4(3):250.

152. Post-mastectomy prosthesis [cited 2020 Dec 11]. Available from: www.hopkinsmedicine.org/health/treatment-tests-and-therapies/postmastectomy-prosthesis#:~:text= Post%2Dsurgical%20camisole%20is%20 often,or%20during%20reconstruction%20breast%20 surgery.&text=Partial%20breast%20prosthesis%2C%20 also%20called%20shaper%20or%20shell%20is%20 a,foam%2C%20fiberfill%2C%20or%20silicone.

153. Post-mastectomy care [cited 2020 Dec 11]. Available from: www.scheckandsiress.com/products-services/post-mastectomy-care/.

154. Thong MY, Manrique YJ, Steadman KJ. Drug loss while crushing tablets: comparison of 24 tablet crushing devices. PLoS One. 2018;13(3):e0193683.

155. Palese A, Bello A, Magee J. Triturating drugs for administration in patients with difficulties in swallowing: evaluation of the drug lost. J Clin Nurs. 2011;20(3-4):587–90.

156. Bain BJ. Morbidity associated with bone marrow aspiration and trephine biopsy—a review of UK data for 2004. Haematologica. 2006;91(9):1293–4.

157. Bain B. Bone marrow aspiration. J Clin Pathol. 2001;54(9):657–63.

158. Bone marrow aspiration and biopsy technique [cited 2020 Dec 11]. Available from: https://emedicine.medscape.com/ article/207575-technique.

159. Bone marrow aspiration & harvesting needles [cited 2020 Dec 11]. Available from: www.mermaidmedical. dk/PDF/Norway/1_Bone%20Biopsy%20&%20Bone%20 Marrow%20Needles/Bone%20Marrow%20Aspiration%20 &%20Harvesting%20Needles.pdf.

160. Hernigou P, Homma Y, Flouzat Lachaniette CH, et al. Benefits of small volume and small syringe for bone marrow aspirations of mesenchymal stem cells. Int Orthop. 2013;37(11):2279–87.

161. Kreidieh FY, Moukadem HA, El Saghir NS. Overview, prevention and management of chemotherapy extravasation. World J Clin Oncol. 2016;7(1):87.

162. Sait MK, Aguam A, Mohidin S, et al. Intravenous site complications for patient receiving chemotherapy: an obsevational study. Ann Short Rep-Oncol. 2019;2:1–4.

163. Peripheral intravenous cannulation & primary care specific medication administration [cited 2020 Dec 12]. Available from: www.ccdhb.org.nz/working-with-us/ nursing-and-midwifery/nursing-at-ccdhb/primary-and-community-nursing/iv-cannulation-drug-administration-primary-care-2017-final.pdf.

164. Farrell C, McCulloch E, Bellhouse S, et al. Peripheral cannulae in oncology: nurses' confidence and patients' experiences. Cancer Nurs Pract. 2017;16:32–8.

165. Nelson R. Lack of protective gear disrupts oncology care. Lancet Oncol. 2020;21(5):631–2.

166. Schieszer J. A call for better use of personal protective equipment among nurses [cited 2020 Dec 11]. Available from: www.oncologynurseadvisor.com/home/cancer-types/ general-oncology/a-call-for-better-use-of-protective-equipment-among-nurses/.

167. Personal protective equipment when working with chemotherapy drugs. Available from: www.halyardhealth.com/ media/128708/c15663_chemo_ppe_brochure.pdf.

168. Driscoll D, Giampietro K, Sanborn M. ASHP guidelines on the safe use of automated compounding devices for the preparation of parenteral nutrition admixtures. Am J Health-Syst Pharm. 2000;57(14):1343–8.

169. Kähler CJ, Hain R. Fundamental protective mechanisms of face masks against droplet infections. J Aerosol Sc. 2020;148:105617.

170. Lai A, Poon C, Cheung A. Effectiveness of facemasks to reduce exposure hazards for airborne infections among general populations. J R Soc Interface. 2012;9(70):938–48.

171. Gates D, Horner V, Bradley L, et al. Temperature measurements: comparison of different thermometer types for patients with cancer. Clin J Oncol Nurs. 2018;22(6).

172. Allegaert K, Casteels K, Van Gorp I, et al. Tympanic, infrared skin, and temporal artery scan thermometers compared with rectal measurement in children: a real-life assessment. Curr Therap Res. 2014;76:34–8.

173. Cook M. Tutorial S—availability of hospital beds for newly admitted patients: the impact of environmental services on hospital throughput. In: Winters-Miner LA, Bolding PS, Hilbe JM, et al., editors. Practical predictive analytics and decisioning systems for medicine. London, UK: Academic Press; 2015. p. 817–31.

174. Petzäll K, Berglund B, Lundberg C. Beds used at a university hospital: a study of functions, problems and requirements. Scand J Caring Sci. 1995;9(3):181–6.

175. Incontinence products to keep handy when providing home healthcare for family [cited 2020 Dec 11]. Available from: www.tena.us/Home-Care-Supplies/home-healthcare-supplies,en_US,pg.html.

176. 10 useful tips about the use of adult diapers [cited 2020 Dec 11]. Available from: www.care4hygiene.com/10-useful-tips-adult-diapers/.

177. Role of the wheelchair [cited 2020 Dec 11]. Available from: www.physio-pedia.com/Role_of_the_Wheelchair.

178. Sedgewick M, Frank A, Kemp P. Improving services for wheelchair users and carers—good practice guide: learning from the Wheelchair Services Collaborative. NHS Modernisation Agency. 2004.

179. Wheelchairs: information and reviews [cited 2020 Dec 12]. Available from: www.disabled-world.com/assistivedevices/mobility/wheelchairs/.

16 Medical Devices for Nephrology

Mohammed Abdelrahim Idris and Ahmed Ibrahim Fathelrahman

CONTENTS

DOI: 10.1201/9781003002345-18

GENERAL BACKGROUND

It has been noticed that the incidence of end stage renal disease (ESRD) has been rising progressively during the last ten to fifteen years. This in turn has led to progressive increase in the incidence rate of renal replacement therapy (RRT). The RRT incidence rate is the product of a complex mix of factors: the incidence and prevalence of diseases that may lead to ESRD, most notably diabetes mellitus[1]; the effectiveness of chronic kidney disease (CKD) management to slow progression to ESRD; the level of kidney function at which RRT is commenced; and, lastly, the availability of resources to provide RRT.

OPTIONS FOR RRT

Options for RRT include the following:[2]

1. Preemptive kidney transplantation, i.e., transplantation before starting dialysis: Transplantation offers survival superior to other modalities of RRTs.[3] Transplantation can be done after the patient starts other modalities of RRTs (e.g., hemodialysis (HD) or peritoneal dialysis (PD).

2. Hemodialysis (HD): This consists of either in-center HD wherein the patient comes to the dialysis center regularly, usually three times per week for the hemodialysis session, usually 4 hours per session; or home hemodialysis (HHD) wherein there is a home HD system, and the patient or a caregiver is the one who is responsible for running the dialysis sessions.

3. Peritoneal dialysis (PD): PD offers patients a type of therapy that can be conducted at home without the need to travel regularly to a dialysis center for dialysis sessions. There is little, if any, need for special water systems and minimal equipment setup time.[4]

The prevalence of each modality of dialysis varies worldwide. It depends on several factors including local experiences, availability of each modality of dialysis, health systems, and governmental policies of supporting certain dialysis modalities. While HD comprises around 80–90% of dialysis population worldwide, in Hong Kong around three quarters of the prevalent dialysis population are on PD and around one third of the prevalent dialysis population in New Zealand are on PD (see Figure 16.1).[5]

1. HEMODIALYSIS

1.1. BACKGROUND

Dialysis is a treatment for patients with advanced kidney diseases by which nitrogenous and other waste products are removed from the blood (Figure 16.2). It allows correction of the electrolyte, water, and acid/base abnormalities associated with renal failure. It involves the passage of the patient's blood through a dialysis machine consisting of a dialyzer with a semipermeable membrane which separates two compartments: the blood compartment and the dialysate fluid compartment. This dialyzer membrane will allow the passage of water and small molecular weight (MW) solutes, but not large molecules (e.g., proteins). For example, MW of urea = 60, creatinine = 113; vitamin B12 = 1355; albumin = 60,000; IgG = 140,000.

The process of dialysis involves the diffusion of solutes across a semipermeable membrane down a concentration gradient. This is the main mechanism of removal of urea and creatinine from blood and replacement of bicarbonate to the blood (derived by the concentration gradient between the two compartments).

Another process is ultrafiltration (UF) which is the convective flow of water carrying with it dissolved solutes down a pressure gradient which is caused either by hydrostatic or

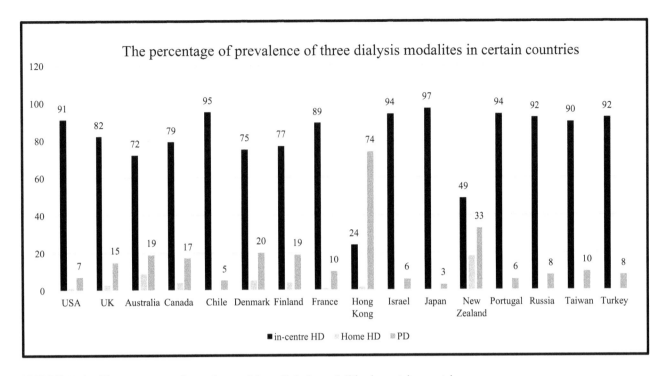

FIGURE 16.1   The percentage of prevalence of three dialysis modalities in certain countries.

Source: Adapted from data by Oxford Handbook of Dialysis. Fourth Edition. 2016

osmotic forces. Water moves freely through the semiper-meable membrane, and small solutes are carried on with water molecules "dragged" along. Large molecules will not pass through the membrane. In HD, it usually occurs because of the negative pressure generated in the dialysate compartment by the dialysate effluent pump (transmembrane pressure [TMP]). Excess fluids from patients can be removed by UF with some solutes that are dragged along with water.

1.2.   DESCRIPTION AND IMPORTANT FEATURES

Vascular Access for Dialytic Therapies

Efficient vascular access is very important for all dialytic therapies, and they represent the lifeline for patients with ESRD who need chronic intermittent HD (Figures 16.3 & 16.4). Ideally, a first choice should be an arteriovenous (AV) fistula placed peripherally (e.g., radiocephalic, brachiocephalic, or brachiobasilic AVFs). Other choices for vascular access for HD include arteriovenous grafts (AVGs), and central venous dialysis catheters (CVCs).

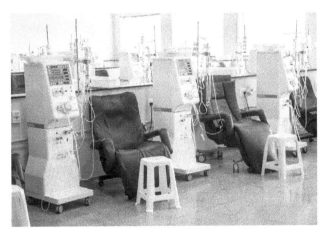

FIGURE 16.2   Hemodialysis room equipment.

Source: www.shutterstock.com/image-photo/hemodialysis-room-equipment-1296544153

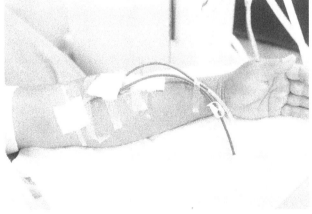

FIGURE 16.3   Vascular access for dialytic therapies 1.

Source: www.shutterstock.com/image-photo/end-stage-renal-disease-364878548

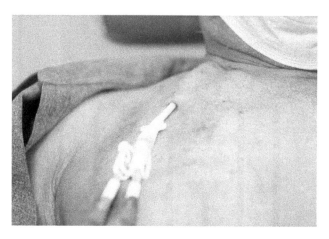

FIGURE 16.4   Vascular access for dialytic therapies 2.

Source: www.shutterstock.com/image-photo/human-vascular-access-594646253

Arteriovenous Grafts AVGs

When the AV fistulas have failed, or creation of AVFs is impossible, graft implantation should be considered as an alternative. Xenografts such as the ovine sheep graft (Omniflow) are well-known materials as an alternative access conduit, with acceptable patency and low rates of infections compared to catheters. The most frequently used implants are prosthetic grafts made of either polyurethane (Vectra) or polytetrafluoroethylene (PTFE). The material is porous, allowing ingrowth of fibroblasts and incorporation of the graft into the subcutaneous tissues. These prosthetic grafts can be implanted in different locations and configurations in the upper limb. AVGs are inferior to AVFs.[6] This is principally due to their lower long-term patency rates and higher need for endovascular interventions to sustain patency.[6] However, AVGs do have certain advantages which include having large surface area for needle positioning, being easily accessible for cannulation, having short maturation time, and having easy surgical handling characteristics.[7] Newer heparin-bonded materials in grafts are being used, but still there are no convincing data that they have any long-term advantages.

AVGs may be positioned in a straight, looped, or curved configuration. The common sites for AVG location are a loop graft in the forearm from the brachial artery to the basilic vein, a straight graft from the radial artery at the wrist to the basilic vein, or an upper arm graft from brachial artery to axillary vein. There are some reports and growing experience with the use of autologous, tissue engineered vascular grafts that showed encouraging results.[8]

The primary patency rates of prosthetic AV grafts range from 60% to 80% and from 30% to 40% at 1 year and 2 years of follow-up, respectively, while secondary patency (i.e., after correction of stenosis or thrombosis) varies from 70% to 90% and from 50% to 70% at 1 and 2 years, correspondingly.[9–12]

Central Venous Catheter Access

Central venous catheters are still widely and frequently used as vascular access for HD. Data from the Dialysis Outcomes and Practice Patterns Study (DOPPS)[13] show that one quarter of HD patients in the US are dialyzed with catheters; and it is even more commonly used in other countries (41% in Belgium and 28% in the UK). Central venous catheters are the favored vascular access only for patients who present with acute kidney injury and for patients with chronic kidney disease with failed vascular access or without permanent AV access.

In practice, there are two types of catheters used: non-tunneled catheters for short-term dialysis, which should be with a limited use only because they are associated with high morbidity; and tunneled cuffed catheters, which can be used up to several months with lower morbidity.

Temporary Vascular Access (Non-Tunneled Catheters)

Temporary percutaneous access should be used when access is required for < 3 weeks. Non-tunneled catheters are single or double lumen catheters made of polymers (polyurethane, polyethylene), which is stiff at room temperature and softens at body temperature. The right internal jugular vein is the preferred site (good evidence) but can be placed in subclavian or femoral veins.

To achieve adequate blood flow rates, the catheter's diameter should preferably be 12 to 14 French. It is advised that the use of non-tunneled catheters not go beyond 7 days.

Temporary dialysis catheters are easy to insert and easy to remove/exchange. They can be used immediately for dialysis after insertion. They are less costly than tunneled catheters. On the other hand, the rates of infection and venous stenosis/thrombosis are higher with temporary dialysis catheters. They are easily dislodged, and their life is shorter than that of tunneled catheters.

Tunneled Dialysis Catheters

These should be used in patients requiring temporary venous access for > 3 weeks. They are often inserted while awaiting permanent access formation or maturation (arteriovenous fistula), but also increasingly used for long-term access in patients who have exhausted all other access options, or sometimes (mostly inappropriately) as first-line, long-term access. Many different lines are available. There is only little objective evidence for major differences (Permcath®, Vascath®, Tesio®, Ash Split Cath®). They can either be duallumen with round or oval cross-sections, or two single-lumen lines inserted in the same vein. These catheters should be able to provide flow rates of at least 300 mL/min (often 400 mL/min). Ingrowth of fibrous tissue into the cuff lowers the rate of infection in the short and long terms and provides subcutaneous tethering. The internal jugular vein and femoral vein routes are preferred because of ease of implantation and low risk of complications, such as central vein stenosis.

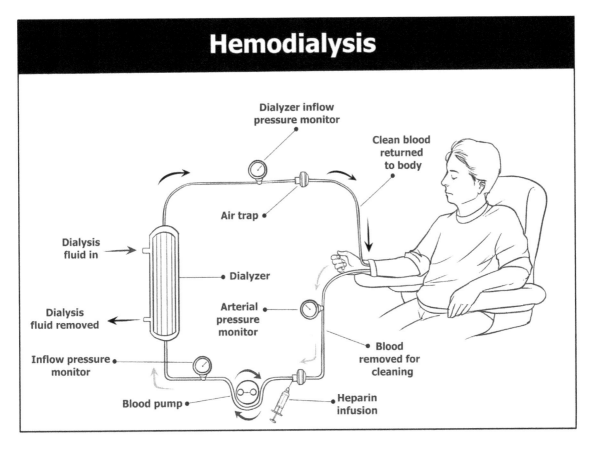

FIGURE 16.5 Illustration of a hemodialysis device.

Source: www.shutterstock.com/image-vector/vector-illustration-hemodialysis-device-1041118396

Dialysis System

The HD system's aim is to deliver blood from the patient to the dialyzer, enable the efficient removal of uremic toxins and excess fluid, and deliver the blood cleared from these toxins back to the patient (Figures 16.5 & 16.6). The dialysis system consists of four main components which are the dialyzer, the dialysis machine, the extracorporeal blood circuit, and the water purification system.[14]

Dialysis Machine

The dialyzer is designed to provide manageable transfer of solutes and water through a semipermeable membrane. The flows of blood and dialysate are separated by the semipermeable membrane and countercurrent (run in two opposite directions). The dialyzer has an inlet and outlet port each for dialysate and blood. The blood compartment and the dialysate compartment in the dialyzer are separated by a semipermeable membrane which allows passage of solutes and fluids between blood and dialysate fluid.

In principle, dialysis machines consist of a blood pump, dialysate delivery system, and safety monitors. Increasingly sophisticated monitors (blood, dialysate, and patient) and sensing software are incorporated to provide real-time management and a continuous record of individual dialysis sessions.

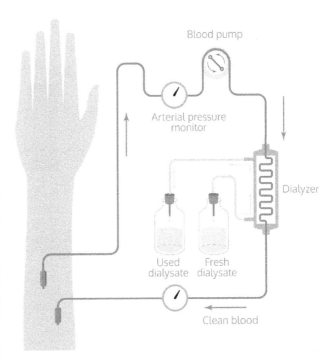

FIGURE 16.6 Dialysis process illustration.

Source: www.shutterstock.com/image-vector/dialysis-process-illustration-767190277

Blood Pump

Usually roller (peristaltic) with a usual blood flow rate 200–600 mL/min.

Bubble Trap

Minimizes risk of air within the circuit returning to the patient, when combined with a distal air detector.

Heparin Administration

Usually provided by the dialysis machine via a syringe pump (Figure 16.7).

Dialysate Delivery

Machines either mix (proportion) dialysate and bicarbonate with pure water individually for the patient, or a single machine performs this centrally before distributing the premixed dialysate to several dialysis machines. Dialysate concentrate is usually liquid (and may contain acetate), while bicarbonate is usually added via a second concentrate either as a solid (to be mixed with water) or as a liquid. Bicarbonate is almost universal now. Individual preparation of dialysate provides greater flexibility, while central proportioning can be cheaper. Water/dialysate must be heated to 37°C and degassed (to remove dissolved gases). The dialysate pump may allow generation of a negative pressure for ultrafiltration (UF).

Ultrafiltration Control

Ultrafiltration control increasingly achieved either by volumetric means or by flow sensors on the dialysate inflow and outflow lines, rather than by measurement of dialysate chamber pressure. Transmembrane pressure (TMP) is adjusted to achieve the desired UF rate. It can achieve accuracies of 99.5% (725 mL/h) and be programmed to occur at different times during dialysis (i.e., not continuously throughout a dialysis session)—sequential UF and dialysis. Maximal UF rates are 74 L/h.

Sodium profiling: Some machines allow the proportion of dialysate concentrate and water to be altered to change the concentration of sodium (predominantly) in the dialysate. This can be preprogrammed or initiated manually.

Hemodiafiltration

High-flux dialyzers can increase convective clearance by allowing high-volume UF during a dialysis session. Requires volumetric control and extremely pure water since large volumes of replacement fluids are used, and there is the possibility of back-filtration through highly permeable membranes. Replacement fluids can be generated centrally within a dialysis unit or, increasingly, by online filtration of standard purified water (within the machine) using two or three ultrafilters to ensure water sterility and purity.

Automatic Chemical or Heat Disinfection

This can be preprogrammed or manual.

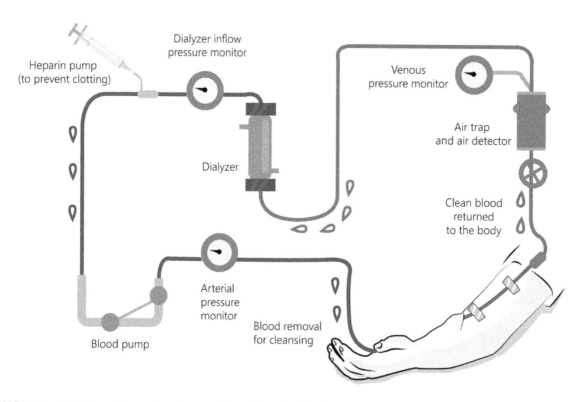

FIGURE 16.7 Dialysis machine and step-by-step flow of cleansing blood.

Source: www.shutterstock.com/image-vector/dialysis-machine-step-by-ste-flow-1419026924

Single- or Double-Needle Dialysis

Almost all machines allow either option. Single-needle dialysis has the advantage of a single venipuncture, but is usually less efficient, and has increased risk of recirculation. A "Y" connector allows arterial blood to be pumped into the machine, and venous blood to be returned to the patient through the same needle, but not at the same time. A defined volume of blood is withdrawn through the arterial circuit, before the previously dialyzed blood is returned to the patient. This requires specialized tubing with an expansion reservoir, since blood withdrawal and return are not synchronous, and usually needs two blood pumps.

Monitors in the Machine

The machine includes three types of monitors which are the blood circuit monitor, pressure monitor, and dialysate monitor.

Blood Circuit Monitors

These are safety monitors to guard against any entry of harmful substances with blood back to the patient during the process of dialysis. One of the important parts of the blood circuit monitor is the air detector.

Air Detectors

Placed distally in the venous circuit together with a bubble trap. Often ultrasonic. Linked to a blood line clamp to stop blood returning to the patient if air is sensed.

Pressure Monitors

Pressure monitors in most machines are integrated to monitor the system pressure in critical positions.

Dialysate Monitors

These are blood leak monitors to detect if there is any blood leak in the dialysate which means there is a rupture in the dialyzer (i.e., detects rupture of the dialyzer). These monitors usually act by infrared or photodetector monitoring. Sensitivity is < 0.5 mL of blood/min.

Temperature

The temperature is continuously monitored to ensure correct dialysate temperature. High temperatures can cause hemolysis. Cold solutions can cause hypothermia. When the monitor alarms, dialysate is diverted to waste. In some cases, this can be used to reduce patient's body temperature (usually by 0.5–1°C), to reduce hypotension, and improve UF.

Conductivity

The electrical conductivity of the dialysate is used to monitor the correct proportioning of concentrate with water. Many machines will use conductivity to allow alterations in the sodium concentration of the dialysate (sodium profiling). When the monitor alarms (high or low conductivity), dialysate is diverted to waste. Pressure:

The usual TMP is around 100–150 mmHg, however, it can vary between patients and treatment sessions. Some machines monitor the pressure in the dialysate outflow line to calculate TMP.

Online Kt/V

By monitoring the urea concentration in the dialysate outflow line, the actual amount of dialysis delivered during each session can be determined. This can also be done by measuring ionic dialysance in the dialysis circuit as a surrogate for urea clearance or measures of ultraviolet absorbance. This provides real-time reporting of delivered dialysis (urea) clearance.

Patients Monitors

Patients monitors in some machines include monitors for automatic monitoring of arterial blood pressure. ECG can be monitored by the machine (e.g., for remotely monitored dialysis).

Blood Volume Monitors

These monitor the hematocrit (Hct) or protein concentration in the arterial blood line by optical or ultrasonic sensors as a surrogate for blood volume (as water is removed from the blood, blood volume falls, and red blood cell and protein concentration increase). They can measure relative blood volume (RBV) reliably and reproducibly and allow automatic feedback. Reduction in blood volume generally precedes hypotension; hence, intervention prior to hypotension can be judged by the reduction in RBV and can reduce the UF rate, increase the dialysate sodium concentration, or infuse normal or hypertonic saline. Most software relies on expert systems, which "learn" the most appropriate time and mode of intervention for an individual patient. They can also measure absolute Hct and oxygen saturation.

In some dialysis machines the rate of blood volume change is used to automatically adjust ultrafiltration rates or to warn of marked reduction in relative blood volume. This technique has been shown to lower the frequency of symptomatic intradialytic hypotension.[15]

Access Recirculation

This can be measured by the change in temperature in the arterial blood line after reducing or increasing the dialysate temperature (by 2.5°C) for a few minutes (thermodilution), or by injecting 5 mL of isotonic or hypertonic saline and measuring change in conductivity. It is non-invasive.

Access Blood Flow

This can be measured by saline injection techniques during Hct monitoring or change in Hct due to a short period of UF.

Delivered Kt/V

This can be calculated from online measurement of urea (or total toxin) removal or change in dialysate conductivity.

Bioimpedance

Bioimpedance devices are increasingly used to determine fluid status in HD patients. A recent RCT in 156 chronic HD patients indicated that assessment of fluid overload with whole-body bioimpedance spectroscopy provides better management of fluid status, leading to regression of left ventricular mass index, decrease in blood pressure, and improvement in arterial stiffness compared with standard care.[16] Calf bioimpedance spectroscopy (cBIS) methods have been developed to identify normal fluid status in HD patients, and a recent study shows that cBIS compares favorably with whole-body bioimpedance methods[17]

Water Treatment System

Patients are exposed to 120–160 liters of water in a 4-hour standard HD session (and more with high-flow hemofiltration). In high-flow hemofiltration, large quantities of replacement solutes are directly infused into the patient, together with whatever contaminants are present in the water. Hence, water quality is of utmost importance to the patient's well-being.

Water from municipal sources is filtered to remove particulate matter. Activated carbon, with high surface area, adsorbs substances such as endotoxins, chlorine, and chloramines. Downstream water softeners use a resin coated with sodium ions, which are exchanged for calcium and magnesium ions, before the water enters the reverse osmosis (RO) system. During RO, water is pumped at high pressure (15 to 20 bar) through a tight membrane. The small pore size of these membranes (0.5 to 0.5 nm) provides an absolute barrier for molecules larger than 100 to 300 Daltons. This process rejects over 99% of all bacteria, viruses, pyrogens, and organic materials. Thereafter water is pumped into the RO storage tank and from there into a loop that supplies the dialysis stations. Common faults include carbon filters with inadequate capacity and recharging with inadequate frequency. Optional ultraviolet irradiation, to be placed upstream of a filter, is used to damage bacteria.

Requirements for chemical quality of water are variable and there is less agreement regarding tolerable levels of bacterial and endotoxin contamination.[18] At the very least, endotoxin concentrations below 0.25 endotoxin units (EU)/ml are suggested, and many support the use of 0.06 EU/ml or lower.

Home Hemodialysis HHD Machines

Until recently most home HD programs used conventional HD equipment designed for home use, e.g., Fresenius 2008K@home™ or Gambro aK96®; however the introduction of the NxStage® technology has led to its rapid uptake in many countries for its ease of use, small footprint, and probable cost- and clinical effectiveness. Sorbent systems were historically used in remote areas but are no longer available. Sorbent systems did not require a water source (just 6 liters of bottled or tap water), had no requirement for a reverse osmosis RO system, filtration, or water

drainage, and were easily transportable. Their dialysis efficacy, however, was limited. Conventional HD machines require permanent plumbing, waste connections, RO systems and filters, and space for storage of consumables, dialyzers, etc. Machines often have a slightly smaller footprint than those used in a center, can allow remote monitoring, and have advanced alarms such as wetness monitoring for patients undertaking overnight dialysis. The NxStage® machine is a compact single-pass system and consists of a cycler which controls the administration and monitoring of the treatment (flow, times, UF rate, etc.) and a single-use disposable drop-in cartridge containing both fluid and blood circuits and dialyzer. Blood flow rates are high but dialysate low in contrast to conventional HD. Dialysate is provided either in sterile bags or generated in a batch using a dedicated system (NxStage® PureFlow™). Ultrapure batches (usually 60 liters, for 2–3 dialysis sessions) are produced from concentrates and tap water, generally containing lactate 45 mmol/l (not bicarbonate), potassium 1 mmol/l, sodium 140 mmol/l, calcium 1.5 mmol/l. It has a very small footprint (38 × 38 × 46 cm; 34 kg) and once the dialysate is made the machine can be disconnected from the water supply. PureFlow™ houses 60 liters of dialysate and requires a little more space (60 × 74 × 80 cm). Patients would generally only use bags when traveling or away from their main home. The machine itself is portable, requires minimal plumbing, is easy and rapid to set up given the cassette-based system containing all lines and filters, does not require RO, and has a reduced carbon footprint. There is a reduced requirement for anticoagulation. The cost of the PureFlow™ system for on-line dialysate generation is significant but overall costs per treatment are probably comparable to conventional home HD systems.

Other new machines are in development for home dialysis therapies.

Wearable Artificial Kidney (WAK)

Wearable artificial kidneys (WAKs) have been successfully tested in clinical trials, proving the concept that this technology is safe and a potential future form of renal replacement therapy.[19] The WAK is light, small, and ergonomic enough to be worn as a belt, allowing patients to ambulate and perform activities of daily life while the WAK delivers sufficient rates of fluids and solute removal. The dialysate is recirculated through a series of sorbent cartilages containing urease, zirconium resins, and charcoal. These purify and regenerate the dialysate so it can be recirculated back into the dialyzer continuously. As a result, the WAK requires only 400 ml of dialysate. At their current stage, though, WAKs are not yet suitable for routine use, facing formidable challenges such as anticoagulation, toxin clearance, and fluid removal.

Continuous Renal Replacement Therapy (CRRT)

CRRT strategies are of a particular usefulness in hemodynamically compromised patients with AKI. They allow slow and gentle removal of solutes and fluid, avoiding major intravascular fluid shifts, and minimizing electrolyte disturbances, hypotension, and arrhythmias. Hypotension occurring during conventional HD may contribute further ischemic insults to the recovering kidney in AKI. Uremia is better controlled by CRRT than HD in catabolic patients with AKI. UF can be achieved continuously to match fluid requirements (especially enteral or parenteral nutrition, and IV drugs). Therapeutic drug levels should be more reliably maintained than with intermittent HD. Inflammatory mediators may also be continuously removed by CRRT, which has (controversially) been suggested might contribute to better hemodynamic stability. Trials do not demonstrate significant improvements in mortality compared with intermittent HD, but studies are not generally randomized, and patients with hypotension, cardiac dysfunction, sepsis syndrome, or hemodynamic instability are usually preferentially treated with CRRT. Clinical experience suggests that critically ill patients with renal failure are more easily managed by CRRT than intermittent HD.

The two most used techniques are:

1. CVVH (F)—continuous venovenous hemofiltration, and
2. CVVHDF—continuous venovenous hemodiafiltration.

CVVHDF combines simple UF and solute replacement with dialysate flow through the hemofilter (dialysis). Dialysate flow is slow. Overall efficiency is increased compared to CVVH and may provide better hemodynamic stability. Most current machines offer this as the first choice of modality.

Hemofiltration vs Hemodialysis

- Hemofiltration relies on convective removal of solutes and fluid (during UF), because of the pressure difference across the membrane, rather than the predominantly diffusive solute removal achieved by intermittent HD. CVVHDF combines both convective and diffusive solute removal.
- Diffusion is very efficient at removing only small MW molecules, while UF removes all plasma molecules passing through a high-flux membrane, regardless of MW.
- Hemodynamic stability is better maintained with convective rather than diffusive solute removal, for ill-defined reasons.
- Hemofiltration does not require dialysate, but does require accurate IV replacement of volume losses, either pre- or postfilter (pre- or postdilution).

Performance

Clearances depend on the membrane, blood flows, and predominantly on extent of UF. Urea clearances vary from 1.7 mL/min for SCUF, 17 mL/min for CVVH, and 30 mL/min for CVVHDF. Weekly urea clearances of 300–350 L/week can be achieved with CVVHDF, compared with 300 L/week for daily HD or 150 L/week for thrice-weekly HD, 100 L/week for CVVH, and 70 L/week for PD.

Standard Prescription

- Will depend on precise modality in use: For CVVHDF both dialysate flow rate and UF volumes are prescribed; in CVVH only UF volume.
- Blood flow 150–400 mL/min (usually 200–250 mL/min). Higher blood flows are needed to achieve higher volume UF rates, and with large filters.
- UF rate 25 mL/kg/h (measured as effluent volume).
- Dialysate flow (in CVVHDF only) 1–2 L/h.
- Heparin to maintain ACT 180–200s (unless contraindicated), or citrate or other anticoagulation.

Ultrafiltration

Controlled either volumetrically or by pressure. Pressure control can be maintained by adjusting the height of the UF collection bag in relation to the hemofilter, or by applying suction to the UF line. Simply adjusting the height of the solute collection bag below the filter will change the rate of UF. Volumetric control relies on a pump to achieve a fixed UF rate. Accurate monitoring of actual UF rate, and the pressures across the hemofilter are important. Total fluid removal of at least 10–15 L/day is required to allow convective solute removal, most of which is replaced (depending on the patient's volume status). UF rate is determined by the difference between UF volume removed per hour and replacement fluid volume returned to the patient. Current recommendations are to aim for an effluent volume (UF rate) of 725 mL/kg/h.

Access for CRRT

Dual-lumen intravascular catheters, or double single-lumen catheters, are placed in the internal jugular or femoral vein. Subclavian access should be avoided (risk of subclavian stenosis). Catheter position should be confirmed radiographically. Tunneled catheters may reduce infection risk but are more difficult to insert in the ICU setting. Complications are the same as for chronic dialysis vascular access. Blood flow is not greatly affected by catheter length but is by the lumen diameter. Catheter malposition, however, affects blood flow rates achieved.

Membrane

High-flux membranes (usually synthetic) are preferentially used for CRRT, given the permeability requirements of hemofiltration, but are not being used in the same manner as in high-flux HD, and have smaller surface areas. Comparisons of biocompatible and incompatible membranes have produced conflicting results on patient survival and renal recovery from AKI. Protein accumulation on membranes reduces efficacy with time.

2. PERITONEAL DIALYSIS

2.1. BACKGROUND

The peritoneal cavity is the biggest space in the body. The peritoneum consists of parietal peritoneum that lines the internal abdominal walls and visceral peritoneum which lines the intra-abdominal viscera. The peritoneum is used in peritoneal dialysis (PD) as a membrane for solute and fluid exchange between the blood in the blood capillaries in contact with the peritoneum and the peritoneal fluids that are instilled inside the peritoneal cavity during the process of PD (Figure 16.8). The dialysis fluid in PD contains glucose as an osmotic agent (or other osmotic agents can be used, like amino acids). The dialysis solution is supplied in plastic bags. During the process of PD, across the peritoneal membrane waste products diffuse to the dialysate, and excess body fluid is removed by osmosis induced by the glucose or another osmotic agent in the dialysis fluid. This process of fluid removal is called ultrafiltration (UF). PD is usually provided 24 h/day and 7 days/week in the form of continuous ambulatory peritoneal dialysis (CAPD) in which there are a few day-time cycles and a long overnight exchange cycle (Figure 16.9). The other type of PD treatment is often referred to as automated peritoneal dialysis (APD), sometimes also called continuous cycling peritoneal dialysis (CCPD), in which nightly exchanges with shorter dwell time are delivered via an automatic PD-cycler.

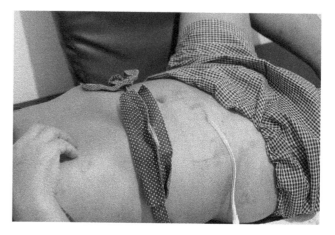

FIGURE 16.9 Continuous ambulatory peritoneal dialysis (CAPD) for acute kidney failure.

Source: www.shutterstock.com/image-photo/continuous-ambulatory-peritoneal-dialysis-capd-acute-1087181063

2.2. DESCRIPTION AND IMPORTANT FEATURES

Principles of Peritoneal Dialysis

In PD, solute and fluid exchange occur between dialysis solutions and peritoneal capillary blood in the peritoneal cavity. The "membrane" lining this cavity consists of a vascular wall, interstitium, mesothelium, and adjacent fluid films. Only about one third of visceral peritoneum is in contact with dialysis fluid, and it is therefore the parietal peritoneum that is primarily involved in peritoneal transport.

Evidence suggests that there are 3 sizes of pores in the capillary wall[20]:

- Small pores (average radius 40–50 Å) for transport of small molecular weight solutes
- Large pores (average radius > 150 Å) for transport of large molecules such as albumin
- Ultrasmall pores (3–5 Å), or aquaporin-1, permeable only to water and are the major water channels

Small Molecular Weight Transfer

Occurs by diffusion down a concentration gradient or by convection.

Diffusion

- Solute transport occurs down a concentration gradient, e.g., phosphate ions diffuse from a high concentration in plasma to dialysate which has no phosphate.
- Occurs through small pores described earlier.
- Small solutes diffuse at a faster rate than larger ones.
- Rate of transport depends on concentration gradient, peritoneal surface area, and number of small pores, i.e., membrane permeability.

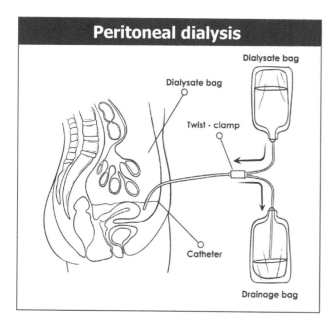

FIGURE 16.8 Illustration of peritoneal dialysis.

Source: www.shutterstock.com/image-vector/peritoneal-dialysis-both-used-treat-kidney-1044714154

- Rate of transport will be quickest at the beginning of a fluid exchange when the concentration gradient is the greatest. With increasing dwell time, equilibration will occur between dialysate and plasma, thereby reducing the concentration gradient and therefore the rate of solute transport. The speed at which this occurs will depend on the rate of transport.
- Concentration gradient can also be from dialysate to plasma, e.g., lactate in dialysate diffuses across the peritoneal membrane from dialysate into plasma.

Convection

- This is also known as solute drag.
- It occurs with UF (i.e., water transport down an osmotic gradient).
- The amount of solute transported by this means depends on the sieving coefficient (ratio of solute concentration in ultrafiltrate compared with plasma).
- Large molecules, e.g., albumin, predominantly cross the peritoneal membrane by convection and utilize the large pores.

Fluid Movement

- Net fluid movement, or UF, is determined by the difference between fluid transferred into the peritoneal cavity by UF and the uptake of fluid out of the peritoneum through peritoneal lymphatics.
- Water transport occurs across both small and ultrasmall pores.
- Ultrasmall pores—or aquaporin-1—account for 40% of total water transport.
- UF rate is governed by Starling's law and is therefore determined by net difference of osmotic and hydraulic pressures:
  - Osmotic pressure is determined by osmotic agent used in dialysate—usually glucose but alternative agents, e.g., amino acids, are used, and more are being developed.
  - Hydraulic pressure is determined by the intraperitoneal pressure which depends on the exchange volume and posture; it is higher when standing upright compared with lying flat.

Peritoneal Access

A safe and permanent access to the peritoneal cavity is the key to successful chronic PD. Most PD catheters are designed in a way with some similarities to catheters originally devised by Tenckhoff and Schechter (Figures 16.10, 16.11 & 16.12).[21] The Tenckhoff catheter is a Silastic tube with side holes alongside its intraperitoneal portion. There are Dacron cuffs, permitting tissue ingrowth that secures the catheter in position and precludes infection and pericatheter leakage (Figure 16.13).

Typical catheters contain two cuffs, one superficial and another deep one. Some catheters contain one cuff, and recently three-cuffed catheters have been developed with a third cuff near the distal end of the catheter to guard against catheter migration after catheter insertion.

The Tenckhoff catheter is straight, having one cuff lying on the peritoneum with the catheter tip pointing in the caudal direction; the outer cuff is close to the skin exit site. Several centimeters of the catheter are thus located transcutaneously in a design to prolong the passage of infective organisms from the outside to decrease incidence of infection. There is no perfect single design of PD catheters and changes in catheter design are continuously appearing. Although several reports showed less common catheter drainage failures with use of the arcuate "swan neck" catheter compared with straight catheters, there is no hard evidence that any of the modified catheters on the market are superior to the original (one- or two-cuff) Tenckhoff catheter.[22] A novel three-cuffed PD catheter has been invented and used successfully (the Saudi catheter). The idea behind a third cuff, which is located near the distal end of the catheter, is to decrease the chance of migration of the distal end of the catheter from its correct place in the pelvis. The initial reports of using this novel catheter are quite promising with significant reduction in the incidence of catheter migration.[23]

PD catheters can be inserted percutaneously using a Seldinger technique (with or without a laparoscope or peritoneoscope) or surgically.

Percutaneous Seldinger Insertion Technique

This technique is simple to learn and can be done easily by physicians. This obviates the need for theater time and general anesthetic.

Laparoscopic PD Catheter Insertion

- A specially designed peritoneoscope or standard laparoscope can be used.
- The peritoneoscope is a small optical instrument (2.2 mm diameter) used to choose the optimal location within the peritoneum, while the catheter is being inserted percutaneously.
- Peritoneoscopic insertion can be performed under local anesthetic, can therefore be done by a physician, and does not require operating theater time.
- Laparoscopic techniques are also used for catheter insertion, using standard 5–10 mm diameter trocars. There is excellent visualization of the peritoneum, allowing the catheter to be sutured into the pelvis, division of adhesions, and omentectomy as required.
- Incisions of both techniques are small, thereby reducing postoperative pain and minimizing the risk of fluid leaks, allowing early use of the PD catheter.

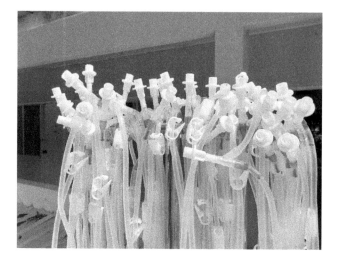

FIGURE 16.10   Peritoneal dialysis catheter.

Source: www.shutterstock.com/image-photo/catheter-peritoneal-dialysis-651263467

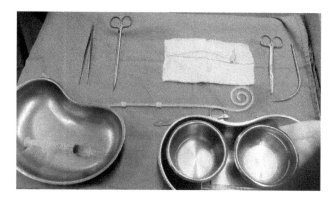

FIGURE 16.11   Tenckhoff catheter on the sterile green towel to be used for peritoneal dialysis.

Source: www.shutterstock.com/image-photo/tenkoff-catheter-on-sterile-green-towel-1044885112

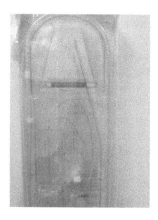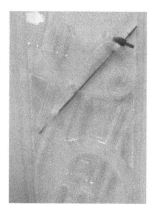

FIGURE 16.12   PD catheter kit.

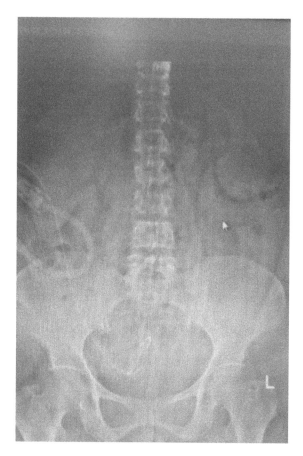

FIGURE 16.13   CXR after PD catheter insertion showing the catheter in its correct place with the coiled distal end in the proper pelvis.

3. TOTAL PLASMA EXCHANGE (PLASMAPHERESIS)

3.1. BACKGROUND

Total plasma exchange (TPE) has been used in a wide range of clinical indication (Figure 16.14). It involves the removal of large-molecular-weight substances which include pathogenic antibodies, cryoglobulins, and lipoproteins from the plasma. It is usually carried out using an automated blood cell separator to ensure fluid balance and maintain a normal plasma volume. This may require the insertion of a femoral or jugular line to allow adequate blood flow from a central vein. Arteriovenous fistulae also can be used for the procedure. Sometimes it is also feasible to execute plasma exchange using peripheral access via large-bore, short, intravenous cannulas, positioned in the antecubital fossa, especially with centrifugal devices because the rates of required blood flow are low. Single-needle access by means of an AV fistula is also reasonably easy to adapt, specifically for centrifugal plasma exchange, because the blood removal and return can be asynchronous.

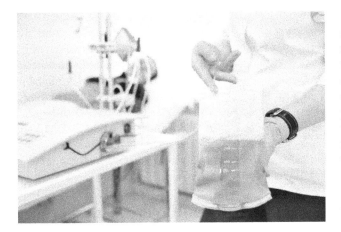

FIGURE 16.14 Plasmapheresis—the procedure of purification of blood and plasma from toxins.

Source: www.shutterstock.com/image-photo/procedure-plasmapheresis-purification-blood-plasma-toxins-1038363271

Typically, 30–40 mL/kg of plasma (1–1.5 plasma volumes) are removed at each procedure and replaced with isotonic 4.5% or 5.0% human albumin solution, with exchange with fresh frozen plasma (FFP) being indicated in certain conditions. A one-plasma volume exchange removes about 66% of an intravascular constituent and a two-plasma volume exchange approximately 85%. Plasma exchange became widely used in the 1970s after early reports of favorable outcomes in Goodpasture disease. Other techniques have also been developed more recently to permit more selective removal of plasma components, such as double-filtration plasma exchange, cryofiltration, and immunoadsorption with or without immobilized ligands.

3.2. Description and Important Features

Plasma exchange can be performed either by centrifugal cell separators or with hollow-fiber plasma filters and standard hemodialysis equipment. The latter is more commonly used in renal units. Centrifugal devices allow withdrawal of plasma from a bowl with either synchronous or intermittent return of blood cells to the patient.[24] The bowls and circuits are disposable and require relatively low blood flow rates (90 to 150 ml/min). A problem with centrifugal devices is platelet loss in which platelet counts can decline by as much as 50%. Membrane plasma filtration uses very permeable hollow fibers with membrane pores 0.2 to 0.5 μm. Plasma easily passes through the membrane while the cells are returned to the patient at the same time. All immunoglobulins will pass through the membrane (IgG more efficiently than IgM); yet, some large immune complexes and cryoglobulins may not be sufficiently cleared, although many membranes permit clearance of molecules up to 3 million daltons.

Membranes used in plasma filters are polysulfone, polypropylene, cellulose diacetate, polymethylmethacrylate, or polyacrylonitrile.

Anticoagulation is almost always needed. There should be careful management in patients with a bleeding risk; for example, those with thrombotic microangiopathy (TMA), recent or ongoing pulmonary hemorrhage, or a recent renal biopsy. In general, citrate is used for centrifugal plasma exchange, and heparin for membrane plasma filtration; however, citrate has particular advantages in patients at higher bleeding risk in view of its regional mode of action that lacks systemic anticoagulation effects.[24]

Both methods of plasma exchange necessitate large volumes of colloid replacement. A single plasma volume exchange lowers plasma macromolecule levels by approximately 60%, and five exchanges over 5 to 10 days clear 90% of the total body immunoglobulin.[25] Replacement with crystalloid is contraindicated because of the need to maintain colloid oncotic pressure. The major disadvantage of albumin solutions is the lack of clotting factors, with the potential development of depletion coagulopathy after plasma exchange. Fresh-frozen plasma (FFP) should be given, usually in addition to human albumin solution, in patients at particular risk of bleeding. If partial replacement is with FFP this should be given late during the exchange so that the constituents are not removed by the ongoing plasma exchange.

Human albumin solution (4% to 5%) must be used for all exchanges except in thrombotic microangiopathies (TMAs), in whom FFP should be used as part of the replacement fluid. FFP also should be part of the replacement fluid in any cases with high risk of bleeding and in cases that serum fibrinogen levels reduce to below 1.25 to 1.5 g/l or prothrombin time is risen 2 to 3 seconds above normal.

Mechanism of Action

Plasma exchange is the procedure through which large-molecular-weight substances are removed from the plasma, such as antibodies, complement components, immune complexes, endotoxin, lipoproteins, and von Willebrand factor (vWF) multimers. The clearance of antibodies from patients is varying and affected by several factors including the macromolecules equilibration rate between the intravascular and extravascular compartments.

Indications for TPE (in Renal Medicine)

1. Anti-glomerular basement membrane antibody (anti-GBM) Disease
2. Small-vessel vasculitis
3. Cryoglobulinemia
4. Recurrent focal segmental glomerulonephritis (FSGS) after kidney transplantation
5. Hemolytic uremic syndrome/thrombotic thrombocytopenic purpura (HUS/TTP)
6. Desensitization for highly sensitized patients of end stage renal disease before kidney transplantation to remove the donor-specific antibodies

4. PHARMACOECONOMIC EVALUATIONS OF DIALYSIS MODALITIES

This chapter did not focus on clinical evidence of the effectiveness of dialysis modalities because pharmacists normally are not involved in the clinical decision to provide a particular modality to a particular patient. This is absolutely a physician-decision practice and is likely to be affected also by the availability of the facility, overall cost, and maybe patient preferences. For example, according to Cruz et al., the Filipino nephrologists considered overall cost to the patient and residual renal function preservation as the most influential factors in dialysis modality choice.[26] However, pharmacists might be involved in policy-making or hospital committees responsible for selecting suitable modalities to be adopted because they are involved directly in purchasing dialysis devices as part of medicines and medical devices supply. Thus, the literature on pharmacoeconomic evaluations of dialysis modalities is more relevant to the pharmacy personnel.

Mushi et al. conducted a systematic review of the cost of dialysis in low- and middle-income countries.[27] They reviewed evidence from studies published during 1998 to March 2013. The review revealed that each year HD cost Int\$3,424 to Int\$42,785, and PD cost Int\$7,974 to Int\$47,971 per patient. Items likely to affect the cost are direct medical cost, particularly medications and consumables for HD, and tubing and dialysis solutions for PD. The authors made a conclusion highlighting the scarcity of economic research evaluating dialysis in low- and middle-income countries. Available research suggests that dialysis is a costly treatment option for the societies in such countries, which increases the burden on the already poor economics and reduces health service coverage. Rosselli et al. from Colombia compared kidney transplantation with chronic dialysis among patients with ESRD using cost-effectiveness study.[28] The study was conducted from the Colombian healthcare system perspective using QALY as a measure of effectiveness. A Markov model was included in analyses covering a period of five years. The study outcomes included deaths prevented, months of dialysis averted, and months of life gained. The study revealed that renal transplantation is a cost-saving option over dialysis and that it improves patients' survival rates and quality of life. Yang et al. from Singapore estimated 10-year period incremental cost-effectiveness ratios (ICERs) of HD, CAPD, and APD from the societal perspective.[29] The study revealed that CAPD is the most cost-effective option to start with for ESRD patients in Singapore.

Afiatin et al. assessed the economics of HD and PD as first policy compared with supportive care choice in ESRD Indonesian patients.[30] They used Markov model-based analysis to compute costs and health-related outcomes in terms of life years (LYs) and QALYs. They found that the most cost-effective alternative first-policy option was that of PD over HD.

Surendra et al. in Malaysia compared HD and CAPD using cost-utility and Markov model analysis from a Ministry of Health perspective.[31] The outcomes were cost/life year (LY), cost/QALY, and ICER. Analyses revealed that beginning with CAPD as the initial dialysis modality in 50% of ESRD patients was very cost-effective over the existing practice of 40%. Decline in CAPD selection resulted in greater costs and a little reduction in QALYs. Findings indicated that offering both modalities is economically viable; however, prioritizing CAPD as the initial modality is more cost-effective.

5. IMPLICATION TO THE PHARMACY PROFESSION AND PHARMACY PRACTICE

1. Various dialysis modalities have been assessed widely from economic side of view in the literature as has been described before. Pharmacists need to be aware of such literature; however, they should interpret it carefully to be sure that a particular evidence is applicable in their setting. An important study characteristic to consider in the interpretation of economic evaluation is the study perspective, whether a healthcare provider (hospital or ministry of health), societal, patient, or a payer. Pharmacists should consider the evidence from a similar setting (similar background and available resources and facilities) and review carefully all aspects of methodology such as types of cost accounted for and the sources of data. Sensitivity analyses are important to understand to what extend the economic evidence might be modifiable according to changing study assumptions.

2. It is important to mention that studies simply calculating the cost of treatment using certain dialysis modalities are not indicating the cost-effectiveness. They are useful only for estimating and securing the required budget. Cost-effectiveness means achieving the required outcomes (clinical, humanistic, or economic) using the least possible cost. An option that looks more expensive might be cost-effective if the increase in outcomes is high enough to justify the increase in cost.

3. Evidence indicates that providing specific care services from healthcare professional to patients undergoing dialysis improves patients' clinical outcomes, satisfaction, and quality of life. Sellars et al. conducted a person-centered decision analysis to determine the outcomes and hospital costs of advance care planning (ACP) intervention led by nurses against usual care during the last 12 months of life for elder patients with ESRD managed with hemodialysis.[32] Their findings indicated that ACP led by nurses got patient preferences but with additional cost. This can be extrapolated to the pharmacy personnel. According to Peter et al., collaborative care models involving pharmacists

improve blood pressure management in patients with CKD.[33] According to Qudah et al., the collaboration between clinical pharmacists and physicians improves the control of BP in patients performing hemodialysis.[34]

6. LESSONS LEARNED/POINTS TO REMEMBER

- Nephrologists and medical practitioners including pharmacists need to be ready to get maximal benefits of the rapidly progressing technology regarding medical devices.
- Well-designed studies are well advised aiming to test potential benefits of new devices in the care and management of patients with kidney diseases, which will help in updating the management guidelines and local policies.
- The economics of dialysis modalities should be considered while adopting the modalities suitable for every setting of practice, and the pharmacists who are involved in such a task should be aware of the available evidence from health economics research.

7. CONCLUSIONS

In the field of nephrology, advances in medical devices technology have played, and continued to play, a major role in patient management and outcome. For example, advances in hemodialysis and peritoneal dialysis machines played a very important role in improving care of the patient with end stage renal diseases. It led to improvement of dialysis efficiency and adequacy which in turn had a good effect on patient care and survival. The continuing advances in medical devices, thus, are expected to continually improve care and outcome of patients with kidney diseases.

REFERENCES

1. Rayner HC, Baharani J, Dasgupta I, et al. Does community-wide chronic kidney disease management improve patient outcomes? Nephrol Dial Transplant. 2014;29:644–9.
2. Devine PA, Aisling EC. Renal replacement therapy should be tailored to the patient. Practitioner. 2014:258:19–22.
3. Kallab S, Bassil N, Esposito L, et al. Indication for and barriers to preemptive kidney transplantation: Transplant Proc. 2010, 42:782–4.
4. Lo WK, Kwan TH, Ho YW, et al. Preparing patients for peritoneal dialysis. Perit Dial Int. 2008:28(suppl 3):S69–S71.
5. Oxford handbook of dialysis. 4th edn. Oxford: Oxford University Press; 2016.
6. Lok CE, Sontrop JM, Tomlinson G, et al. Cumulative patency of contemporary fistulas versus grafts (2000–2010). Clin J Am Soc Nephrol. 2013;8:810–18.
7. Maya ID, Oser R, Saddekni S, et al. Vascular access stenosis: comparison of arteriovenous grafts and fistulas. Am J Kidney Dis. 2004,44:859–65.
8. Wystrychowski W, McAllister TN, Zagalski K, et al. First human use of an allogeneic tissue-engineered vascular graft for hemodialysis access. J Vasc Surg. 2014.
9. Glickman MH, Stokes GK, Ross JR, et al. Multicenter evaluation of a polyurethane vascular access graft as compared with the expanded polytetrafluoroethylene vascular access graft in hemodialysis applications. J Vasc Surg. 2001;34:465–72.
10. Kaufman JL, Garb JL, Berman JA, et al. A prospective comparison of two expanded polytetrafluoroethylene grafts for linear forearm hemodialysis access: does the manufacturer matter? J Am Coll Surg. 1997;185:74–9.
11. Lenz BJ, Veldenz HC, Dennis JW, et al. A three-year follow-up on standard versus thin wall ePTFE grafts for hemodialysis. J Vasc Surg. 1998;28:464–70.
12. Garcia-Pajares R, Polo JR, Flores A, et al. Upper arm polytetrafluoroethylene grafts for dialysis access. Analysis of two different graft sizes: 6 mm and 6–8 mm. Vasc Endovasc Surg. 2003;37:335–43.
13. Ethier J, Mendelssohn DC, Elder SJ, et al. Vascular access use and outcomes: an international perspective from the dialysis outcomes and practice patterns study. Nephrol Dial Transplant. 2008;23:3219–26.
14. Misra M. The basics of hemodialysis equipment. Hemodial Int. 2005;9:30–6.
15. Santoro A, Mancini E, Basile C, et al. Blood volume controlled hemodialysis in hypotension-prone patients: a randomized, multicenter controlled trial. Kidney Int. 2002;62:1034–45.
16. Hur E, Usta M, Toz H, et al. Effect of fluid management guided by bioimpedance spectroscopy on cardiovascular parameters in hemodialysis patients: a randomized controlled trial. Am J Kidney Dis. 2013;61:957–65.
17. Liu L, Zhu F, Raimann J, et al. Determination of fluid status in haemodialysis patients with whole body and calf bioimpedance techniques. Nephrology (Carlton). 2012;17:131–40.
18. Glorieux G, Neirynck N, Veys N, Vanholder R. Dialysis water and fluid purity: more than endotoxin. Nephrol Dial Transplant. 2012;27:4010–21.
19. Gura V, Rivara MB, Bieber S, et al. A wearable artificial kidney for patients with end-stage renal disease. JCI Insight. 2016;1(8).
20. Rippe B, Stelin G. Simulations of peritoneal solute transport during continuous ambulatory peritoneal dialysis (CAPD). Application of two-pore formalism. Kidney Int. 1989;35:1234–44.
21. Tenckhoff H, Schechter H. A bacteriologically safe peritoneal access device. Trans Am Soc Artif Intern Organs. 1973;10:363–70.
22. Flanigan M, Gokal R. Peritoneal catheters and exit-site practices toward optimum peritoneal access: a review of current developments. Perit Dial Int. 2005;25:132–9.
23. Hwiesh AKAI, Rahman ISA, Audah NAI, et al. A Novel three cuff peritoneal dialysis catheter with low entry technique: three years single center experience. Urol Nephrol Open Access J. 2017;4(5):150–6.
24. Kaplan AA. Therapeutic plasma exchange: a technical and operational review. J Clin Apher. 2013;28:3–10.
25. Derksen RH, Schuurman HJ, Meyling FH, et al. The efficacy of plasma exchange in the removal of plasma components. J Lab Clin Med. 1984;104:346–54.

26. Cruz DN, Troidle L, Danguilan R, et al. Factors influencing dialysis modality for end-stage renal disease in developing countries: a survey of Filipino nephrologists. Blood Purif. 2011;32(2):117–23.

27. Mushi L, Marschall P, Fleßa S. The cost of dialysis in low and middle-income countries: a systematic review. BMC Health Serv Res. 2015 Jun;15(1):1–0.

28. Rosselli D, Rueda JD, Diaz CE. Cost-effectiveness of kidney transplantation compared with chronic dialysis in end-stage renal disease. Saudi J Kidney Dis Transplant. 2015 Jul 1;26(4):733.

29. Yang F, Lau T, Luo N. Cost-effectiveness of haemodialysis and peritoneal dialysis for patients with end-stage renal disease in Singapore. Nephrology. 2016 Aug;21(8):669–77.

30. Afiatin, Khoe LC, Kristin E, et al. Economic evaluation of policy options for dialysis in end-stage renal disease patients under the universal health coverage in Indonesia. PLoS ONE. 2017 May 18;12(5): e0177436.

31. Surendra NK, Abdul Manaf MR, Hooi LS, et al. Cost utility analysis of end stage renal disease treatment in Ministry of Health dialysis centres, Malaysia: hemodialysis versus continuous ambulatory peritoneal dialysis. PLoS One. 2019 Oct 23;14(10): e0218422.

32. Sellars M, Clayton JM, Detering KM, et al. Costs and outcomes of advance care planning and end-of-life care for older adults with end-stage kidney disease: a person-centred decision analysis. PLoS One. 2019 May 31;14(5): e0217787.

33. Peter WL, Farley TM, Carter BL. Role of collaborative care models including pharmacists in improving blood pressure management in chronic kidney disease patients. Curr Opin Nephrol Hypertens. 2011 Sep 1;20(5):498–503.

34. Qudah B, Albsoul-Younes A, Alawa E, et al. Role of clinical pharmacist in the management of blood pressure in dialysis patients. Int J Clin Pharm. 2016 Aug;38(4):931–40.

17 Medical Devices for Orthopedics

Binaya Sapkota, Sunil Shrestha, Salina Sahukhala, and Rishi Ram Poudel

CONTENTS

GENERAL BACKGROUND

Immobility may be caused by Parkinson's disease (PD), spinal cord injury (SCI), cerebral palsy (CP), traumatic brain injury, multiple sclerosis (MS), or muscular dystrophy (MD).[1,2] Lower-extremity orthopedic conditions such as hip fracture, femur fracture, or lower-extremity amputation may also lead to mobility impairment.[1] Impaired gait is characterized by decreased walking speed, shorter stride (i.e., step in walking) length, and enhanced gait variability.[3]

Pain on weight-bearing results in antalgic gait wherein stance phase is significantly shortened as compared to the swing phase. Restricted mobility reduces learning ability and socialization, and has other negative consequences.[4] Uses of proper assistive devices (AD) lead to physiologic benefits such as improved cardiorespiratory function, increased circulation, and prevention of osteoporosis. On the other hand, continued repetitive improper use may lead to excessive stress on upper-extremity joints and cause tendinopathy and even osteoarthritis. Still, high-quality studies are not sufficient to evaluate the impact of specific AD on mobility outcomes and fall prevention.[5] McSweeney et al. (2017) studied the most common causes of mobility impairment in 29 low-income countries and reported that those were road traffic accidents (RTAs), war, congenital malformation, leprosy, and polio.[6] Allen et al. (2001) studied the substitutability of mobility equipment for human (i.e., caretaker) involvement or assistance such as complete or partial substitution and reported that substitution of equipment for human assistance results in lower out-of-pocket (OOP) expenditure.[7]

There are various types of orthopedic devices available on the market specific to various orthopedic conditions. The global medical device market is expanding by leaps and bounds since these devices are non-medicinal alternatives for various musculoskeletal problems. Various lightweight as well as eco-friendly materials are given priority by the manufacturers these days. Designs are also continuously evolving based on experiences and clinical trials. We have discussed the ambulatory assistive devices (e.g., canes, crutches, walkers), seating assistive technology (e.g., wheelchairs, commodes), arm sling pouches, cervical collars, lumbar braces, chest braces, elbow and wrist immobilization orthoses (e.g., wrist braces, elbow braces), finger splints, knee braces, ankle braces, and compression gloves since these are widely implicated from the pharmacy's and pharmacist's points of view. The devices within each category may be of different types depending on their shape, size, or purpose of use. Physicians, pharmacists, and other concerned health professionals should select the appropriate device for the patients' conditions and counsel them on their appropriate application. Here, we have discussed in depth those devices which are applicable from the pharmacy's or pharmacist's point of view.

CHAPTER OBJECTIVES

At the end of the chapter, the readers will be able to understand the details of the following devices:

1. Ambulatory assistive devices: Canes; Crutches; Walkers
2. Seating assistive technology: Wheelchairs; Commodes
3. Arm sling pouches
4. Cervical collars
5. Lumbar braces
6. Chest braces
7. Elbow and wrist immobilization orthoses: Hand and wrist braces; Elbow and arm braces
8. Finger splints
9. Knee braces
10. Ankle braces
11. Compression gloves

DEVICE 1: AMBULATORY ASSISTIVE DEVICES (AAD) (ASSISTIVE TECHNOLOGY DEVICES [ATDS]/WALKING AIDS, MOBILITY ASSISTIVE TECHNOLOGY [MAT]/DEVICES): CANES, CRUTCHES, AND WALKERS

DEVICE 1.1: CANES (WALKING STICKS)

a) Background

Ambulatory assistive devices (AADs) such as canes, crutches, and walkers are mainly useful for older people, especially with gait disorders, because they are not usually treated either surgically or medically.[5,8,9] Even if they are treated, these devices provide them with further ambulatory support. They help stabilize and enhance muscle action, reduce weight-bearing load, and help in ambulation.[8,9] They enhance gait safety and prevent falls and trauma. Nevertheless, there is little information about how their use modifies gait parameters.[3] Detailed information on these devices is still insufficient despite widespread prescription. Because these devices are mainly used by the disabled or mentally impaired, their adherence is generally compromised.[8]

Selection of Ambulatory Assistive Devices

Before selecting a device for an individual patient, the patient should be evaluated for whether he/she requires one or both upper extremities to achieve a balance of the body or bear weight. Patients requiring only one upper extremity can use a cane, while those requiring both upper extremities can use forearm crutches or walkers.[9]

b) Device Description/Important Features

Canes are simply walking sticks and are made up of a variety of materials such as wood (especially walnut, oak), metal (mostly aluminum), plastics (such as acrylics), and fiberglass.[10] They are adjustable in length to fit the users'

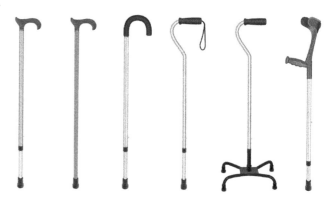

FIGURE 17.1 An assortment of canes, crutches, and walking sticks.

Source: www.shutterstock.com/image-vector/set-walking-sticks-crutches-telescopic-metal-786130408>

heights and needs and are available with varieties of handles and handgrips as per the user's needs and preferences, e.g., a spade handle decreases pressure on the user's hand and helps in better grip. A three- or four-legged pyramid cane enhances the total base of support preventing falls. Persons with bone and joint impairments apply more force to the cane compared to the patients with neuropathy.[8] Canes were initially used only for balance and not weight-bearing, but their modified designs (such as offset, multiple-legged, and walking canes) help in various degrees of weight-bearing. Significantly few researches have compared the efficacy of different types of canes.[8,9] A cane is usually the first assistive device used by multiple sclerosis (MS) patients to increase their walking speed.[10]

Adjusting the height of the cane as per user's need is crucial. If the cane is too short, the user may feel increased stress on the lumbosacral region whereas if it is too long, the user has to lean forward during the gait cycle. Hence, optimum height is a must while using the cane.[8,10]

Cane Designs[10]

Cane shafts may be straight, offset, folding, or height-adjustable. Straight shafts are the least expensive and most durable while the folding canes are more comfortable to store. An adult-size cane can be folded to about 30 cm height. A single rubber tip, broad with deep grooves, is present on the base of the cane to enhance the support area.

Types of Canes[5,8,9]

  i. Standard canes
 ii. Offset canes
iii. Multiple-legged canes (quad canes, quadruped canes)
 iv. Walking canes (Hemi-walkers)

i. Standard Canes   Standard wooden canes are inexpensive, lightweight devices whereas their aluminum versions are more expensive, but they have an adjustable length. They have an umbrella handle in general.

ii. Offset Canes   Offset canes are made of aluminum and have an adjustable length. These are useful for painful gait disorders caused by hip or knee osteoarthritis as well as for the elderly population. They usually have a shotgun handle which is flat in shape and helps distribute pressure throughout the hand.

iii. Multiple-Legged Canes (Quad Canes)   Multiple-legged canes provide an increased base of support and allow more weight-bearing than the standard one. These are useful for osteoarthritis.

iv. Walking Canes   Walk canes are broad-based aluminum devices compared to the standard, offset, or multiple-legged canes. They have two components: a vertical component with a handle and two legs, and also two additional legs angled away from the user. They are useful for cases of stroke with hemiparesis and moderate to severe loss of lower extremity function.

Measuring Canes[11]

While measuring a cane height, the cane must be placed approximately 6 inches (15.24 cm) from the lateral border of the toes. During this, the patient should be wearing appropriate, comfortable shoes.

These are the various ways to determine the appropriate cane length:

  i. Method 1 (floor to the greater trochanter): The patient should stand erect with the top of cane at the same level as the greater trochanter. The length of the cane is measured through distance from the floor to the greater trochanter.
 ii. Method 2 (distal wrist crease to the floor): The patient should stand erect with arms hanging loosely by the side. The length of the cane is measured through distance from the distal wrist crease to the floor.

Formula: Length of cane = height of the individual (meters) x 0.45 + 0.87 m. (L = H x 0.45 + 0.87 m)

c) Purpose/How to Use[12]

Walking with a Cane

- Hold the cane in your hand at your side to support the opposite lower limb.
- Make a tight grip and stand with the cane.
- Take a step with the injured leg and simultaneously bring the cane forward. Move the cane and injured leg forward together.
- Then step the cane with your noninjured leg.
- Repeat these steps while moving forward with the cane.

Stepping Up and Down with a Cane[12]

To go upstairs:

- First, step up with your noninjured leg.
- Bring the cane and injured leg level with the non-injured leg.

To go downstairs:

- First, step down the stair with the cane with your injured leg.
- Simultaneously step down with your noninjured leg level with the injured leg.
- Use the cane to maintain balance and support while stepping downstairs.

d) Important Safety Issues (Cautions and Common Adverse Effects)

- Standard cane generally has an umbrella handle, which may increase pressure on the palm of the hand.[5]
- One demerit of the multi-legged cane is that all its legs must simultaneously be in contact with the ground for its optimal function.[8,9]
- Patients with hemiplegia may not comfortably use the 4-footed cane compared to a single tip.[10]

e) Storage Conditions and Maintenance

- Improper storage may lead to maintenance problems in assistive devices such as loose rubber caps or handgrips.[5]
- Store the canes in an upright position near the user's bed to be used even in the middle of the night, but you may store the cane in the cupboard if the user does not need at night.
- Do not store the cane flat on the floor because this can make the user fall and possibly suffer injury while picking it up.
- Clean the cane with soap and water, and dry with a cloth at least once a week.
- Ensure that all caps are appropriately fitted to the bottom of the cane and that there are no cracks on the cane. Inspect the cane at least once a week to confirm whether there are any cracks or bends in the rubber fittings.[13]

f) Important Features (Capabilities and Limitations) and Special Advantages

- Canes are useful in case of sensory, vestibular, and visual ataxia. Standard canes are useful for the management of mild arthritis.[8]
- The multi-leg (multiple-legged) cane can stand upright on the floor; even when it is not in use. This helps the user freely move his/her hand to perform other activities. This is useful for the management of moderate arthritis.[8,9]
- A hemiwalker is mainly applicable for patients requiring continuous weight-bearing with only one arm, such as patients with right-sided hemiparesis or hemiplegia and moderate-to-severe loss of right lower-extremity function.[8,9]

g) Special Tips for Patient Counseling

- Detailed understanding of the patient's gait, cognitive function, physical endurance capacity, living condition, and preference is a must while choosing the appropriate ambulatory assistive device.[5,8,9] Patients' thorough examination of neuromuscular, cardiopulmonary, and orthopedic function status, as well as their home environment, should also be performed while selecting the device.[10]

- Users have to improve their exercise tolerance to walk with an assistive aid.[8]
- All the assistive devices must be appropriately fitted or used. Otherwise, musculoskeletal and neurovascular complications may appear due to the nerve and vascular compressions.[10] Properly fitted devices increase walking safety and reduce the risk of falling.[3]

h) Evidence of Effectiveness and Safety

Assistive devices enhance, maintain, and improve functional capabilities of patients with neurologic disorders.[10] Hardi et al. (2014) studied the effect of various walking aids on quantitatively measured gait parameters in community people and concluded that the assistive device users have better gait performance than when walking without it. They reported that the gait performances significantly improved when assessed with versus without the walking aid. They reported enhanced stride time and length, reduced cadence (i.e., number of steps per minute) and stride length variability for cane and crutches users, and enhanced gait speed and stride length, and reduced double support in the case of walker users.[3] Esch et al. (2003) from the Netherlands showed that use of walking aids results in reduced joint stiffness and disability as well as better pain control among patients with rheumatoid arthritis (RA) and osteoarthritis (OA).[14] Interestingly, Allen et al. (2001) found that the use of canes and crutches decreased overall hours of both formal and informal care compared to the walkers and wheelchairs.[7]

i) Economic Evaluation

Assistive devices reduce healthcare costs in the case of older adults by facilitating mobility and daily activities.[10] Impaired gait adversely affects work performance and efficiency, socialization, and quality of life. This leads to dependence on others and increases the risk of falling as well. These fall injuries may increase healthcare costs. These all have adverse implications on the household economy.[3] Wolff et al. (2005) reported that the average annual per capita spending for canes was low, ranging from US$0.17 to $0.85.[15]

j) Implication to the Pharmacy Profession and Pharmacy Practice

Since improper use of assistive devices, lack of sufficient user information and education, and duration of use may cause problems to the patients,[16] pharmacists have a prime role in bridging the gap. Pharmacists should instruct and train the users on how to fit crutches, how to walk with them, how to go up and down stairs with crutches, and how to sit and stand with them.

k) Challenges to Pharmacists and Users

Many patients and users are generally unaware of their proper uses. Bradley and Hernandez (2011) also reported that most patients with assistive devices are never instructed on the proper use and use inappropriate, damaged, or improperly fitted devices. They reported that most patients bought and used the devices at their discretion or the suggestion of their family members or friends. Only one third of patients usually get their device after consulting with a health professional, and only 20% obtain education on their proper use. Providing adequate education on their proper use may improve mobility and reduce disability.[5] Since improper uses of canes may lead to musculoskeletal and neurological complications and pharmacists are the first point of contact for community people, they have to instruct the patients on the proper use of the devices. Orthopedic surgeons, physiotherapists, and other related healthcare providers also have a role in instructing the patients regarding their appropriate use. Consultant pharmacists can also provide routine home visits to evaluate the patients' usage status of the assistive devices in terms of height, fit, and maintenance of the device.

l) Recommendations: Ways Forward

- Pharmacists should instruct and train the users on fitting and walking with crutches even up and down stairs with practical demonstrations.
- Pharmacists should instruct the patients on the proper uses of canes because their improper uses may lead to musculoskeletal and neurological complications.
- Orthopedic surgeons and physiotherapists should also instruct the patients on their appropriate use in their levels.
- Consultant pharmacists may make home visits to evaluate the patients' usage patterns of canes.

m) Conclusions

Canes are useful for older people suffering from gait disorders which are not treated surgically or medically. Although these were initially used only for balance and not weight-bearing, their modified designs are useful to provide various degrees of weight-bearing supports. Pharmacists have an essential front-line role in instructing patients on proper uses of canes to avoid untoward musculoskeletal and neurological complications.

n) Lessons Learned

- Canes reduce healthcare costs for geriatric patients with gait disorders because these facilitate mobility and assist in daily activities.
- Different types of canes such as standard, offset canes, multiple-legged, and hemiwalkers are available on the market to assist people in mobility.
- Canes, if not appropriately used for long periods, may lead to musculoskeletal and neurological problems for the users.
- Consultant pharmacists may provide home visit services to evaluate the patients' usage status of canes.

DEVICE 1.2: CRUTCHES

a) Background

Lower-extremity injuries limit mobility and functional abilities, making some patients permanently dependent on walking aids.[17,18] Crutches are one of the most frequently used assistive devices (like canes, walkers, and wheelchairs) and are used to provide ambulation support. When selecting an appropriate assistive device, many factors such

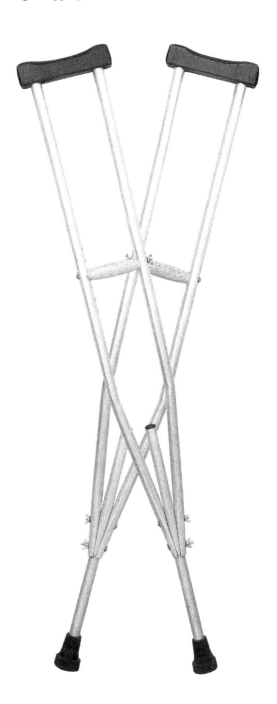

FIGURE 17.2 A pair of crutches.

Source: www.shutterstock.com/image-photo/crutches-made-aluminum-wood-leather-isolated-413207020

as weight-bearing restriction, ambulation, fitness, and cognitive level, as well as the user's environmental condition, are taken into consideration. Axillary crutches are widely applied assistive devices for temporary ambulation.[18] Walking aids such as crutches may have physical, psychological, and functional implications including boosting the users' confidence, safety, and daily activity. Appropriate walking aids must be chosen for existing neurological conditions associated with walking[16] because it affects the weight-bearing status and depicts a significant effect on muscle activity.[19]

b) Device Description/Important Features

Crutches are appropriate to transfer more weight to the user's arms than with a cane. Crutches generally provide more lateral stability to the user. A single crutch provides up to 80% of weight-bearing of the body whereas two crutches allow for 100% in swing-through gait pattern.[5,8] Wooden or metal with a molded plastic covering can be used as a handgrip. Height of the handgrip and overall height of the crutch are adjustable using nuts and bolts in wooden crutches, and through spring-loaded buttons in metal crutches. Wooden crutches are suitable for short-term use, whereas metal axilla crutches are more appropriate for long-term use.[20]

Types of Crutches[5,8,9,10,21]

    i. Axillary (Underarm or German) crutches
    ii. Triceps crutches
    iii. Forearm (Elbow or Lofstrand or Canadian) crutches
    iv. Platform crutches

i. Axillary Crutches Axillary crutches (ACs) are simple assistive devices used temporarily or permanently to support the mobility of patients. ACs are so named because the top of the crutch is sometimes known as the axillary piece. These are inexpensive and are adjustable for both hand height and overall length. They provide weight-bearing ambulation support but are challenging to use because these are energy-requiring devices.[22]

ii. Triceps Crutches Triceps crutches are made of aluminum and were developed at the Roosevelt Institute for Rehabilitation during the twentieth-century poliomyelitis epidemic. These are used for patients suffering from paralyzed shoulder muscles.

iii. Forearm (Lofstrand) Crutches Forearm crutches (FCs) are made of aluminum and are useful for providing bilateral upper-extremity support to the users.

iv. Platform Crutches Platform crutches enhance forearm weight-bearing in case of the upper extremity weight-bearing difficulties.

Axillary Crutch Measurements
- Standing: Measured from the anterior axillary fold to a point 15.2 cm from the heel of the footwear.

During measurement, the elbow should be slightly flexed (approximately 20–30°). Alternative methods for measurements include subtracting 40 cm from a patient's height or equal to 77% of the patient's height.[8,23]

c) Purpose/How to Use

- Place the end of the crutch about 5 cm from the side of the shoe and about 15 cm in front of the toe, and the top of the crutch should be about two finger widths (about 5 cm) below the axilla.[8] Hold the top of the crutches (also known as crutch pads) close to your sides.[24]
- Adjust the handgrip in a pattern that elbows bends 20° to 30° keeping the grip at hip level when your arms are at your sides.[8,10,24]
- Optimize the crutches to the users' heights. If these are too short, the user has to lean forward, whereas if these are too long, the user has to force the shoulders up and this increases the compression of nerves.[8,10]
- Put one crutch under each arm while you are standing.
- When you go up and down stairs, hold both crutches under the arm that is away from the handrail and use the other hand to hold the handrail.[20]

d) Important Safety Issues (Cautions and Common Adverse Effects)

Crutches demand high energy (about double) from the users and more coordination, requiring their proper fit. So, these are generally not suitable for frail older adults.[5,20,25]

- If the axillary crutch is improperly fitted, it causes nerve compression or axillary artery compression.[5]

e) Storage Conditions and Maintenance[26]

- Store the crutches in a dry place with a temperature between 5°C and 41°C and relative humidity of the air between 30% and 70%.
- Do not store the crutches by exposing to extreme heat or cold places (> 37°C or < 0°C). If hand grips are exposed to extreme temperature, high humidity, and/or moisture, damage to the crutches may occur. If exposed to extreme temperature (e.g., > 41°C), the crutches will be hot and need to be cooled before using.
- Protect the crutches from dust or grease by securely packaging them.
- Regularly clean the crutches, especially grips (handle) or base (ferrule) with clear water and dry the surface with a cloth.

- Do not use any abrasive or corrosive chemical, cleanser, or bleaching agent or greasy product because these can make the crutches slippery.
- Regularly check the condition of the crutch bases because these get worn out quickly.

f) Important Features (Capabilities and Limitations) and Special Advantages

- Axillary crutches are inexpensive and are used to provide weight-bearing ambulation support to the user with compromised ambulatory status.
- Forearm crutches allow for free movement of hands without releasing the crutch from the forearm. They are useful for paraplegia.[8,9]
- In platform crutches, body weight is borne on the forearm instead of the hand. This makes them useful in cases of elbow contractures and painful wrists or hands.[8]
- Crutches provide more relief than a standard walking stick (i.e., canes) during mobility or activity. They provide partial or complete relief when used for fractures of the legs and severe arthritis affecting lower limb joints.
- Crutches are used postoperatively after an operation on the muscles or joints or after amputation of a part of the leg. They can also be used for patients with neurological disturbance, such as ataxia.[20]

g) Special Tips for Patient Counseling

- Crutches are generally used in pairs. Otherwise, body balance may be hampered. Crutches enable patients to walk with a faster gait compared to a walker.[10]
- Keep the rubber tips of crutches dry which can become slippery when they are wet, and never remove the rubber tips.
- Look ahead while you walk with your crutches; do not look down.
- Take short steps and rest frequently and even request support at any time when you feel the need.
- Wear properly fitted and low-heeled shoes. Take care while walking on uneven or slippery surfaces.[24]
- Reduce the crutch use gradually as muscle strength increases.[19]
- Use crutches only on even ground and take special care while stepping up and down the stairs.[20]

h) Evidence of Effectiveness and Safety

Spring-loaded crutches are more comfortable than the standard axillary crutches.[27,28] If the spring is too stiff, initial ground contact produces a large impulse back to the body, whereas if the spring is too soft, the stored energy is not sufficient for propulsion.[28] The patient's height, the distance between the top of the crutch and axilla, and angle of the elbow should be considered while fitting axillary crutches.[21]

i) Economic Evaluation

Axillary crutches are the most widely used crutches in the United States, and cost ranges from US$20 to $50, whereas forearm crutches cost from US$30 to $200.

j) Implication to the Pharmacy Profession and Pharmacy Practice

Sadowski et al. (2015) found that 45% of pharmacists in Alberta, Canada had no training in fitting or providing instruction about canes, crutches, or walkers.[29] If the pharmacists themselves are not properly trained, the patients may not get accurate information on the device use. Patients should be well trained on climbing and descending stairs with the crutches.[22] More energy (about 60% more than normal) is consumed while using crutches and so these are not a good choice for patients with cardiac and chronic chest problems. Warnings of potential complications from the crutches should always be delivered to the patients. A short practical demonstration on walking with crutches is beneficial for the patient.[20]

k) Challenges to Pharmacists and Users

Crutches (mainly axillary crutches), if misused, may induce life-threatening complications such as embolism due to crutch-induced trauma, and non-life-threatening complications such as thoracic and radial nerve palsies. These complications are usually preventable. Thus, patients should be counseled on the risk of crutches use.[22] Crutches that are too tall can pull the shoulders up, and crutches that are too short force the patient to lean forward and cause instability.[21] Inaccurate use of crutches, lack of user awareness and education, usage frequency, duration, and pattern generate problems for patients.[16] Patients who have multiple sclerosis, stroke, and low vision may face difficulties in using crutches. Some patients may not tolerate the weight transferred through the arms during the use of crutches and may experience instability of the joint.[20]

l) Recommendations: Ways Forward

- Pharmacists should have the proper idea of the types of crutches available and should select appropriate ones for the target users.
- Pharmacists should counsel the patients that any crutch may have advantages and disadvantages based on their usage patterns.
- Pharmacists should counsel the patients and take their consent whenever they change crutches from one type to another.

m) Conclusions

Crutches are one of the most frequently applied assistive devices used to support mobility and daily activities.

Appropriate walking aids, including crutches, are necessary because they affect muscle activity. Axillary crutches, if misused, may induce embolism or thoracic and radial nerve palsies, which are usually preventable. Therefore, pharmacists should counsel the patients on the pros and cons of crutch use.

n) Lessons Learned

- Crutches provide more relief than a standard walking stick (i.e., canes) during mobility or activity.
- Crutches are mainly of four types: axillary, triceps, forearm, and platform crutches. Their appropriate selection for the particular mobility-related problem is essential for better clinical outcomes and patient satisfaction.
- Wooden crutches are mainly meant for short-term use, whereas metal axilla crutches are meant for long-term use.
- Patients suffering from multiple sclerosis, stroke, and poor vision may face problems while using crutches.

DEVICE 1.3: WALKERS

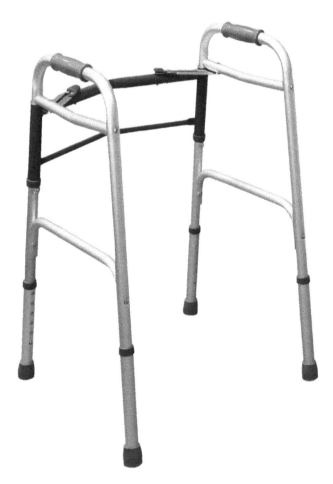

FIGURE 17.3 A classic walker.

Source: www.shutterstock.com/image-photo/medical-special-equipment-walkers-crutches-walkingsticks-1015315015

a) Background

The population of people aged 65 years and older is rapidly growing all over the world, among which 30–40% have gait disorders, leading to falls.[30] Each year, around one third of adults aged 65 years and older fall, accounting for 70% of physical injuries, morbidity and mortality, functional inabilities, dependence, and compromised quality of life (QoL); additionally, falls are the second leading cause of accidental death.[31–33] Need and use of assistive devices rise with age, ranging from 14–18% among the healthy elderly to 45–96% in frail older adults.[30] Walkers improve stability and posture in patients with lower extremity weakness or poor balance.[5,34] Assistive devices (e.g., walkers and canes) help the patients maintain balance during day-to-day activities.[35]

b) Device Description/Important Features

Walkers are usually aluminum frames used to provide bilateral support. They relieve the patients of the need to control a pair of canes or crutches.[10] They improve the user's posture by enhancing the base of support, supporting the user's body weight, and enhancing stability.[8,9] Varieties of walkers such as standard, folding, reciprocal, rolling, front-wheeled, and four-wheeled are available on the medical market. Gait patterns are variable while using the walkers, and these depend on the user's needs and the type of walker used.[8]

Types of Walkers[5,8,9,36]
- i. Standard walkers
- ii. Front-wheel walkers
- iii. Four-wheel walkers

i. Standard Walkers Standard walkers provide the most stability to the user, but because the user must pick these up off the ground before advancing, this renders a slow, controlled gait pattern. They have four legs with rubber tips that should simultaneously come into contact with the floor. These are useful for patients with moderate to severe cerebellar ataxia but less useful for cognitively impaired patients because these require more attention.

ii. Front-Wheeled Walkers Front-wheeled walkers are useful for patients who have difficulty lifting a standard walker. These are useful for moderate to severe Parkinson's disease, or moderate ataxia.

iii. Four-Wheeled Walkers Four-wheeled walkers are used if the patients require a broader base of support to help them walk long distances. They are useful for mild to moderate Parkinson's disease, and ataxia.

c) Purpose/How to Use[37]

How to Walk with Walker
- Raise the walker a few inches or centimeters, or up to one arm's length in front of you.

- Ensure that all four tips or wheels of the walker are in touch with the ground.
- Step forward with your weak leg and then with the other leg, placing it in front of the weak leg.
- Repeat these steps while moving forward.

Stepping Up or Down Stairs

- Place the walker on the step in front of you if you are going up and beneath the step if you are going down.
- Ensure that all four tips or wheels are touching the ground.
- To go up, step up with non-injured leg first and then bring your weak leg up to the step.
- To go down, step down with your weak leg first and bring your strong leg down.

d) Important Safety Issues (Cautions and Common Adverse Effects)

- Walkers reduce the normal arm swing and cause an abnormal flexion of the back while walking.
- They should not be used on stairs.[8,9]

e) Storage Conditions and Maintenance

- Keep the walker within reach of the user to decrease unnecessary efforts to search for the device. Fold the walker and store in a cupboard if not used for an extended period.
- Examine the walker monthly for wear-and-tear or damage. If the walker is used in more outdoor settings, wear may occur quickly.
- Ensure that rubber tips are clean and even; replace these with new ones if they are worn.
- Wipe the walker with an antibacterial cleanser and allow to dry. If the walker is wet, dry it off completely to prevent it from rusting. Thoroughly clean the walker at least weekly.[13]
- Check the wheels of the rollator walker, height, and brakes regularly to ensure they are functioning properly.

f) Important Features (Capabilities and Limitations) and Special Advantages

- Standard walker is useful in cases of myopathy or neuropathy, paraplegia, Parkinsonism, cerebellar ataxia, cerebrovascular disease, and hydrocephalus.[9]
- Walkers prevent the user from accidental falls and maintain the posture of the body.

g) Special Tips for Patient Counseling

- Use the appropriate walker type because the inappropriate type may cause an imbalance in the user's body. This can cause the walker to roll away and may result in a fall.[8]
- Flex the elbows at 15° while using a walker.[10]

h) Evidence of Effectiveness and Safety

Walkers offer a more comprehensive and stable base than other assistive devices such as canes and crutches, and are available in various adjustable sizes. Walkers reduce the weight load on the affected limbs, improve balance, decrease pain, and increase mobility and during ambulation. Walkers can be optimized to the needs of the users to consume less expenditure of energy with good outcomes.[30]

i) Economic Evaluation

Wolff et al. (2005) reported that the average annual per capita expenses for walkers ranged from US$2.04 to $2.57.[15]

j) Implication to the Pharmacy Profession and Pharmacy Practice

Walkers facilitate independence and improve quality of life with assistive mobility. Wheeled walkers may have limitations, including the need to reduce gait speed while avoiding an obstacle or while changing direction. Walkers should be selected depending on the patient's clinical criteria and degree of collaboration.[30]

k) Challenges to Pharmacists and Users

Luz et al. (2015) reported that many users might not consistently use their canes or walkers in homes, leading to the risk of falls although they were aware of preventing falls with the walkers.[32] Such intentional or any other type of primary or secondary nonadherence to walker use may promote falls, leading to high healthcare costs and public health implications.

l) Recommendations: Ways Forward

- Pharmacists should select appropriate walkers that the target users can comfortably and effectively use for day-to-day mobility activities.
- Pharmacists should appreciate the differences among various walkers to get their optimum clinical output.
- Pharmacists should not switch to a new type of walkers without the target users' involvement, consent, and follow-up review and demonstration on the proper use of the device.

m) Conclusions

Around one third of adults aged 65 years and older fall, and these falls are the second leading cause of accidental death. Walkers improve stability and posture in case of lower-extremity weakness and help the patients maintain balance during day-to-day activities. Still, many patients may not consistently use these in homes, which increases the risk of falls, ultimately leading to augmented healthcare costs. Pharmacists should counsel the patients about the differences among various walkers to get their optimum clinical output.

n) Lessons Learned

- Walkers improve the user's posture by enhancing the base of support, supporting the user's body weight, and enhancing stability.
- Varieties of walkers are available on the medical market, out of which standard, front-wheeled, and four-wheeled are the most common ones.
- Appropriate walker type should be used because the inappropriate one may cause stress in the body.

DEVICE 2: SEATING ASSISTIVE TECHNOLOGY (SAT): WHEELCHAIRS AND COMMODES

2.1 WHEELCHAIRS

a) Background

Wheelchair and seating-assistive technology (WSAT) is a device providing wheeled mobility and seating support for a person with difficulty in walking or moving around.[38] It is one of the lifesaving strategies to gain recovery and independence in cases of brain injury, spinal cord injury (SCI), or cerebral vascular accident (CVA). Around 20 to 100 million people worldwide, especially in low- and lower-middle-income countries (LLMIC) need a wheelchair, of which around 95% lack access to proper wheelchair provision. The term "wheelchair provision" was defined as a general term used for wheelchair design, production, supply, and service delivery.[6] Ultra-lightweight wheelchairs, which are manual wheelchairs weighing < 13.6 kg and having an adjustable position, are being common in the US.[39]

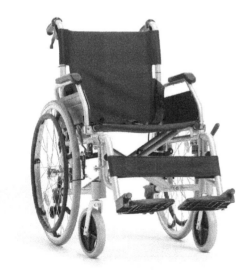

FIGURE 17.4 A wheelchair.

Source: www.shutterstock.com/image-photo/wheelchair-507404446

Criteria for an Appropriate Wheelchair[6]

- Satisfies the user's needs and environmental conditions
- Should be the right match for the user
- Provides proper fit and postural support (helps the user to sit upright)
- Can be maintained and repaired locally

b) Device Description/Important Features

Wheelchairs have a variety of customizable design specifications as per the individual's needs such as weight, durability, and cost; because of this, the notion of "one size fits all" does not fit.[6] Wheelchairs may be manual or power. Every wheelchair has the following parts as an integral component of the design[40,41]:

  i. Seat length: Seat length should be 2–3 cm wider than the seat of the user.
  ii. Seat depth: Anterior side of the seat should be 4 cm.
  iii. Seat height: Knees should be flexed at 90°. Seat height should be measured from the bottom of the heel of the shoe.
  iv. Back height: Back height may be longer or shorter depending on the trunk control.
  v. Headrest: Required if the patient does not have proper neck control and has cervical spinal cord injury (SCI).
  vi. Armrest: Distance from elbow to the seat when the elbow is flexed is 90°.
  vii. Belt: Required if the patient does not have sitting balance.
  viii. Cushion: All patients should use an appropriate and cleanable cushion to relieve pressure. Air cushions may be used in cases of seat sores. A flat seat cushion is generally preferred because it can be placed in any direction.
  ix. Footrest: Footrest should be about 5 cm high from the floor.
  x. Wheels: Wheels should have adequate dimensions based on the patient's needs.

Out of these parts, seat length, depth, and height are the three essential parts for the sitting position. Wheelchairs with at least three parts missing are not appropriate for use.[40] Wheelchair adjustments may be required in cases of neuropathies, skin integrity, reduced strength, and amputations seen as the late complications of diabetes mellitus.[42]

c) Purpose/How to Use

Sitting Down into a Wheelchair

- Lock the brakes and raise the footplates on both sides.
- Hold the arm rests with both hands and sit down into the seat gently.
- Put your feet on the foot plates.

Standing Up from a Wheelchair
- Lock the brakes on both sides and take your feet off the footplates.
- Hold the armrests with both hands and stand up from the seat gently.

How to Fold the Wheelchair
- Rotate and lift the footplates in the direction of the arrows indicated on the device.
- Lift the front and back parts in the middle of the seat and push inward to fold.

d) Important Safety Issues (Cautions and Common Adverse Effects)
- Use of a wheelchair while not meeting the criteria may have many harmful consequences such as physiological complications, compromised performances and independence, pressure injuries leading to reduced quality of life (QoL), and ultimately death.[6]
- If the appropriate sitting position is not maintained in the wheelchair, spinal cord injury (SCI) patients may face musculoskeletal problems.[43]

e) Storage Conditions and Maintenance
- Keep the wheelchair near the user when it is in regular use or store in a designated area (when not in use for a long period), protecting it from moisture to avoid rusting.
- Keep oil on moving parts for smooth movement.
- Check all nuts and bolts on the chair to verify that they are securely tightened. Check the wheel lock so that it does not rub against the tire.
- Wipe the wheel chair surfaces and cushion with a clean cloth at least once a month. Use a detergent or cleansing agent for stains and spots.[13]
- Pump up tires from time to time.
- Regular check-up must be done for rust and upholstery.

f) Important Features (Capabilities and Limitations) and Special Advantages
- An appropriate wheelchair has multiple functions such as assisting in breathing, drinking, eating, going to the toilet, and avoiding pressure injuries.[6]
- Wheelchairs are very useful for mobility in patients with SCI, and make users independence in physical functioning, mobility, and home life.[2,44]
- These are used as the base of support for day-to-day activities.[41]

g) Special Tips for Patient Counseling
- Keep the wheelchair on flat ground.
- Users have a fundamental human right to get education and training to improve posture and mobility with the wheelchair and seating assistive technology (WSAT).[6,45]

- Insufficient education and training may lead to improper wheelchair provision with adverse effects on the user's physical health, safety, and quality of life.[6]
- Always make sure that the brakes are locked before sitting down or standing up from the wheelchair.
- Do not stand up or sit down while your feet are on the footplates to avoid an accident due to rolling of the wheels.

h) Evidence of Effectiveness and Safety
Although some users may perceive wheelchairs as the evil necessity, this improves their mobility and helps the users in social participation as well.[6] Wheelchair users generally travel 1.5 to 2.5 km/day. This is possible for the people who use wheelchairs only with its help.[39] Assistive devices such as wheelchairs enhance QoL and mobility of persons with disabilities, and this parameter is considered the marker of the success of the impact of wheelchair intervention.[46] Wheelchairs are also vital for rehabilitation purposes[47] and help patients with impaired mobility to engage in personal, professional, and social activities.[48]

i) Economic Evaluation
Wolff et al. (2005) reported that annual per capita spending ranged from US$28.80 to $40.49 for manual wheelchairs and from US$23.06 to $138.81 for power wheelchairs.[15]

j) Implication to the Pharmacy Profession and Pharmacy Practice
Once WSAT is delivered to the users, they must be trained on their proper use.[6] Therefore, pharmacists can disseminate information on their proper use to the target users. If a wheelchair is used inaccurately, the user may not achieve the optimum benefit of all of its features, even leading to an accident. Pain and discomfort to the user are often regarded as an indicator to improve the wheelchair design or technology and seating environment.[41] Once the wheelchair is prescribed to the patient, he/she should be trained in its proper use and maintenance.[43]

k) Challenges to Pharmacists and Users
Ekiz et al. (2017) reported that more than half of spinal cord injury (SCI) patients misuse wheelchairs. Since wheelchair components such as seat height and seat depth may vary in different periods, the pharmacists and users must be up to date about the recent advancements.[40] When the wheelchair is delivered to the users for the first time, they may not get the right training in wheelchair operation, cleaning, and maintenance.[47]

l) Recommendations: Ways Forward
- Pharmacists and healthcare providers should check and train patients on the correct uses of the wheelchairs.
- Pharmacists and health professionals need to review the patient's adherence to wheelchairs at each visit.

- Pharmacists should give priority to the wheelchairs approved by the concerned regulatory authorities.

m) Conclusions

The wheelchair is one of the lifesaving strategies to gain recovery and independence in cases of brain injury, spinal cord injury (SCI), and/or cerebral vascular accident (CVA). Wheelchairs may be manual or power. Pharmacists should review the patient's adherence to wheelchairs at each visit.

n) Lessons Learned

- Wheelchairs have a variety of customizable design specifications, meaning that "one size fits all" does not fit.
- Wheelchair users generally travel 1.5 to 2.5 km/ day from the level of their complete loss of activity.
- If the appropriate sitting position is not maintained in the wheelchair, musculoskeletal problems may be potentiated significantly among the spinal cord injury (SCI) patients.
- Use of a broken wheelchair may deteriorate the quality of life by hampering mobility.

DEVICE 2.2   COMMODES (SANICHAIRS, SHOWER CHAIRS, TECHNOLOGY-ASSISTED TOILETS [TATs])

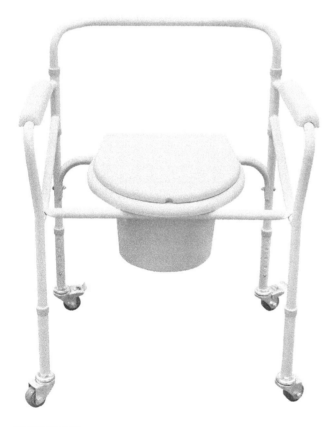

FIGURE 17.5

Source: www.shutterstock.com/image-photo/invalid-toilet-isolated-under-white-background-170129315

a) Background

Commodes are a type of assistive device specially used in toilets for mobility-impaired people. Commode chairs in the bathroom help prevent falls.[49] Commodes boost the users' safety at night by removing their fear about falling at the toilet.[50] Although commodes, sanichairs and shower chairs are used synonymously, they are slightly different. A sanichair has no pan, whereas a mobile commode has a permanent or disposable pan. A shower chair is similar to a commode if a pan is inserted in it and is only used while taking a shower or bath.[51]

Selection of Commode[51]

Following are the important considerations for the selection of commode:

i. Functional considerations
ii. User and caretaker considerations
iii. Environmental considerations

i. Functional Considerations
- Adjustable in terms of length of footrests and height
- Made of cleanable material
- Proper fit of the disposable pan to the commode
- Rustproof and waterproof

ii. User and Caretaker Considerations
- Acceptable appearance
- Comfortable in terms of design and height of the seat
- Stable when brakes are applied in the mobile commode
- Removable pan for cleaning purposes
- Transferable in terms of removable armrests/ footrests

iii. Environmental Considerations
- Sufficient storage facility when not used

b) Device Description/Important Features

Folding commode chairs with adjustable seat height are preferred in orthopedic settings.[49] Commodes are made of plastic material, stainless steel, or ceramics, or combination of these. Previously, these used to be made of leather, which is obsolete these days due to their foul smell when in contact with microorganisms. Commode chairs may or may not be fitted with a plastic bowl or pan to collect urine and feces. If bowls are fitted, users can urinate or defecate over the bowl, whereas, in the absence thereof, the users or caretakers have to keep the chair over the toilet pan so that the users can urinate or defecate over it. Commodes can be mobile, armchair, folding, or bed-attached. Each type is suitable for different users and environments. However, mobile commodes are widely used in hospital wards,[51] but since these are portable and foldable, these are also the preferred mode of toileting in household levels.

Design and Performance Standards or Specifications for Commodes[52]

Commode frames are usually made of aluminum, stainless steel, or PVC and lightweight but durable. Frame design and seat design are commonly considered design characteristics and their performance must be tested while evaluating the safety and effectiveness of commodes.

Frame Design
- Designs allowing access to the body for cleaning
- Frame shape to fit over a toilet
- Arm supports for leaning or repositioning
- Backwards-sloping seat angles to support positioning
- Rust- or water-proofing
- Folding frames to help in storage and transport
- Stability and safety during transferring, propelling (transporting), and washing

Seat Design
- Cut-outs or full openings to help access to the perianal area
- Seat shapes to maximize seating surface area and distribute pressure through the thighs
- Positioning within the aperture of the seat
- Seat materials and construction in terms of sufficient cushioning, and no joints on the inner edge of the aperture

Performance Evaluation of MSC
- Backwards-sloping seat angles
- Proper fit over a toilet
- Locking arm supports
- Removable or mobile arm supports

c) **Purpose/How to Use**
- Ensure that the commode is within the easy access of the user. Properly fit the commode to accommodate the individual shape and size of the user.
- Adjust the height of the seat and armrests to make these supportive and easy to reach without the unnecessary need of bending.
- Fit the commode in private so that the user may feel comfortable while toileting.
- Clear the area surrounding the commode of unnecessary clutter to avoid potential fall.
- Ensure that the commode's rubber feet are securely locked into place so that it remains stable during use.

d) **Important Safety Issues (Cautions and Common Adverse Effects)**
- Some users feel it unsafe or uncomfortable to sit on for any length of time. If the commode chair height is too low, users may feel difficulty while standing up after using it.

- Users may fall while getting on and off the commode.[50]
- Healthcare-associated infections (HCAIs) are essential concerns for the health professionals, users, and caretakers while using assistive devices such as commodes, especially in hospitals and also in the households. Therefore, environmental cleanliness and decontamination procedures are required to prevent and minimize the risk of the spread of infection in the community.
- Risks of the spread of *Clostridium difficile*, methicillin-resistant *Staphylococcus aureus* (MRSA), and vancomycin-resistant *enterococci* (VRE) are particularly severe with commode use.[53]
- Although decontamination procedures are followed, especially in hospital settings, still physical decontamination (i.e., removing dirt but not necessarily microorganisms) is the most standard method employed. This may not necessarily reduce the bioburden. Therefore, appropriate disinfectants, in terms of the nature of the material of the commode, should be used.[53]

e) **Storage Conditions and Maintenance**
- Store the commode chairs in a designated storage area after they are used and cleaned.[49] Commodes are generally supplied to the patients without any instruction on maintenance or without any information about the contact address during the occurrence of problems.[50]
- Check at least monthly for signs of cracks. Regularly replace the rubber stoppers on the legs to prevent the chair from shifting or moving.
- Proper check should be done for rust.
- Rinse the commode thoroughly with warm water to avoid skin irritation and then dry it using a towel to prevent molds, bacteria, and fungi. You may use a solution of ammonia and water (1/3 ammonia to 2/3 warm water) to clean the commode.[13]

f) **Important Features (Capabilities and Limitations) and Special Advantages**
- Commodes are mainly used for persons with impaired mobility, difficulty in climbing stairs, and/or urinary incontinence, and also for comfort in defecation at the bedside.[50]
- Adults with spinal cord injury (SCI) find mobile shower commodes (MSC) useful for bowel care, showering, and other daily activities. MSC frame and seat design should be customized to the individual user.[52]

g) **Special Tips for Patient Counseling**
- Use commodes that are suitable for them in terms of seating position and height.
- Maintain proper hand hygiene after its use.
- Clean and disinfect the commodes properly with alcohol or detergent wipes after each use.

h) Evidence of Effectiveness and Safety

Main concern for the commode use is the spread of infection in the community. Otherwise, it has lots of beneficial actions for mobility-impaired people for toileting. If proper disinfectant such as sodium hypochlorite solutions diluted to 1,000 ppm is used, it kills many of the microorganisms due to its broad spectrum of antimicrobial activity. This is also inexpensive, but the main disadvantage with this disinfectant is that it is corrosive at concentrations > 500 ppm. Its excessive and harmful corrosive effects can be minimized with the two-stage process of application and rinsing, but adequate contact time should be ensured before rinsing. Otherwise, its effectiveness cannot be experienced in terms of reduction of the bioburden. The person handling this disinfectant should apply personal protective equipment (PPE) as well. Chlorine dioxide has been proposed as an alternative to sodium hypochlorite since half the contact time compared to the latter is sufficient for it and is not corrosive to surfaces. Moreover, it does not need any rinsing.[53]

i) Economic Evaluation

TATs cost from CAD$400 to CAD$2,500, making them an affordable assistive device. Price may vary depending on the brand and its associated features.[54]

j) Implication to the Pharmacy Profession and Pharmacy Practice

Health professionals should be aware of the privacy concerns of the commode users when counseling them about the safe storage of their commode.[50] Pharmacists, users, and caretakers can work together to make its use comfortable and friendly, and they need to perform regular follow-ups as well. Hospital pharmacists should purchase a safe, functional, cost-effective commode that is also acceptable to the users.[51]

k) Challenges to Pharmacists and Users

Naylor and Mulley (1993) investigated the use of commodes and attitudes of users (140 users) and caretakers (105 caretakers) towards the users and found problems with commode use, such as lack of privacy, unpleasant smells, lack of follow-up after its supply, and others. They reported that most people used the commode only for urination but not for defecation, whereas only 16 used it for both urination and defecation. Some users applied deodorants, disinfectants, air purifiers, and ionizers to mask the fecal odor.[50]

l) Recommendations: Ways Forward

- Pharmacists should instruct patients to clean and maintain commodes properly and should ensure that they follow the instructions correctly.
- Pharmacists need to ensure that patients follow appropriate techniques for using commodes.
- Pharmacists should counsel the patients or caretakers to apply proper disinfection measure after

the commode use since inappropriate disposal of excreta after its use may spread infection in the community.

m) Conclusions

Commodes are specially designed technology-assisted toilets used mainly for mobility-impaired people. Folding commode chairs with adjustable seat height are preferred in orthopedic cases. Appropriate disinfection after commode use is suggested to prevent the spread of healthcare-associated infections (HCAIs).

n) Lessons Learned

- Commodes are mainly used for persons with impaired mobility for defecation at the bedside.
- *Clostridium difficile*, methicillin-resistant *Staphylococcus aureus* (MRSA), and vancomycin-resistant *enterococci* (VRE) may be spread with inappropriate commode use.
- The commode is to be fitted in a private area to make the user feel comfortable while toileting.
- Commodes can be mobile, armchair, folding, and bed-attached; mobile commodes are mainly used in hospital wards.

DEVICE 3: ARM SLING POUCH (ARM SLING/ POUCH, SHOULDER SLING/IMMOBILIZER)

A) BACKGROUND

Slings or braces help patients avoid physical activities involving the affected shoulder.[55] An arm sling helps realign scapular symmetry and support the forearm in a flexed arm position.[56] Usually, a splint, brace, or cast is first applied to the injured arm before using an arm sling. Arm slings are used to alleviate pain caused by a strain, surgery, dislocation, fracture, or injury in the shoulder, arm, elbow,

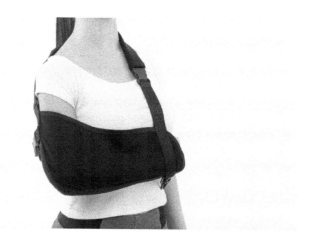

FIGURE 17.6 An arm sling.

Source: www.shutterstock.com/image-photo/broken-hand-wearing-arm-brace-1234385740

or wrist in adults and children. An arm sling is very easy to wear and adjust and has shoulder straps with pads and a thumb loop. The lightweight fabric used for its production is a breathable blend of nylon, polyester, and cotton mesh fabric which permits the users to feel relaxed in the parts used. Different types of arm slings are helpful for different injuries like fracture, sprain, strain, or dislocation due to an accident. Physicians suggest an appropriate arm sling for a particular condition. Hwang and An (2015) reported improvements in walking velocity with the use of elastic arm sling and found it useful for gait training for stroke patients.[57]

B) DEVICE DESCRIPTION/IMPORTANT FEATURES

A shoulder immobilizer is a soft foam support consisting of four parts: large chest strap, upper arm cuff/strap, hand/wrist cuff/strap, and shoulder strap.[58] The thumb loop provides support and stability for the arm and shoulder. The front-facing buckle allows the user to tighten or loosen the sling by adjusting the length of the sling straps. Arm sling is reversible for use on the left or right arm, i.e., the wearer can use it on both arms as per his/her requirements. Minimum and maximum lengths of the strap are around 17 and 34 inches respectively, and the sling itself is 16 inches long. Since it is latex-free, the users do not feel any allergic reactions after use. An elastic arm sling consists of four plastic rings made of thin, flexible polyethene and three elastic bandages. Four plastic rings improve the arm position of the affected arm and provide shoulder stability without the complete restriction of the arm motion.[57]

C) PURPOSE/HOW TO USE[58,59]

- Place arm in a sling and pull rings together.
- Hold the arm close to the body, keeping the elbow at 90°.
- Pull the shoulder strap through the double rings and secure.
- Bring waist strap around back.
- Pull waist strap through the ring and secure.
- Place thumb in thumb strap or thumb loop for comfort.
- Adjust the shoulder and waist straps to ensure a comfortable fit.

D) IMPORTANT SAFETY ISSUES (CAUTIONS AND COMMON ADVERSE EFFECTS)

- Immobilization slings may also lead to impaired gait and falls among some users.[55]
- Immobilization can also lead to pain, functional restrictions, and patient discomfort due to the delayed recovery phase.[55] If the users experience increased pain, swelling, skin irritation, or any adverse reactions with its use, they need to consult health professionals for its remedy immediately.

E) STORAGE CONDITIONS AND MAINTENANCE

- Hand or machine wash the arm sling in cold or warm (but not hot) water and lay flat to dry. Wash the sling separately if machine washing.
- Do not use an automatic dryer since the immobilizer is made of foam material.

F) IMPORTANT FEATURES (CAPABILITIES AND LIMITATIONS) AND SPECIAL ADVANTAGES

- An arm sling helps to treat clavicle fracture, relieve pain, and provide support during the first four weeks, usually a period of intense pain. Initial healing of a clavicle fracture occurs in around 6–8 weeks when the soft tissue (callus) bridges the fracture.[60]
- It provides support to shoulder, elbow, arm, or wrist injuries and stabilizes these parts following the surgery.

G) SPECIAL TIPS FOR PATIENT COUNSELING

- Use the sling to support the injured arm until the fracture heals sufficiently.[61]
- Wear the sling during waking hours except when toileting, dressing, bathing, and engaging in activities with risk of fall.
- Carefully read fitting instructions and warnings before use to ensure proper performance of the brace.
- Be aware that the device alone will not prevent or reduce all injuries. Therefore, excessive dependability on it and stopping all movements will not alleviate pain. Proper rehabilitation and activity modification are also essential.
- Do not share your used sling to others because it is for single patient use only.
- Hand wash in warm water using a mild detergent before and after use and lay flat for air drying.
- Remove the sling if the physician suggests small movement or during rehabilitation.
- Do not apply the immobilizer directly over the skin since it may cause rashes and fungal infection due to excessive build-up of moisture. Instead, apply the sling over the light cloth.[58]

H) EVIDENCE OF EFFECTIVENESS AND SAFETY

Whelan et al. (2014) reported that adherence with the brace or sling wear was good with 85% (51 of 60) for at least 3 weeks.[62] Myint et al. (2008) found the adherence of patients to the sling during waking hours to be 87.3% ± 12.9% with a range of 57.7–100%.[63]

I) ECONOMIC EVALUATION

Still, conclusive evidence of the effects of an arm sling on the physiological costs of walking is lacking. However,

Jeong et al. (2017) conducted a randomized crossover trial among 57 hemiplegic patients with chronic stroke in Korea and found that walking with an arm sling was more efficient compared to walking without an arm sling. They found that the energy cost and oxygen expenditure were lower among the hemiplegic patients with a single cane who used arm sling compared to the non-users of the arm sling. These improved the walking endurance among the arm sling users.[56]

J)   IMPLICATION TO THE PHARMACY PROFESSION AND PHARMACY PRACTICE

Tirefort et al. (2019) compared clinical and radiographic outcomes up to 6 months with and without postoperative sling immobilization among 80 randomly selected patients (40 with sling and 40 without sling). They found that postoperative immobilization with a sling may not be required for patients for a small or medium rotator cuff tear.[55] Seybold et al. (2009) found that sling immobilization was not tolerated more than 1 week in case of traumatic anterior shoulder dislocation by toddlers and pediatric patients due to the absence of pain and free range of motion.[64]

K)   CHALLENGES TO PHARMACISTS AND USERS

For adults, an arm sling can be used for the first three weeks at all times except during dressing, showering, and mild exercises. After three weeks, the users may gradually deprive (i.e., wean) from the sling but they should not immediately lift objects with the injured arm.

L)   RECOMMENDATIONS: WAYS FORWARD

- Pharmacists should instruct patients to clean and use the arm pouches properly.
- Health professionals should ensure that the patients properly understood the instructions provided.
- Pharmacists should counsel the patients that they do not apply the immobilizer directly over the skin to avoid rashes and fungal infection.

M)   CONCLUSIONS

An arm sling helps the patients avoid physical activities involving the affected shoulder and also reduces pain from injuries and surgeries. An arm sling is very easy to wear and adjust and has shoulder straps with pads and a thumb loop. The lightweight fabric used for its production is breathable, allowing the user's cool environment in the parts used. The users should carefully read and follow the instructions to ensure proper performance of the sling.

N)   LESSONS LEARNED

- Shoulder immobilizer consists of a broad chest band, upper arm cuff, handcuff, and shoulder strap.

- An elastic arm sling consists of four plastic rings made of flexible polyethene and three elastic bandages.
- Adults can continuously use an arm sling for the first three weeks except during dressing, showering, and mild exercises.
- Immobilization with sling use can also lead to pain, functional restrictions, and patient discomfort due to the delayed recovery phase.

DEVICE 4: CERVICAL COLLAR (CERVICAL COLLAR BRACE, C-COLLAR, NECK COLLAR/BRACE)

A)   BACKGROUND

Patients with head trauma may also simultaneously have a cervical spine injury. Therefore, cervical spine immobilization (spinal motion restriction) has been incorporated into the first aid management for unconscious trauma patients.[65] Today's modernized world has made almost everyone habituated and/or dependent on technology and the related devices such as computers and smartphones, chronic usage of which in a wrong and unhealthy posture may lead to cervical spine problems. Kuo et al. (2019) reported that stress on the cervical spine reaches up to 60 lb when the neck is tilted forward at 60°, and gravitational pressure on the cervical spine during tablet or computer use becomes 3–5 times higher in the neck flexion posture compared to the neutral position.

Similarly, a drooping posture during chronic smartphone use enhances gravitational pressure on the cervical spine, leading to neck pain and degeneration. Such chronic mobile device usage may lead to musculoskeletal complaints (1% to 67.8%), neck complaints (17.3% to 67.8%), and early cervical degeneration for which a cervical collar may serve as a support. The chronic users of such technological devices suffer from "text neck" (i.e., cervical spinal degeneration caused by the repeated stress of forwarding head flexion while looking down at the screens of mobile devices and "texting" for a chronic period). Head and neck posture can be maintained and improved by wearing a neck collar.[66]

B)   DEVICE DESCRIPTION/IMPORTANT FEATURES

Cervical collars may be rigid or soft depending on the requirement and preference of the users. Support to the head weight provided by the collar varies with the different materials and designs used for collar manufacturing, as well as patient adherence to it.[66]

Types of Cervical Collars[66,67]
- i.   Hard (rigid) collars
- ii. Soft collars (non-rigid cervical collar [nRCC])
- iii. Adjustable collars
- iv. Extrication collars (field collars)

i. Hard Collars

Hard collars are made of plastics and foams, which cover the neck region to support the users. They are applied until spinal stability is ensured.

ii. Soft Collars

Soft collars are constructed of foams and centered on the cervical spine. They do not sufficiently immobilize the cervical spine compared to the rigid collars.

iii. Adjustable Collars

Adjustable collars have straps and buttons that fit different neck lengths.

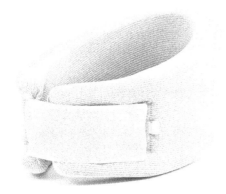

FIGURE 17.7 A soft cervical collar.

Source: www.shutterstock.com/image-photo/neck-support-brace-on-white-background-201719987

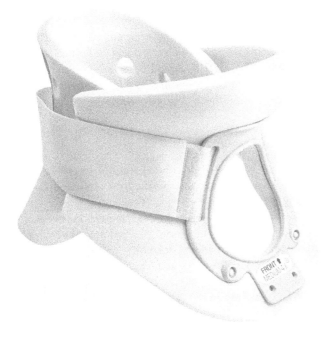

FIGURE 17.8 An extrication cervical collar.

iv. Extrication Collars (Field Collars)

Extrication cervical collars are stiff collars positioned pre-hospital before transferring patients from the site of the traumatic event. Because these are fitted at the field level, these are also known as field collars. Extrication collars may include Stifneck, Philadelphia, and Miami J collars.

c) Purpose/How to Use[68]

- Open the sides of the front panel outward.
- Make sure the top of the collar supports the jawbone.
- Hold firmly with one hand and push the sides of the front panel around the neck.
- Place the back panel on the back of your neck.
- Attach both sides of the back panel to the front with the straps.

d) Important Safety Issues (Cautions and Common Adverse Effects)

- Cervical collar in trauma patients decreases lung capacity or pulmonary volumes and spirometry parameters. The case becomes even more severe for children. Therefore, special care needs to be taken for patients suffering from lung diseases and respiratory distress to avoid hypoxia with the use of a cervical collar.[69,70]Also, a ventilation monitor should be present while applying a neck collar to multiple trauma patients.[70]
- Endotracheal intubation is difficult for patients during cervical collar use due to the difficulty in glottic visualization.[71]
- Cervical collars can also limit the mouth opening so that aspiration may result from vomiting in the supine position.[71–73]
- Long term improper use may lead to atrophy of muscles around the neck.
- Hard collars may obstruct venous outflow and increase intracranial pressure (ICP) by around 4.5 mmHg via jugular venous compression.[65,73,74] This may deteriorate the clinical outcome due to the subsequent secondary traumatic brain injury (TBI).[65]
- If not worn properly, the collar may cause neurological and respiratory complications.[73] Longer time of its application may result in a pressure ulcer, and a cervical collar-related pressure ulcer (CRPU) is a serious concern to be managed.[67]

e) Storage Conditions and Maintenance

- Clean your collar (i.e., pads within the collar) with warm soapy water when it is dirty or smells to prevent skin irritation and sores.
- Wipe the collar with a cloth with warm soapy water if the plastic part of the collar is dirty and dry air pads on a flat surface for about 6 to 8 hours.

- Replace the pads with new pads if they are damaged.

F) IMPORTANT FEATURES (CAPABILITIES AND LIMITATIONS) AND SPECIAL ADVANTAGES

- Cervical collars limit cervical motion or movements between head and thorax and reduce physiologic stress and gravitational stress by supporting a portion of the head weight.[66]
- They support the patient's head and reduce cervical injury caused by spinal movements.[75]
- Cervical braces decrease the forward head position and thoracic kyphosis, which relieves the users from unnecessary stress on their neck.[66]

G) SPECIAL TIPS FOR PATIENT COUNSELING

- Remain in a neutral position, rather than the excessive neck flexion posture, when using electronic devices to prevent musculoskeletal problems including muscle fatigue, pain, and neck disorders.[66]
- Do not drive or lift heavy things while wearing the collar.
- The cervical collar may limit your neck range of motion (RoM), from side to side and up and down.
- Wear a collar for 6 to 8 weeks to get the most benefit for your recovery, and then afterwards you may gradually reduce the time.

H) EVIDENCE OF EFFECTIVENESS AND SAFETY

Advanced Trauma Life Support (ATLS) guidelines from the American College of Surgeons (ACS) and the prehospital Trauma Life Support (PHTLS) guidelines from the National Association of Emergency Medical Technicians (NAEMT) recommend that cervical collars be applied for trauma patients with head and neck injuries from the time of the event to prevent permanent neurologic damages.[69,71,73] Application of collars has also been emphasized as a first measure along with the establishment of free airways in the ABCs of major trauma.[73]

I) ECONOMIC EVALUATION

Collars were launched into the clinical practice to prevent secondary injury to the spinal cord because it helps immobilize the spine. It has been well accepted even in prehospital care. Millions of trauma patients use collars each year.[73]

J) IMPLICATION TO THE PHARMACY PROFESSION AND PHARMACY PRACTICE

Health professionals, including pharmacists, can train collar users to maintain proper posture while wearing it.

K) CHALLENGES TO PHARMACISTS AND USERS

Both the soft and rigid braces reduce neck movement compared with no brace. There are contrasting reports for the clinical effectiveness of soft cervical collars in cases of whiplash injury because it cannot sufficiently immobilize the cervical spine. There is even a similar type of contrasting report in cases of the rigid brace as well for severe cervical injuries compared to usual or active mobilization.[76] Therefore, pharmacists need to be aware of the recent advancements and also need to communicate with the users to know about their necessities. Most patients do not want to apply the collar due to its appearance and limited ventilation. Medical device manufacturers need to manufacture more aesthetic collars to achieve patient acceptability. Ghorbani et al. (2016) found that patients preferred an open-design collar due to its simple open structure and aesthetic design. The open-design collar has minimum skin contact and less covering, making it more acceptable to wear.[75]

L) RECOMMENDATIONS: WAYS FORWARD

- Health professionals should instruct patients to clean the cervical collar according to the manufacturer's directions.
- Pharmacists should counsel and demonstrate for patients how to use the cervical collar properly.
- Pharmacists should review the patients' cervical collar usage and seek the users' cooperation to optimize its effects.

M) CONCLUSIONS

Cervical spine immobilization with the cervical collar has been incorporated into first aid management of unconscious traumatized patients. Chronic mobile device usage may lead to musculoskeletal and neck problems and early cervical degeneration for which a cervical collar may serve as a support. Pharmacists should be aware of the recent advancements in a cervical collar and should counsel the user about the importance of proper use.

N) LESSONS LEARNED

- Collars were used in clinical settings to prevent secondary injury to the spinal cord by immobilizing the spine.
- Cervical collars limit cervical motion between head and thorax and minimize physiologic stress.
- Special care should be taken for patients suffering from lung diseases and respiratory distress to avoid hypoxia with the use of a cervical collar.
- Many patients do not want to apply the collar due to its appearance and limited ventilation. So, the health technology product (HTP) manufacturers should manufacture more aesthetic collars to achieve patient acceptability.

DEVICE 5: LUMBAR BRACES (ABDOMINAL/LUMBAR/BACK BELTS, PELVIC/BACK SUPPORT BELTS)

A) BACKGROUND

Low back pain (LBP) is one of the most prevalent public health concerns all over the world.[77] It is the most prevalent occupational hazard among people < 45 years of age.[78] It may be caused by increased spinal compression due to the lifting of heavy objects.[79] Lumbosacral braces (LBs) restrict lumbar motion and reduce compression of the lumbar spine, thus helping in conditions with pain and instability of the lumbosacral spine. Although LBs increase compression over the skin as well, mechanical and physiological effects of LBs are yet to be confirmed.[80] Although LBs are not helpful for primary prevention, they have secondary prophylactic advantages for the patients suffering from LBP.[81,82] Boutevillain et al. (2019) found that rigid lumbar braces worn for 3 months may decrease pain associated with chronic LBP (cLBP) by 30%.[83] These days, back belts are also worn to minimize occupational low back pain (LBP).[84] Psychological, neuromuscular, and biomechanical benefits of LBs have been inconclusively suggested. Psychological benefits are the perceived mechanical support by the LBs, neuromuscular benefits include lumbar stability, and biomechanical benefits include decreased compression stresses in the lumbar spine due to reduced lumbar range of motion (ROM).[82]

B) DEVICE DESCRIPTION/IMPORTANT FEATURES

Lumbar belts are also known by several other names. The term "back belt" refers to a therapeutic device used for a back injury and includes spinal braces, supports, corsets, and orthoses. The term "abdominal belt" refers to the device used by truck drivers, storekeepers, warehouse workers, and porters for the prevention of LBP. Back belts

have shoulder straps or braces to affix them and to give support to the back. Lightweight belts made of synthetic materials with many elasticized layers are designed these days. Previously, these were also made of leather but less these days due to the risk of degradation with adverse environmental conditions like moisture. Proper fitting is a must for belts, but manufacturers usually adopt the one-size-fits-all approach, and this can be possible with its elastic nature and multilayered design.[85]

Types of Lumbar Belts[77,81,86,87]

There were already more than 70 types of lumbar belts, which can be broadly categorized under the following three types based on their design features[85]:

    i. Extensible LBs (Flexible LBs)
    ii. Semi-rigid LBs
    iii. Non-extensible LBs (Rigid LBs)

i. Extensible LBs (Flexible LBs)

Extensible LBs are both flexible and elastic and are made of soft material, such as cotton/elastic material, or neoprene (synthetic, flexible rubber).

ii. Semi-Rigid LBs

These belts have partial flexibility or extensibility and are mainly used for mild or moderate pain.

iii. Non-Extensible LBs (Rigid LBs)

Non-extensible LBs are flexible but not elastic and do not expand with the outward expansion of the abdomen. Therefore, they increase lumbar stiffness due to high intra-abdominal pressure (IAP). This would ultimately increase spinal stability without increasing spine compression. These are mainly used for moderate to severe pain and to promote healing of spinal fractures or back surgery.

C) PURPOSE/HOW TO USE

- Wear the back support belt around the lower or middle back by wrapping the brace around the back.
- Connect the two ends of the brace across the abdomen.
- Adjust the pressure in the brace tightly and adequately using two pull tabs on either side of the brace.

D) IMPORTANT SAFETY ISSUES (CAUTIONS AND COMMON ADVERSE EFFECTS)

- Regular use of a brace may cause skin rashes or lesions, which can be prevented with the regular cleaning of both the brace and skin. If skin irritation persists, stop wearing the brace for few days while the skin heals.

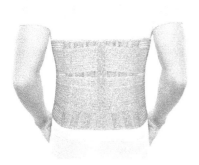

FIGURE 17.9 A back support belt.

Source: www.shutterstock.com/image-photo/orthopedic-lumbar-support-corset-products-belts-1701763618

- Do not use a lumbar brace for more than a few hours a day to avoid muscle weakening and atrophy.

E) Storage Conditions and Maintenance

- Follow the cleaning instructions provided by the brace manufacturer to preserve the brace's durability and effectiveness.
- Remove any dirt or dust particles on the brace and clean the brace by handwashing with soap water since most back braces are not designed to be machine washed or dried.
- Rinse the brace thoroughly and dry completely before wearing, because a soapy or wet brace may cause skin irritation.

F) Important Features (Capabilities and Limitations) and Special Advantages

- Lumbar belts help prevent back strain and injury by maintaining a proper posture of the spine.
- Back support improves the posture of the user since bad posture may cause spinal weakness and result in deformities and injuries.
- It is comfortable to wear, and the user can wear this even under clothes.
- Although a back brace is no cure, it helps manage symptoms of osteoporosis, back muscle sprains, spinal cord injuries, tumor metastasis, and fractures.

G) Special Tips for Patient Counseling

- Wear a lumbar belt only for the first few days or weeks after a severe back injury.
- Avoid using a belt if you do not have a back injury.
- You may use it to lift heavy objects and remove or loosen it when not lifting weight.
- Always consult with the physician to get an idea about the proper size and fit of the belt to ensure its safety and effective pain relief.

H) Evidence of Effectiveness and Safety

A back brace works by improving the posture, supporting, strengthening, and removing stress from the back muscles. This also prevents the back from worsening, keeping the user at low risk of injury and developing spine problems.

I) Economic Evaluation

A lumbar brace is used as the primary (i.e., to prevent the onset and treat) or secondary preventive measure (i.e., to prevent recurrences) of low back pain economically.[88]

J) Implication to the Pharmacy Profession and Pharmacy Practice

There are controversial reports on the use of back belts to prevent musculoskeletal injuries, and this fact has even been accepted by the National Institute of Occupational Safety and Health (NIOSH), and Agency for Health Care Policy and Research reports.[89] NIOSH does not recommend back belts for uninjured persons for the prevention of injuries[90,91] and also does not regard them as personal protective equipment (PPE) from any injuries.[90] Health professionals, including pharmacists, need to keep themselves abreast of the latest advancements and select the best belt for a few weeks based on the severity of the LBP. Back belts are used in occupational settings as nonprescription devices[91] for which pharmacists have a definite role in patient counseling and dispensing. The lumbar brace can be used to prevent low-back pain in employees in the workplace.[88]

K) Challenges to Pharmacists and Users

Patients should keep in mind that the back support belt alone cannot decrease back injury. Maintaining proper posture while sitting, standing, sleeping, walking, and weight lifting positions is a must to prevent back pain. Patients should never use it to enhance their weight lifting capacity.

L) Recommendations: Ways Forward

- Uninjured persons need not use a back belt for the prevention of injuries.
- Pharmacists should keep up-to-date information on the latest advancements and select the belt based on the severity of the LBP.
- Use the lumbar brace as the primary or secondary preventive measure of low-back pain.

M) Conclusions

Low back pain (LBP) is one of the most prevalent public health problems all over the world even among people below the age of 45 years, for which lumbar belt plays a significant pain-alleviating role. A lumbar belt restricts lumbar motion and reduces compression of the lumbar spine and relieves the lumbar pain. Usually, manufacturers follow the one-size-fits-all approach for the lumbar belt due to its elastic nature and multilayered design. However, proper fitting is essential.

N) Lessons Learned

- Lumbar belts can be flexible, semi-rigid, or rigid types, and they are selected based on the need and severity of lumbar pain.
- Regular use of the brace may cause skin rashes which can be prevented with the regular cleaning of both the brace and skin.

- Back belts need not be used if one does not have a back injury.
- Health professionals, including pharmacists, should counsel the patients to apply the belt for a few weeks based on severity of the LBP.

DEVICE 6: CHEST BRACES (EXTERNAL STERNUM BRACES/ORTHOSES, DYNAMIC COMPRESSION BRACES, PECTUS BRACES)

A) BACKGROUND

Pectus carinatum (pigeon chest) is a congenital deformity characterized by outward protruding of the chest.[92–96] Male-to female ratio of the condition has been documented to be 4 or 5:1 and is noticed especially around the age of 11.[92,93,96–98] Its exact pathogenesis is yet to be known.[92] It may present with or without symptoms. Common symptoms are chest pain, chest wall tenderness, shortness of breath, palpitations, wheezing, and exercise intolerance.[96] It causes a prominence of the sternum or breastbone. Pectus carinatum has a prevalence of 0.3 to 0.7 and is not covered even by clothing. Patients suffer from cosmetic issues with decreased self-esteem and a lower quality of life (QoL) compared with those without this problem.[92,99] The mainstay of treatment for this is surgical procedure until now, but it also has other complications. Patients have also been treated with chest braces since the 1970s because it helps restore normal thoracic shape with the help of external pressure on the thoracic wall.[92,93,99]

B) DEVICE DESCRIPTION/IMPORTANT FEATURES

A chest brace compresses the rib cage, chest muscles, sternum, and upper back. It is suitable for strains, sprains, or tenderness or post-surgery to support the rib cage. It has adjustable hook and loop chest straps for compression adjustment and is designed for all activities.

C) PURPOSE/HOW TO USE

- Loosen the buckle on one side and open the buckle on the other side. Wrap the brace around the torso.
- Insert the opened strap back into the buckle while standing.
- Tighten the brace symmetrically.
- Follow the break-in schedule for the first two weeks and then wear the brace 24/7 to obtain the best results.

D) IMPORTANT SAFETY ISSUES (CAUTIONS AND COMMON ADVERSE EFFECTS)

- Skin lesions, abrasion, and breakdown may be occasionally encountered mostly at the beginning of chest brace application.

- Children cannot tolerate chest brace intervention for a long period and may develop skin breakdown and lesions if the bracing pressure is > 2.5 psi.[100]

E) STORAGE CONDITIONS AND MAINTENANCE

- Hand wash the foam pads on the brace with soapy water and allow to dry.
- You may rub the interior with alcohol every 1–2 weeks, but a daily rinse of water is sufficient to clean the brace.
- Do not dry the brace with heat or heating device.
- Do not wear the brace during strenuous physical exercise or showering.

F) IMPORTANT FEATURES (CAPABILITIES AND LIMITATIONS) AND SPECIAL ADVANTAGES

- Athletes can wear for preventative measures and extra support during physical exercise and training.
- It provides extra protection to soft tissue injuries and also remodels the chest shape with the help of external compression.

G) SPECIAL TIPS FOR PATIENT COUNSELING

- Patients should learn how to attach and detach the brace and get instructions on the frequency of wear.[92] If patients are adherent, it gives rapid correction of the pectus carinatum protrusion with excellent patient satisfaction.[95]
- Begin bracing as the child enters puberty. Complete correction may take up to 8 months. After the shape has normalized, it is still worn at night only for 3–6 months to prevent a relapse. After this, the chest should remain in a normal shape.
- Wear according to the physician's instructions and do not share the used brace with others.
- Monitor the skin for pressure areas. Redness may occur but should disappear within 0.5–1 hour of the removal of the brace. If you have painful redness that is not disappearing, contact the physician.

H) EVIDENCE OF EFFECTIVENESS AND SAFETY

After completing the brace treatment, patients are followed every 6 months until the age of 18 years.[92] The child should wear the brace at least 20 hours a day, except during showering or sports, to get its optimum effects. After the chest regains its normal shape, the child should still wear the brace 8 hours a day. If the child does not show progress after wearing the brace for at least one year, they should go for surgical intervention. Children should remain in the hospital for 3 to 5 days after surgery and should restrict activities for 2 to 3 months post-surgery.

I) ECONOMIC EVALUATION

Chest wall deformities were previously managed or repaired with operative procedures but these days brace therapy is gaining popularity among surgeons. Chest bracing, when appropriately used for about 2 years, usually restricts chest expansion.[100]

J) IMPLICATION TO THE PHARMACY PROFESSION AND PHARMACY PRACTICE

Brace therapy helps to avoid surgical complications in most of the cases. Therefore, it is adopted as the first-line treatment for pectus carinatum, the surgical treatment being the second-line treatment for those who are nonadherent to it. Patient adherence is the most critical factor for its favorable outcomes, and poor adherence can be improved by its design improvement and patient counseling about its importance.[93]

K) CHALLENGES TO PHARMACISTS AND USERS

The brace pressure created by the chest bracing may lead to patient discomfort and nonadherence at the beginning of the application.[100] Patients should wear the brace for 14 to 23 hours a day for several months. Once the clinically significant level of correction of chest deformity has been achieved, the child can wear the brace only at nighttime to maintain the corrected shape. It is difficult or challenging for the pharmacists to counsel the patients about maintaining the break-in schedule and revising the adherence status of the patients as follows:

> Day 1: 1–2 hrs
> Day 2: 2–3 hrs
> Day 3: 3–4 hrs
> Day 4: 4–5 hrs
> Day 5: 6–7 hrs
> Day 6: 8+ hrs (try sleeping in brace)
> Day 7: 10–12 hrs
> Day 8: 12–14 hrs
> Day 9: 14–16 hrs
> Day 10: 16–18 hrs
> Day 11: 18–20 hrs
> Day 12: 20–22 hrs
> Day 13: 23–24 hrs

L) RECOMMENDATIONS: WAYS FORWARD

- Children or their caretakers should learn how to apply the chest brace from the pharmacists or physicians or other health professionals.
- Since brace therapy helps to avoid surgical complications, it is adopted as the first-line treatment for pectus carinatum.
- It is essential to follow the break-in schedule for the first two weeks and then wear the brace 24/7 to obtain optimum results.

M) CONCLUSIONS

Pectus carinatum (pigeon chest) is a congenital deformity characterized by outward protruding of the chest, for which chest bracing therapy has been recognized as the first-line management these days. The chest brace compresses the rib cage, chest muscles, sternum, and upper back and is useful for strains, sprains, or tenderness or post-surgery to support the rib cage. Patients should wear the brace for 14 to 23 hours a day for several months to achieve optimum correction in the chest wall deformity.

N) LESSONS LEARNED

- Traditionally, surgical correction of the chest deformity was the mainstay therapeutic intervention, whereas these days chest bracing has been accepted as the first-line management of the same.
- A chest brace has adjustable hook and loop chest straps for compression adjustment and is designed for all activities by the user.
- It is essential to follow the break-in schedule for the first two weeks while on chest brace therapy, although it is challenging to manage.
- Brace therapy helps to avoid surgical complications in many cases.

DEVICE 7: ELBOW AND WRIST IMMOBILIZATION ORTHOSES: HAND AND WRIST BRACES; ELBOW AND ARM BRACES

7.1 HAND AND WRIST BRACES (WRIST WRAP/ SPLINT/SLEEVE, CARPAL TUNNEL BRACE)

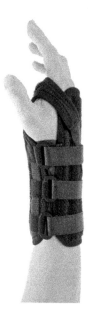

FIGURE 17.10 A wrist brace as indicated for carpal tunnel syndrome and other wrist problems.

Source: www.shutterstock.com/image-photo/close-person-wearing-supportive-black-brace-367445312

a) Background

Wrist pain is a common problem and is caused by tendinitis, sprain, carpal tunnel syndrome (CTS), arthritis, and fractures. CTS is characterized by pain in the wrist and hand and paresthesia (numbness, tingling sensation) in the fingers. CTS is the most typical compressive neuropathy, in which the median nerve is compressed within the carpal tunnel of the wrist and has a prevalence of 4–12%.[101–105] CTS is more common among women and the elderly population.[106,107] Diabetes, pregnancy, hypothyroidism, rheumatoid arthritis, and wrist trauma are common conditions causally associated with CTS. CTS may also be caused by prolonged use of a computer or laptop keyboard, playing particular sports, driving, sewing, painting, and writing continuously for several hours. Patients with CTS may suffer from progressive loss of strength in the hand (especially in the thumb), paresthesia, and pain in the palm, which is aggravated usually at night and disturbs sleep.[11] CTS may cause pain in the hands, weakness, and loss of sensation (LOS) with restrictions in daily activities, and deteriorating quality of life (QoL).[108] Wrist braces are helpful to maintain the affected wrist in a neutral position, thereby reducing the pressure within the tunnel and thereby relieving the associated pain.[109] Finger, hand, or wrist injuries mainly occur during sports activities, machinery work-related tasks, and accidental falls, and appropriate bracing has a pivotal role in the management of those injuries. Thumb/wrist splints are useful in managing certain inflammatory conditions such as De Quervain's tenosynovitis and tendinitis as well as in Keinbock's disease (avascular necrosis of lunate bone).

b) Device Description/Important Features

The brace contains a metal or plastic splint under the wrist to stabilize the same and is also topped with different metal or plastic for additional support and stabilization. It comes in a left or right wrist orientation but can be used for both left and right hands if reversible. Wrist braces are usually designed in a one-size-fits-all approach. The material is lightweight and is made of rubber, cotton, neoprene blend, polyester, nylon, polycarbonate, polyurethane, and polypropylene. It is breathable so that the users can wear it while working or sleeping throughout all seasons of the year. The fabric is further treated with an antimicrobial agent to prevent it from deterioration by microbial invasion. It is comfortable to wear and easy to adjust because it has adjustable straps to control compression.

Types of Wrists Braces
  i. High-protection level braces
  ii. Medium-protection level braces
  iii. Low-protection level braces

i. High-Protection Level Braces   These are made of plastic or metal and have foam or soft material inside to make it comfortable for the user. These are used for patients with severe conditions.

ii. Medium-Protection Level Braces   These are made of neoprene, which provides comfort and warmth to the user.

iii. Low-Protection Level Braces   These are simple neoprene supports, which allow free movement at the wrist joint. These provide heat retention and compression, and reduce inflammation.

c) Purpose/How to Use

- Remove or unwrap the outer covering of the straps.
- Place the splint in contact with the palm of your hand.
- Ensure that your thumb is in contact with the material if there is a thumb section.
- Wrap the straps loosely (but not too tight), starting with the strap nearest your elbow.

d) Important Safety Issues (Cautions and Common Adverse Effects)

- Generally, splints are to be used for the short term since excessive or continuous use can lead to chronic pain, itching, stiffness of a joint, muscle weakness, loss of circulation, and numbness in hands.[110]
- Wearing a wrist brace all the time can weaken muscles. Thus, it is good to increase the wearing duration gradually, starting from 1–2 hours in the initial period.
- Braces (especially hard ones) may make it difficult to engage in some activities.

e) Storage Conditions and Maintenance

- Regularly clean the wrist brace by hand washing in warm soapy water and dry it before wearing because it may become dirty with sweat, dust, or dropped bits of food. Hand wash the brace with warm soapy water or disinfectant to keep your braces clean. Always close the straps before washing.
- Rinse well, and air dry the wrist braces after washing but do not keep them in the direct sunlight. Also, do not use an oven to dry even in an emergency condition.
- Read the instructions about machine washing, available on the package or the label of the braces, since most of the wrist braces available on the market cannot be machine washed or dry cleaned. Place the brace inside a cloth bag or a cushion cover before putting it into the washing machine if it is to be machine washed.
- Do not use any chemical while washing the wrist braces because it damages the elasticity or the material or tarnishes the color of the brace.
- Frequently check for any signs of wear or damage to the wrist brace.
- Do not use bleach or fabric softeners to wash the brace unless indicated on the label.

- Always wear rubber gloves over the wrist braces while gardening to prevent them from getting dirty.

f) Important Features (Capabilities and Limitations) and Special Advantages

- A wrist brace helps eliminate the range of motion in one direction.[103] It helps relieve wrist pain by stabilizing the wrist in a neutral position.
- Hand and wrist braces are used for injuries including sprains and after surgical procedures of the hand or wrist because they promote healing by reducing joint mobility.
- Wrist braces help patients recover from an injury and improve the quality of life (QoL) in cases of chronic conditions such as arthritis.
- Wrist braces restrict excessive movement of the joint by stabilizing the same and allow the user to function and perform daily activities. Such immobilization of the wrist with a brace also helps reduce inflammation and pain.

g) Special Tips for Patient Counseling

- Always use the correct size of brace for your hand or wrist because wearing a tight wrist brace may cause too much pressure around the wrist.
- Remove the splint from the brace if you need a full range of motion (ROM) of the wrist. This will enable you to complete other activities as well while the brace is on.
- Wear the brace throughout the day even while using a computer or doing other tasks.
- Consult the physician if you feel pain, numbness, or discomfort in your wrist or hand.
- Also, consult the doctor to understand the type of brace, frequency, and duration of wear. A wrist brace is not a sharable item.
- Check for breaks or blisters in the skin due to excessive wear of a wrist brace. Also, check for redness, soreness, or swelling of the skin around the wrist and change in color of the wrist. Immediately consult your physician if such problems occur.

h) Evidence of Effectiveness and Safety

Wrist splints (or braces) are used to limit or restrict wrist motion and provide support, especially during the night and/or inactive periods.[111] Wrist splints worn full-time improve symptoms of carpal tunnel syndrome and acute and chronic injuries. The braces also improve physical activities, slow disease progression, and ameliorate pain.[110]

i) Economic Evaluation

The wrist brace is comfortable and not too rigid and also relieves the patient from wrist pain at an affordable price.[110] Hypoallergenic or latex- or neoprene-free braces are preferred if the patient is allergic to neoprene or latex material.

j) Implication to the Pharmacy Profession and Pharmacy Practice

There must be accurate diagnosis of the injury to confirm whether a brace or splint is indicated along with the close follow-up after bracing or splinting to improve adherence by the target users.[110] The pharmacist should ensure that wrist brace is fitted accurately to avoid it from rubbing, straining the used part. Health professionals, including pharmacists, should review the usage pattern to confirm whether patients are feeling discomfort, and counsel them about the solution. The pharmacist can counsel the patients to try a different type of brace or additional cushioning around the bony areas of the wrist to provide the patients with comfort. Pharmacists, orthopedic surgeons, or sports medicine professionals should ensure that the patient is using the brace accurately and for the prescribed period of time.

k) Challenges to Pharmacists and Users

Many patients may feel that orthopedic supports, including the brace which they are using, will hinder their daily activities and they will hesitate to wear it altogether. When the patient discontinues using the brace too early, this may hinder the healing process and delay recovery. Wearing clean braces prevents foul smell, infections, and skin rashes, but the users may not clean the brace appropriately most of the time.

l) Recommendations: Ways Forward

- Pharmacists or sports medicine professionals should ensure that the patient is using the brace accurately for the prescribed time.
- The users should regularly clean the wrist brace by hand washing in warm soapy water and dry it before wearing.
- Pharmacists should counsel the patients that chronic use of wrist braces may lead to itching, loss of circulation, and numbness in hands.

m) Conclusions

Wrist pain is one of the most common problems caused by tendinitis, sprain, carpal tunnel syndrome (CTS), arthritis, and fractures and is usually managed with the wrist brace. The brace contains a metal or plastic splint under the wrist to stabilize the same. Splints should be used for the short term since excessive or continuous use can lead to chronic pain and joint stiffness and muscle weakness.

n) Lessons Learned

- Wrist braces can be high-, medium-, or low-protection level braces.
- Hand and wrist braces maintain the affected wrist in a neutral position to get relief from the wrist pain.
- Hypoallergenic or latex-free braces are preferred if the patient is allergic to neoprene or latex.

- Many patients feel that wrist braces may hinder their daily activities and so they hesitate to wear it altogether.

DEVICE 7.2: ELBOW AND ARM BRACE/SLEEVE (ELBOW/ARM BAND, ELBOW STRAP/SUPPORT, TENNIS ELBOW STRAP, ARM COMPRESSION SLEEVE)

a) Background

Elbow stiffness is one of the complications of elbow trauma[112,113]; a 50% reduction of elbow range of motion can reduce upper extremity function by about 80%.[112] The elbow is the second most commonly dislocated joint in the body after the shoulder among adults.[114–116] Elbow motion helps position the hands in space and also helps to move them at various distances from the body.[117,118] Elbow injuries (e.g., sprains, dislocations) may occur during a fall, and the prophylactic elbow braces help restrict the joint's extension limit.[119] Elbow stiffness commonly occurs due to elbow trauma involving bone and soft-tissue injury. To prevent the stiffness of elbow joint, it is important to start the elbow motion early after injury or surgery. However, in occasions wherein the elbow cannot be mobilized early, the elbow should be splinted in extension, which helps to minimize bleeding and extravasation of fluid, thus minimizing elbow stiffness.[120,121] Elbow dislocations can be simple or complex. Simple dislocations are without fracture, while complex dislocations have a concomitant fracture.[114,115]

Restriction of elbow mobility and elbow stiffness are commonly experienced complaints after elbow trauma or surgery. A range of motion of 100° (30° to 130°) indicates proper elbow function whereas a loss of 50° of motion results in 80% functional loss in daily activities.[122] Gripping and holding is difficult during elbow stiffness,

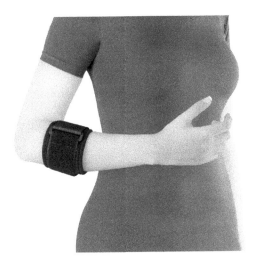

FIGURE 17.11 An elbow strap brace.

Source: www.shutterstock.com/image-photo/elbow-strap-support-tennis-isolated-on-1883622277

and strengthening the muscles helps reduce pain in 80–95% of cases. Infections of the skin or elbow joint due to the bacterial invasion via wounds may also cause elbow pain. Surgery or tumor growth may necessitate the use of an elbow brace for protection. If a patient finds that computer typing hurts his or her elbow, he/she should try to reduce the daily amount of typing and/or split the typing into short bursts (known as work pacing).

Tennis elbow is the inflammation of the tendons attached to the lateral side of the elbow and occurs in 1–3% of the general population. The prevalence may increase to > 50% among tennis players, who use regular repetitive hand functions.[123] The source of the pain is always on the outside of the arm but the pain and tenderness radiate down the arm towards the wrist. Patients may feel difficulty with twisting activities during sports or even opening the lid of a jar. Another similar condition known as golfer's elbow (also known as climber's elbow or pitcher's elbow) occurs on the bony inside portion of the elbow.

b) Device Description/Important Features

An elbow brace is designed especially for tennis or golfer's elbow and has adjustable compression straps for a customized fit. It provides compression, protection, and relief. It has breathable, dual-stretch soft knit material and is lightweight for all-day comfort while wearing. It is easy to wear and take off, and it can be used on the left or right elbow. It is made of cotton, nylon, polyester, neoprene blend, polyurethane, cotton, silicone, and polycarbonate. Based on the circumference diameter around the forearm, it usually has the following sizes:

   i. Extra Small: 20–23 cm
   ii. Small: 23–25 cm
   iii. Medium: 25–28 cm
   iv. Large: 28–31 cm
   v. Extra Large: 31–33 cm

Size may slightly vary company-wise, and extra-large size may come up to 36+. Circumference measurement around the forearm is taken 3 cm below the elbow joint. Compression arm sleeves are selected based on the measurements of wrist, elbow, and upper arm circumference, and length.

Types of Elbow Braces[118]
   i. Protective braces
   ii. Braces with an adjustable range of motion (ROM)
   iii. Mobilization braces

i. Protective Braces Elbows may be immobilized in flexion or extension with the elbow braces. These braces help protect the elbow by preventing its movement during the postinjury or postoperative periods. They also help repair the damaged ligament and bone and are indicated in the initial phases of management of the fracture or dislocation.

ii. Braces with an Adjustable Range of Motion (ROM) These braces allow protected flexion-extension movement and are used after an injury or in the postoperative period. Treatment with braces should consider the histological healing phase. Unrestrained mobilization can be gradually initiated in the flexion-extension pattern after 1–7 days. After 7–15 days, the brace can be removed, and mobilization exercises can be continued until the recovery of complete ROM.

iii. Mobilization Braces Mobilization braces exploit the elastic properties of soft tissues, and small increases in ROM with these braces for a long-time help alter the soft tissues.

c) **Purpose/How to Use**

- Position the elbow brace on the upper forearm around 1 inch (2.5 cm) below the elbow
- Place the brace and secure with the hook-and-loop closure. The support should fit comfortably.

d) **Important Safety Issues (Cautions and Common Adverse Effects)**

- These mobilization braces demand the physician take time to instruct the patient about using the brace appropriately and assessing the results.
- Patient nonadherence to the bracing may sometimes be problematic.[118]

e) **Storage Conditions and Maintenance**

- Elbow braces and supports are machine washable in cold water.
- Wash regularly to maintain the shape and compression of the fabric but wash separately with a laundry detergent with no additives.
- Lay the brace flat and let it air-dry; do not dry it via dryer. Proper washing and drying help maintain its elasticity and fit.

f) **Important Features (Capabilities and Limitations) and Special Advantages**

- A compression sleeve protects the arm against wounds and injuries and reduces inflammation from lymphedema, injury, or general swelling.[124]
- An elbow brace is used for sprains, strains, arthritis, swelling, tendinitis, and tennis/golfer's elbow.
- It provides stability, pain relief, and comfort for the elbow and forearm.
- It is used in cases of restricted range of motion (ROM) due to soft tissue contractions and/or joint stiffness after surgery.
- It provides compression and serves as the muscle and joint stabilizer.

g) **Special Tips for Patient Counseling**

- Wear the elbow brace directly against your skin. Choose a washable elbow brace.
- Wearing it at bedtime is not effective; wear it during the daytime when you're active and let your elbow relax at night.
- You can wear sleeves even under clothing to keep arms insulated in cold weather.

h) **Evidence of Effectiveness and Safety**

Effectiveness of elbow joint bracing can be confirmed by the range of motion protection it offers.[120] Braces are useful in elbow rehabilitation after an acute injury or surgical fixation to decrease the risk of venous stasis and to allow mobility within a safe ROM.[118] Runners, bikers, golfers, and athletes get UV protection from the arm sleeves or braces.

i) **Economic Evaluation**

Price of the tennis elbow braces ranges from US$15 to $80, with an average of US$50. Braces made of neoprene generally cost US$15.

j) **Implication to the Pharmacy Profession and Pharmacy Practice**

Although elbow braces can be worn the whole day, pharmacists have to counsel the patients to remove them during rehabilitation.[118]

k) **Challenges to Pharmacists and Users**

Patient adherence is greater using this brace (but still not 100%) since it is more comfortable to wear, it is lightweight, and can be used even at nighttime.[118] Surgery is only considered if symptoms are present for > 6 months and have not responded to traditional treatments with the bracing.

l) **Recommendations: Ways Forward**

- Pharmacists should counsel the patients to remove the elbow brace during elbow movement exercises.
- Patients should separately wash the brace with a laundry detergent with no additives to maintain the shape and compression of the fabric.
- Pharmacists should counsel the patient to initiate unrestrained mobilization after 1–7 days and stop bracing after 7–15 days, but to continue mobilization exercises till the recovery of complete ROM.

m) **Conclusions**

Elbow injuries (e.g., sprains, dislocations) may occur during a fall, and the prophylactic elbow braces help restrict the joint's extension limit. An elbow brace is designed especially for tennis or golfer's elbow and has adjustable compression straps for easy customization. Braces are useful after an acute injury or surgical fixation to decrease the risk of venous stasis and to allow mobility within a safe range of motion.

n)   Lessons Learned

- Elbow braces are available in different sizes and are of three main types: protective braces, braces with adjustable ROM, and mobilization braces.
- The brace is made of cotton, nylon, polyester, neoprene blend, polyurethane, cotton, silicone, and polycarbonate.
- The brace helps repair the damaged ligament and bone and helps manage the fracture or dislocation.
- Effectiveness of elbow joint bracing can be confirmed by the range of motion protection it offers.

DEVICE 8: FINGER SPLINT (FINGER ORTHOSIS/ IMMOBILIZER, MALLET FINGER SPLINT)

A)   BACKGROUND

Splints and orthoses support, align, position, immobilize, prevent or correct deformity, assist weak muscles, or improve function.[125] An orthosis is an external device used to modify the structural or functional characteristics of the neuro-musculoskeletal system. It controls the abnormal motion of one or more body segment(s) around a joint(s) by applying forces to either side of a joint, and by controlling its position and movements and limiting or preventing unnecessary movements and positions.[126] Orthoses permit the patient some hand movements.[127]

Trigger Finger (Trigger Digits) and Prevalence

Trigger finger is a disease of the tendons of the hand which leads to triggering (locking) of affected fingers, dysfunction, and pain during flexion or extension movement. It affects women more compared to men and appears mostly in the latter decades of life. Trigger finger is usually seen in the case of osteoarthritis, rheumatoid arthritis, and carpal tunnel syndrome and metabolic disorders (e.g., diabetes). Thumb, long, and ring fingers are affected more

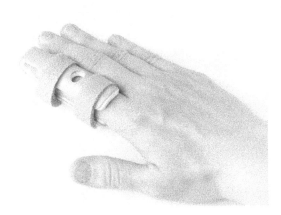

FIGURE 17.12   A finger splint.

Source: www.shutterstock.com/image-photo/grey-plastic-twosided-finger-splint-two-1732238134

commonly than the index and small fingers.[128] It occurs more commonly in patients with diabetes mellitus (due to glucose-induced collagen modifications), carpal tunnel syndrome (CTS), rheumatoid arthritis (RA), hypothyroidism, mucopolysaccharide storage disorders, and congestive heart failure. Its lifetime prevalence among nondiabetics aged above 30 years is about 2.2%. It is more common among women than men, and the age distribution is bimodal with one group below 6 years of age and the other above 40 years of age. Most patients experience a problem in a single finger while some experience problems in multiple fingers. The thumb is the most commonly affected finger, followed by the ring finger and the little finger. The right hand is the commonly affected part, and spontaneous recovery may also occur in 20–29% of the cases.[129] Incidence rate among children is 0.33% (i.e., 3.3 per 1,000) and the thumb is almost always the affected finger.[129,130]

Diagnosis of Trigger Finger

This diagnosis is made only by history and physical examination, since there are no specific diagnostic tests. Laboratory tests and radiographic examination techniques are not indicated unless an underlying cause (such as infection) is suspected. Treatment modalities are operative and nonoperative (corticosteroid injections and splinting). Operative therapy is effective with cure rates of 89–97% in nonrandomized studies but has a higher cost, extended absence from work, and surgical complications. Splinting is effective in 70% of cases compared with 82% receiving an injection.[129]

Mallet Finger (Drop or Baseball Finger)

Mallet finger is a condition in which the end of a finger cannot be actively straightened due to injury. It is commonly treated with the splinting of the finger for six or more weeks and less occasionally by surgical fixation.[131,132]

Finger Splint

A finger splint is used for tendinitis in the hands or fingers, trigger finger, broken fingers, or knuckles, and also used postoperatively. It supports and reduces the pain of the weak fingers by immobilizing the fingers. It also prevents the development of arthritic and neuromuscular deformities.

B)   DEVICE DESCRIPTION/IMPORTANT FEATURES

The splint is made of polyethene, neoprene, polypropylene, and polylactic acid (PLA).[133] Splints and casts immobilize fingers and decrease musculoskeletal injuries by reducing pain and promoting healing.[134] The malleable, lightweight aluminum interior and customizable straps help in proper fitting and promote breathability with the neoprene material. It can be worn on any finger on any of the hands. The adjustable straps provide a custom fit and proper compression and are made of eco-friendly materials. Splints can vary in terms of size (such as small, medium, and up to extra-large), shape or curvature (e.g., curved or straight), and degree of immobility. Rounded or curved splints are best for bone fractures whereas straight splints are best for fingertip injuries.

c) Purpose/How to Use[135]

- Always place the tape and splint securely in place.
- Wear consistently the whole day for a minimum of 6–8 weeks.
- Keep the splinted finger clean and dry at all times to avoid soreness in the skin.
- Wash both your finger and splint daily by gently resting the fingertip on the edge of the table or similar surface. Remove the tape and carefully slide the splint off and wash the skin with soapy water, and dry thoroughly.

d) Important Safety Issues (Cautions and Common Adverse Effects)

- Any immobilizer may cause ischemia, heat injury, pressure sores, infection, dermatitis, and/ or neurologic injury regardless of the duration of application.[134]
- Prolonged application of immobilizers such as casts or splints may lead to chronic pain, joint stiffness, and muscle atrophy.[134]
- The splint is not useful for definitive care of unstable fractures.[134]

e) Storage Conditions and Maintenance

- Firmly secure the splint with fresh tape.
- Always store the splint in its carry case to prevent it from getting damaged.
- You can use sodium hypochlorite (bleach) solutions to clean the splint but avoid high and prolonged concentrations of bleach to avoid discoloration of the splint.
- Completely dry the splint and the straps and then keep these in their storage/carry case.

f) Important Features (Capabilities and Limitations) and Special Advantages

- The splint is worn at all times to promote healing and is worn during periods of inactivity for its analgesic, anti-inflammatory, and protective effects on the joints (e.g., rheumatoid arthritis, osteoarthritis).
- It stabilizes one or more joints in cases of deformity and improves the position in case of RA.[133]
- It decreases pain in cases of carpal tunnel, trigger finger, and tendon inflammation.

g) Special Tips for Patient Counseling

- Limit application of casts and splints to the short term to avoid complications.[134]
- Wear the splint even during nighttime since it is comfortable and you do not notice even if you sleep while wearing it.
- Properly fit the splint to improve patient adherence and minimize risk.

h) Evidence of Effectiveness and Safety

A splint generally interferes very little with the normal movement of the user's hand.[135] Most mallet finger injuries are managed with immobilization of the affected joint in extension with the splint.[136]

i) Economic Evaluation

Finger splints generally do not need individuals to be vigorously trained in their application. Thus, these are powerful tools to provide first aid and also avoid the high costs of medical care.

j) Implication to the Pharmacy Profession and Pharmacy Practice

Splinting is helpful for acute orthopedic conditions such as fractures, joint dislocations, sprains, and soft tissue injuries.[134]

k) Challenges to Pharmacists and Users

Most mallet finger injuries heal with 6–8 weeks of splinting, whereas a few cases may need a referral to the higher centers.[132] There is no consensus over the best design and/ or wearing schedule. Patient adherence to splinting is a concern for most users.

l) Recommendations: Ways Forward

- Pharmacist should counsel the users that prolonged use of the splint may lead to chronic pain, joint stiffness, and muscle atrophy.
- Patients should be counseled well enough to fit the splint correctly to improve their adherence and minimize risk.
- High concentration of sodium hypochlorite (bleach) solutions should not be used to prevent discoloration of the splint.

m) Conclusions

Trigger finger is a disease of the tendons of the hand, leading to triggering (locking) of affected fingers, dysfunction, and pain during flexion or extension movement. Finger splinting is used for tendinitis in the hands or fingers, trigger finger, broken fingers, and also used postoperatively. The splint can be worn the whole day to promote healing with its analgesic, anti-inflammatory, and protective effects on the joints.

N) Lessons Learned

- Finger splints immobilize fingers and minimize musculoskeletal injuries by reducing pain and promoting healing.
- Finger splints are made of polyethene, neoprene, polypropylene, and polylactic acid (PLA).
- Rounded or curved splints are best for bone fractures whereas straight splints are best for fingertip injuries.
- Any immobilizer like a finger splint may cause ischemia, heat injury, pressure sores, infection, dermatitis, and/or neurologic injury regardless of the duration of application.

DEVICE 9: KNEE BRACES (ARTHRITIS KNEE BRACE, KNEE STABILIZER/IMMOBILIZER/SLEEVE/SUPPORT)

A) Background

Knee pain, primarily associated with knee osteoarthritis (OA), is common in the elderly and usually has a nontraumatic and insidious onset. In contrast, knee trauma and sports injuries are common in the younger population.[137] Knee OA is mainly related to ageing and obesity and causes pain, inflammation, and reduced range of motion (ROM), functional disability, and QoL. Although the pathophysiology of knee OA is not known, it usually involves degenerative joint disease with damage to the articular cartilage.[138] OA has a significant economic burden on the healthcare delivery system.[139] Knee OA is more common among women and 6% of the population 30+ years and 12% of the population aged 65+ generally have knee OA.[140] Proper care of knee injuries is vital for any sports medicine and includes the application of braces.[141]

Orthoses are recommended by the third recommendation of the European League Against Rheumatism (EULAR) and American College of Rheumatology (ACR) for the non-pharmacological management of knee OA.[142] Knee braces or sleeves are elastic nonadhesive orthoses and can be used for individuals with osteoarthritis (OA) of the knee.[142,143] A knee brace supports, positions, immobilizes, prevents or corrects the deformity, supports weak muscles, and improves physical function.[140,143,144] It reduces disease progression and pain and improves functional impairment.[143]

B) Device Description/Important Features

A knee brace is made of nylon, cotton, polyester, silicone, polyurethane, polyethene, polypropylene, neoprene blend, aluminum, and/or steel, and is breathable and lightweight.

TYPES OF KNEE BRACES

A. Based on the Application or Purpose of Use[141,145]

i. Prophylactic Braces (Anderson Knee Stabler)

These have unilateral or bilateral bars, hinges, and adhesive straps and prevent injury or reduce the severity of knee injury during sport.

ii. Postoperative (Rehabilitative) Braces

These braces have full-length rigid bars with adjustable hinges at the knee which allow a controlled range of motion (ROM) and 6 to 8 non-elastic straps to keep the brace in place. They protect injured ligaments and control knee flexion and extension angles during healing. They are used for a short period (usually 2–8 weeks) after acute injury or surgery and also for nonsurgical ligament injuries or nondisplaced fractures along with crutches.

iii. Functional Knee Braces

These are made of a composite of metal and plastic material with vertical hinges to control hyperextension. They provide stability for patients with an unstable knee (e.g., ACL tear) and also minimize future injuries without deteriorating function. They prevent extra injuries and protect a surgically repaired knee (e.g., post ACL reconstruction).

iv. Unloader Knee Braces

These are effective in osteoarthritis of knee in that they help to reduce the load/pressure on the affected/damaged compartment of the knee. They relieve pain, improve function, and delay need for surgical intervention (knee replacement).

B. Based on Design[141]

i. Compression sleeves: plain sleeves, sleeves with pads, or sleeves with buttress
ii. Wraparound (dual-wrap) braces
iii. Hinged knee braces
iv. Knee straps

i. Compression Sleeves

These are made of neoprene with a nylon cover and can be used even under clothing. These are available as plain sleeves, sleeves with pads, or sleeves with buttress. Sleeves with pads provide more protective cushioning to the patella and anterior knee. Sleeves with buttress have opening for the patella (i.e., a buttress). The buttress may be circular, C-shaped, J-shaped, or H-shaped. Whatever may be the special design, these sleeves increase warmth and provide even compression on the knee to relieve swelling and pain. They are useful for mild knee pain, and also minimize arthritis. They compress the tissue and limit the movement of the patella. Thus, they are beneficial for athletes with an unstable patella.

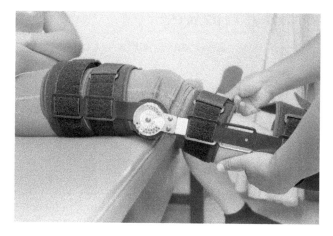

FIGURE 17.13 A hinged knee brace.

Source: www.shutterstock.com/image-photo/orthopedist-secures-leg-brace-on-knee-426898519

ii. Wraparound (Dual-Wrap) Braces

These provide more support than sleeves, so they are useful for athletes who face mild to moderate knee pain.

iii. Hinged Knee Braces

These are mainly used post-surgery, and also by the athletes requiring a higher level of protection and support. They help maintain proper alignment of the knee even while bending and this helps heal and avoid extra injuries. They are also preferred in post-surgery settings.

iv. Knee Straps

These can also be worn even under clothes. They prevent patella injuries and knee pain by compressing the patellar tendon. Thus, they are most preferred for runner's knee or jumper's knee (patellar tendinitis).

c) Purpose/How to Use[146]

- Use the knee braces as directed by the physician or pharmacists.
- Take care when putting the brace on to make sure the knee bends on the hinge region.
- Fasten straps, tapes, or loop around your leg.
- Ensure that braces have not moved during activities because poorly positioned braces can hurt rather than support the knee.
- Wear the knee brace during all activities liable to cause injury to the knee.

d) Important Safety Issues (Cautions and Common Adverse Effects)

- Knee sleeves do not provide support to the ligament and are not useful for the treatment of an unstable knee.

- Knee sleeves can cause swelling due to the heat retention around the knee or due to the obstruction of venous and lymphatic return below the sleeve. If these complications appear, they should only be used during sports.
- Functional brace users have higher energy expenditures compared to the nonusers and never substitute for surgical management and rehabilitation. Functional braces are not useful for prophylaxis.[141]
- When the brace is applied very tightly, it may cut off blood circulation to the leg, which ultimately may lead to discoloration, inflammation, or tingling in the leg.

e) Storage Conditions and Maintenance

- Knee braces may be damaged even during regular use, so always inspect your brace for wear and tear and replace it if it is worn out.
- Regular machine washing with soap and water is good for its fabric.
- Cover any exposed metal to prevent it from scratching or injuring you or other people.

f) Important Features (Capabilities and Limitations) and Special Advantages

- A knee brace is used for sprains, strains, arthritis, tendinitis, and/or irritation of the kneecap.
- Postoperative or rehabilitative braces are used for acute knee ligament injuries or after surgery of ligament.

g) Special Tips for Patient Counseling

- Tighten the brace optimally until you feel comfortable.
- Loosen the straps or choose optimally sized brace because if the brace is too tight, it may block circulation.
- You may choose rigid braces to gain more support or compression sleeves to achieve more mobility but with less support.
- Choose the right knee brace based on the level of support required and the physician's suggestion.
- Remember that the brace alone is not sufficient to treat or protect the injured knee. Knee braces complement but do not replace surgery or rehabilitation.

h) Evidence of Effectiveness and Safety

The only nonpharmacological therapies recommended by the EULAR guidelines for the management of knee pain are the use of appliances such as sticks, knee bracing, and other assistive devices. In the UK, the National Institute for Health and Care Excellence (NICE) guideline recommends the application of local heat and cold, braces, joint supports, and assistive devices for the same.[147] Yeung and Yeung (2001) also found that knee braces are effective in reducing knee injuries.[148]

I) ECONOMIC EVALUATION

Some knee braces cost hundreds of dollars, and some medical insurance companies may cover these costs, relieving the patients of their cost burden. It should be noted that the most expensive brace is not always the best one.

J) IMPLICATION TO THE PHARMACY PROFESSION AND PHARMACY PRACTICE

Choice of treatment for knee pain depends on the condition, site, and severity of the pain. Also, a combination of education, advice, and physical therapy serve as first-line treatment for knee pain.[137]

K) CHALLENGES TO PHARMACISTS AND USERS

Physical exercise and rehabilitation alone have not been effective for managing traumatic knee pain in younger patients.[137] Wearing the brace, ensuring a good fit, helps the users relieve pain. Users can wear the brace the whole day or only for certain activities, because wearing it excessively can cause compression problems, leading to stasis of circulation.

L) RECOMMENDATIONS: WAYS FORWARD

- Pharmacists should counsel the patients that wearing the brace, ensuring a good fit, helps them find relief from pain.
- The users should not apply the brace too tightly to avoid the blockage of circulation.
- Health professionals should counsel the patients to wear the knee brace during all activities liable to cause injury to the knee but simultaneously also inform them that the knee brace alone is not sufficient to treat or protect the injured knee.

M) CONCLUSIONS

Knee pain is common in adolescents and adults and usually has a nontraumatic and insidious onset. Knee braces are elastic nonadhesive orthoses used for individuals with osteoarthritis (OA) of the knee to support, position, immobilize or correct deformity, and improve physical function. Knee bracing and other assistive devices are the only nonpharmacological therapies recommended by the EULAR guidelines for the management of knee pain.

N) LESSONS LEARNED

- Knee braces are made of nylon, cotton, polyester, silicone, polyurethane, polypropylene, neoprene blend, and/or aluminum, and are breathable and lightweight.

- Knee braces may be prophylactic, rehabilitative, or functional depending on their purpose of the application, and maybe categorized into compression sleeves, wraparound braces, hinged knee braces, or knee straps based on their design.
- Knee braces are used for sprains, strains, arthritis, or tendinitis, but do not provide support to the ligament and unstable knee.
- If the knee sleeves cause inflammation in the knee region due to the heat retention or obstruction of venous and lymphatic return, they should only be used during sports.

DEVICE 10: ANKLE BRACES (ANKLE GUARDS/SUPPORTS/SPLINTS)

A) BACKGROUND

Ankle sprains (injury to ankle ligaments) are one of the most common sports-related injuries (seen in 15–20% of cases).[149–153] Around 35% of these cases lead to functional ankle instability (FAI).[151,154] Patients with ankle sprains suffer from pain, loss of function, and poor quality of life (QoL).[150,151] The severity of ankle sprains can be categorized as mild (grade I), moderate (grade II), and severe (grade III).[151,155]

i. Mild (grade I) sprains are characterized by stretching or minor tearing of ligaments causing the ankle to loosen.

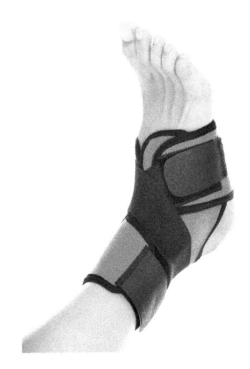

FIGURE 17.14 An ankle brace.

Source: www.shutterstock.com/image-photo/trauma-ankle-brace-isolated-84875062

ii. Moderate (grade II) sprains are characterized by tearing of ligaments and increased ankle loosening.

iii. Severe (grade III) sprains are characterized by a complete tear of ligaments causing the ankle to be very loose and unstable.[155]

The mainstay of initial treatment of ankle arthritis is nonsurgical management of symptoms with nonsteroidal anti-inflammatory drugs (NSAIDs), bracing, joint injection, and/or shoe modifications. Braces are useful for adherent patients who are not concerned with cosmetic appearances.[156] Ankle orthoses prophylactically protect ligaments from excessive stresses and recurrent ankle sprains in patients with chronic ankle instability (CAI).[149,151,154,157–159]

B)   DEVICE DESCRIPTION/IMPORTANT FEATURES

Rigid, semi-rigid, elastic, and non-rigid ankle braces are available on the market. Generally, a rigid or semi-rigid brace or device is preferred for clinical use.[160] Rigid braces provide a higher level of support, whereas soft ones provide more comfort. Semi-rigid braces support and stabilize the injured foot.[155]

Types of Ankle Braces[161–163]

i. Elastic compression (neoprene) braces

ii. Semi-rigid braces (SRB): lace-up ankle braces and hinged ankle braces

iii. Rigid braces

i.   Elastic Compression Braces

Elastic compression braces are used to manage mild ankle sprains and tendinitis. These are made of lightweight stretchable (i.e., compressible) material to support the ankle joint with compression. These braces can be easily fitted by measuring ankle joint size and can be used on either the left or right ankle. These braces provide ankle joint warmth, decrease muscle stiffness, inflammation, and discomfort during mobility.

ii.   Semi-Rigid Braces

These are made of thermoplastic material and are used for sports purposes.

A.   LACE-UP ANKLE BRACES

These are semi-rigid ankle braces made of lightweight material and are used for mild to moderate ankle sprains and also for prevention of repeat ankle sprains. These braces provide more support and better fit than the compression brace and are reusable, but take more time to put on and take off than the semi-rigid hinged brace. These can also be applied on either the left or right ankle as can compression braces.

B.   HINGED ANKLE BRACES

These semi-rigid braces with ROM increase side-to-side support compared to the lace-up brace and can perform the movement with required ROM.

iii.   Rigid Braces

Rigid braces are made of hard plastic material and are mainly used by sports personnel because they are effective in treating ankle sprains, fractures, and repeated ankle sprains. These braces provide more side-to-side support and compression, which reduces swelling, compared to the semi-rigid braces but are challenging to fit.

C)   PURPOSE/HOW TO USE

- Select comfortable brace fit by tightening straps or laces to tolerable compression level. Walk around and recheck brace fit and adjust brace fit during activity.[155]
- Wrap the ankles for compression or support to relieve from inflammation.
- Bind the tape around the foot, beginning from the inside wrapping to the outside.
- Cross the front of the foot at 45° angles. Then wrap the brace back to the inside of the heel from where you began for better fitting and effectiveness.

D)   IMPORTANT SAFETY ISSUES (CAUTIONS AND COMMON ADVERSE EFFECTS)

- An ankle brace may impair the athletic performance by reducing the functional range of motion of the ankle joint.[164]
- Wearing an ankle brace is not a 100% cure for all ankle injuries. This means ankle pain may persist despite the ankle brace application.
- Regularly check the condition of the ankle brace since it may get damaged due to frequent wear and tear incidents.

E)   STORAGE CONDITIONS AND MAINTENANCE

- Check regularly for holes, cracks, and wear-and-tear, and replace any damaged braces.
- Wash the brace in cold water with mild detergent and air-dry.[155]
- Keep your ankle brace in good condition by regularly cleaning it as directed by the medical experts or the manufacturers on the product leaflet.

F)   IMPORTANT FEATURES (CAPABILITIES AND LIMITATIONS) AND SPECIAL ADVANTAGES

- An ankle brace reduces recurrent sprains and functional ankle instability (FAI), and is used for initial ankle sprains. It improves abnormal ankle gait.[154]

- Recurrent ankle sprain is very common (around 60%) among sportspersons and the external ankle brace prevents such reinjury.[165]
- It supports bones and muscles and keeps them in place after surgery.
- Functional ankle braces are suitable for the treatment of acute ankle sprains, whereas semi-rigid ones decrease the risk of future ankle sprains.[110]
- Ankle braces support the ankle joint via compression, stabilization, and warmth, and also prevent the ankle from further injury or damage.

G) SPECIAL TIPS FOR PATIENT COUNSELING

- Support the ankle with tape or a brace to prevent ankle sprains.[153]
- You can use an ankle brace for prophylactic purposes to avoid future sprains.[158]
- Get the usage guidance from a physician, physical therapist, or pharmacist because the brace choice is guided by the ankle condition. Some patients may wear the brace for shorter durations whereas others may need to wear it the whole day.

H) EVIDENCE OF EFFECTIVENESS AND SAFETY

Healing for first-time acute ankle sprains generally takes 6–12 weeks after which patients may resume work or sports activities.[150] The PRICE (Protection, Rest, Ice, Compression, Elevation) strategy is used for acute ankle sprain for which an ankle brace causes compression on the injured part. Similarly, the Dutch College of General Practitioners guideline also recommended the ICE (Immobilization, Compression, and Elevation) approach during the first week, followed by ankle taping for 6 weeks and ankle bracing after that during sports activities to prevent recurrences.[151]

I) ECONOMIC EVALUATION

Fatoye and Haigh (2016) reported that the cost of semi-rigid ankle brace was £184 and quality-adjusted life years (QALY) gained with this 0.72. They concluded that semi-rigid ankle brace is a cost-effective modality for ankle sprains.[150] Usually, an ankle brace may cost from US$2 to $360, and this may vary with the brand, materials used in manufacturing, and the purpose of the brace. For example, rehabilitative ankle braces may cost more compared to the ones used for basic ankle compression and support.

J) IMPLICATION TO THE PHARMACY PROFESSION AND PHARMACY PRACTICE

An ankle brace should be just tight enough to restrict motion of the ankle but not be so tight as to halt blood circulation. Thus, patients are instructed to check their blood circulation status by pinching the nail of the big toe and observing whether color quickly returns to the nail or not. The pharmacist should counsel the patients to wear the ankle brace any time they are doing something. They may take it off during periods of resting or sitting down and may put it back on when they get up. If the patients wear it even during rest, it should not feel uncomfortable with them.

K) CHALLENGES TO PHARMACISTS AND USERS

Users may have the misconception that the ankle brace may slow performance, but there is minimal to no effect on activity. In reality, an ankle brace (if properly applied) improves performance even after an ankle injury and helps prevent reinjury.[155]

L) RECOMMENDATIONS: WAYS FORWARD

- Patients should obtain the relevant usage instruction from a physician, physical therapist, or pharmacist because the brace choice is guided by the ankle condition.
- Pharmacists should counsel the patients to wear the ankle brace when they are doing something that needs ankle stability.
- Pharmacist should counsel the patients that wearing an ankle brace is not a 100% guaranteed cure for all ankle injuries because ankle pain may persist despite wearing it.

M) CONCLUSIONS

Patients with ankle sprains suffer from pain, loss of function, and low quality of life (QoL), and such sprains can be mild (grade I), moderate (grade II), or severe (grade III). Ankle orthoses such as braces protect ligaments from recurrent ankle sprains and are one of the nonsurgical management modalities of the same. Ankle braces reduce functional ankle instability (FAI), and improve abnormal ankle gait. However, tight ankle braces that are too tight may obstruct the blood circulation.

N) LESSONS LEARNED

- Ankle braces may be soft, semi-rigid, or rigid, out of which rigid or semi-rigid is preferred for patient use.
- Rigid braces provide a higher level of support, whereas a soft one is more comfortable. Semi-rigid braces support and stabilize the injured foot.
- Wearing an ankle brace does not ensure a 100% cure for all ankle injuries and ankle pain may still persist despite brace use.
- The ankle brace should be just tight enough to immobilize the ankle movement or motion but not be so tight as to halt blood circulation.

DEVICE 11: COMPRESSION GLOVES (ARTHRITIS/STRETCH/EDEMA/PRESSURE/ THERAPY GLOVES, A-GLOVES, C-GLOVES, COPPER COMPRESSION ARTHRITIS GLOVES, ARTHRITIS COMPRESSION GLOVES)

A) BACKGROUND

Rheumatoid arthritis (RA) is a systemic disease with chronic inflammation of synovial tissues of joints and tendons causing synovitis, joint pain, and stiffness around the affected joints.[166–168] RA affects 0.5–1% of the population all over the world.[167] The inflammatory reaction may lead to cartilage destruction, bone erosion, joint instability, dislocation, deformities, and loss of function of the affected part including hands (e.g., reduced grip strength, range of motion).[166,169] Peak onset of RA is generally in the age of 40–60 years, and if left untreated, it causes significant disability and reduced quality of life (QoL).[168] Compression gloves provide relief from the hand synovitis such as morning stiffness and/or night pain in arthritis by applying external compression (pressure) and warmth to the hand and mobilizing local edema.[166,168] Compression therapy provided by the gloves is based on the principle of pressure around the affected extremity to reduce the edema volume.[170]

B) DEVICE DESCRIPTION/IMPORTANT FEATURES

Compression gloves are custom-made elastic garments made of nylon, elastane, wool, and acrylic.[166,168,171] These days, compression gloves are being manufactured with grip-enhancing material (e.g., rubber, silicone) on the

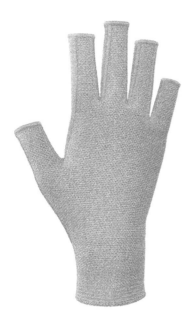

FIGURE 17.15 A compression glove.

Source: www.shutterstock.com/image-photo/gloves-open-fingers-compression-pressure-on-1905611863

palmar surface to provide a better grip for the patients who have arthritis. The gloves are made of 90% cotton, 5% copper, and 5% spandex. The following five designs are popular to enhance the grip:

i. Rectangular rubber tabs
ii. Honeycomb-pattern silicone adhered to fabric
iii. Wave-pattern silicone adhered to fabric
iv. Line-pattern silicone beads adhered to fabric
v. Line-pattern silicone beads embedded into the fabric[172]

Types of Arthritis Gloves

i. Open-finger gloves (fingertip gloves)
ii. Wrist wraps
iii. Heated gloves (thermal gloves, infrared arthritis gloves that use infrared light)
iv. Thermoskin arthritic gloves

i. Open Fingers Gloves

These help the users feel items without much constriction.

ii. Wrist Wraps

These also have a thumb loop for easy adjustments and are useful when patients need extra wrist support.

iii. Heated Gloves

These cover the entire wrist, hand, and fingers, except the fingertips, to support movement during physical activities. These can be worn even on sunny days to allow the sun's rays to activate the infrared heat.

iv. Thermoskin Arthritic Gloves

These are available in small to extra-large sizes, so patients requiring variable glove size prefer these. They have an adjustable strap for the optimum size and also have soft materials to achieve maximum comfort and breathability.

C) PURPOSE/HOW TO USE

- Properly fit the glove(s) but do not wear too tightly.
- Use for short periods initially during the day to become accustomed to them.
- Do not wear the gloves the whole day.
- Remove gloves frequently to wash and dry hands to maintain hand hygiene.
- You may wear the gloves whole night to get pain relief but ensure that they should not disturb sleep.
- Make sure your gloves fit well, not too tight or too loose to allow the required level of degree of compression.
- Wear the gloves continuously for about 8 hours a day to gain optimum relief from pain.
- Don't keep your hands idle all day, and engage in some hand movement activities to alleviate arthritis symptoms.

- Don't wear these gloves if you have carpal tunnel syndrome, because arthritis gloves can exacerbate CTS; consult with your doctor about treatment options.

D) IMPORTANT SAFETY ISSUES (CAUTIONS AND COMMON ADVERSE EFFECTS)

- Compression gloves should be cautiously used in cases of bilateral carpal tunnel syndrome.[166]
- Do not wear gloves continuously.[168]
- Stop using the gloves and contact the physician if you find any problems with the continuous glove use such as numbness, paresthesia, overly tight compression, allergic reaction, and/or skin irritation.
- Remove the gloves if the fingertip becomes discolored (e.g., red, white, or blue coloration of fingers) or numb or tingling.

E) STORAGE CONDITIONS AND MAINTENANCE

- Store gloves properly to prevent their degradation and maintain reliability.
- Store these gloves in a cool, dry environment at a temperature between 10°C and 22°C to maintain their good performance. High temperatures may accelerate hypothermic chemical reaction on the chlorinated gloves and cause the latex to ignite.
- Avoid too much inventory of powder-free latex gloves in extreme heat, and periodically check such gloves for deterioration, brittleness, or chemical odor.
- Do not store these gloves near chemicals, heat, humidity, ultraviolet light, high-energy radiation, or ozone to maintain product integrity.
- Machine wash the gloves in cold water or hand wash them using nonbiological detergent and lay them flat to dry.
- Do not dry on direct heat such as with a radiator and do not use fabric conditioner.

F) IMPORTANT FEATURES (CAPABILITIES AND LIMITATIONS) AND SPECIAL ADVANTAGES

- Heated (infrared) gloves increase blood circulation in hands and relieve arthritic pain with the continuous pressure on the parts used.
- Even if the gloves did not relieve the arthritic pain, it improves the user's grip.
- The gloves relieve stiffness and soreness in the wrists, palms, and fingers by supporting muscles and joints.
- These reduce inflammation in hands and fingers, alleviate pain in these regions, and also improve the strength of handgrip.

G) SPECIAL TIPS FOR PATIENT COUNSELING

- Wear the compression gloves to get pain relief during the day or nighttime, and to improve hand function during the daytime.
- Wear arthritis gloves based on your needs, and you may even wear a glove only on a single hand.[168]
- Wear these gloves while sleeping for 8 hours for best results.
- Proper fit of the gloves is a must since the severity of arthritic hand swelling can vary every day.

H) EVIDENCE OF EFFECTIVENESS AND SAFETY

The pressure applied by the gloves may relieve the users from hand pain, inflammation, and stiffness in the affected muscles.

I) ECONOMIC EVALUATION

Compression gloves generally cost US$19.90 for any of the small, medium, or large sizes. If patients do not have access to or budget for any of the sophisticated arthritis gloves, even wearing cotton gloves regularly can alleviate their problems. They may apply medicated ointment or creams to their hands before bedtime and immediately use gloves.

J) IMPLICATION TO THE PHARMACY PROFESSION AND PHARMACY PRACTICE

Since patients' preferences related to glove composition, their budget, and fit are vital,[166] pharmacists should be alert to promote adherence. It is a wise decision to rotate the powder-free latex glove inventory using the "first in, first out" approach in the pharmacy. If the glove deteriorates, it should be discarded because compromised gloves may not sufficiently protect the affected parts.

K) CHALLENGES TO PHARMACISTS AND USERS

Most people experience hand pain during the active periods in the day, so they need to wear gloves during active periods. However, if the patients feel hand pain is disturbing their sleep at night, they may wear gloves even at nighttime.[168,169] Many users usually get the beneficial effects of these gloves when wearing them at nighttime. The users may even type on the computer keyboard and use their phones with the fingerless arthritis gloves.

L) RECOMMENDATIONS: WAYS FORWARD

- Pharmacists should instruct the patients to wear the compression gloves to get pain relief during the whole day and to engage in hand mobility activities during the daytime.
- Pharmacists should be vigilant to promote adherence by reviewing the usage patterns of the patients.

- Pharmacists should counsel the patients to store the arthritis gloves in a cool, dry environment at a temperature between 10°C and 22°C to maintain their good performance.

M) CONCLUSIONS

Rheumatoid arthritis (RA) is a chronic inflammatory condition of joints and tendons causing synovitis, joint pain, and stiffness around the affected joints, for which arthritis gloves or compression gloves are usually applied. These gloves relieve morning stiffness and/or night pain in arthritis by applying external compression or pressure and warmth to the hand. Pharmacists should counsel the patients not to use these gloves and contact the physician if they face problems with their continuous use such as paresthesia, overly tight compression, hypersensitivity, and skin irritation.

N) LESSONS LEARNED

- Compression gloves are made of nylon, elastane, wool, and acrylic, and these days they are being manufactured with grip-enhancing material such as rubber or silicone.
- Arthritis gloves may be available on the market in open-finger gloves, wrist wraps, heated gloves, or thermoskin arthritic gloves types.
- High temperatures may cause a hypothermic reaction on the chlorinated gloves and cause the latex to ignite.
- The users may even type on the computer keyboard and use the phone with the fingerless arthritis gloves.

DEVICE 12: OTHER DEVICES USED IN ORTHOPEDIC PRACTICE

Besides the aforementioned orthopedic devices of importance to the pharmacy practice in clinical, hospital, community, or household settings, other orthopedic devices are also crucial from orthopedic practitioners' point of view. Some of these devices are listed here:

1. Extramedullary fixation devices (plates and screws: dynamic compression plate [DCP], limited contact dynamic compression plate [LC-DCP], locking compression plate [LCP], screws)
2. Intramedullary fixation devices (nails: k-nail, elastic nail, interlocking nail)
3. Implants for joint replacement (knee replacement, hip replacement, endoprosthesis)
4. Synthetic bone grafts and bone cement
5. Materials such as Gelfoam and Surgicel (absorbable hemostats) used to fill the dead space or minimize bleeding intraoperatively

6. Orthopedic plaster material: cast tape (fiberglass, polyester); cast padding (natural, synthetic, cotton blend, absorbent); orthopedic stockinette (synthetic, cotton)
7. Orthopedic bandages: elastic light support bandage; elastic adhesive bandage; tubular support bandage; cast bandages; plaster of Paris bandages
8. Metallic sutures (silver sutures)

Since these are mainly applicable to the orthopedic practitioners more than to the pharmacists, these are out of the scope of the present chapter. The interested readers are suggested to refer to the relevant literature.

REFERENCES

1. Demers J, Fuhrer MJ, Jutai JW, et al. Tracking mobility-related assistive technology in an outcomes study. Asst Technol. 2008;20(2):73–83. https://doi.org/10.1080/10400435.2008.10131934.
2. Gray DB, Morgan KA, Gottlieb M, et al. Person factors and work environments of workers who use mobility devices. Work. 2014;48:349–59. https://doi.org/10.3233/WOR-141907.
3. Hardi I, Bridenbaugh SA, Gschwind YJ, et al. The effect of three different types of walking aids on spatiotemporal gait parameters in community-dwelling older adults. Aging Clin Exp Res. 2014;26:221–8. https://doi.org/10.1007/s40520-014-0204-4.
4. Krey CH, Calhoun CL. Utilizing research in wheelchair and seating selection and configuration for children with injury/dysfunction of the spinal cord. J Spinal Cord Med. 2004;27:S29–S37. https://doi.org/10.1080/10790268.2004.11753782.
5. Bradley SM, Hernandez CR. Geriatric assistive devices. Am Fam Physician. 2011;84(4):405–11.
6. McSweeney E, Gowran RJ. Wheelchair service provision education and training in low and lower middle income countries: a scoping review. Disabil Rehabil: Assist Technol. 2017:1–13. https://doi.org/10.1080/17483107.2017.1392621.
7. Allen SM, Foster A, Berg K. Receiving help at home: the interplay of human and technological assistance. J Gerontol: Soc Sci. 2001;56B(6):S374–S382.
8. Faruqui SR, Jaeblon T. Ambulatory assistive devices in orthopaedics: uses and modifications. J Am AcadOrthop Surg. 2010;18:41–50.
9. Hook FWV, Demonbreun D, Weiss BD. Ambulatory devices for chronic gait disorders in the elderly. Am Fam Physician. 2003;67(8):1717–24.
10. Edelstein JE. Assistive devices for ambulation. Phys Med Rehabil Clin N Am. 2013;24:291–303. https://doi.org/10.1016/j.pmr.2012.11.001.
11. Alves MPT, Araújo GCS. Low-level laser therapy after carpal tunnel release. Rev Bras Ortop. 2011;46(6):697–701.
12. Vorvick LJ, Zieve D. Using a cane. U.S. National Library of Medicine. 2020. Available from: https://medlineplus.gov/ency/patientinstructions/000343.htm (accessed 19 Sept 2020).
13. DDS. Adaptive equipment maintenance protocols. The D.C. Developmental Disabilities Administration Adaptive

Equipment Task Force. District of Columbia Department on Disability Services. 2012:1–44.

14. Esch MVD, Heijmans M, Dekker J. Factors contributing to possession and use of walking aids among persons with rheumatoid arthritis and osteoarthritis. Arthritis Rheum (Arthritis Care & Research) 2003;49(6):838–42. https://doi.org/10.1002/art.11463.

15. Wolff JL, Agree EM, Kasper JD. Wheelchairs, walkers, and canes: what does medicare pay for, and who benefits? Health Affairs. 2005;24(4):1140–9. https://doi.org/10.1377/hlthaff.24.4.1140.

16. Demir YP, Yildirim SA. Different walk aids on gait parameters and kinematic analysis of the pelvis in patients with Adult Neuromuscular Disease. Neurosciences. 2019;24(1):36–44. https://doi.org/10.17712/nsj.2019.1.20180316.

17. Fischer J, Nüesch C, Göpfert B, et al. Forearm pressure distribution during ambulation with elbow crutches: a cross-sectional study. J Neuro Eng Rehabil. 2014;11:61. https://doi.org/10.1186/1743-0003-11-61.

18. Kocher BK, Chalupa RL, Lopez DM, et al. Comparative study of assisted ambulation and perceived exertion with the wheeled knee walker and axillary crutches in healthy subjects. Foot Ankle Int. 2016:1–6. https://doi.org/10.1177/1071100716659748.

19. Maguire C, Sieben JM, Scheidhauer H, et al. The effect of crutches, an orthosis Thera Togs, and no walking aids on the recovery of gait in a patient with delayed healing post hip fracture: a case report. Physiother Theory Pract. 2016;32(1):69–81. https://doi.org/10.3109/09593985.2015.1075640.

20. Potter BE, Wallace WA. Crutches. Br Med J. 1990;301:1037–9.

21. Kujath AS. Crutch fitting. Orthopaedic Nursing. 2018;37(4):262–4. https://doi.org/10.1097/NOR.0000000000000469.

22. Ogunlusi JD, Davids T, Edward S, et al. Bilateral wrist drop complicating axillary crutches mobilization in a young adult. West Indian Med J. 2013;62(6):548–51.

23. Odebiyi DO, Adeagbo CA. Ambulatory devices: assessment and prescription. Prosthesis. 2020:1–29. https://doi.org/10.5772/intechopen.89886.

24. Curti B. Using crutches. University Health Network. 2018. Available from: www.uhnpatienteducation.ca (accessed 5 Aug 2020).

25. Hügle T, Arnieri A, Bünter M, et al. Prospective clinical evaluation of a novel anatomic cuff for forearm crutches in patients with osteoarthritis. BMC Musculoskelet Disord. 2017;18:110. https://doi.org/10.1186/s12891-017-1459-7.

26. Bonnier N. User manual: elbow crutches. Version EN 01–06/2018. FDI France Medical 2018:1–7.

27. Segura A, Piazza SJ. Mechanics of ambulation with standard and spring-loaded crutches. Arch Phys Med Rehabil. 2007;88:1159–63. https://doi.org/10.1016/j.apmr.2007.05.026.

28. Zhang Y, Liu G, Xie S, et al. Biomechanical evaluation of an innovative spring-loaded axillary crutch design. Assistive Technol. 2011;23(4):225–31. https://doi.org/10.1080/10400435.2011.614676.

29. Sadowski CA, Li JC, Pasay D, et al. Interprofessional peer teaching of pharmacy and physical therapy students. Am J Pharm Educ. 2015;79(10):1–6.

30. Lopes S, Filipe L, Silva R, et al. An innovative concept for a walker with a self-locking mechanism using a single mechanical approach. Int J Environ Res Public Health. 2019;16:1671. https://doi.org/10.3390/ijerph16101671.

31. Liu H. Assessment of rolling walkers used by older adults in senior-living communities. Geriatr Gerontol Int. 2009;9:124–30. https://doi.org/10.1111/j.1447-0594.2008.00497.x.

32. Luz C, Bush T, Shen X. Do canes or walkers make any difference? Non-use and fall injuries. Gerontologist. 2015:1–9. https://doi.org/10.1093/geront/gnv096.

33. Stevens JA, Thomas K, Teh L, et al. Unintentional fall injuries associated with walkers and canes in older adults treated in U.S. emergency departments. J Am Geriatr Soc. 2009;57:1464–9. https://doi.org/10.1111/j.1532-5415.2009.02365.x.

34. Poole M, Simkiss D, Rose A, et al. Anterior or posterior walkers for children with cerebral palsy? A systematic review. Disabil Rehabil: Assist Technol. 2017:1–12. https://doi.org/10.1080/17483107.2017.1385101.

35. Bateni H, Heung E, Zettel J, et al. Can use of walkers or canes impede lateral compensatory stepping movements? Gait Posture. 2004;20:74–83. https://doi.org/10.1016/S0966-6362(03)00098-5.

36. Sloan HL, Haslam K, Foret CM. Teaching the use of walkers and canes. Home Healthcare Nurse. 2001;19(4):241–6.

37. Vorvick LJ, Zieve D. Using a walker. U.S. National Library of Medicine. 2020. Available from: https://medlineplus.gov/ency/patientinstructions/000342.htm#:~:text=Place%20the%20walker%20in%20front,to%20help%20you%20stand%20up (accessed 19 Sept 2020).

38. WHO. Guidelines on the provision of manual wheelchairs in less resourced settings. World Health Organization; 2008. Available from: https://www.who.int/publications/i/item/9789241547482 (accessed 26 Oct 2020).

39. Sonenblum SE, Sprigle S. Wheelchair use in ultra-lightweight wheelchair users. Disabil Rehabil: Assist Technol. 2016:1–6. https://doi.org/10.1080/17483107.2016.1178819.

40. Ekiz T, Demir SO, Sümer HG, et al. Wheelchair appropriateness in children with cerebral palsy: a single center experience. J Back Musculoskelet Rehabil. 2017;30:825–8. https://doi.org/10.3233/BMR-150522.

41. Sprigle S. Measure it: proper wheelchair fit is key to ensuring function while protecting skin integrity. Adv Skin Wound Care. 2014;27(12):561–72.

42. Scherrer S, Chee JCY, Vu N, et al. Experts' opinion on manual wheelchair adjustments for adults with diabetes. Disabil Rehabil: Assist Technol. 2017:1–9. https://doi.org/10.1080/17483107.2017.1283543.

43. Ekiz T, Demir SO, Ozgirgin N. Wheelchair appropriateness in patients with spinal cord injury: a Turkish experience. Spinal Cord. 2014;52:901–4. https://doi.org/10.1038/sc.2014.128.

44. Worobey L, Oyster M, Nemunaitis G, et al. Increases in wheelchair breakdowns, repairs, and adverse consequences for people with traumatic spinal cord injury. Am J Phys Med Rehabil. 2012;91:463Y469. https://doi.org/10.1097/PHM.0b013e31825ab5ec.

45. Gowran RJ, Clifford A, Gallagher A, et al. Wheelchair and seating assistive technology provision: a gateway to freedom. Disabil Rehabil. 2020:1–12. https://doi.org/10.1080/09638288.2020.1768303.

46. Devitt R, Chau B, Jutai JW. The effect of wheelchair use on the quality of life of persons with multiple sclerosis.

Occup Therapy Health Care. 2004;17:63–79. https://doi.org/10.1080/J003v17n03_05.

47. Toro ML, Eke C, Pearlman J. The impact of the World Health Organization 8-steps in wheelchair service provision in wheelchair users in a less resourced setting: a cohort study in Indonesia. BMC Health Serv Res. 2016;16:26. https://doi.org/10.1186/s12913-016-1268-y.

48. Henderson GV, Boninger ML, Dicianno BE, Worobey LA. Type and frequency of wheelchair repairs and resulting adverse consequences among veteran wheelchair users. Disabil Rehabil: Assist Technol. 2020:1–7. https://doi.org/10.1080/17483107.2020.1785559.

49. Tzeng H. A feasibility study of providing folding commode chairs in patient bathrooms to reduce toileting-related falls in an adult acute medical-surgical unit. J Nurs Care Qual. 2011;26(1):61–8.

50. Naylor JR, Mulley GP. Commodes: inconvenient conveniences. BMJ. 1993;307:1258–60.

51. Ballinger C, Pain H, Pascoe J, et al. Choosing a commode for the ward environment. Br J Nurs. 1996;5(8):485–8.

52. Friesen E, Theodoros D, Russell T. Clinical assessment, design and performance testing of mobile shower commodes for adults with spinal cord injury: an exploratory review. Disabil Rehabil: Assist Technol. 2013;8(4):267–74.

53. Cousins G. Role of environmental cleanliness and decontamination in care homes. Nurs Standard. 2016;30;19:39–43.

54. Yachnin D, Gharib G, Jutai J, et al. Technology-assisted toilets: improving independence and hygiene in stroke rehabilitation. J Rehabil Assist Technol Eng. 2017;4:1–8. https://doi.org/10.1177/2055668317725686.

55. Tirefort J, Schwitzguebel AJ, Collin P, et al. Postoperative mobilization after superior rotator cuff repair: sling versus no sling—a randomized prospective study. J Bone Joint Surg Am. 2019;101:494–503. https://doi.org/10.2106/JBJS.18.00773.

56. Jeong YG, Jeong YJ, Koo JW. The effect of an arm sling used for shoulder support on gait efficiency in hemiplegic patients with stroke using walking aids. Eur J Phys Rehabil Med. 2017;53(3):410–15. https://doi.org/10.23736/S1973-9087.17.04425-2.

57. Hwang Y, An D. Immediate effects of an elastic arm sling on walking patterns of chronic stroke patients. J. Phys. Ther. Sci. 2015;27(1):35–7.

58. Johns Hopkins Hospital Patient Information. Instructions for wearing your shoulder immobilizer brace. 2010 May 10. Available from: www.hopkinsmedicine.org/orthopaedic-surgery/_documents/specialty-areas/shoulder/ShoulderImmobilizer.pdf (accessed 10 Aug 2020).

59. King S, Graham A, Bagaoisan C. How to get dressed after shoulder surgery with a shoulder immobilizer. University Health Network. 2019. Available from: www.uhnpatient-education.ca (accessed 10 Aug 2020).

60. Lenza M, Faloppa F. Conservative interventions for treating middle third clavicle fractures in adolescents and adults. Cochrane Database Syst Rev. 2016, Issue 12. Art. No.: CD007121. https://doi.org/10.1002/14651858.CD007121.pub4.

61. Handoll HHG, Ollivere BJ. Interventions for treating proximal humeral fractures in adults (Review). Cochrane Database Syst Rev. 2010, Issue 12. Art. No.: CD000434. https://doi.org/10.1002/14651858.CD000434.pub2.

62. Whelan DB, Litchfield R, Wambolt E, et al. External rotation immobilization for primary shoulder dislocation: a randomized controlled trial. Clin OrthopRelat Res. 2014:1–7. https://doi.org/10.1007/s11999-013-3432-6.

63. Myint JMWW, Yuen GFC, Yu TKK, et al. A study of constraint-induced movement therapy in subacute stroke patients in Hong Kong. Clin Rehabil. 2008;22:112–24. https://doi.org/10.1177/0269215507080141.

64. Seybold D, Schildhauer TA, Muhr G. Rare anterior shoulder dislocation in a toddler. Arch Orthop Trauma Surg. 2009;129:295–8. https://doi.org/10.1007/s00402-007-0546-x.

65. Mobbs RJ, Stoodley MA, Fuller J. Effect of cervical hard collar on intracranial pressure after head injury. ANZ J. Surg. 2002;72:389–91.

66. Kuo Y, Fang J, Wu C, Lin R, Su P, Lin C. Analysis of a customized cervical collar to improve neck posture during smartphone usage: a comparative study in healthy subjects. Eur Spine J. 2019:1–11. https://doi.org/10.1007/s00586-019-06022-0.

67. Lacey L, Palokas M, Walker J. Preventative interventions, protocols or guidelines for trauma patients at risk of cervical collar-related pressure ulcers: a scoping review. JBI Database System Rev Implement Rep. 2019;17(12):2452–75.

68. Magtoto R, Sloman H. How to use the Aspen™ cervical collar. University Health Network. 2019. Available from: www.uhn.ca/PatientsFamilies/Health_Information/Health_Topics/Documents/How_to_use_the_Aspen_Cervical_Collar.pdf (accessed 6 Aug 2020).

69. Ala A, Shams-Vahdati S, Taghizadieh A, et al. Cervical collar effect on pulmonary volumes in patients with trauma. Eur J Trauma EmergSurg. 2015:1–4. https://doi.org/10.1007/s00068-015-0565-1.

70. Rahmani F, Pouraghaei M, Moharamzadeh P, et al. Effect of neck collar fixation on ventilation in multiple trauma patients. Trauma Mon. 2016;21(4):e21866. https://doi.org/10.5812/traumamon.21866.

71. Yuk M, Yeo W, Lee K, et al. Cervical collar makes difficult airway: a simulation study using the LEMON criteria. Clin Exp Emerg Med. 2018;5(1):22–8.

72. Irwin M, Foley AL. Cervical collar placement algorithm for triage nurses. J Emerg Nurs. 2018;44(6):668–70. https://doi.org/10.1016/j.jen.2018.08.009.

73. Sundstrøm T, Asbjørnsen H, Habiba S, et al. Prehospital use of cervical collars in trauma patients: a critical review. J Neurotrauma. 2014;31:531–40. https://doi.org/10.1089/neu.2013.3094.

74. Yard J, Richman PB, Leeson B, et al. The influence of cervical collar immobilization on optic nerve sheath diameter. J Emerg Trauma Shock. 2019;12(2):141–4.

75. Ghorbani F, Kamyab M, Azadinia F, et al. Open-design collar vs. conventional Philadelphia collar regarding user satisfaction and cervical range of motion in asymptomatic adults. Am J Phys Med Rehabil. 2016;95:291–9.

76. Whitcroft KL, Massouh L, Amirfeyz R, et al. A comparison of neck movement in the soft cervical collar and rigid cervical brace in healthy subjects. J Manipulative Physiol Ther. 2011;34:119–22.

77. Ludvig D, Preuss R, Larivière C. The effect of extensible and non-extensible lumbar belts on trunk muscle activity and lumbar stiffness in subjects with and without

low-back pain. Clin Biomech. 2019;67:45–51. https://doi.org/10.1016/j.clinbiomech.2019.04.019.

78. Mokhtarinia H, Ghamary J, Maleki-Ghahfarokhi A, et al. The new "Tehran Back Belt": design then testing during a simulated sitting task improved biomechanical spine muscle activity. Health Promotion Perspect. 2019;9(2):115–22. https://doi.org/10.15171/hpp.2019.16.

79. Kingma I, Faber GS, Suwarganda EK, et al. Effect of a stiff lifting belt on spine compression during lifting. Spine. 2006;31(22):E833–E839.

80. Bonnaire R, Molimard J, Calmels P, et al. Biomechanical analysis and modelling of lumbar belt: preliminary study. Comput Methods Biomech Biomed Eng. 2013;16(S1):219–21. https://doi.org/10.1080/10255842.2013.815880.

81. Boucher J, Roy N, Preuss R, et al. The effect of two lumbar belt designs on trunk repositioning sense in people with and without low back pain. Ann Phys Rehabil Med. 2017;60;306–11. https://doi.org/10.1016/j.rehab.2017.03.002.

82. Larivière C, Caron J, Preuss R, et al. The effect of different lumbar belt designs on the lumbopelvic rhythm in healthy subjects. BMC Musculoskelet Disord. 2014;15:307. https://doi.org/10.1186/1471-2474-15-307.

83. Boutevillain L, Bonnin A, Chabaud A, et al. Short-term pain evolution in chronic low back pain with Modic type 1 changes treated by a lumbar rigid brace: a retrospective study. Ann Phys Rehabil Med. 2019;62:3–7. https://doi.org/10.1016/j.rehab.2018.06.008.

84. Ammendolia C, Kerr MS, Bombardier C. Back belt use for prevention of occupational low back pain: a systematic review. J Manipulative Physiol Ther. 2005;28:128–34. https://doi.org/10.1016/j.jmpt.2005.01.009.

85. Hodgson EA. Occupational back belt use: a literature review. AAOHN J. 1996;44(9):438–43.

86. Shahvarpour A, Preuss R, Sullivan MJL, et al. The effect of wearing a lumbar belt on biomechanical and psychological outcomes related to maximal flexion-extension motion and manual material handling. Appl Ergonomics. 2018;69:17–24. https://doi.org/10.1016/j.apergo.2018.01.001.

87. Shahvarpour A, Preuss R, Larivière C. The effect of extensible and non-extensible lumbar belts on trunk postural balance in subjects with low back pain and healthy controls. Gait Posture. 2019;72:211–16. https://doi.org/10.1016/j.gaitpost.2019.06.013.

88. van Duijvenbode I, Jellema P, van Poppel M, et al. Lumbar supports for prevention and treatment of low back pain. Cochrane Database Syst Rev. 2008, Issue 2. Art. No.: CD001823. https://doi.org/10.1002/14651858.CD001823.pub3.

89. Smith DL, Dainoff MJ, Mark LS, et al. Effect of a back belt on reaching postures. J Manipulative PhysiolTher. 2004;27:186–96. https://doi.org/10.1016/j.jmpt.2003.12.028.

90. Bobick TG, Belard J, Hsiao H, et al. Physiological effects of back belt wearing during asymmetric lifting. Appl Ergonomics. 2001;32:541–7.

91. Minor SD. Use of back belts in occupational settings. Phys Ther. 1996;76(4):403–8.

92. Beer SA, Blom YE, Lopez M, et al. Measured dynamic compression for pectus carinatum: a systematic review. Sem Pediatr Surg. 2018;27:175–82. https://doi.org/10.1053/j.sempedsurg.2018.06.001.

93. Jung J, Chung SH, Cho JK, et al. Brace compression for treatment of pectus carinatum. Korean J Thorac Cardiovasc Surg. 2012;45:396–400. https://doi.org/10.5090/kjtcs.2012.45.6.396.

94. Kravarusic D, Dicken BJ, Dewar R, et al. The Calgary protocol for bracing of pectus carinatum: a preliminary report. J Pediatr Surg. 2006;41:923–6. https://doi.org/10.1016/j.jpedsurg.2006.01.058.

95. Lee RT, Moorman S, Schneider M, et al. Bracing is an effective therapy for pectus carinatum: interim results. J Pediatr Surg. 2013;48:184–90.

96. Shaul D, Phillips JD, Gilbert J, et al. Pectus Carinatum Guideline. Am Pediatr Surg Assoc (APSA). 2012:1–4. Available from: www.eapsa.org/apsa/media/Documents/Pectus_Carinatum_Guideline_080812.pdf (accessed 14 Aug 2020).

97. Al-Githmi IS. Clinical experience with orthotic repair of pectus carinatum. Ann Saudi Med. 2016;36(1):70–2. https://doi.org/10.5144/0256-4947.2016.70.

98. Martinez-Ferro M, Fraire C, Bernard S. Dynamic compression system for the correction of pectus carinatum. Sem Pediatr Surg. 2008;17:194–200. https://doi.org/10.1053/j.sempedsurg.2008.03.008.

99. Beer SA, Gritter M, Jong JR, et al. The dynamic compression brace for pectus carinatum: intermediate results in 286 patients. Ann Thorac Surg. 2017;103:1742–9. https://doi.org/10.1016/j.athoracsur.2016.12.019.

100. Ates O, Karakus OZ, Hakgüder G, et al. Pectus carinatum: the effects of orthotic bracing on pulmonary function and gradual compression on patient compliance. Eur J Cardio-Thorac Surg. 2013;44:e228–e232. https://doi.org/10.1093/ejcts/ezt345.

101. Fernández-De-Las-Peñas C, Cleland J, Palacios-Ceña M, et al. The effectiveness of manual therapy versus surgery on self-reported function, cervical range of motion, and pinch grip force in carpal tunnel syndrome: a randomized clinical trial. J Orthop Sports Phys Ther. 2017;47(3):151–61.

102. Fernandez-de-las-Penas C, Cleland J, Palacios-Cena M, et al. Effectiveness of manual therapy versus surgery in pain processing due to carpal tunnel syndrome: a randomized clinical trial. Eur J Pain. 2017;21:1266–76. https://doi.org/10.1002/ejp.1026.

103. Martins RS, Siqueira MG. Conservative therapeutic management of carpal tunnel syndrome. ArqNeuropsiquiatr. 2017;75(11):819–24. https://doi.org/10.1590/0004-282X20170152.

104. Meems M, Oudsten BD, Meems B, et al. Effectiveness of mechanical traction as a non-surgical treatment for carpal tunnel syndrome compared to care as usual: study protocol for a randomized controlled trial. Trials. 2014;15:180. https://doi.org/10.1186/1745-6215-15-180.

105. Middleton SD, Anakwe RE. Carpal tunnel syndrome. BMJ. 2014;349:g6437. https://doi.org/10.1136/bmj.g6437.

106. Elwakil TF, Elazzazi A, Shokeir H. Treatment of carpal tunnel syndrome by low-level laser versus open carpal tunnel release. Lasers Med Sci. 2007;22:265–70. https://doi.org/10.1007/s10103-007-0448-8.

107. Page MJ, Massy-Westropp N, O'Connor D, et al. Splinting for carpal tunnel syndrome. Cochrane Database Syst Rev. 2012; Issue 7. Art. No.: CD010003. https://doi.org/10.1002/14651858.CD010003.

108. Atroshi I, Tadjerbashi K, McCabe SJ, et al. Treatment of carpal tunnel syndrome with wrist splinting: study

protocol for a randomized placebo-controlled trial. Trials. 2019;20:531. https://doi.org/10.1186/s13063-019-3635-6.

109. O'Connor D, Marshall SC, Massy-Westropp N, et al. Non-surgical treatment (other than steroid injection) for carpal tunnel syndrome. Cochrane Database Syst Rev. 2003, Issue 1. Art. No.: CD003219. https://doi.org/10.1002/14651858. CD003219.

110. Gravlee JR, Durme DJV. Braces and splints for musculo-skeletal conditions. Am Fam Physician. 2007;75(3):342–8.

111. Domizio JD, Mogk JPM, Keir PJ. Wrist splint effects on muscle activity and force during a handgrip task. J Appl Biomech. 2008;24:298–303.

112. Attum B, Obremskey W. Posttraumatic elbow stiffness: a critical analysis review. JBJS Rev. 2016;4(9):e1. http://doi.org/10.2106/JBJS.RVW.15.00084.

113. Trehan SK, Wolff AL, Gibbons M, et al. The effect of simulated elbow contracture on temporal and distance gait parameters. Gait Posture. 2015;41:791–4. https://doi.org/10.1016/j.gaitpost.2015.02.010.

114. Chang ES, Bishop ME, Dodson CC, et al. Management of elbow dislocations in the national football league. Orthop J Sports Med. 2018;6(2):2325967118755451. https://doi.org/10.1177/2325967118755451.

115. de Haan J, Hartog D, Tuinebreijer WE, et al. Functional treatment versus plaster for simple elbow dislocations (FuncSiE): a randomized trial. BMC Musculoskelet Disord. 2010;11:263. https://doi.org/10.1186/1471-2474-11-263.

116. Kesmezacar H, Sarikaya IA. The results of conservatively treated simple elbow dislocations. Acta Orthop Traumatol Turc. 2010;44(3):199–205. https://doi.org/10.3944/AOTT.2010.2400.

117. Fradet L, Liefhold B, Rettig O, et al. Proposition of a protocol to evaluate upper-extremity functional deficits and compensation mechanisms: application to elbow contracture. J Orthop Sci. 2015;20:321–30. https://doi.org/10.1007/s00776-014-0679-z.

118. Fusaro I, Orsini S, Sforza T, et al. The use of braces in the rehabilitation treatment of the post-traumatic elbow. Joints. 2014;2(2):81–6.

119. Lake AW, Sitler MR, Stearne DJ, et al. Effectiveness of prophylactic hyperextension elbow braces on limiting active and passive elbow extension prephysiological and postphysiological loading. J Orthop Sports Phys Ther. 2005;35:837–43.

120. Charalambous CP, Morrey BF. Posttraumatic elbow stiffness. J Bone Joint Surg Am. 2012;94:1428–37. https://doi.org/10.2106/JBJS.K.00711.

121. Mittal R. Posttraumatic stiff elbow. Indian J Orthop. 2017;51(1):4–13. https://doi.org/10.4103/0019-5413.197514.

122. Muller AM, Sadoghi P, Lucas R, et al. Effectiveness of bracing in the treatment of nonosseous restriction of elbow mobility: a systematic review and meta-analysis of 13 studies. J Shoulder Elbow Surg. 2013;22:1146–52.

123. Sadeghi-Demneh E, Jafarian F. The immediate effects of orthoses on pain in people with lateral epicondylalgia. Pain Res Treatment. 2013, Article ID 353597. https://doi.org/10.1155/2013/353597.

124. Devoogdt N, Kampen MV, Geraerts I, et al. Different physical treatment modalities for lymphoedema developing after axillary lymph node dissection for breast cancer: a review. Eur J Obstetr Gynecol Reprod Biol. 2010;149:3–9. https://doi.org/10.1016/j.ejogrb.2009.11.016.

125. Egan M, Brosseau L, Farmer M, et al. Splints and orthosis for treating rheumatoid arthritis. Cochrane Database Syst Rev. 2001, Issue 4. Art. No.: CD004018. https://doi.org/10.1002/14651858.CD004018.

126. Tyson SF, Kent RM. The effect of upper limb orthotics after stroke: a systematic review. Neuro Rehabil. 2011;28:29–36. https://doi.org/10.3233/NRE-2011-0629.

127. Silveira AT, Souza MA, Fernandes BL, et al. From the past to the future of therapeutic orthoses for upper limbs rehabilitation. Res Biomed Eng. 2018;34(4):368–80. https://doi.org/10.1590/2446-4740.170084.

128. Tarbhai K, Hannah S, von Schroeder HP. Trigger finger treatment: a comparison of 2 splint designs. J Hand Surg. 2012;37A:243–9. https://doi.org/10.1016/j.jhsa.2011.10.038.

129. Peters-Veluthamaningal C, van der Windt DAWM, Winters JC, et al. Corticosteroid injection for trigger finger in adults. Cochrane Database Syst Rev. 2009, Issue 1. Art.No.: CD005617. https://doi.org/10.1002/14651858.CD005617.pub2.

130. Farr S, Grill F, Ganger R, et al. Open surgery versus nonoperative treatments for paediatric trigger thumb: a systematic review. J Hand Surg (European Volume) 2014;39E(7):719–26. https://doi.org/10.1177/1753193414523245.

131. Handoll HHG, Vaghela MV. Interventions for treating mallet finger injuries. Cochrane Database Syst Rev. 2004, Issue 3. Art. No.: CD004574. https://doi.org/10.1002/14651858.CD004574.pub2.

132. Wang QC, Johnson BA. Fingertip injuries. Am Fam Physician. 2001;63:1961–6.

133. ICRC. Manufacturing guidelines: upper limb orthoses. Geneva, Switzerland: International Committee of the Red Cross (ICRC) Physical Rehabilitation Programme; 2014:1–63.

134. Boyd AS, Benjamin HJ, Asplund C. Splints and casts: indications and methods. Am Fam Physician. 2009;80(5):491–9.

135. Hand Therapy Team. Rehabilitation following mallet finger: patient information. Middlesbrough, North Yorkshire, England: The James Cook University Hospital; 2016 Nov. p. 1–2.

136. Cheung JPY, Fung B, Ip WY. Review on mallet finger treatment. Hand Surg. 2012;17(3):439–47. https://doi.org/10.1142/S0218810412300033.

137. Afzali T, Fangel MV, Vestergaard AS, et al. Cost-effectiveness of treatments for non-osteoarthritic knee pain conditions: a systematic review. PLoS ONE. 2018;13(12):e0209240. https://doi.org/10.1371/journal.pone.0209240.

138. Mine K, Nakayama T, Milanese S, et al. The effectiveness of braces and orthoses for patients with knee osteoarthritis: a systematic review of Japanese-language randomised controlled trials. Prosthet Orthot Int. 2016;1–12. https://doi.org/10.1177/0309364616640926.

139. Gohal C, Shanmugaraj A, Bedi A, et al. Effectiveness of valgus offloading knee braces in the treatment of medial compartment knee osteoarthritis: a systematic review. Sports Health. 2018;10(6):500–14. https://doi.org/10.1177/1941738118763913.

140. Raja K, Dewan N. Efficacy of knee braces and foot orthoses in conservative management of knee osteoarthritis: a systematic review. Am J Phys Med Rehabil. 2011:247–62. https://doi.org/10.1097/PHM.0b013e318206386b.

141. Martin TJ. Technical report: knee brace use in the young athlete. Pediatrics. 2001;108(2):503. https://doi.org/10.1542/peds.108.2.503.

142. Beaudreuil J, Bendaya S, Faucher M, et al. Clinical practice guidelines for rest orthosis, knee sleeves, and unloading knee braces in knee osteoarthritis. Joint Bone Spine. 2009;76:629–36. https://doi.org/10.1016/j.jbspin.2009.02.002.

143. Duivenvoorden T, Brouwer RW, van Raaij TM, et al. Braces and orthoses for treating osteoarthritis of the knee. Cochrane Database Syst Rev. 2015, Issue 3. Art. No.: CD004020. https://doi.org/10.1002/14651858.CD004020.pub3.

144. Chew KTL, Lew HL, Date E, et al. Current evidence and clinical applications of therapeutic knee braces. Am J Phys Med Rehabil. 2007;86:678–86. https://doi.org/10.1097/PHM.0b013e318114e416.

145. Yang X, Feng J, He X, et al. The effect of knee bracing on the knee function and stability following anterior cruciate ligament reconstruction: a systematic review and meta-analysis of randomized controlled trials. Orthop Traumatol: Surg Res. 2019;105:1107–14. https://doi.org/10.1016/j.otsr.2019.04.015.

146. American Academy of Family Physicians. Knee bracing—what works? Am Fam Physician. 2000 Jan 15;61(2):423.

147. Woods B, Manca A, Weatherly H, et al. Cost-effectiveness of adjunct non-pharmacological interventions for osteoarthritis of the knee. PLoS ONE. 2017;12(3):e0172749. https://doi.org/10.1371/journal.pone.0172749.

148. Yeung EW, Yeung SS. A systematic review of interventions to prevent lower limb soft tissue running injuries. Br J Sports Med. 2001;35:383–9.

149. Benca E, Ziai P, Hirtler L, et al. Biomechanical evaluation of different ankle orthoses in a simulated lateral ankle sprain in two different modes. Scand J Med Sci Sports. 2019;29:1174–80. https://doi.org/10.1111/sms.13455.

150. Fatoye F, Haigh C. The cost-effectiveness of semi-rigid ankle brace to facilitate return to work following first-time acute ankle sprains. J Clin Nurs. 2016;25:1435–43. https://doi.org/10.1111/jocn.13255.

151. Kemler E, Port I, Backx F, et al. A systematic review on the treatment of acute ankle sprain: brace versus other functional treatment types. Sports Med. 2011;41(3):185–97.

152. Simon J, Donahue M. Effect of ankle taping or bracing on creating an increased sense of confidence, stability, and reassurance when performing a dynamic-balance task. J Sport Rehabil. 2013;22:229–33.

153. Willeford K, Stanek JM, McLoda TA. Collegiate football players' ankle range of motion and dynamic balance in braced and self-adherent—taped conditions. J Athletic Train. 2018;53(1):66–71. https://doi.org/10.4085/1062-6050-486-16.

154. Zhang G, Cao S, Wang C, et al. Effect of a semirigid ankle brace on the in vivo kinematics of patients with functional ankle instability during the stance phase of walking. BioMed Res Int. 2019:1–10. https://doi.org/10.1155/2019/4398469.

155. VUMC. What you need to know about ankle bracing. Vanderbilt University Medical Center. 2010:1–7. Available from: www.vumc.org/sports-medicine/sites/vumc.org.sports-medicine/files/public_files/documents/anklebracing_webbooklet2010.pdf (accessed 18 Aug 2020).

156. Hayes BJ, Gonzalez T, Smith JT, et al. Ankle arthritis: you can't always replace it. J Am AcadOrthopSurg. 2016;24:e29–e38. https://doi.org/10.5435/JAAOS-D-15-00354.

157. Feger MA, Donovan L, Hart JM, et al. Effect of ankle braces on lower extremity muscle activation during functional exercises in participants with chronic ankle instability. Int J Sports Phys Therapy (IJSPT) 2014;9(4):476–87.

158. Hall EA, Simon JE, Docherty CL. Using ankle bracing and taping to decrease range of motion and velocity during inversion perturbation while walking. J Athletic Train. 2016;51(4):283–90. https://doi.org/10.4085/1062-6050-51.5.06.

159. Newman TM, Vairo GL, Buckley WE. The comparative effects of ankle bracing on functional performance. J Sport Rehabil. 2018;27(5):491–502. https://doi.org/10.1123/jsr.2016-0136.

160. Frey C, Feder KS, Sleight J. Prophylactic ankle brace use in high school volleyball players: a prospective study. Foot Ankle Int. 2010;31(4):296–300. https://doi.org/10.3113/FAI.2010.0296.

161. Alfuth M, Klein D, Koch R, et al. Biomechanical comparison of 3 ankle braces with and without free rotation in the sagittal plane. J Athletic Train. 2014;49(5):608–16. https://doi.org/10.4085/1062-6050-49.3.20.

162. Lang B. Types of ankle braces for sports injuries. Medical University of South Carolina (MUSC) Health Sports Medicine. 2018 Nov 12. Available from: https://muschealth.org/blog/2018/november/ankle-brace (accessed 22 Sept 2020).

163. Maeda N, Urabe Y, Tsutsumi S, et al. Effect of semi-rigid and soft ankle braces on static and dynamic postural stability in young male adults. J Sports Sci Med. 2016;15:352–7.

164. Bot SDM, van Mechelen W. The effect of ankle bracing on athletic performance. Sports Med. 1999;27(3):171–8. https://doi.org/10.2165/00007256-199927030-00003.

165. Agres AN, Chrysanthou M, Raffalt PC. The effect of ankle bracing on kinematics in simulated sprain and drop landings: a double-blind, placebo-controlled study. Am J Sports Med. 2019;47(6):1480–7. https://doi.org/10.1177/0363546519837695.

166. McKnight PT, Kwoh CK. Randomized, controlled trial of compression gloves in rheumatoid arthritis. Arthritis Care Res. 1992;5(4):223–7.

167. Nasir SH, Troynikov O, Massy-Westropp N. Therapy gloves for patients with rheumatoid arthritis: a review. Ther Adv Musculoskel Dis. 2014;6(6):226–37. https://doi.org/10.1177/1759720X14557474.

168. Prior Y, Sutton C, Cotterill S, et al. The effects of arthritis gloves on people with Rheumatoid Arthritis or Inflammatory Arthritis with hand pain: a study protocol for a multi-centre randomised controlled trial (the A-GLOVES trial). BMC Musculoskelet Disord. 2017;18:224. https://doi.org/10.1186/s12891-017-1583-4.

169. Hammond A, Jones V, Prior Y. The effects of compression gloves on hand symptoms and hand function in rheumatoid arthritis and hand osteoarthritis: a systematic review. Clin Rehabil. 2015;1–12. https://doi.org/10.1177/0269215515578296.

170. Gustafsson L, Patterson E, Marshall K, et al. Efficacy of compression gloves in maintaining edema reductions after application of compression bandaging to the stroke-affected

upper limb. Am J Occup Ther. 2016;70:7002290030. https://doi.org/10.5014/ajot.2016.017939.

171. Miller-Shahabar I, Schreuer N, Katsevman H, et al. Efficacy of compression gloves in the rehabilitation of distal radius fractures: randomized controlled study. Am J Phys Med Rehabil. 2018;97:904–10. https://doi.org/10.1097/PHM.0000000000000998.

172. Dewey WS, Richard RL, Hedman TL, et al. A review of compression glove modifications to enhance functional grip: a case series. J Burn Care Res. 2007;28:888–91. https://doi.org/10.1097/BCR.0b013e318159e076.

18 Medical Devices for Gastroenterology and Hepatology

Syed Furrukh Jamil and Haafiz Allah-Bakhsh

CONTENTS

INTRODUCTION

Contemporary gastrointestinal (GI) practice has seen unprecedented progress during the last 30–40 years. Conventional one-size-fits-all management approaches are losing ground to evidence-based personalized care, gaining momentum in all aspects of clinical practice. Apart from advances in basic and clinical sciences, these headways have been made possible due to perpetual refinements in diagnostic and therapeutic devices—a testament to sustained breakthroughs in material sciences, electronics, and computational sciences. As laid out in the manuals, these instruments' structural and operational details are complex and esoteric and generally beyond the comprehension of otherwise integral elements of the healthcare delivery teams such as the pharmacy personnel. The dual purpose of this chapter is to demystify this information and present it in the context of clinical application so that all those involved in patient care could obtain reasonable familiarity with this rapidly advancing field. Thus, the discussion focuses on clinically relevant structural features, indications, pertinent operational details, and the well-accepted limitations of these devices. Pathophysiological nuances of the diseases and the technical details of the devices are omitted. Both the text and the accompanying illustrations remain engaged with the contextual discussion of the therapeutic principles and the procedural details.

The chapter follows the normal anatomical layout of the GI system; each subsection provides essential clinical information such as the anatomy, common pathologies, and diagnostic and therapeutic challenges; and, how individualized application of advanced imaging, motility assessment, endoscopic interventions, and the utilization of specific point-of-care tools have revolutionized a modern GI practice. Although the chapter is framed for a broader audience, the relevance of the covered devices for a clinical pharmacist is further reinforced by a dedicated subsection that also contains tables outlining online reference resources with additional academic and technical details related to the covered devices.

ESOPHAGUS

The esophagus, a muscular tube, is the first segment of the gastrointestinal tract (Figure 18.1), starting from the pharynx and joining the stomach after passing through an opening in the diaphragm. It is approximately 25 cm long and 2 cm in diameter in an adult, with the primary function of transporting the bolus of food from the oral cavity to the

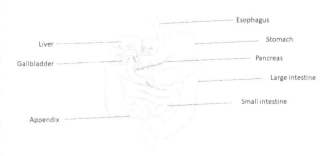

FIGURE 18.1 Topology of the gastrointestinal system.

DOI: 10.1201/9781003002345-20

stomach. This function depends on exquisite neuromuscular coordination between swallowing mechanisms and an aboral propagation of esophageal contraction-relaxation waves culminating in lower esophagal sphincter relaxation and bolus passage into the stomach.

Common Pathologies: Esophageal dysfunction can result from primary esophageal pathologies or the surrounding organs' diseases. Most common primary esophageal pathologies include gastroesophageal reflux disease (GERD), eosinophilic esophagitis, motility disorders such as achalasia, cricopharyngeal incoordination, and diffuse esophageal spasm. Similarly, diverticula, hiatus hernia, viral and fungal esophagitis, and bleeding from Mallory-Weiss syndrome are common.

The digestive system starts from the mouth and ends at the anus. As outlined in this cartoon diagram, significant organs of the system include the esophagus, stomach, small intestine, large intestine, rectum, and anus. The accessory organs, including the liver, gallbladder, and pancreas, are linked at the level of the duodenum.

Gastroesophageal Reflux Disease (GERD): Gastroesophageal reflux disease (GERD) is a very common cause of a visit to a physician. Patients usually present with symptoms of heartburn with or without regurgitation of fluid or food. GERD is often diagnosed based on history and treated with concurrent lifestyle modification and pharmacotherapy

such as proton pump inhibitors.[1-3] For symptoms refractory to these measures or when the diagnosis is uncertain, an upper GI endoscopy, or an esophageal manometry with esophageal pH testing may be required. Ambulatory pH monitoring is the best test to quantify acid reflux along with the patient's reported symptoms. The procedure entails placing a transnasal catheter or a wireless probe in the esophagus, which measures pH for 24 to 48 hours.[4]

Motility Disorders: Patients with esophageal motility disorders usually present with dysphagia (difficulty swallowing food).[5] Although various esophageal and non-esophageal pathologies can cause dysmotility, achalasia is the prototype esophageal motility disorder resulting from a lack of relaxation of the lower esophageal sphincter. Diagnostic modalities for motility disorders have evolved over the years. High-resolution manometry with esophageal pressure topography has taken the center stage versus the traditional reliance on low-yield barium swallowing studies[6-8] These advances result from the availability of sophisticated manometry related equipment.

High-resolution manometry (Figure 18.2) with esophageal pressure topography has streamlined the diagnosis of esophageal motility disorders. As shown in Figure 18.3, a thin catheter with a series of closely spaced pressure sensors is placed through an anesthetized nostril and advanced through the esophagus to the stomach. With each requested

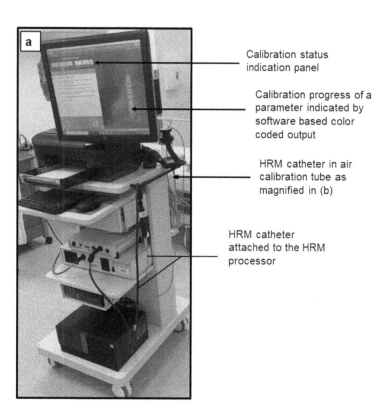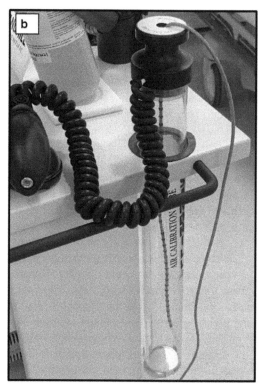

Calibration status indication panel

Calibration progress of a parameter indicated by software based color coded output

HRM catheter in air calibration tube as magnified in (b)

HRM catheter attached to the HRM processor

FIGURE 18.2 High-resolution manometry equipment setup: (a) HRM catheter is calibrated before esophageal intubation. The calibration method varies according to the type of probe to be used and the manufacturer's specifications. In this system, as an example, the HRM catheter is shown placed in an airtight pressure chamber (magnified in [b]) in which a set pressure is produced against which software-based calibration is accomplished. Separate calibration is done for water in a separate container, and validation is confirmed by the system. HRM: high-resolution manometry.

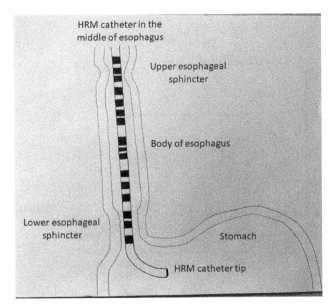

FIGURE 18.3 Cartoon drawing illustrating the position of high-resolution esophageal manometry catheter: The HR esophageal manometry catheter is a flexible tube that is inserted in the patient's esophagus in such a way that the distal tip of the catheter lies in the stomach. Black bands represent susceptible and accurate pressure sensors that detect event-specific pressure changes in the entire esophagus, including upper and lower esophageal sphincters.

swallow, a manometer measures the strength, relaxation, and coordination of esophageal muscles in the body and both upper and lower sphincters. High-resolution manometry gathers data from a more closely spaced pressure sensor (1 cm apart); hence, it offers much-enhanced resolution over conventional manometry.[9,10]

STOMACH

The stomach is a J-shaped organ with four anatomic regions: cardia, fundus, body, and pylorus, connecting the esophagus with the duodenum, the first part of the small intestine. Apart from its reservoir function, it initiates the digestion of the food through its rhythmic contractions and relaxations, releases vital secretions (acid and enzymes), and controls gastrointestinal motility. For example, to facilitate the break-up and the digestion of the macronutrients, the stomach can accommodate a significant increase in its luminal contents without any appreciable rise in intragastric pressure through adaptive relaxation. Apart from its role in digestion, acid secretion plays a vital role in defense against pathogens gaining access through the gastrointestinal system. Similarly, the stomach is also an important endocrine organ producing peptide hormones such as ghrelin and leptin, central to both enteric and nonenteric physiology.

Common Pathologies: Like that of the esophagus, stomach dysfunction commonly results from primary gastric diseases, although secondary gastric dysfunction is not uncommon. Common gastric pathologies include acid peptic disorders, dysmotility such as gastroparesis, functional dyspepsia, and gastric neoplasms.

Gastric Motility Disorders: Gastric motility disorders include gastroparesis (delayed emptying), dumping syndrome (rapid gastric emptying), and functional dyspepsia. Historically these disorders were diagnosed by typical symptoms in the context of regular endoscopic and radiographic examinations. However, during the last two decades, gastric emptying scan gained widespread acceptance.[11–13] Although the protocol may vary from center to center, the typical procedure involves consuming food with added radioactive material that enables monitoring of the rate at which the tracer leaves the stomach and enters the small intestine. For example, (99Tc) containing an egg-white based meal with adequate fat content is offered to the patient, and the imaging is performed after one, two, and four hours after the meal ingestion.[14] More recently, the FDA approved a wireless motility capsule, which provides an additional advantage of being utilized as an outpatient procedure.[15,16] After the capsule is swallowed, it travels through the GI tract and simultaneously records the transit time, luminal pH, and pressure, thus furnishing vital information for diagnosing specific motility disorders.[17]

Acid Peptic Disorders: Despite widespread public awareness of the everyday lifestyle triggers, acid peptic disease remains a common GI disorder of our time. Apart from the dietary triggers, drugs such as NSAIDs and *H. pylori* infection remain the most important modifiable risk factors for acid peptic disorders.[18,19] Endoscopic examination plays a pivotal role in establishing the diagnosis, documenting the response to therapeutic interventions and managing the complications such as bleeding gastroduodenal ulcers.[20]

Conventional Endoscopy: Modern endoscopes (Figure 18.4) have evolved over the years and endoscopy has become the procedure of choice for the diagnosis of most of the upper and lower GI disorders.[21,1,19,21,22] Apart from allowing the operator to examine the macroscopic appearance, this procedure provides access to perform the biopsy of the suspected areas of the gut mucosa for microscopic examination (Figure 18.5). Similarly, various therapeutic procedures are standard of care, including foreign body removal, restoration of vascular homeostasis through injections, energy-based coagulation, or the delivery of hemostatic clips (Figure 18.6). The scope of these therapeutic procedures can be imagined by the catalogue of the commonly utilized specific add-on equipment including clips, knives, hooks, biopsy forceps, applicators, injection needles, coagulation probes, balloon catheters, retrieval devices (extraction bags, extraction baskets, graspers), balloon dilators, esophageal stents, guide wires, polypectomy snares, a variety of energy-delivery catheters, balloon dilators, and stents.[23,24]

ERCP: Endoscopic retrograde cholangiopancreatography (ERCP) is a further refinement of endoscopy. A specialized side-viewing upper endoscope is advanced into the duodenum to advance specific diagnostic and therapeutic accessories into the bile and pancreatic ducts. Once the

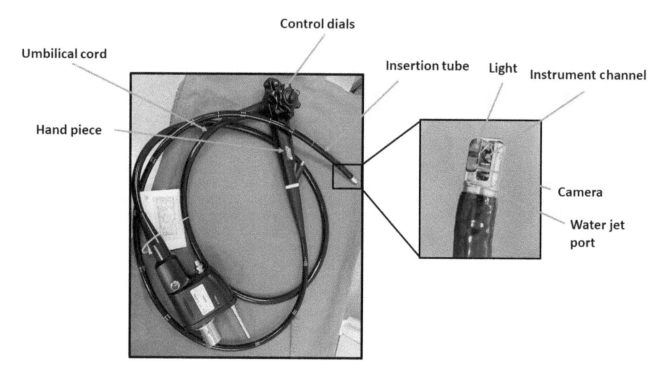

FIGURE 18.4 A typical endoscope: As an example of a typical endoscope, a side-viewing duodenoscope is shown, which is used for performing ERCP for the diagnosis and therapy of pancreaticobiliary pathologies. In the inset, elements of side-viewing assembly are illustrated, which include a camera, light source, water jet port, and a working (instrument) channel. The channel elevator (not depicted) can be used to direct instruments independent of the scope tip movements. ERCP: endoscopic retrograde cholangiopancreatography.

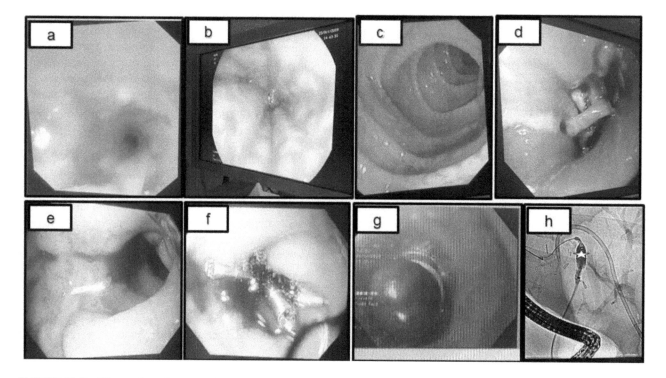

FIGURE 18.5 Diagnostic and therapeutic application of endoscopy in gastroenterology and hepatology.

(a) Esophageal stricture following a corrosive ingestion; (b) candida esophagitis; (c) mucosal scalloping of duodenal mucosa typically seen in celiac disease; (d) esophageal foreign body (button battery); (e) duodenal bleeding ulcer before therapy; (f) duodenal ulcer as in (e) after endoclip application; (g) esophageal variceal band ligation, and Hh) balloon (*) dilation of biliary stricture through ERCP.

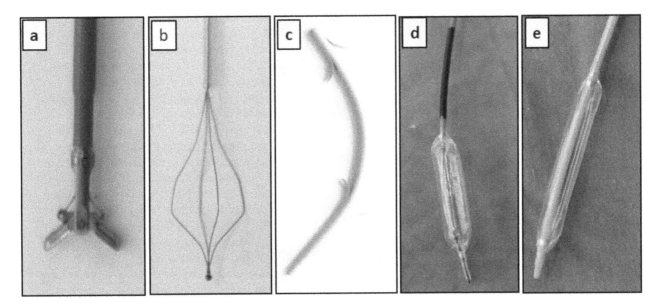

FIGURE 18.6 Accessories utilized through instrument channel of an endoscope: Out of a plethora of these tools, a few are shown as examples, including (a) disposable hot biopsy forceps; (b) retrieval basket; (c) pancreatic stent; (d) endoscopic esophageal/pyloric balloon dilatation catheter; (e) biliary dilation balloon.

intended duct is cannulated, further advancement is guided by the contrast medium-based radiologic visualization and application of any therapeutic interventions. One of the most common indications of ERCP is the extraction of stones in the common bile duct. Other indications include elucidation of the etiology of obstructive jaundice, tissue sampling from biliary or pancreatic ducts, workup of the pancreatitis of unknown etiology, biliary stenting (Figure 18.5h), drainage of the pancreatic pseudocyst, and nasobiliary drainage.[25,26] Although this procedure provides instantaneous access and relief of biliary colic, additional training and skills are needed to perform an ERCP. Similarly, ERCP has a higher potential for serious complications such as pancreatitis than conventional endoscopic examinations.[27,28,29,30]

Although sedation is required, most endoscopic examinations are performed as outpatient procedures and are very well tolerated. After careful discussion of the procedure and informed consent, the patient is made comfortable, and sedation is provided usually by the anesthesia team. Using advanced endoscopy system set-up (Figure 18.7), the intended procedure (esophagoscopy, gastroscopy, gastroduodenoscopy, ERCP, colonoscopy, flexible sigmoidoscopy, or proctoscopy) is performed, and the required samples are collected for appropriate diagnostic evaluations. After the procedure, the endoscope is withdrawn, and the sedation is discontinued. The patient is observed and supported in the postoperative observation station until neurologic status returns to normal and enteral intake is established and tolerated. The patient is discharged.

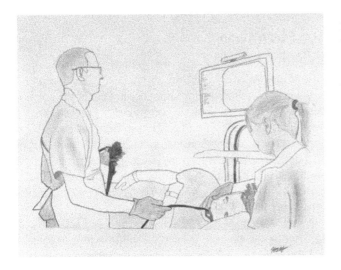

FIGURE 18.7 Endoscopy procedure setup. An upper endoscopic examination is depicted in this sketch drawing. Usually, an intravenous line is inserted, IV sedation and oropharyngeal local anesthetic spray are utilized, and the patient is made comfortable. A plastic mouthpiece is inserted, and the endoscope is advanced under direct visualization, usually to the last part of the duodenum. Apart from careful inspection, desired biopsies and other interventions are performed under direct observation on the display monitor. Whereas the patient's position may vary, the setup for other endoscopic examinations such as ERCP and colonoscopy remains similar to EGD, as shown in this drawing.

THE WIRELESS MOTILITY AND PH CAPSULE (WMC)

The main advantages of the wireless motility and pH capsules include their utility in the outpatient setting and concurrently assessing regional and whole-gut transit times. The US Food and Drug Administration (FDA) has approved its application to evaluate gastroparesis and colonic transit in chronic idiopathic constipation.[31] The wireless capsule is easy to swallow (26 x 13 mm) and non-digestible with a battery life of five days; it measures pressure, pH, and temperature as it traverses the GI tract.[32]

NUTRITIONAL DEVICES

A. ENTERAL TUBES

Enteral tubes (Figure 18.9) are medical devices widely used for providing nutritional supplements through the gastrointestinal tract for patients who cannot eat at all or eat enough to meet their nutritional requirements.[33,34,35] These are also frequently utilized for the administration of medication, especially in acute care settings. Likewise, in the setting of significant gastrointestinal dysfunction, these tubes become essential for removing air and fluids from the stomach.

The choice of the enteral tube depends on the purpose for its use and on whether the tube is needed in the short or long term. Short-term enteral tubes include the orogastric (OG), nasogastric (NG), nasoduodenal (ND), and nasojejunal (NJ) tubes. Tubes intended for more long-term use include the gastrostomy tube (PEG, G-tube), gastrojejunostomy tubes, and jejunostomy tubes.[36]

1. Orogastric (OG) and Nasogastric (NG) tubes: These types of tubes are inserted either through the mouth (OG tube) or the nose (NG tube) and advanced through the esophagus into the stomach. Typically, an OG tube is utilized for up to 2 weeks, while an NG tube can be utilized as long as 4 to 6 weeks.

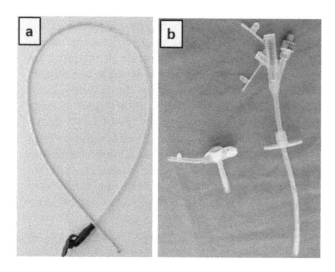

FIGURE 18.8 Feeding tubes: (a) Nasogastric or orogastric insertion tubes come in different sizes as expressed in French (Fr) units; smaller French sizes have a larger diameter. Plastic tubes are usually utilized for a shorter duration, whereas silicone tubes can last for weeks and thus are preferred over plastic tubes when jejunal feeds are planned; (b) Gastrostomy tubes: Shown are a tri-funnel gastrostomy tube (longer tube on the right) available in different French sizes; And the smaller tube on the left is the MIC-KEY button gastrostomy tube (low profile) which is also available in different French sizes.

Suppose the need for tube-based nutritional support lasts longer than this period. In that case, OG or NG can be replaced with a long-term tube typically inserted directly into the stomach, usually through transcutaneous access [37] (*vide quid sequitur*).

2. Nasoduodenal (ND) and Nasojejunal (NJ) tubes: These tubes are relatively more flexible and narrower compared to OG and NG tubes. ND and NJ tubes are inserted like OG/NG but rest either in the duodenum (ND) or in the jejunum (NJ). These can be inserted endoscopically or manually with radiological monitoring to confirm the position. These can remain in place for up to 4 to 6 weeks.

3. Gastrostomy Tube (GT): This is commonly known as a percutaneous endoscopic gastrostomy (PEG) tube when secured endoscopically. These are also frequently inserted by surgeons laparoscopically or by an interventional radiologist under fluoroscopic guidance. A long catheter-type tube (picture) is used at initial insertion, converted into a short tube (Mic-Key Button) in about eight weeks to be less obtrusive and easy to conceal for regular daily schedules.

4. Gastrojejunostomy Tube: A gastrojejunostomy tube is inserted through a gastrostomy and advanced to the jejunum. These tubes have gastric ports used for decompression, whereas a jejunal port is used for feeding and medication administrations.

5. Jejunostomy Tube: This tube is inserted directly into the jejunum. Like gastrojejunostomy tubes, this tube is utilized for continuous feeding since the small intestine is not suitable for bolus feeds.

SMALL INTESTINE

The small intestine connects the stomach with the large intestine and is approximately 20 feet long. It comprises the duodenum, jejunum, and ilium. Functions of the small intestine include modulation of global gastrointestinal physiology; digestion of carbohydrates, fats, and proteins; and absorption of all nutrients, vitamins, trace elements, and bile salts. These functions are carried out by well-coordinated interactions of the pancreas, gallbladder, and an array of specialized secretory and absorptive functions of the small intestinal mucosa.

Common Pathologies: Pathologies of the small intestine are diverse, ranging from acute self-limiting or acute viral enteritis to chronic diseases such as inflammatory bowel disease and neoplasia. Some common gastrointestinal diseases with predominant small intestinal involvement include celiac disease, short bowel syndrome, small bowel bacterial overgrowth, and specific disorders of epithelial integrity, transport, metabolism, absorption, and digestion.

1. Short Bowel Syndrome: Chronic intestinal failure or short bowel syndrome is a disorder in which the small intestine cannot provide optimal digestive

and absorptive functions either due to intestinal volume loss from surgical interventions, an underlying congenital intestinal mucosal deficit, or a motility disorder.

2. Crohn's Disease: Crohn's disease is an inflammatory bowel disease that can affect any part of the gastrointestinal system, although terminal ileum and colon involvement are the classic presentations. Usually, the patient presents with chronic abdominal pain, diarrhea, and weight loss. However, although axial imaging such as CT scans is commonly done, endoscopic examination and microscopic examination of the biopsies from the affected area necessary to establish the diagnosis.

LARGE INTESTINE

The large intestine is an inverted U-shaped structure that incompletely surrounds the small intestine. It comprises the appendix, caecum, ascending, transverse, descending, and sigmoid colon, and the rectum. It is one fifth (1.5 meters) of the whole GI tract. Its primary function is water absorption, keeping what remains as waste before it is collected in the rectum and then defecated through the anal canal, an area with the specialized organization of muscles and nerves enabling an intricate regulation of bowel movements.

Common Pathologies: Like the small intestine, the pathologies of the large intestine range from short-lived acute illnesses to chronic relapsing diseases such as IBS, IBD, functional constipation, polyps, diverticulosis, and neoplasia. Ulcerative colitis is the most familiar large bowel disease after constipation. It is an inflammatory bowel disease like Crohn's disease. Patients usually present with alternative diarrhea and constipation, hematochezia, weight loss, lower abdominal pain, and tenesmus. Colonoscopy is the best diagnostic modality for colonic diseases.

Anorectum: Normally, the tone of the anal sphincter muscle increases as the stool enters the rectum preventing the passage of stool until a socially acceptable environment is available for a voluntary evacuation of the rectum. If the sphincter muscle is weak or neural mechanisms are not contracted timely, fecal incontinence may occur. Common causes of sphincter dysfunction include spinal cord injuries, sphincter muscle weakness, obstetric trauma, and damage sustained during prior interventions in the rectoanal area.

Anorectal Manometry: Anorectal manometry is most commonly indicated for patients suffering from fecal incontinence or when dysmotility is suspected to be the primary etiology of constipation.[38,39] It can also be utilized as an aid in biofeedback-based colon retraining programs.[40] Anorectal manometry's specific electrophysiologic objectives include assessing rectal sensation, compliance, anal sphincter tone, and anorectal inhibitory reflex. These are determined using a small balloon with the manometry catheter in the rectum to distend the rectum; the catheter

records the intended parameters. Anorectal manometry plays a vital adjunctive role in the workup of children with ultrashort-segment Hirschsprung disease, a rare but consequential cause of encopresis in this age group. This disorder results from an absence of ganglion cells in the submucosa and myenteric plexuses of the distal colon resulting in failed relaxation of the internal anal sphincter in response to the distention by balloon inflation.

ANORECTAL MANOMETRY: EQUIPMENT AND PROCEDURE

The electrophysiological principles of RM are the same as those of esophageal manometry: aiming to elucidate rectal sensation and compliance, anal sphincter pressure, and anorectal inhibitory reflex. After explaining the procedure, the patient is asked to lie on the left lateral position with hips and knees kept flexed. A balloon-deflated lubricated probe is gently advanced into the rectum. Anal resting pressure is measured over 20 seconds. Afterwards, sequentially, the patient is asked to squeeze the anus, bear down as if to defecate, and cough to measure rectoanal reflex activity. Finally, the balloon is slowly inflated, and the patient is asked to indicate when he/she experiences a feeling of fullness or distension in the rectum.

COMMONLY USED COLON CARE ACCESSORIES

Ostomy Bags: Elective or emergent small or large bowel resection due to various underlying diseases may become necessary as a part of a short- or intermediate-term care plan. Once an ostomy (bowel opening to the abdominal surface) has been created, it requires a collection bag (ileostomy or colostomy), as shown in Figure 18.9.

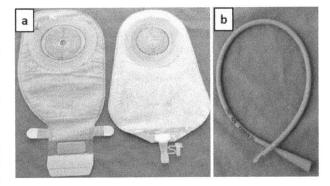

FIGURE 18.9 Colon care accessories: Ostomy bags are used to collect ileostomy or colostomy output. As shown in the photograph (a), these come in drainable (right) or closed single-use forms (left). The opening of the bag can be adjusted according to the stoma size. (b) Rectal tubes are used for multiple purposes such as rectal washout and administering enemas and other drugs, including contrast medium for imaging purposes.

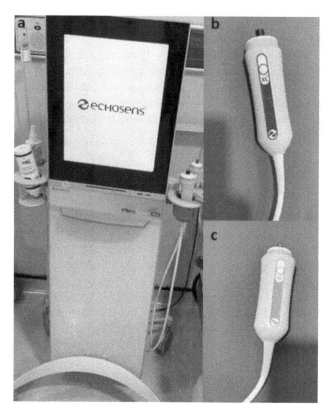

FIGURE 18.10   Fibroscan: This is also known as liver ultrasonographic elastography and transient elastography.

Enemas: Enemas are products given through anal opening. Most indications of enemas are for bowel preparation before colonoscopy or constipation. Phosphate enemas (Fleet®) are widely used for these purposes, but they should be used cautiously in the elderly population since they could lead to hypotension and electrolyte imbalance. Contrast enema and air enema, respectively, are used for diagnostic and therapeutic purposes.

Noninvasive Assessment of Hepatic Fibrosis: Fibroscan (figure 18.10) is a noninvasive point-of-care scan that helps to grade hepatic fibrosis through ultrasonic shear wave (vibration) velocity determination. Typically, through an ultrasonic probe, a 50 MHz wave is passed through the liver, and the velocity of the shear wave is recorded in meters per second units by a transducer present in the same probe. These data are then converted into liver stiffness and expressed as kilopascals (kPa). Apart from being noninvasive, the equipment is easy to use, and the study usually takes less than 10 minutes to be completed. However, the Fibroscan test is not feasible for patients with morbid obesity or those with ascites. Similarly, a minimum of eight to ten successful measurements is needed for the results to be valid. Despite these limitations, Fibroscan has made its place reliable as an easy-to-use test for the presence or absence of significant hepatic fibrosis, especially when supported by clinical examination and other investigations.

EQUIPMENT USED IN GASTROENTEROLOGY AND HEPATOLOGY CARE: IMPLICATION FOR A PHARMACIST

Apart from the contemporary issues related to indications, contraindications, pharmacokinetics, and pharmacodynamics of the drugs utilized before, during, and after GI procedures, the tools and equipment discussed in this chapter have direct relevance to the pharmacy practice in many ways, including the following:

1. The pharmacist may have a first-responder role for both the practitioner and the patient, providing consultative services for the availability and relative benefits of the accessories such as nasogastric tubes, ileostomy and colostomy bags, and gastrostomy tubes. Similarly, a pharmacist may be asked to help troubleshoot malfunctions of these accessories.
2. The pharmacist may play a vital role in guiding the consumers for the available resources on the merits of a particular product. Such information is usually available in the form of product manuals issued by the manufacturers and sometimes crystallized in guidelines produced by professional societies such as those outlined in Table 18.1.
3. A pharmacist is usually a leading member of the institutional committees charged with selecting all new and any upgrades of the competing systems. These include inclusive endoscopy and high-resolution manometry systems and a catalogue of noninvasive instruments that are part and parcel of modern GI and hepatology practices.
4. In various capacities, pharmacists may also play a vital role as an advisor to the manufacturers, from the inception of a new product to the upgrades of the existing equipment and accessories.

CONCLUSIONS

1. Contrary to all other organ systems, the gastrointestinal system provides a unique host-environment matrix along its entire length with specific regional specializations. As a result, many sophisticated diagnostic and therapeutic devices have been designed and successfully incorporated into routine clinical care.
2. Most of the commonly utilized devices in a modern gastroenterology practice, such as endoscopy, high-resolution manometry, and elastography, need significant time commitment to comprehend the principal equipment's structural and functional properties and the associated accessories.
3. Spurred by the ongoing expansion of clinical indications and the commercial competition, very frequent upgrades of the existing devices is the norm, mandating all involved healthcare personnel to

TABLE 18.1

Online Resources for Approved Guidelines and GI-Related Technology Assessment Reviews

NICE	National Institute for Health and Care Excellence	Provides guidance to improve health and social care in the UK	www.nice.org.uk/
AHRQ	Agency for Healthcare Research and Quality	A US agency that develops cohesive knowledge tools and data required to improve the healthcare system	www.ahrq.gov/
BSG	British Society of Gastroenterology and Hepatology	The voice of the British gastroenterology and hepatology communities	www.bsg.org.uk/medical-interest/
ESGE	European Society of Gastroenterology and Endoscopy	European gastroenterology organization which issues guidelines and recommendations	www.esge.com/publications/guidelines/
AGA	American Gastroenterology Association	AGA's clinical guidelines are evidence-based recommendations to help guide clinical practice and decision making based on rigorous systematic reviews of the medical literature	https://gastro.org/guidelines/

TABLE 18.2

Online Resources from Commercial Companies Producing Gastroenterology- and Hepatology-Related Products

Online Resources from Commercial Companies Producing Gastroenterology- and Hepatology-Related Products.

Olympus	A well-known worldwide manufacturer of different types of endoscopes, endotherapeutic devices, capsule endoscopy solutions, etc.	www.olympus-europa.com/
Medtronic/Covidien	Covidien is an arm of Medtronic focused on various GI related equipment.	www.medtronic.com
PANTAX Medical	One of the main manufacturers of endoscopy systems	www.pentaxmedical.com/
LABORIE	A leading developer and manufacturer tools used in colorectal other gastrointestinal procedures	www.laborie.com/
Given Imaging	Manufactures and markets diagnostic products for the diagnosis of the gastrointestinal tract	www.givenimaging.com/
Diversatek healthcare	Supplier of a wide range of tools used in diagnostic and therapeutic GI practice	www.diversatekhealthcare.com/

remain familiar with the evolution of at least the most relevant aspects of these devices.

4. As a vital member of the healthcare delivery teams, a pharmacist plays a prime role in delivering modern gastrointestinal care. Familiarity with key structural and functional aspects of the devices covered in this chapter will prepare the pharmacy staff for a vital contribution along the continuum of clinical practice.

ACKNOWLEDGMENTS

Authors are thankful to Huzaifa for drawings used in Figures 18.3 and 18.7; materials used in Figure 18.5a, b, c, e, and f are a kind courtesy of Dr. Al-Hamwa Moudi. Dr Ahmad Abdullah kindly provided material used in Figure 18.5d.

REFERENCES

1. Fass R. Therapeutic options for refractory gastroesophageal reflux disease. J Gastroenterol Hepatol. 2012;27(Suppl. 3):3–7. https://doi.org/10.1111/j.1440-1746.2012.07064.x.

2. Dean BB, Gano AD, Knight K, et al. Effectiveness of proton pump inhibitors in nonerosive reflux disease. Clin Gastroenterol Hepatol. 2004;2(8):656–64. https://doi.org/10.1016/S1542-3565(04)00288-5.

3. Hunter JG, Kahrilas PJ, Bell RCW, et al. Efficacy of transoral fundoplication vs omeprazole for treatment of regurgitation in a randomized controlled trial. Gastroenterology. 2015;148(2):324–33.e5.https://doi.org/10.1053/j.gastro.2014.10.009.

4. Ripoll C, Groszmann R, Garcia-Tsao G, et al. Hepatic venous pressure gradient predicts clinical decompensation in patients with compensated cirrhosis. Gastroenterology. 2007;133(2):481–8. https://doi.org/10.1053/j.gastro.2007.05.024.

5. Pandolfino JE, Kahrilas PJ. AGA technical review on the clinical use of esophageal manometry. Gastroenterology. 2005;128(1):209–24. https://doi.org/10.1053/j.gastro.2004.11.008.

6. Murray JA, Clouse RE, Conklin JL. Components of the standard oesophageal manometry. Neurogastroenterol Motil. 2003;15(6):591–606. https://doi.org/10.1046/j.1365-2982.2003.00446.x.

7. Wong U, Person EB, Castell DO, et al. Improving high-resolution impedance manometry using novel viscous and super-viscous substrates in the supine and upright positions: a pilot study. J Neurogastroenterol Motil. 2018;24(4):570–6. https://doi.org/10.5056/jnm18010.

8. Schizas D, Kapsampelis P, Tsilimigras DI, et al. The 100 most cited manuscripts in esophageal motility disorders: a bibliometric analysis. Ann Transl Med. 2019;7(14):310. https://doi.org/10.21037/atm.2019.06.34.

9. Clouse R, Prakash C. Topographic esophageal manometry: an emerging clinical and investigative approach. Dig Dis. 2000;18(2):64–74. https://doi.org/10.1159/000016967.

10. Kahrilas PJ. Esophageal motor disorders in terms of high-resolution esophageal pressure topography: what has changed. Am J Gastroenterol. 2010;105(5):981–7. https://doi.org/10.1038/ajg.2010.43.

11. Jielani A, Fatima T, Hussain JA, et al. Gastric emptying scintigraphy in assessment of chronic vomiting. J Ayub Med Coll Abbottabad. 2018;30(2):295–7.

12. Levin AA, Levine MS, Rubesin SE, et al. An 8-year review of barium studies in the diagnosis of gastroparesis. Clin Radiol. 2008;63(4):407–14. https://doi.org/10.1016/j.crad.2007.10.007.

13. Sharma A, Coles M, Parkman HP. Gastroparesis in the 2020s: new treatments, new paradigms. Curr Gastroenterol Rep. 2020;22(5). https://doi.org/10.1007/s11894-020-00761-7.

14. Abell TL, Camilleri M, Donohoe K, et al. Consensus recommendations for gastric emptying scintigraphy: a joint report of the American Neurogastroenterology and Motility Society and the Society of Nuclear Medicine. J Nucl Med Technol. 2008;36(1):44–54. https://doi.org/10.2967/jnmt.107.048116.

15. Farmer AD, Scott SM, Hobson AR. Gastrointestinal motility revisited: the wireless motility capsule. United Eur Gastroenterol J. 2013;1(6):413–21. https://doi.org/10.1177/2050640613510161.

16. Saad RJ, Hasler WL. A technical review and clinical assessment of the wireless motility capsule. Gastroenterol Hepatol. 2011;7(12):795–804.

17. Maqbool S, Parkman HP, Friedenberg FK. Wireless capsule motility: comparison of the smartPill® GI monitoring system with scintigraphy for measuring whole gut transit. Dig Dis Sci. 2009;54(10):2167–74. https://doi.org/10.1007/s10620-009-0899-9.

18. Clarrett DM, Hachem C. Gastroesophageal reflux disease aff ects millions of people worldwide with significant clinical implications. Mo Med. 2018;115(3):214. Available from: /pmc/articles/PMC6140167/?report=abstract (accessed 7 Apr 2021).

19. Badillo R. Diagnosis and treatment of gastroesophageal reflux disease. World J Gastrointest Pharmacol Ther. 2014;5(3):105. https://doi.org/10.4292/wjgpt.v5.i3.105.

20. Sandhu DS, Fass R. Current trends in the management of gastroesophageal reflux disease. Gut Liver. 2018;12(1):7–16. https://doi.org/10.5009/gnl16615.

21. Loughrey MB, Shepherd NA. The indications for biopsy in routine upper gastrointestinal endoscopy. Histopathology. 2021;78(1):215–27. https://doi.org/10.1111/his.14213.

22. Balart LA. Endoscopy in gastrointestinal disease. Procedures that offer an alternative to surgery. Postgrad Med. 1985;77(6):179–85. https://doi.org/10.1080/00325481.1985.11698990.

23. Advances in diagnostic and therapeutic endoscopy—PubMed. Available from: https://pubmed.ncbi.nlm.nih.gov/11026918/ (accessed 7 Apr 2021).

24. Nabi Z, Reddy DN. Advanced therapeutic gastrointestinal endoscopy in children—today and tomorrow. Clin Endosc. 2018;51(2):142–9. https://doi.org/10.5946/ce.2017.102.

25. Meseeha M, Attia M. Endoscopic retrograde cholangiopancreatography. In: StatPearls. Treasure Island, FL: StatPearls Publishing; 2021. Available from: www.ncbi.nlm.nih.gov/pubmed/29630212 (accessed 7 Apr 2021).

26. Tso DK, Almeida RR, Prabhakar AM, et al. Accuracy and timeliness of an abbreviated emergency department MRCP protocol for choledocholithiasis. Emerg Radiol. 2019;26(4):427–32. https://doi.org/10.1007/s10140-019-01689-w.

27. Bleeding complications and clinical safety of endoscopic retrograde cholangiopancreatography in patients with liver cirrhosis—PubMed. Available from: https://pubmed.ncbi.nlm.nih.gov/31016905/ (accessed 7 Apr 2021).

28. Balmadrid B, Kozarek R. Prevention and management of adverse events of endoscopic retrograde cholangiopancreatography. Gastrointest Endosc Clin N Am. 2013;23(2):385–403. https://doi.org/10.1016/j.giec.2012.12.007.

29. Ishii S, Fujisawa T, Ushio M, et al. Evaluation of the safety and efficacy of minimal endoscopic sphincterotomy followed by papillary balloon dilation for the removal of common bile duct stones. Saudi J Gastroenterol. 2020;26(6):344–50. https://doi.org/10.4103/sjg.SJG_162_20.

30. Ishii S, Isayama H, Ushio M, et al. Best procedure for the management of common bile duct stones via the papilla: literature review and analysis of procedural efficacy and safety. J Clin Med. 2020;9(12):3808. https://doi.org/10.3390/jcm9123808.

31. Saad RJ. The wireless motility capsule: a one-stop shop for the evaluation of GI motility disorders. Curr Gastroenterol Rep. 2016;18(3):1–7. https://doi.org/10.1007/s11894-016-0489-x.

32. Kuo B, McCallum RW, Koch KL, et al. Comparison of gastric emptying of a nondigestible capsule to a radio-labelled meal in healthy and gastroparetic subjects. Aliment Pharmacol Ther. 2008;27(2):186–96. https://doi.org/10.1111/j.1365-2036.2007.03564.x.

33. Enteral feeding. Nasogastric, nasojejunal, percutaneous endoscopic gastrostomy, or jejunostomy: its indications and limitations. Postgraduate Medical Journal. Available from: https://pmj.bmj.com/content/78/918/198 (accessed 7 Apr 2021).

34. Pearce CB, Collett J, Goggin PM, et al. Enteral nutrition by nasojejunal tube in hyperemesis gravidarum. Clin Nutr. 2001;20(5):461–4. https://doi.org/10.1054/clnu.2001.0484.

35. Fulbrook P, Bongers A, Albarran JW. A European survey of enteral nutrition practices and procedures in adult intensive care units. J Clin Nurs. 2007;16(11):2132–41. https://doi.org/10.1111/j.1365-2702.2006.01841.x.

36. Paine P, McMahon M, Farrer K, et al. Jejunal feeding: when is it the right thing to do? Frontline Gastroenterol. 2020;11(5):397–403. https://doi.org/10.1136/flgastro-2019-101181.

37. Rahnemai-Azar AA, Rahnemaiazar AA, Naghshizadian R, et al. Percutaneous endoscopic gastrostomy: indications, technique, complications and management. World J Gastroenterol. 2014;20(24):7739–51. https://doi.org/10.3748/wjg.v20.i24.7739.

38. Mitrani C. Anorectal manometric characteristics in men and women with idiopathic fecal incontinence. J Clin Gastroenterol. 1998;26(3):175–8. https://doi.org/10.1097/00004836-199804000-00005.

39. Camilleri M, Thompson WG, Fleshman JW, et al. Clinical management of intractable constipation. Ann Intern Med. 1994;121(7):520–8. https://doi.org/10.7326/0003-4819-121-7-199410010-00008.

40. Rao SSC, Seaton K, Miller M, et al. Randomized controlled trial of biofeedback, sham feedback, and standard therapy for dyssynergic defecation. Clin Gastroenterol Hepatol. 2007;5(3):331–8. https://doi.org/10.1016/j.cgh.2006.12.023.

19 Medical Device Issues

Albert I. Wertheimer

It would be so good if everyone were diligent, honest, and responsible, but unfortunately, that is not always the case. Medical devices in developed countries are rigorously tested and licensed by some governmental agency that specifies who may purchase the device, who may use it, and under what circumstances. But human nature as it exists sometimes leads us astray. So, we know of examples of fraud, deceit, and greed involving medical devices. In this brief chapter, we will look in detail at some of these problems and hopefully take away some lessons to guide our future behaviors.

Just as drugs, women's purses, and designer wrist watches are counterfeited, that is also found in the medical device area. It occurs most frequently with replacement parts which may be produced by some illegal operation, and not the company whose name appears on the outer carton. Some spare parts are made to look like the original branded product, but are, in actuality—fakes, or what we call unauthorized copies. Some parts are not new at all, but are recycled, used parts that were intended to be disposed of after the recommended period of service. Some parts are not exactly the same and may have lower specifications or are unable to perform the full range of functions with the same accuracy as the legitimate product.

But even if the correct legitimate replacement parts are used, that is not the end of potential problems. Some unscrupulous persons or organizations may elect to use parts and machines well beyond their listed expiration or replacement dates. Consider an X-ray machine that should have a critical component replaced every six months, and the owner decides to stretch that time period to nine months or even twelve months. He or she cannot be sure that the machine is giving accurate readings after the six-month period. In fact, they would in all likelihood be unable to know how misleading their device's results were. Then, there is the matter of the proper care and maintenance of medical devices. Many manufacturers suggest that machines be recalibrated and tested once a year. It saves money to skip this step, but it can be dangerous if a miscalibrated device is used for medical or surgical decision-making. Just as an automobile should have an oil change at some specified interval, there are maintenance issues associated with many devices.

Let us assume that we purchased a fine device and care for it properly, using legitimate parts and having technicians check the device every six months. Unfortunately, we still cannot be assured that there will be no problems. Think of the time when you visited a shop and the clerk could not locate the item that you have routinely purchased frequently in the past. This is most probably due to the use of a newly hired person who was not sufficiently trained. That analogous situation can take place with device use.

Consider the newly employed technician who understood most but not all of his training on the new laser device. We can expect to find that every job has a learning curve. Some are longer than others, but it is a fact of life that some poorly trained or inexperienced personnel may make mistakes when they are just beginning their new jobs. We expect them to become more proficient over time with the benefit of actual experience. But that does not provide much comfort to their earliest patients. Again, to save money, it can be assumed that some persons will hire persons off the street with no educational background or experience to learn a task "on the job." That might be okay for patients after several months but our sympathies are due to their earliest patients.

There was a scandal several years ago when an endoscopy piece intended for single use was cleaned and reused multiple times. The cleaning was not sufficient and GI infections were spread from one patient to the next. It is understandable when there is no budget for single-use products that repeated use might be permitted, but the cleaning and sterilization would have to be quite thorough.

Periodically we learn about devices that make fraudulent claims. Perhaps, the most well known case is of the Theranos System. The device was promoted as being able to perform numerous tests on a blood sample requiring only the tiny amount of blood from a skin prick, like what is used by diabetics for blood glucose testing using a small lancet on one of the fingers. The device did not work and the faulty results were kept secret. This example is similar to the many useless or dangerous devices that were sold in the late 1800s and early twentieth century before national food and drug agencies were established by governments throughout the world. Some devices emitted radium or other ionizing radiation or simply did nothing beyond making sounds or having blinking lights.

Today's devices are miraculous in what they contribute to accurate diagnoses, detection of abnormalities, presence of drugs of abuse, identification of pregnancy, ovulation, and the visualization of the inner workings of the body as with functional MRIs, or ultrasound, for example. But an unchecked X-ray device in a dentist's office that leaks radiation should not be permitted to exist today. So then, how do we use these wonderful devices wisely? The answer is through the utilization of common sense. We should know enough about the devices we use to know the typical values they yield and the range of numbers they reveal. If those

DOI: 10.1201/9781003002345-21

numbers change in any significant way and a new pattern is being formed, it would probably be wise to have that device checked by an expert. Similarly, if a device tells us that the last six persons tested had low blood glucose levels, one should be suspicious because that is not a likely situation.

There is an adage that if something is too good to be true, then it probably is too good to be true. If CAT scanners cost $0.5 million, and you are offered one for half that amount, something is wrong. The device was either stolen, damaged in a flood, used but repainted to look like new, or was headed to the scrap yard due to malfunctioning. New models of devices may cost a little more than previous models but generally, they offer improved features such as great precision or definition, the ability to connect to the internet, internal digital memories, etc. One must be certain that they are receiving the model they are paying for.

There is a special concern in some lesser-developed countries. Some countries have perpetual budget problems and in the device field, this is seen as either a shortage of regulators and/or inspectors. Oftentimes, there is a sufficient number of inspectors, but they either receive a miniscule salary, or in some places, they have not been paid for several months. As one might imagine, this financial situation is an invitation for fraud and corruption. We have seen this for decades: inspectors have been bribed to approve imports of pharmaceuticals that were found to be subpotent or contaminated, and which should have gone to the incinerator or land fill. Instead, some unscrupulous group decided to sell the drugs where there was a possibility of making additional profit at the expense of unknowing, innocent people. A bribe as low as $25 or $50 goes a long way when an inspector has not been paid his or her salary for some months, or when the monthly salary is only $50 in the first place. We can see then how easy it might be to take advantage of this situation and pay for the inspector to look the other way when inspecting a bad batch of drugs.

There is an analogous situation found with medical devices in lesser-developed countries when, for example, a device is banned in Europe or North America or removed from the market due to faulty results, radiation leakage, or unreliable results, lack of precision, etc. Again, dishonest persons might attempt to export those medical devices into countries where the regulatory agencies are lacking in personnel, or where the regulatory agencies do not have the resources or capability to test the devices and forbid their importation.

It is indeed unfortunate that such unscrupulous behavior continues in the twenty-first century, but its existence is a fact of life and will be with us until we make it too difficult or costly for this criminal behavior to continue. Then the criminals can go back to making fake women's purses or DVDs. Pharmacists will probably not play the major role in detecting device crime, but, nevertheless, should be aware always of its possibility and be vigilant in the case that some clues or tips arouse their suspicions.

Okay, what can pharmacists do? The answer is simple and straightforward. For one thing, they can learn everything they can about the devices used in their areas of specialization or from the physicians with whom they have the greatest amount of professional contact. They can offer to assist in the training of new hires who will be using medical devices and make their expertise available if those device operators have questions or problems. And just as in the case of pharmacovigilance with drug products, pharmacists should always be on the lookout for signals or patterns of potential device problems. That contribution by the pharmacist is of immense value.

Index

Note: Page numbers in *italics* refer to figures; page numbers in **bold** refer to tables.

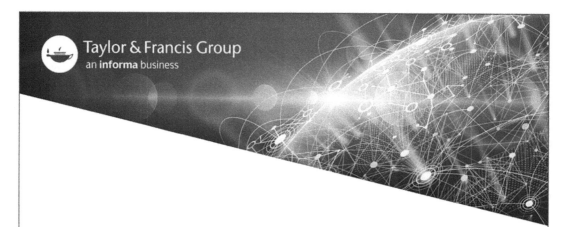
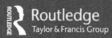
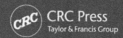

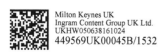

9 781032 168241